Handbook of Kinesiology

Functional anatomy • Biomechanics
Assessment of joints and muscles

Vincenzo Pirola

Handbook of Kinesiology

Functional anatomy • Biomechanics
Assessment of joints and muscles

edi·ermes

edra
PUBLISHING

HANDBOOK OF KINESIOLOGY
Functional anatomy • Biomechanics • Assessment of joints and muscles
by Vincenzo Pirola

ISBN 978-1-962679-08-4

eISBN 978-1-962679-17-6

Book Publishing Manager: Costanza Smeraldi

Paper, printing and Binding Manager: Paolo Ficicchia

Proofreading of Translation: Sandra A. Calarota

Layout: Edi.Ermes srl

Cover: Roberta Bordoli

Drawings: Andrea Rossi Raccagni, Marco Fanuli and Raffaella Stilo/Archive Edi.Ermes

edra
PUBLISHING

Edra Publishing US LLC
3309 Northlake Boulevard, Suite 203
Palm Beach Gardens, FL, 33403
EIN: 844113980
info@edrapublishing.com
www.edrapublishing.com

Printed in Italy in March 2024 by "Rotomail Italia" S.p.A., Vignate (MI)

Preface

The *Handbook of Kinesiology* is provided as a comprehensive text, even if it is inevitably concise. As well as the fundamental basics of functional anatomy, neurophysiology and biomechanics, it also includes the main elements for being able to perform an evaluation of the articulation of the joints of the human body and force of the primary muscles.

Obviously, the latter description may also be affected by a lack of depth, especially in relation to the methods of fixation (stabilization) and on how to avoid the compensatory movements which can render functional evaluation less accurate. For the related insights, we direct you to texts concerned exclusively with the evaluative aspects.

However, a firm stabilization of the body segments that are not subject to evaluation does not require any particular functional anatomical knowledge, however the description in the *Handbook of Kinesiology* seems to us sufficient for a good functional examination.

the Author

Contents

1. Bones, joints, muscles

2. Movements and biomechanics

6. Thorax and thoracic column

7. Shoulder and pectoral girdle

12. Ankle and foot

13. Application aspects

Bones

Definition: organs of different morphology, of whitish or yellowish color, of solid consistency, endowed with great mechanical resistance.

The bones are connected by joints and give origin or insertion to the muscles. The adult skeleton is composed of approximately 206 bones. The shape of each bone is related to the static and dynamic mechanics of the locomotor system.

Classification of bones

- Long bones – one dimension prevails over the other two (length compared to width and thickness)
- Flat bones – two dimensions (length and width) prevail over the third (thickness)
- Short bones – all dimensions are equivalent.

Characteristics of long bones

- Diaphysis – elongated shaft (or body) of the long bone
- Epiphysis – more or less enlarged ends of the long bone.

Descriptive terminology of bone morphology

- Projections and reliefs
  - apophyses (processes) – well-defined projections
  - tuberosities – less well-defined projections
  - tubercles – defined reliefs
  - spines – pointed reliefs
- Depressions
  - sulci – thin depressions
  - fossae – rounded depressions
  - canals – elongated depressions.

Bones are made up of bone tissue:

- spongy – made up of more or less dense trabeculae, irregularly oriented, that surround the small cavities known as areolae
- compact – dense layer of bone tissue.

In addition to the areolae of the spongy bone tissue, there is another type of bone cavity represented by the medullary cavity of the long bones (within the diaphysis). The external surface of the bones is covered by the

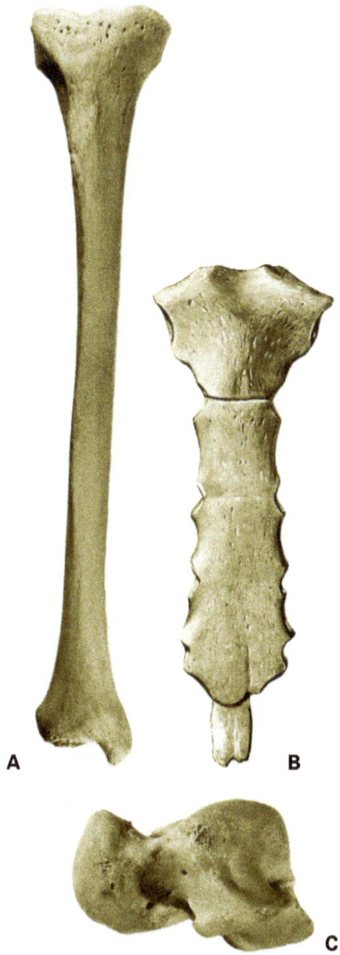

Bone structure. The prevalence of length and width over thickness, or the relative equivalence of the dimensions allow bones to be classified as long (**A**), flat (**B**) and short (**C**).

periosteum, a fibrous membrane, and the internal cavities of the compact and spongy bone substance are covered by endosteum, also fibrous in nature.

The long bones are formed by compact bone tissue at the diaphysis (which delimits the medullary cavity) and of spongy bone at the epiphysis, surrounded by compact bone tissue.
The flat bones are formed by spongy bone tissue surrounded by two layers of compact bone tissue.
The short bones are formed by spongy bone tissue surrounded by compact bone tissue.

Bone tissue

It is formed by:
- cells – osteoblasts, osteocytes and osteoclasts
- intercellular matrix or substance – collagen fibers, amorphous substance (organic matrix) and mineral salts.

Osteoblasts

- Function – they synthesize intercellular substance
- Location – layer of cells adhering to the support (fibrous, cartilaginous or bone connective tissue) on which the intercellular substance is deposited.

Osteocytes

- Function – they are derived from osteoblasts and can transform back into osteoblasts
- Location – in the cavities of the bone matrix (called bone lacunae), each occupying a lacuna (bone canaliculi).

Osteoclasts

- Function – they reabsorbed intercellular substance
- Location – erosion cavities of intercellular substance (resorption lacunae).

Collagen fibers

- Bundles of tropocollagen filaments with a high elastic modulus and high breaking load.

Amorphous substance

- Hyaluronic acid and hexosamine polymers with little water and electrolytes.

Mineral salts

- Calcium (99% of the body's calcium; 26% of the dry weight of the bone)
- Phosphorus (90% of the body's phosphorus; 12% of the dry weight of the bone)
- Sodium (25% of the body's sodium)
- Chloride
- Fluoride.

Structure of bone tissue

Both the trabeculae of the spongy tissue and the continuous layer of the compact bone tissue are formed of bone lamellae.

Definition of bone lamellae: thin layer (with a thickness of 5-10 μm) formed of collagen fibers, amorphous substance, mineral salts and a row of lacunae containing osteocytes.

Characteristics of bone lamellae

- In each bone lamella, the collagen fibers run parallel to each other, the orientation of the fibers differing from one lamella to the other
- In infancy, the lamellae of compact bone tissue are arranged concentrically
- Starting from puberty, the concentric organization of the lamellae of compact bone tissue is rearranged, creating a new arrangement known as interlocking fragments (lamellar bone tissue with osteons and breccia).

Definition of osteons (concentric haversian system): fragment of lamellar bone tissue with concentric arrangement of the lamellae within a central canaliculus (haversian canal).

Definition of breccia: fragment of lamellar bone tissue formed from non-concentric lamellae without a central canaliculus.

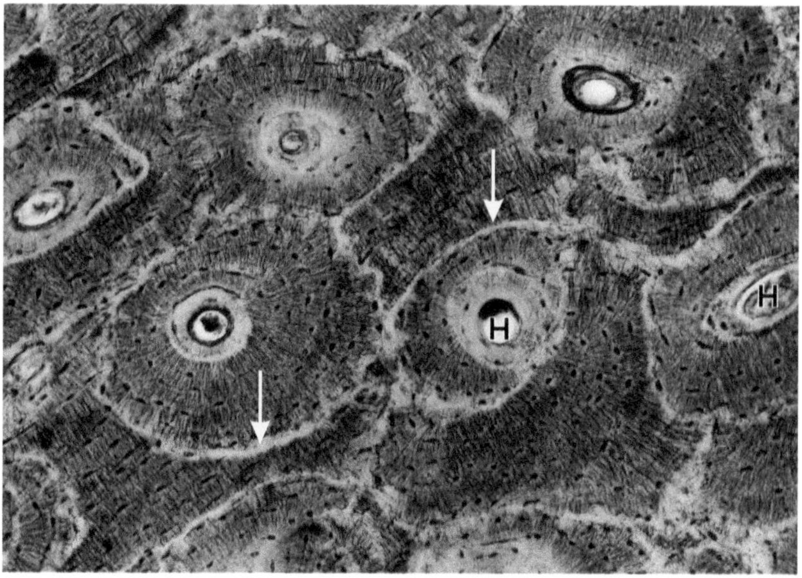

Section of a human compact bone (adult femoral diaphysis). Many osteons can be seen with a haversian canal (**H**) in a central position. Among the osteons there are fragments of bone breccia. The boundary between the osteons and the bone breccia is represented by the cementing lines indicated by **arrows**.

Levels of bone tissue organization

1st level structure → compact and spongy arrangement of the bone

2nd level structure → lamellar (concentric or with osteons and breccia) and non-lamellar composition

3rd level structure → different spatial orientation of collagen fibers

4th level structure → submicroscopic arrangement of the collagen fibers, mineral salts and amorphous substance

5th level structure → molecular arrangement of the bone constituents

There is a relationship between the 1st level structure and the mechanical engagement of a bone:

- in the diaphysis of the long bones there is a fixed relationship between the external diameter and internal diameter, which gives an optimal mechanical resistance
- in the spongy bone, the trabeculae follow the lines of greater mechanical engagement (load trajectories)

Mechanical resistance of the bone (dependent on the levels of bone tissue arrangement)	
Traction	10-20 kg/mm^2
Compression and flexion	15 kg/mm^2
Torsion	18 kg/mm^2

Joints

Definition: structures formed of two or more different or even similar contact surfaces whose shape and mode of contact depend on one or more possibilities of movement of the bone segments they are part of.

Joint appendages

- Articular cartilage
- Joint capsule
- Synovial membrane (or synovium)
- Synovial bursae
- Marginal labra
- Articular menisci (discs)
- Ligaments
- Connective tissue.

Articular cartilage

- Covers the articular surfaces of the bones
- It is a connective tissue
- It is of hyaline type
- It is formed of cell groups (which give it a state of tension and determine its elasticity) immersed in an amorphous substance called chondrin (or matrix), rich in three-dimensionally arranged collagen fibers and a ground substance composed of polysaccharides; it does not contain vessels and nerves, so the intake of nutritious substances and the elimination of waste products occurs through exchanges between the chondrin and the synovial fluid
- It is 0.2-6 mm thick (the increase in thickness is due to swelling of the ground substance):
  - dependent on pressure and extension stresses
  - greater at the periphery than at the center (due to the action of the ligaments)
- Improves the contact of the articular surfaces
- Reduces joint wear caused by stresses
- Undergoes:
  - thinning, if the motor stresses are reduced (articular ankylosis)
  - thickening (long-lasting), if the motor stresses are increased (for example, through training).

Joint capsule

- It is formed of a fibrous layer and a synovial membrane.

Synovial membrane

- It is rich in vessels and nerves

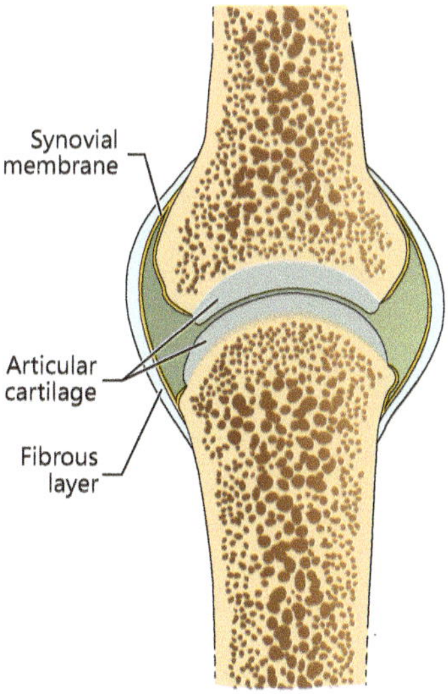

Articular cartilage, macroscopic aspect.

- Secretes a fluid (synovial fluid) containing albumin with the following functions:
  - nutrition of the articular cartilage
  - lubrication of the internal walls of the articular cavity
- Its inactivity causes it to thicken, reducing joint mobility.

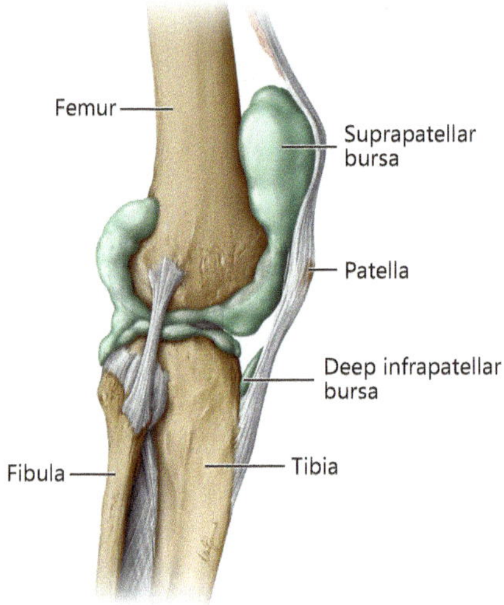

Two important mucous bursae. Above, the suprapatellar bursa, the largest in the human body. Below on the right, the deep infrapatellar bursa.

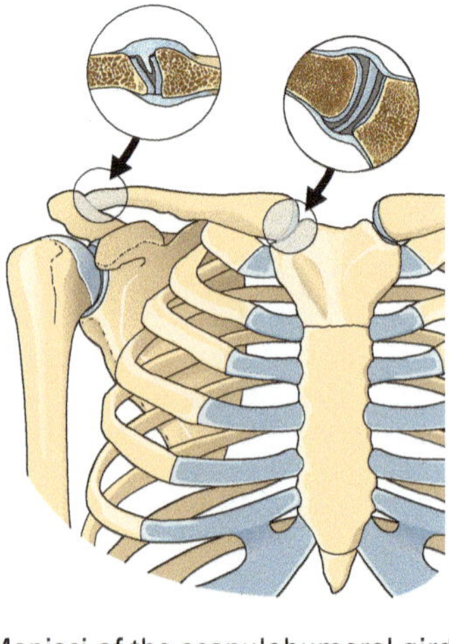

Menisci of the scapulohumeral girdle.

Sinovial bursae

- Contain synovial fluid
- Allow the tendons and muscles to slide over the bones and connective tissue or other muscles
- Facilitate choice of direction of a muscle or group of muscles
- Make muscle action more efficient by increasing the corresponding lever arm.

Marginal labra

- Are formed of fibrous cartilage
- Lack vessels and nerves
- Increase concordance between the articular surfaces (examples of these are the marginal labra that extend the glenoid and acetabular cavities).

Articular menisci

- Are formed of fibrous cartilage
- Lack vessels and nerves
- Improve articular concordance
- Act as shock absorbers
- Increase the articular surface
- They can be complete or incomplete.

Ligaments

- Are formed of numerous collagen fibers and scarce elastic fibers
- Have few vessels and nerves
- Their elongation does not exceed 20% of their resting length
- Are very resistant to traction, but not to torsion
- Reinforce the joint capsule
- Maintain articular concordance
- Precede muscle action
- Reduce muscle fatigue.

Connective tissue

- Is interposed between muscles and joint capsule
- Is rich in sensory receptors.

Classification of joints

Synarthrosis (continuity joints)

Syndesmosis (fibrous synarthrosis)
- Joining the articular surfaces through collagen or elastic fibers
- Examples:
  - interosseous membrane (between the radius and ulna)
  - proximal and distal tibiofibular joints
  - gomphoses (joint between tooth and bone)
  - sutures
  - ligamenta flava.

Synchondrosis (cartilaginous synarthroses)
- Joining the articular surfaces through hyaline cartilage
- Examples:
  - sternocostal joints (first, sixth and seventh rib)
  - bone metaphysis.

Symphysis (fibrocartilaginous synarthrosis)
- Joining the articular surfaces through fibrous cartilage and connective tissue
- Examples:
  - joint between the pubic bones
  - joint between the vertebral bodies (disc plus anterior and posterior longitudinal ligaments).

Synostosis (bone synarthroses)
- Consequence of bone fusion at the end of growth
- Examples:
  - joints between the pelvic bones.

Diarthrosis (contiguity joints)

Hinge joint (trochlea)
- Concave surface congruent with the convex surface
- 1 degree of freedom (flexion-extension)
- Horizontal rotation axis
- Examples:
  - humeroulnar joint
  - interphalangeal joints
  - knee joint.

Pivot joint (trochoid joint)
- Concave surface congruent with the convex surface
- 1 degree of freedom (external and internal rotation)
- Vertical rotation axis
- Examples:
  - proximal and distal radioulnar joints
  - atlantoaxial joint.

Condylar joint (ellipsoid joint)
- Concave ellipsoidal surface congruent with the convex ellipsoidal surface
- 2 degrees of freedom (flexion-extension and abduction-abduction)
- 2 rotation axes (horizontal and sagittal)
- Examples:
  - metacarpophalangeal joint
  - radiocarpal joint.

Saddle joint
- Ellipsoidal surfaces each with two curvatures – concave and convex (saddle)
- 2 degrees of freedom
- 2 rotation axes
- Examples:
  - carpometacarpal joint of the thumb.

Ball and socket joint (spheroidal joint)
- Partially spherical surfaces, concave and convex
- 3 degrees of freedom (all movements)
- 3 rotation axes
- Examples:
  - glenohumeral joint
  - hip joint.

Plane joint
- Has no axes of movement
- The articular surfaces are mainly flat and irregular
- Allows limited sliding movements

- Examples:
  - carpal joints
  - tarsal joints
  - sternocostal joints (second, third, fourth and fifth rib)
  - intervertebral joints.

Amphiarthrosis

- Little mobility
- Very tense joint capsules and ligaments
- Poorly congruent articular surfaces
- Examples:
  - sacroiliac joint
  - proximal tibiofibular joint.

Main types of synarthrosis

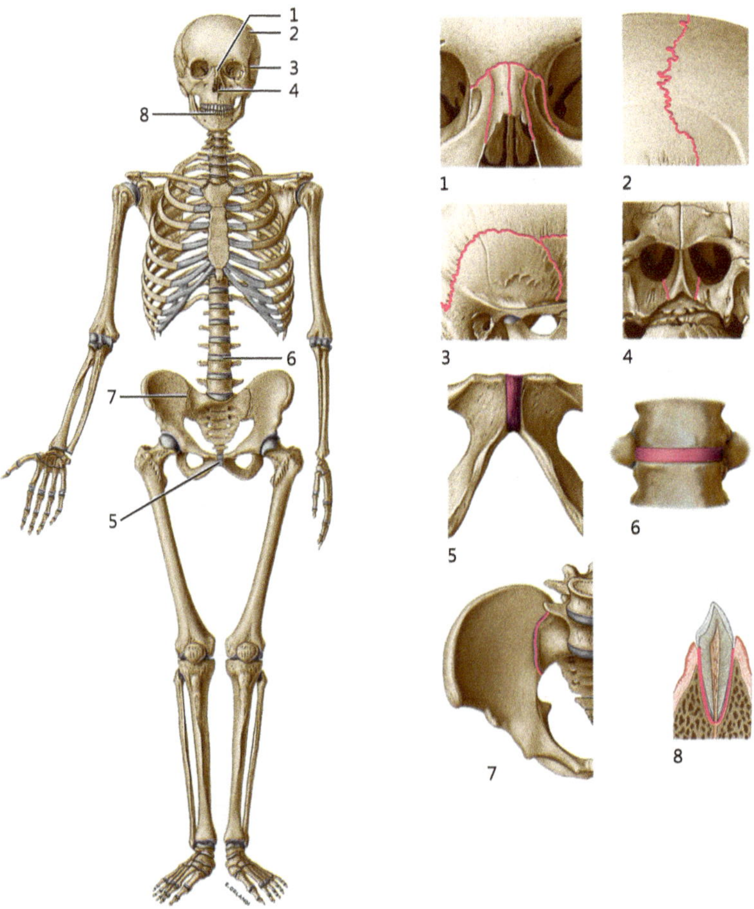

Main types of diarthrosis

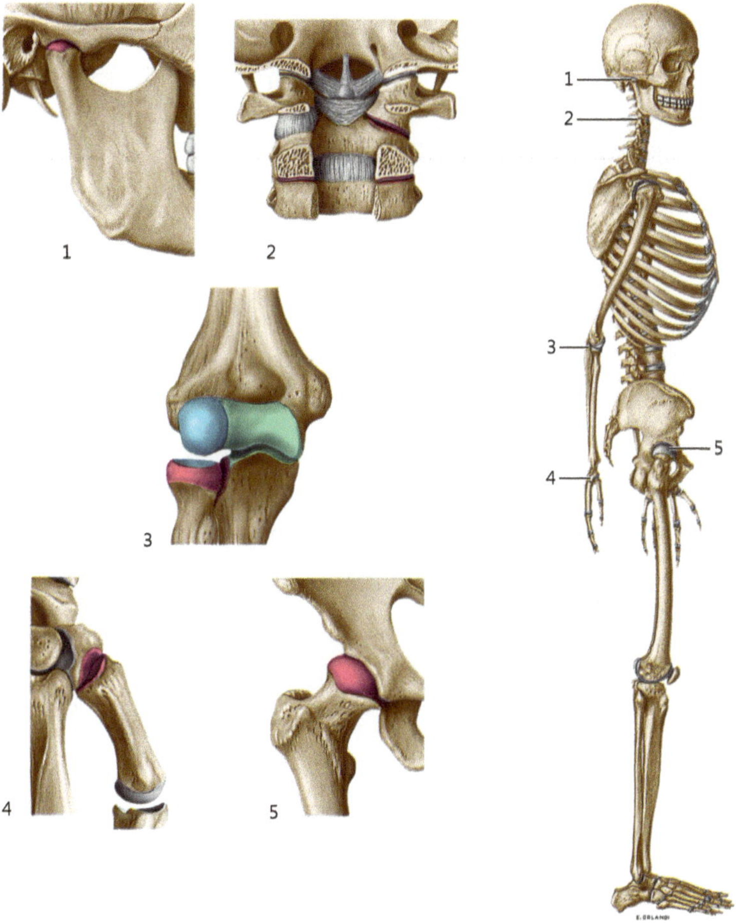

Main types of *diarthrosis*: **1**, condylar joint; **2**, plane joint; **3**, pivot or trochoid joint (in *red*), hinge joint or trochlea (in *green*), condylar joint (in *blue*); **4**, saddle joint; **5**, ball and socket (or spheroidal) joint.

◁ Main types of *synarthrosis*: **1**, plane suture; **2**, serrate suture; **3**, squamous suture; **4**, wedge-and-groove suture or schindylesis; **5-6**, symphysis; **7**, amphiarthrosis; **8**, gomphosis.

Articular surfaces of the diarthroses

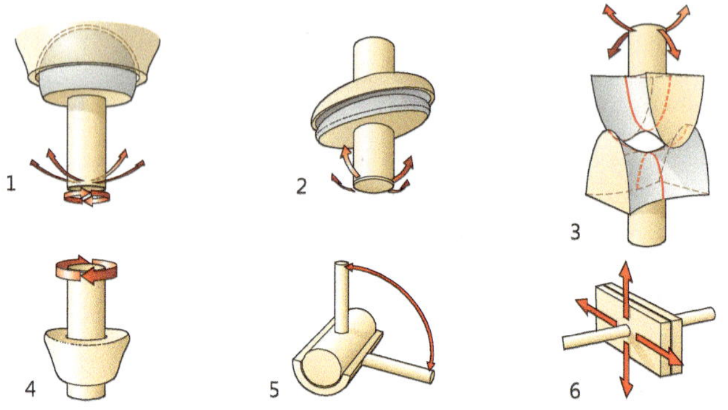

Schematic drawing of the shape of the articular surfaces of the diarthroses: **1**, enarthrosis (semispherical shape); **2**, condylar joint (ellipsoidal shape); **3**, saddle joint (the two meeting surfaces are concave on one axis and convex on the axis orthogonal to it); **4**, pivot or trochoid joint (cylindrical shape); **5**, hinge joint (cylindrical shape); **6**, plane joint (flat surfaces).

Example of amphiarthrosis: sacroiliac joint

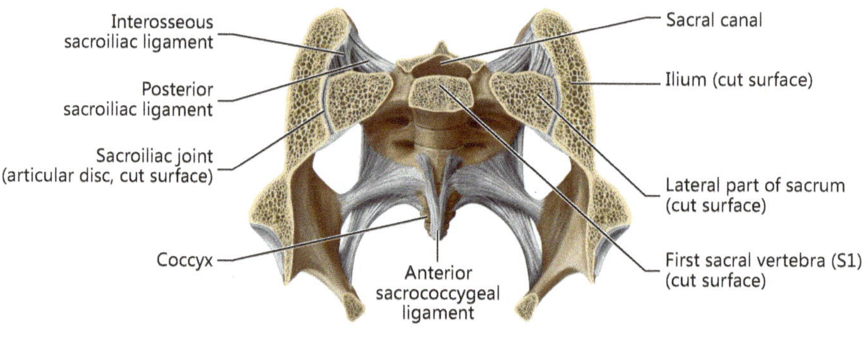

Transverse section passing through the first sacral segment showing the relations between sacrum and hip bones at the level of the sacroiliac joints.

Joint movements

See section "Reference system", page 47.

Kinematic chains

The arrangement of bones in series (typical of the limbs and vertebral column), in parallel (characteristic of the phalanges, metacarpal and metatarsal bones), in a group (such as the carpal, tarsal and pelvic bones), and the arrangement of the resulting joints, considered from a functional perspective, i.e., from the point of view of movements allowed, constitute a kinematic chain (the sequence of muscle actions constitutes a kinetic chain).

Characteristics of kinematic chains:

- degree of freedom (sum of the degrees of freedom of each joint in the chain)
- open kinematic chain (the distal joint is free in the space); examples include the limbs and vertebral column (an open kinematic chain appears closed when it is opposed by a force that acts against its movement, for example, the thrust of the ground against the load of the foot)
- closed kinematic chain (the chain is closed on itself; examples include the pelvis and the thoracic cage)

Kinematic chain of the upper limb

Joints*	Degrees of freedom
Glenohumeral or shoulder (ball and socket joint)	3
Sternoclavicular (double plane joint)	3
Acromioclavicular (double plane joint)	3
Scapulothoracic (pseudo joint)	1
Elbow (pivot or trochoid joint and hinge joint or trochlea)	2
Wrist (condylar joint)	2
Metacarpophalangeal (condylar joint)	2
Proximal interphalangeal (hinge joint or trochlea)	1
Distal interphalangeal (hinge joint or trochlea)	1
Total degrees of freedom of the upper limb	18

* Excluding the sternocostal and costovertebral joints.

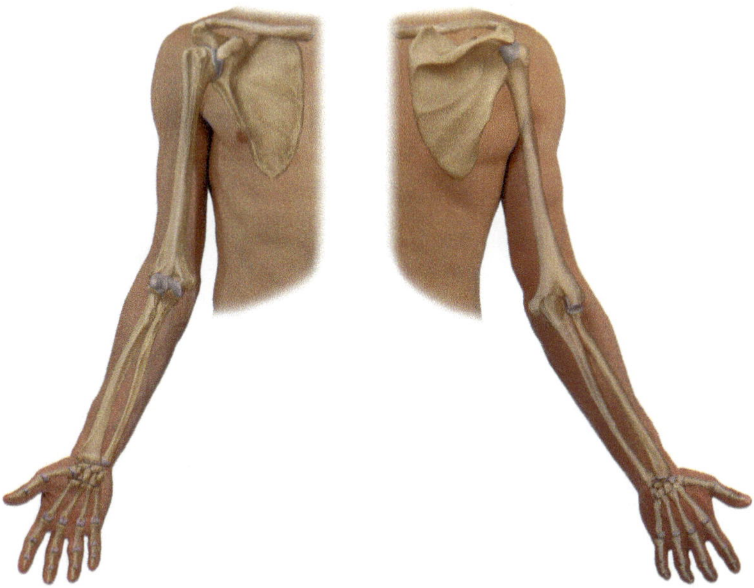

Joints of the upper limb.

Kinematic chain of the lower limb

Joints*	Degrees of freedom
Hip (ball and socket joint)	3
Knee (hinge joint or trochlea)	2
Ankle (complex hinge joint)	2
Metatarsophalangeal (condylar joint)	2
Proximal interphalangeal (hinge joint or trochlea)	1
Distal interphalangeal (hinge joint or trochlea)	1
Total degrees of freedom of the lower limb	11

* Excluding the subtalar (talocalcaneal), transverse tarsal, tarsometatarsal and intermetatarsal joints.

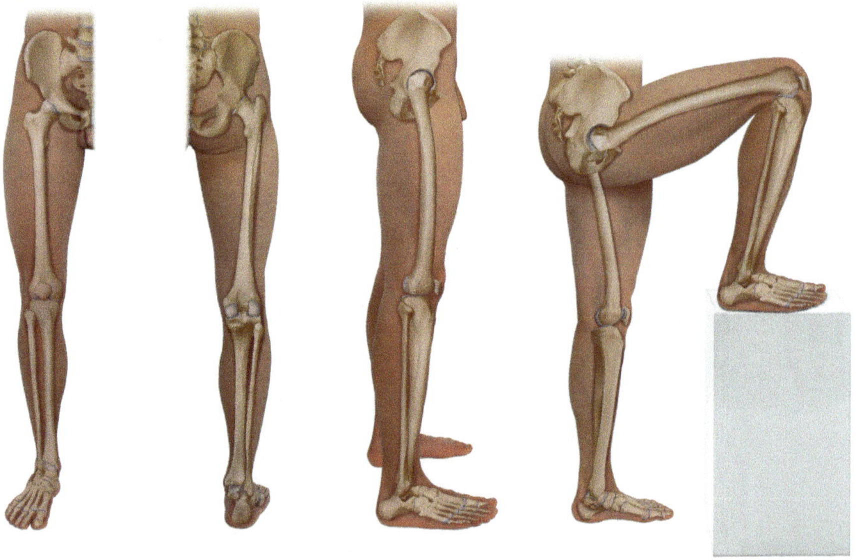

Joints of the lower limb.

Both in the kinematic chain of the upper limb and in that of the lower limb, the number of degrees of freedom of each joint tends to decrease in the distal direction. As a result, gripping and manipulation are favored by the upper limb, also facilitated by the parallel arrangement of the phalanges and the metacarpals, whose joints can be moved individually. In the lower limb, however, the flexion-extension of the toes is total, favoring above all the transmission of the load to the ground.

Muscles

Definition: terminal elements responsible for the executive phase of movements.

Anatomical structure

Each muscle is formed of:
- connective tissue lining fascia (epimysium)
- muscle fibers, the number of which depends on:
  - size of the transverse diameter of the muscle
  - trophism of the muscle fibers
  - orientation of the muscle fibers
- supporting connective tissue layer (to the epimysium – the outermost connective tissue layer – are added the perimysium – which wraps groups of muscle fibers – and the endomysium – which covers each muscle fiber).

The muscle fasciae compact and protect the muscle fibers, giving them their elasticity, maintaining their trophism (through vessels and nerves that run along the fasciae) and preserving muscle tone.

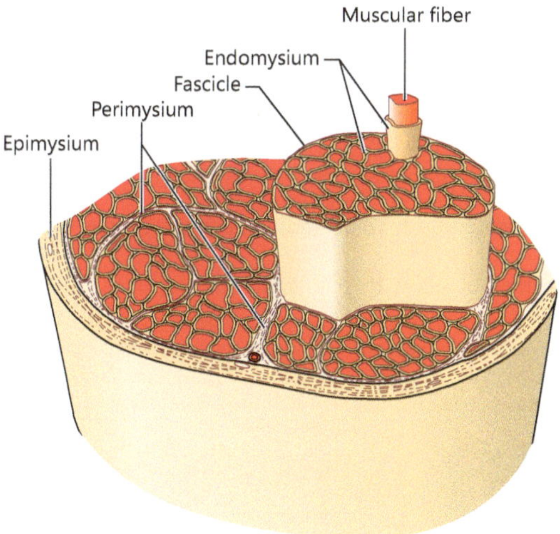

Diagram of the transverse section of skeletal muscle showing the connective tissue layer.

Each muscle fiber:
- has a diameter between 10 and 100 μm
- is coated in a connective tissue fascia (endomysium)
- is characterized by sarcoplasm (cytoplasm) and sarcolemma (plasma membrane)
- has a certain number of fibrils (myofibrils).

Each myofibril:
- has a diameter between 1 and 2 μm
- is formed of myofilaments (actin and myosin) that are contiguous to each other or in contact in relation to the functional state and aligned parallel to the axis of the muscle.

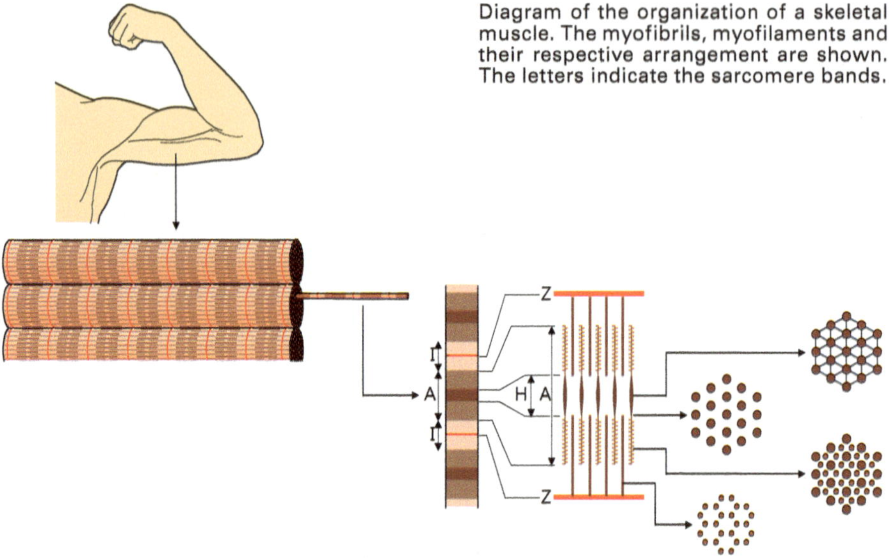

Diagram of the organization of a skeletal muscle. The myofibrils, myofilaments and their respective arrangement are shown. The letters indicate the sarcomere bands.

Ultrastructure of the myofibrils

The myosin filaments (formed of myosin molecules) are thicker and have pedunculated expansions (heads).
The actin filaments (formed of actin, tropomyosin and troponin molecules) are thinner.

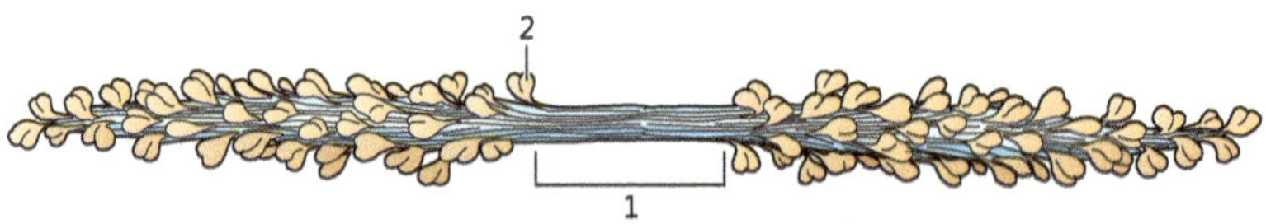

Diagram illustrating the arrangement of the myosin molecules within a filament (in this case a thick filament). **1**, Bare area; **2**, myosin heads (from VV.AA. *Citologia e istologia funzionale.* Milan, Edi.Ermes, 2005).

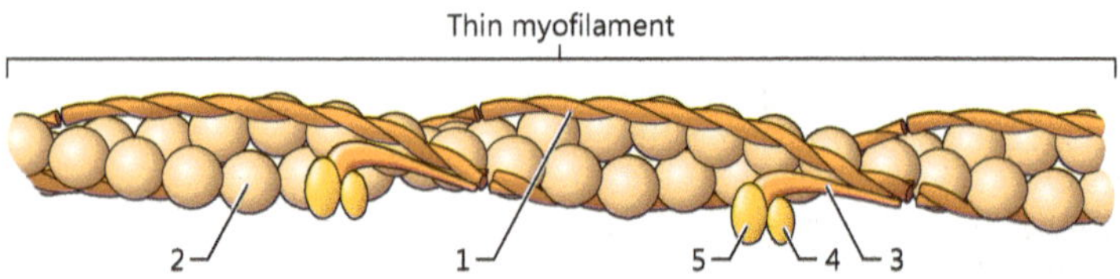

Diagram of a thin myofilament. **1**, Tropomyosin; **2**, actin; **3**, troponin A; **4**, troponin C; **5**, troponin T (modified from Colombo R, Olmo E. *Biologia della cellula.* Milan, Edi.Ermes, 2007).

Muscle contraction

During contraction, the heads of the myosin filaments bind to the actin filaments (with a cogwheel mechanism through which, when a head loses contact, this is achieved by the next one and so on until contraction ends).

Morphological and molecular events of muscle contraction

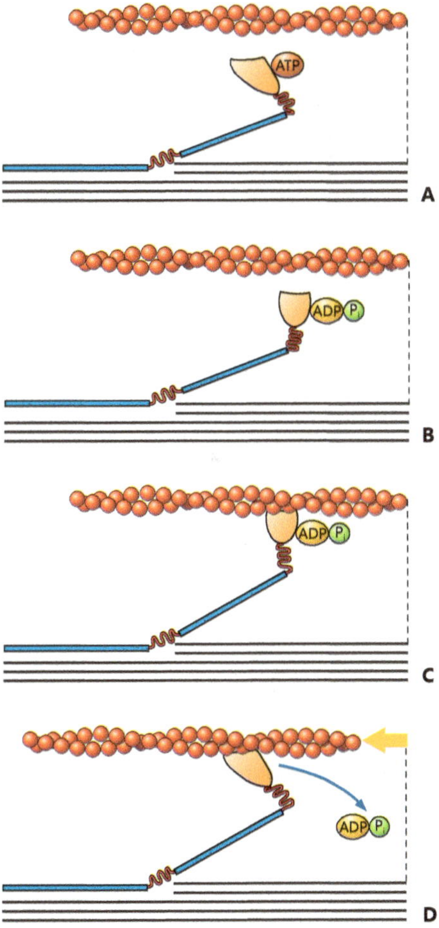

Diagram illustrating the relationship between "molecular events" and "morphological events" during muscle contraction. **A**, At rest, the myosin heads always bind to an ATP molecule; they are separated from the actin filament and form an angle of 45° with respect to the latter; **B**, with the arrival of calcium, the myosin heads hydrolyze ATP, exploiting the energy released to take on a 90° configuration with respect to the actin filament. The hydrolysis products, ADP and Pi, remain bound to the head; **C**, the myosin head (90°) binds to the actin filament; **D**, the actin/myosin bond favors the release of the ATP hydrolysis products from the myosin head. This allows the head to return to the 45° configuration. During the latter phenomenon, myosin pulls the actin filament towards the center of the sarcomere (modified from Rosati P, Colombo R. *Istologia.* 4th ed. Milan, Edi.Ermes, 2001).

The energy required for muscle contraction is derived from degradation of glycogen and from the oxidation reactions that lead to the formation of substances such as ATP and creatine phosphate.
During muscle contraction, chemical energy is transformed into mechanical energy.

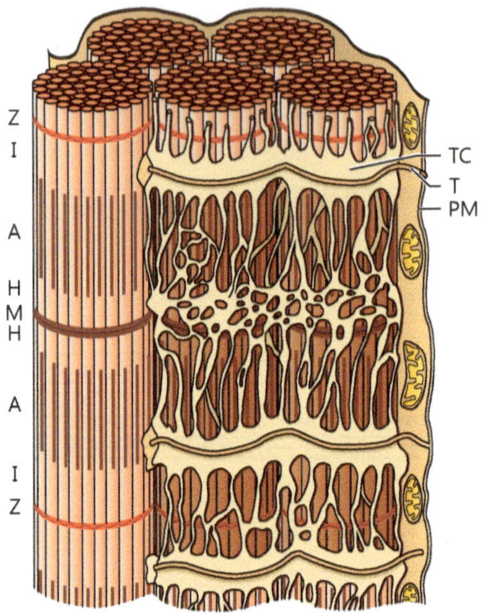

Three-dimensional diagram of the arrangement of the sarcoplasmic reticulum in a skeletal striated muscle fiber. The letters on the left indicate the sarcomere bands. The plasma membrane (**PM**) forms tubular invaginations (**T**) in relation to which the terminal cisternae (**TC**) of the reticulum are associated. The association of two terminal cisternae and the interposed tubule **T** is called a "triad", and is always located between **A**-band and **I**-band.

Sarcomere

Observation of a muscle in longitudinal section shows transverse striations (hence the term striated muscle) known as bands or zones, produced by the particular alignment of the actin and myosin filaments.

The alternation of a light band (I-band), divided in half by a dark line (Z-line), and a dark band (A-band), divided in half by a light zone (H-zone), which in turn is divided in half by a dark line (M-line), can be observed.

The sarcomere (basic contractile unit or functional contractile unit) is bounded by two Z-lines, thus comprising an A-band and two I-semibands.

Activity of the muscle fibers

The transmission of the motor stimulus to the muscle, responsible for the excitation or inhibition of the muscle fiber activity, occurs through axons that originate from the motor neurons α and γ of the anterior horns of the spinal cord and from the cells of the somatic motor nuclei of the cranial nerves. Through the peripheral nerves, the axons reach the muscle fibers, with which they then come into contact through particular synaptic devices called neuromuscular junctions.

Neuromuscular junction

It is composed of:

- synaptic vesicles within the terminal part of the axon (synaptic bouton)
- presynaptic membrane
- synaptic space (cleft or gap)
- postsynaptic membrane.

When the synaptic terminal bouton is reached by a nerve impulse, the synaptic vesicles release acetylcholine into the synaptic space, which binds to the receptors of the postsynaptic membrane, causing a variation in their action potential (depolarization), which gives rise to the action potential that propagates to the system of sarcotubules and T-tubules. Sarcotubules are longitudinal canaliculi of the smooth endoplasmic reticulum of the sarcoplasm that give rise to the transverse cisternae called terminal cisternae, whereas the T-tubules are invaginations of the sarcolemma of the muscle fiber. This system of cisternae and canaliculi is in contact with the myofibrils.

Upon arrival of the depolarization wave, the transverse cisternae release calcium ions into the myofibrils, which activate the bond between actin and myosin. Acetylcholine, synthesized by choline acetyltransferase, is degraded by acetylcholinesterase immediately after

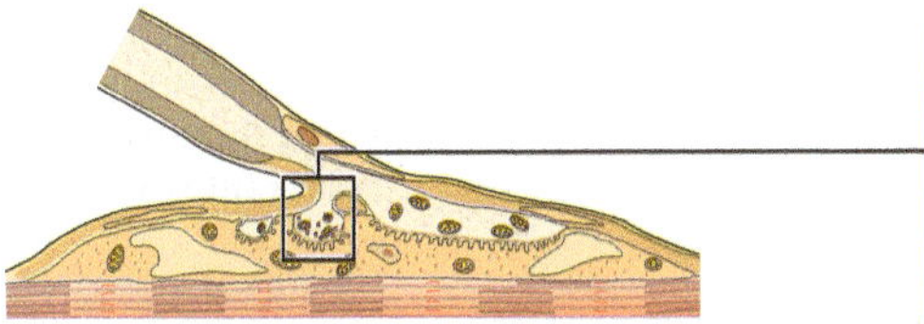

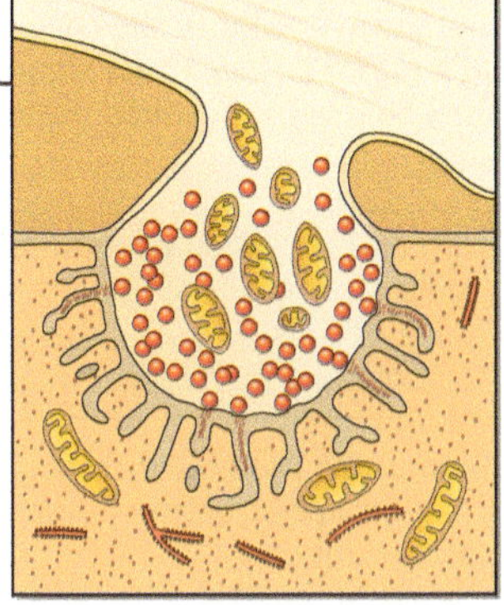

Schematic drawing of an expansion of the motor end plate showing its ultrastructural characteristics. Note that, unlike the synapse, the muscle fiber membrane (postsynaptic membrane) forms numerous invaginations. The synaptic space is also occupied by the basal lamina. The vesicles of the boutons on the motor end plate contain acetylcholine.

the arrival of the impulse, simultaneously with the reabsorption of calcium ions in the terminal cisternae through a calcium pump.

Mechanical muscle model

It expresses the relationship between muscle fiber and elastic structures, which are components of the connective tissue. The elastic structures are arranged:

- in series – tendons and their extensions inside the muscles
- in parallel – sarcolemma, connective fasciae and connective tissue interposed between muscle fibers.

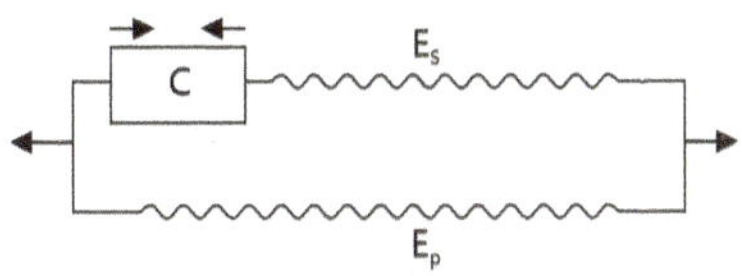

Mechanical muscle model.

Function of the elastic structures:

- in series – to cushion the stresses produced by stretching and muscle contractions
- in parallel – to cushion the stresses produced by muscle stretching.

Representing the contractile elements with C, the elastic ones in series with Es and the elastic ones in parallel with E_p, if only C were present, after stretching, the entire process necessary for the contraction would be carried out only actively, thus requiring additional energy. The elastic contribution to muscle stretching allows a saving in contractile energy, due precisely to the elastic return of the muscle. In addition, E_s and E_p resist traction and muscle contraction by protecting the muscle internally.

Motor unit

It is the functional unit of the neuromuscular system, consisting of:

- motor neuron
- nerve fiber
- a variable number of muscle fibers innervated by the nerve fiber (from 5-6 to 1000-2000, almost always in the same muscle).

Muscle contraction is a process defined as the "all-or-none law", in the sense that if the stimulus exceeds a certain threshold, the whole muscle will respond by contracting. This law is not always valid in the case of motor units; i.e., it may occur that not all the muscle fibers of a motor unit contract simultaneously. It is in fact possible that there is a difference in the threshold value between the muscle fibers (or the neuromuscular junctions) of a single motor unit.

The degree of precision of a muscle's movements depends on the ratio between muscle fibers to motor neurons of that muscle: the greater the number of motor neurons relative to the number of muscle fibers, the greater the degree of precision of the muscle (this is the case, for example, in the short muscles of the thumb and index finger).

In addition to the possible threshold difference within a single motor unit, there is a difference in the threshold between motor units, which are therefore distinguished into the following motor units:

- low threshold
  - with rapid rise in discharge rate (I)
  - with slow rise in discharge rate (II)
- high threshold
  - with rapid rise in discharge rate (III)
  - with slow rise in discharge rate (IV).

Muscular force (tension) depends on the number of motor units activated and their discharge rate. The threshold is the fundamental element for recruiting a greater or smaller number of motor units (and therefore muscle fibers) based on the amount of muscle effort required. In muscle activity, low-threshold motor nerve fibers are recruited first, followed by high-threshold fibers (the former have a greater discharge rate than the latter). The high-threshold fibers are recruited only when a high tension is required.

Motor neurons α (that innervate the extrafusal muscle fibers, i.e., the true muscle fibers, whereas motor neurons γ innervate the intrafusal muscle fibers, i.e., the fibers of the muscle spindle) of the anterior horn of the spinal cord are distinguished as:

- tonic α motor neurons (low threshold)
- phasic α motor neurons (high threshold)

It is the tonic α motor neurons that first activate the muscle fibers through the tonic α nerve fibers (being recruited before the phasic α one, due to the low threshold). However, the tonic α nerve fibers have a lower conduction velocity than the phasic α nerve fibers.

At birth, all the motor units are tonic (i.e., slow) and so are the corresponding muscle fibers, defined as red due to their histological staining. Over the course of development, in relation to the predominantly static or dynamic function of the muscle, they differentiate into phasic (or fast) motor units corresponding to white muscle fibers. Each muscle is therefore formed of red and white fibers, the numerical prevalence of which is related to the function it performs. For example, among the posterior muscles of the leg, the soleus, which has a predominantly postural function, is formed primarily of red fibers, whereas the gastrocnemius, more closely linked to dynamic functions, is formed primarily of white fibers. Among the muscles with a prevalence of red fibers is the diaphragm, which is characterized by its continuous and repetitive action.

Muscle function

The muscle function consists of moving, slowing and stopping a body segment.
The greater or lesser excursion of the body segment, in addition to the characteristics of the joint, depends on the biomechanical factors represented by:
- mass of the body segment
- moment of force
- action of the force of gravity.

(See Chapter 2 "Movements and biomechanics").

Muscular force

Contractile force, as well as neural factors (number of motor units activated and their discharge rate), depends on muscle factors represented by:
- reciprocity of muscle action
- type of muscle contraction
- shape and diameter of the muscles
- shortening (contraction), elongation (stretching) and contraction velocity of the muscle fibers
- muscle power
- moment of force
- angle of insertion of the muscle.

Reciprocity of muscle action

The body segments on which a muscle has origin and insertion tend to get closer during muscle contraction. This tendency due to the muscle action is called reciprocity and occurs when both body segments are free (not blocked).

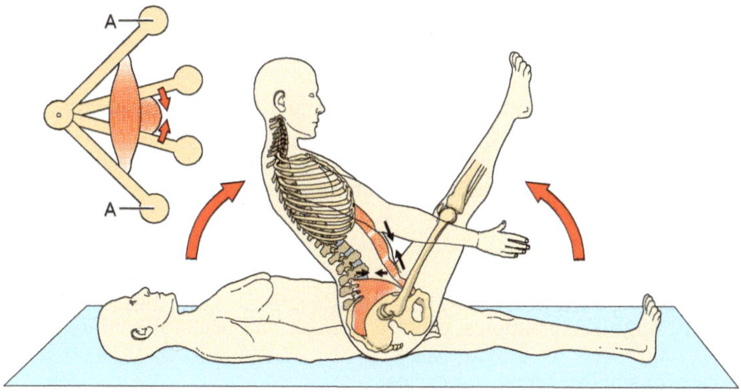

Muscle reciprocity.

Type of muscle contraction

- Isometric (static):
  - resistance (opposed by the two muscle insertion heads) is equal to the force expressed by the muscle fibers

- at the macroscopic level there is no variation in the length of muscle fibers (at the ultrastructural level there is shortening of the sarcomeres – contractile components – and elongation of the elastic elements in series)
- the work is zero
- the energy expended is used to balance the resistance produced by the body segment in question with the muscular force and is less than that used in concentric isotonic contraction and greater than that used in eccentric isotonic contraction.

- Concentric isotonic (in shortening):
  - the force exerted is greater than the resistance
  - the work is positive (movement occurs)
  - the energy expended is used to overcome the resistance and to shorten the muscle (therefore, it is maximal compared to isometric and eccentric isotonic contractions).
- Eccentric isotonic (elongation):
  - the force exerted is lesser than the resistance
  - the work is negative
  - the energy expended is used to slow and gradually stop the stretching of the muscle fibers (therefore, it is minimal compared to isometric and concentric isotonic contractions).
- Isokinetic (does not exist in nature):
  - resistance is self-adapting (i.e., an increased resistance is applied to the joint involved in the movement, taking into account the subject's ability to move the joint at a fixed velocity, which can vary gradually from 0 to 300-500 degrees/second; the velocity and resistance applied are established in relation to the subject's ability, assessed using computerized diagnostic-therapeutic tests; in normal human movement, resistance is fixed)
  - it is used for recovery from muscle deficits.

Shape and diameter of the muscles

The quality of muscular work almost always depends on the shape and diameter of the muscles.

Shape of the muscles

- Parallel or fusiform fibers (greater shortening and elongation, lesser force) (examples: sartorius and biceps brachii)
- Oblique fibers (lesser shortening and elongation, greater force) (examples: gluteus maximus and acromial part of the deltoid) that can be divided into:
  - semipennate (or unipennate)
  - pennate (or bipennate)
  - multipennate
- Orbicular (example: orbicularis oculi)
- Fan-shaped (triangular) (examples: pectoralis major and pectoralis minor, gluteus medius)
- Multipennate (examples: serratus muscles)
- Straight fibers (examples: rectus abdominis and digastric)
- Quadrilateral fibers (four-sided) (example: quadratus lumborum)
- Multi-tendons (examples: biceps brachii, triceps brachii and quadriceps femoris).

The more muscle fibers a muscle contains, the more force it can exert (the greater force of the pennate muscles depends on the greater number of fibers they have, obtained thanks to the oblique orientation of the fibers).

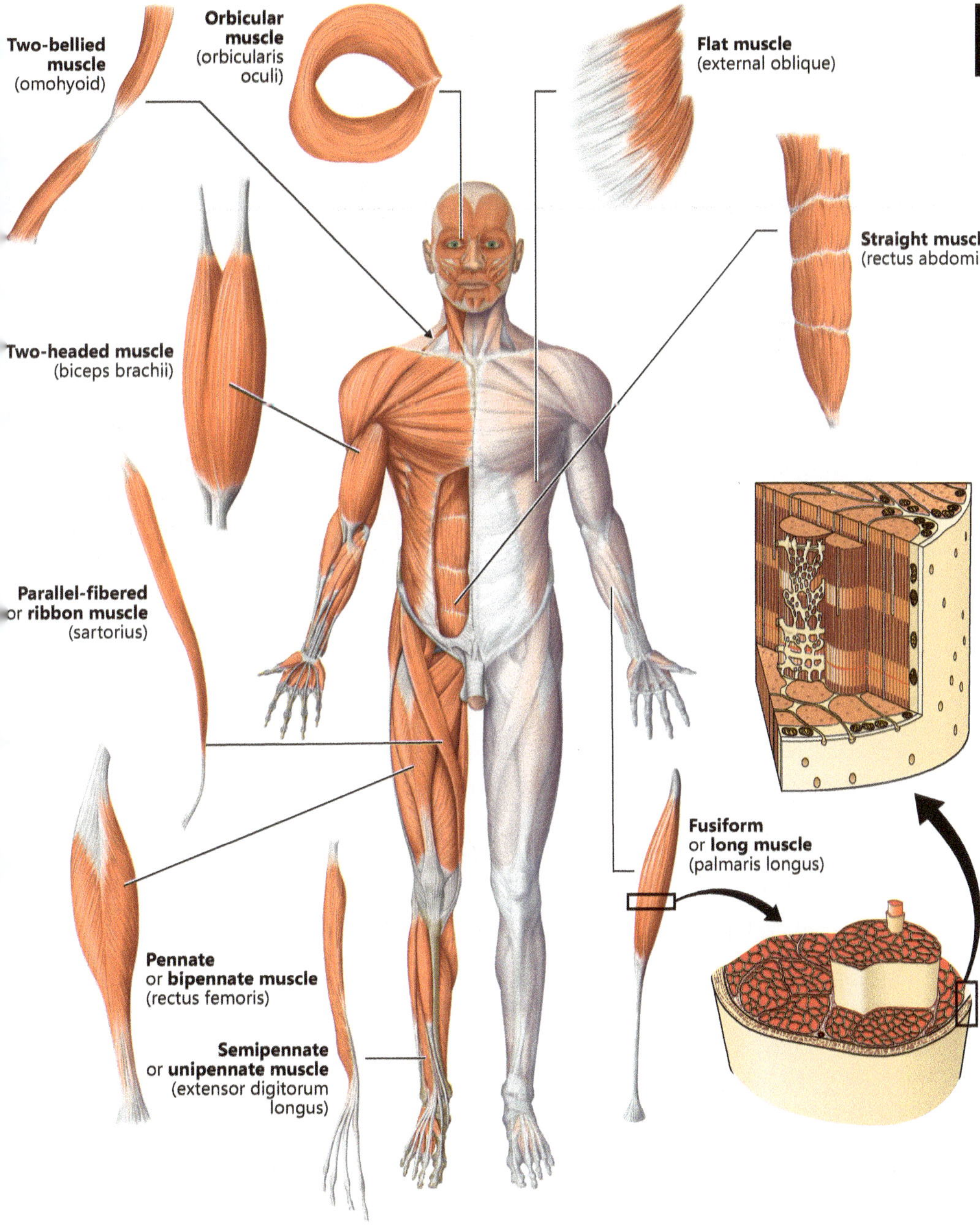

Types of muscles according to their shape.

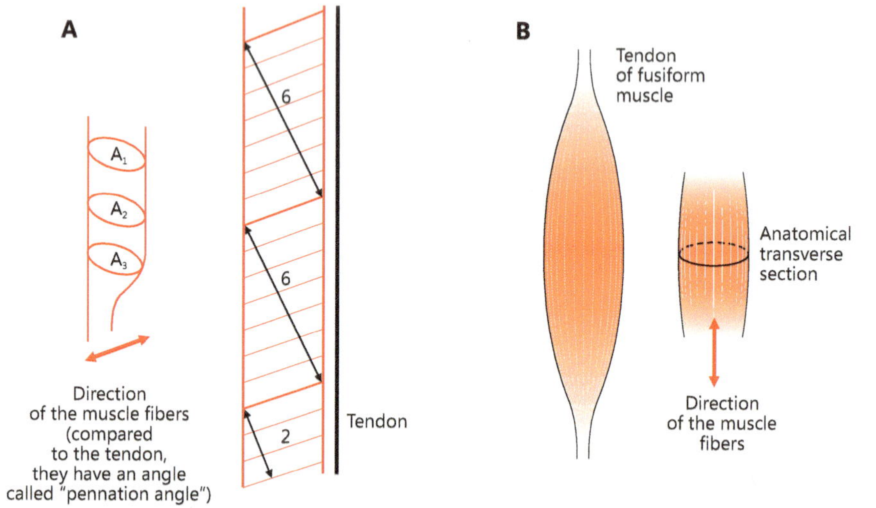

A, Semipennate muscle. Physiological transverse section: 6 + 6 + 2 = 14 x 2.5 = 35 cm². (**Note**: the mean muscle thickness is 2.5 cm). Trigonometry must be used for greater precision when indicating muscular force. **B**, Fusiform muscle. Anatomical transverse section: 3 x 3 = 9 cm². (**Note**: the mean transverse diameter is 3 cm).

Diameter of the muscles

The potential force of a muscle can be assessed from a quantitative point of view by two methods:

- measuring the diameter in anatomical transverse section:
  - this is only possible in fusiform muscles
  - the point of the muscle where the diameter has the greatest amplitude is selected (the area of the section is the square of the diameter)
- measuring the diameter in physiological transverse section:
  - in the pennate muscles and when it is not possible to measure the diameter at its mid-point
  - the sum of the length of the lines that cut the muscle fibers perpendicularly (the transverse section area is obtained by multiplying this data by the average thickness of the muscle, obtained from the anatomical section).

The muscular force, referring to diameter, is between 30 and 50 Newton $\times$ cm^2.

Shortening (contraction), elongation (stretching) and contraction velocity of the muscle fibers

The contractile function is influenced by the following mechanical properties of the muscle:

- stiffness (rigidity) – the muscle's reaction to elongation produced by the contractile (active) and elastic (passive) elements: it is directly proportional to the increase in elongation
- viscosity – the muscle's reaction to the contraction velocity and elongation for which small frictions between the elastic elements in series and large frictions between the contractile elements (actin and myosin filaments) are responsible: the former are propor-

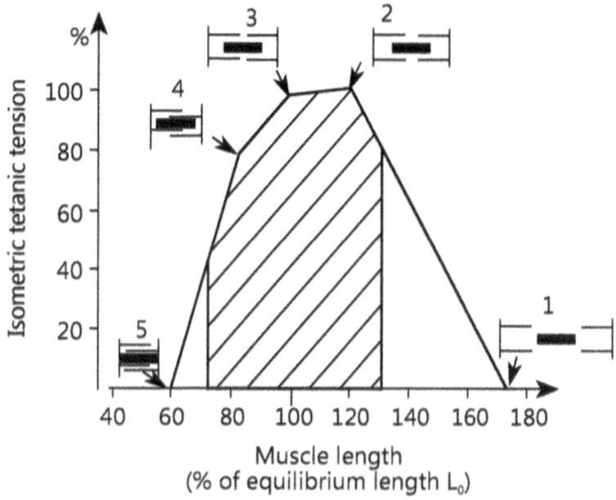

Active tension/length curve. When the muscle has a length greater than 100% (L_0 = length of equilibrium of the isolated muscle) this depends on stretching. Stretching imparts a passive tension that has been subtracted. The curve therefore expresses the active tension developed by the muscle stimulated at various lengths (from Cremaschi D. *Fisiologia generale. Principî.* Milan, Edi.Ermes, 1996).

tional to the increase in contraction velocity, and the latter are not (the consequence of the viscosity is the dissipation of part of the energy used for muscle action).

Tension/length curve

Stiffness is well highlighted by the tension/length curve, which relates the force applied with the elongation undergone by the fibers.

Elongation of the muscle from the resting length. In this case:
- muscle tension begins just after the resting length (when the muscle was previously elongated, the stimulus necessary for the contraction may be smaller)
- for values greater than 190% of the resting length, the muscle breaks.

Elongation of the muscle from 50% of the resting length, in the contraction phase (contraction is not possible below 50% of the resting length). In this case:
- for values between 50 and 100% of the resting length, tension is supported by the contractile structures (at 50% of the resting length there is an overlap of the actomyosin cross-bridges, which corresponds to a lower contractile efficiency)
- for values between 100 and 130% of the resting length, the tension is also supported by the elastic structures (the maximum number of actomyosin cross-bridges is determined at values equal to 120-130% of the resting length)
- for values greater than 130% of the resting length, the tension is supported only by the elastic structures (in fact, separation of the actin and myosin filaments occurs, with a reduction in the contractile force until it disappears)
- for values greater than 190% of the resting length, the muscle breaks.

The force exerted by a muscle is proportionally equal to:
- 0 for values 50% of the resting length
- 20 for values 100% of the resting length
- 25 for values 120% of the resting length
- 10 for values 120-130% of the resting length.

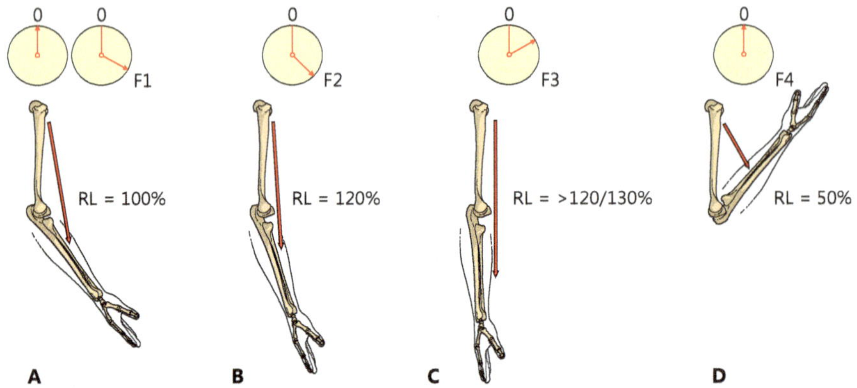

Extent of the forced exerted by the muscle stimulated to contract at four different starting lengths: **A**, at RL = its resting length; **B**, at 120% of its RL; **C**, at values greater than 120% of its RL; **D** at values equal to 50% of its RL. The extent of the different force values are obtained as a result of muscle electrical stimulation (neural factor) and the state of the elastic forces (mechanical factor). In the different quadrants above, the force can be verified (maximum in F2 and zero in F4).

Muscle tone

Definition: slight tension of the relaxed muscle fibers (with a length equal to the resting length) produced by the tension of the elastic elements in series and by intermittent active contractions in response to stresses such as palpation and passive mobilization.

Tension/velocity curve

It relates the force exerted by the muscle with the contraction velocity.

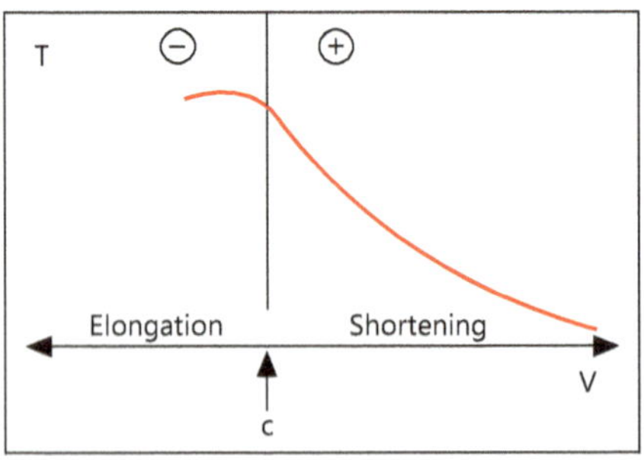

Tension/velocity (T/V) curve. *In the center* (c): zero overall muscle shortening velocity (isometric contraction). The contractile component is shortened, whereas the elastic component is elongated. *On the left*: the velocity is negative because the work is negative in the eccentric contraction. *On the right*: concentric contraction always exerts positive work.

Elongation (stretching) of the muscle:
- increased contraction velocity (eccentric) corresponding to an increase in tension, which then stabilizes.

Shortening (contraction) of the muscle:
- increased contraction velocity corresponding to a reduction in tension, until zero (i.e., the contraction force is reduced to the point of exhaustion).

The reduction in tension (contractile force) is due to the friction (viscosity) caused during sliding of the actin and myosin filaments (contractile elements). Therefore, a greater contraction force corresponds to a lesser contraction velocity.

Maintenance of the contraction velocity without reducing the contractile force is obtained by the intervention of non-muscular factors (neural) represented by:

- recruitment (spatial summation) – activation of an increasing number of motor units with the increase of the load to be sustained or overcome
- summation (temporal summation) – greater frequency of stimulation of the activated motor units (greater discharge rate or greater number of neural stimuli directed at the activated motor units)
- synchronization – greater number of muscle fibers activated at the same time (simultaneous activation of motor units that normally work asynchronously).

The simultaneous intervention of these factors allows efficient contraction for brief periods of time.

Muscle power

Definition: product of muscular force and contraction velocity ($P = F \times V$).

The maximum muscle power (the greatest force and contraction velocity possible with minimum energy expenditure, i.e., the maximum function corresponding to optimal F and V values) is obtained for intermediate values of contraction and shortening velocity. It can be maintained by varying the contraction velocity in relation to the load:

- with small loads (lower F), V can be high (reduced V in the presence of small loads causes maintenance of F for very long periods)
- with large loads (higher F), V can be reduced (high V in the presence of large loads requires an excessive number of muscle fibers to be recruited and therefore more motor units to be activated).

Moment of force

The rigid body segment (bone), on which the muscle is inserted, which as a result of the muscle action rotates around one or more axes of the corresponding joint, constitutes a lever. The muscle insertion represents the point of application of the power (P) (which here assumes the simplest meaning of "muscular force"), the center of gravity of the body segment represent the point of application of resistance (R) and the axis around which the movement is carried out (usually the center of the joint) is the fulcrum (f). The distances from f of P and R constitute the P and R arms, respectively. The location of f in relation to P and R, with greater or lesser length of the P and R arms, conditions the muscular force (see sections "Forces", page 57, and "Lever", page 69).

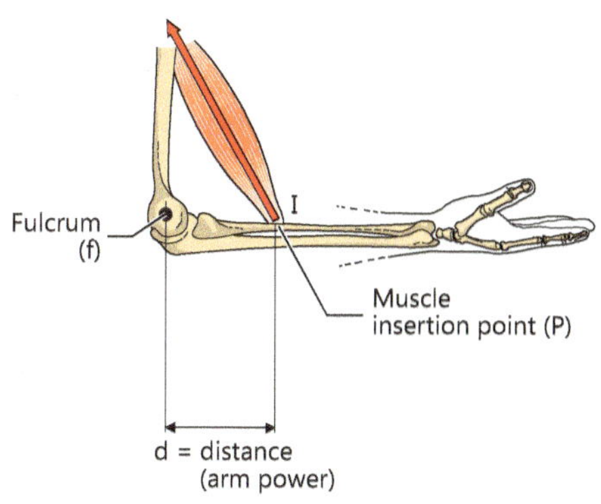

Illustration of the variation of muscular force according to the distance from the point of insertion.

Angle of insertion of the muscle

It is the angle formed by the axis of the muscle with the axis of the body segment of the insertion, of variable width during the various degrees of joint excursion. There are angles of insertion that depend on certain positions of the body segment in which the muscle is inserted, from which the movement can begin by improving the contractile capacity (see figure on page 24).

The muscle axis is the resultant force (A) of two component forces R (rotary or motor component, orthogonal to the body segment) and S (stabilizing component, directed along the axis of the body segment). Although each muscle has its own behavior, the biceps brachii can be taken as an example, for which, based on biomechanical analyses, when the width of the angle of insertion is:

- 0-45°, S tends to prevail
- = 45°, → S = R
- 45-120°, R tends to prevail (it is from these angles that it is convenient to start the contraction).

(See section "Lever", page 69).

Muscle role

Definition: specific function assumed by a muscle (or by a muscle group) in relation to an aspect of the movement carried out.

Types of roles:

- agonist (motor or activator)
  - primary (examples: iliopsoas and rectus femoris, main hip flexors)
  - accessory (example: sartorius, which assist the flexion of the hip)
  - emergency (example: brachioradialis, innervated by the radial nerve, which intervenes in the flexion of the elbow when the other two main flexor muscles are unable to do so, for example, because of a musculocutaneous nerve injury)
- antagonist (muscle or muscle group that opposes movement, stopping it initially and then releasing it)
- neutralizer (muscle that neutralizes another muscle or its action to allow the execution of a movement; for example: the inhibition of the clavicular and spinal parts of the deltoid allows abduction of the shoulder)
- fixator (stabilizer: muscle that contracts isometrically by fixing one or more body segments to avoid destabilizing factors such as gravity, traction by other muscles or rebounds produced by very fast movements)
- support (general stabilization against gravity, especially in dynamic movements such as throwing a weight, kicking a ball, etc.)
- synergistic (muscle that works together with other muscles by fulfilling the same role as, for example, the agonist role in the flexion movement of the elbow).

Polyarticular muscles

Definition: muscles that cross multiple joints.

The amplitude of a movement can vary depending on the different positions assumed by the body segments of the affected joints.

Example: flexion-extension of the wrist and the digits of the hand (the movements of flexion of the hand and its digits, as well as the movements of extension of these body segments, are carried out by the same muscles). When the wrist is flexed whilst the fingers are flexed, the joint excursion of the wrist is reduced, as is the excursion of the metacarpophalangeal and interphalangeal joints when the fingers are flexed whilst the wrist is flexed. This occurs because the traction of the muscles is exerted both at the origin and at the insertion with:

- consequent shortening of the agonist muscles (state of active insufficiency due to incomplete contraction of the flexor muscles)
- consequent elongation of the antagonist muscles (state of passive insufficiency due to incomplete stretching of the extensor muscles).

This tension mechanism, during both shortening and elongation, is defined as countercurrent (or non-cooperating).

However, if a joint is positioned contrary to the movement that the other joint(s) must perform, the movement carried out will be considered concurrent or cooperative. For example, using the extension of the wrist to fully flex the fingers, the flexion movement of the fingers will be facilitated through the defined concurrent mechanism. Instead, extending the fingers will facilitate flexion of the wrist. In this way there is alternation of tension between shortening and stretching (alternating between shortening and stretching in the two joints).

An example of concurrent and countercurrent mechanisms in walking occurs in the flexion of the knee associated with flexion of the hip and extension of the knee associated with flexion of the hip, respectively.

A further advantage of the polyarticular muscles (associated with concurrent mechanism) compared to monoarticular muscles is exemplified by movements of the lower limbs during walking, when the left leg (with hip and knee flexed) surpasses the right (with hip and knee extended). In this case there will be:

- left limb (concurrent mechanism) in the oscillatory advancement
  - rectus femoris – shortening at the hip and elongation at the knee (figure 1)

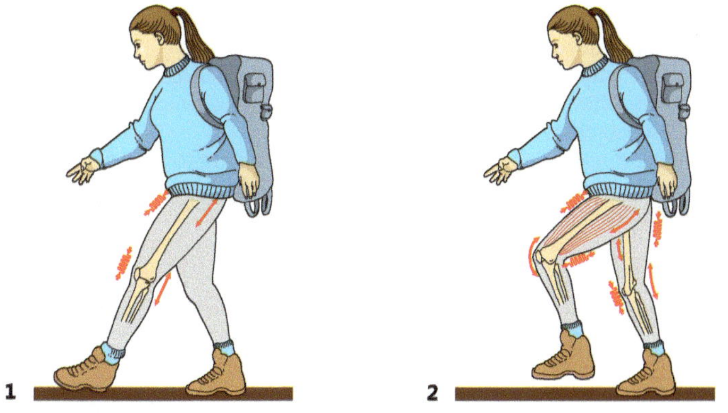

The right leg extended on the heel support, performing the countercurrent mechanism of both the rectus femoris (contraction of the two insertions) and the hamstring muscles (stretching of the two insertions), produces a state of active and passive insufficiency that leads, due to the excess tension caused, the leg to be brought back into knee flexion and hip flexion. ←——→ = Elongated insertion. →∿∿∿← = Shortened insertion.

  - hamstring muscles (semimembranosus, semitendinosus and biceps femoris) – elongation at the hip and shortening at the knee
- left limb (countercurrent mechanism) when leaning on the heel (figure 2)
  - opposite situation compared to the previous position of the rectus femoris and hamstring muscles.

The gait movement (alternating the two limbs) occurs through the transfer of elastic and muscular tensions from the antagonist to the agonist and from one joint to the other, with considerable energy savings compared to the monoarticular muscles (2nd advantage of polyarticular muscles).

Biarticular muscles

Definition: muscles that cross two joints.

Biarticular muscles are characterized by two different force arms (related to the two joints they cross). The diversity of the two force arms allows one movement to be privileged over the other.

Examples: the hamstring muscles have a major force arm at the hip (6.7 cm) and a minor force arm at the knee (3.4 cm), favoring the extension movement of the hip over flexion of the knee. The rectus femoris, however, has a major force arm at the knee (4.4 cm) and a minor force arm at the hip (3.9 cm), favoring the extension movement of the knee over flexion of the hip. When the hamstring muscles and rectus femoris work together, it is easier to obtain extension of the hip and simultaneous extension of the knee rather than opposing movement.

Neural stimulation of muscle contraction

The excitability of muscle tissue in response to a neural stimulus is achieved through the production of an action potential at the level of the sarcolemma (plasma membrane of the muscle fiber) that, by propagating along the membrane, reaches the sarcotubule system (longitudinal canaliculi of the smooth endoplasmic reticulum that give rise to transverse cisternae) and T-tubules (invaginations of the sarcolemma of the muscle fiber) in contact with the myofibrils. It depends on:
- the adequate intensity of the neural impulse (corresponding to the threshold value or liminal value of excitation, i.e., the minimum intensity sufficient to produce the contraction), which can be achieved:
  - gradually (accommodation phenomenon), corresponding to a modest contractile action
  - quickly, corresponding to a greater contractile efficiency
- the sufficient duration of the neural impulse.

Simple muscle twitch

Definition: excitation of a muscle due to a single stimulus of short duration.

The duration of the simple muscle twitch is 5-10 hundredths of a second and can be subdivided into three phases:
- initial phase (mechanical latency) – time between the action of the stimulus and the beginning of the muscle contraction (1 hundredth of a second)
- contraction phase (4 hundredths of a second)
- relaxation phase (5 hundredths of a second).

The simple muscle twitch represents the lowest level of neuromuscular excitation. It corresponds to a minimal contractile force, which can be increased up to the maximum contractile capacity through:

- the activation of an ever-increasing number of motor units (recruitment of spatial summation)
- the greater stimulation rate greater of the motor units activated (temporal summation)
- the simultaneous activation of the motor units normally activated asynchronously: stimulation asynchrony consists of the alternate partial use of the muscle fibers during the execution of a movement (synchronization).

These mechanisms depend on:

- the refractory nature of the muscle fibers
- the discharge frequency of the neural stimuli.

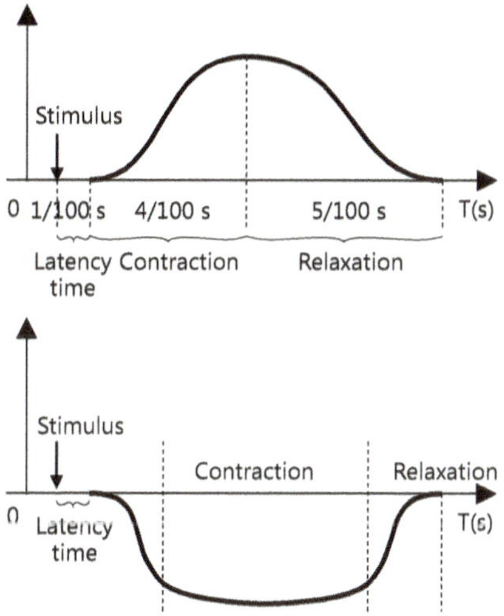

Simple muscle twitch. Above, isotonic contraction. Below, isometric contraction.

Refractory nature of the muscle fibers

Definition: period of time in which the capacity of the muscle to respond to neural stimuli is diminished or hindered (it is included in the mechanical latency phase of muscle contraction).

It can be divided into:

- absolute (the contraction is not possible even with maximal neural stimulus)
- relative (the contraction is possible only if the intensity of the stimulus is higher than normal due to an increase in the activation threshold).

Discharge frequency of the neural stimuli

Starting from a succession of simple twitches, the increase in the discharge frequency of neural stimuli may be such that the next stimulus is found:

- in the relaxation phase of the muscle – incomplete tetany (frequency between 20 and 40 Hz; more frequent mode of muscle contraction)
- in the contraction phase of the muscle – complete tetany.

Note: The force developed in the tetanic contraction (4) is around twice that produced by the simple muscle twitch (1).

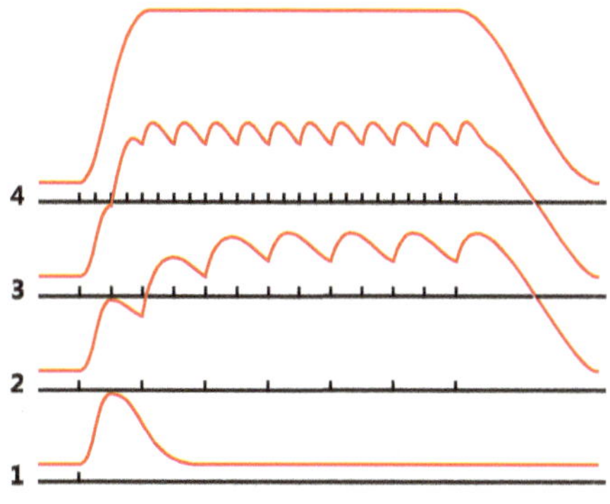

Isotonic myogram of: **1**, a simple muscle twitch; **2-3**, incomplete tetany; **4**, complete tetany. The stimuli are indicated in the abscissa.

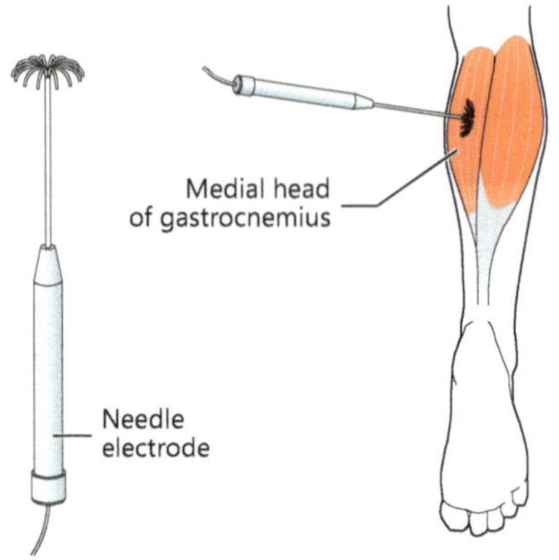

Electromyography.

Electromyography

Definition: recording of the electrical activity of a muscle (at rest or during activity) expressed by the potential difference between an indicator electrode (needle electrode inserted into a muscle belly) and a reference electrode (fixed potential chemical electrode, consisting, for example, of a needle lining cannula).

The potential difference between the two electrodes is amplified and visualized by a cathode oscilloscope that can be connected to a camera that photographs the trace, a magnetic tape recorder and an amplification system for sound made audible by an external source.

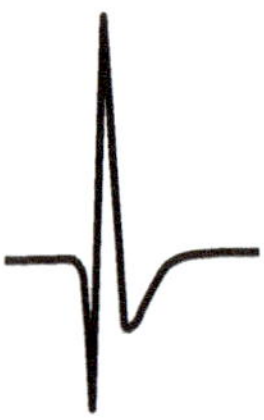

Normal triphasic action potential of a motor unit.

Recording normal electrical activity

- The introduction of the needle generates a discharge potential that is rapidly extinguished (duration of 2-3 s)
- At rest, no electrical activity is recorded (electrically silent muscle).

Slow voluntary contraction of the muscle causes activation of a reduced number of motor units with the onset of compound action potentials (resulting from the action potentials generated by all the muscle fibers of the activated motor units that are within the recording radius of the electrode), called motor unit potentials, represented by biphasic or triphasic waves.

Parameters of motor unit action potentials under normal conditions:

- variable in relation to muscle and age of the patient
- in general:
  - duration of 5-15 ms
  - amplitude of 0.2-2 millivolts
  - frequency of 5/s.

When the contraction force increases:

- the discharge rate of the individual motor units increases
- the number of motor units recruited increases, which corresponds to increases in amplitude and frequency of motor unit action potentials, maintaining the characteristics of biphasic or triphasic waves.

In case of maximum contraction, the number of motor units recruited is so high that, if the needle electrode is not very selective, it is no longer possible to distinguish the motor unit action potentials (interference trace).

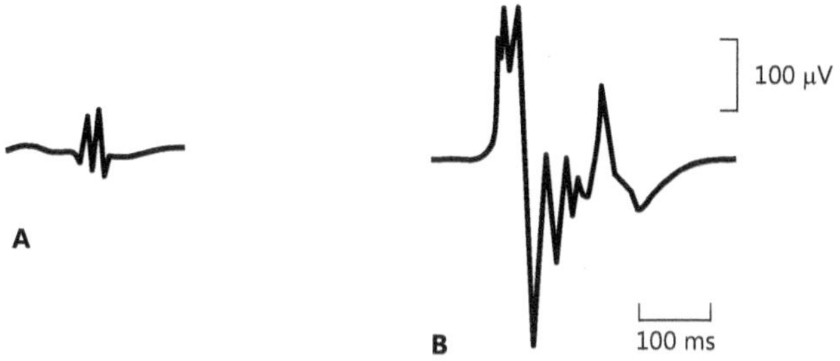

A, Reduced motor unit action potential, of short duration, polyphasic, as often observed in myopathies. **B**, Motor unit action potential, long-lasting, polyphasic, that can be present in neuropathies.

Recording pathological electrical activity

Onset at rest (complete relaxed muscle) of:

- fibrillation potentials and positive pointed waves
- repetitive discharge complexes (in the case of denervation or muscle trauma, but also in the course of inflammatory myopathies)
- fasciculation potentials (in chronic neuropathies)
- myotonic discharges (in muscle tone disorders).

Motor unit action potentials:

- of short duration and polyphasic (in myopathies)
- of long duration and polyphasic (in neuropathies).

The electromyogram can detect motor unit abnormalities and characterized them as neurogenic or myogenic.

Electromyography of an individual muscle fiber

A needle electrode is inserted into the slightly contracted muscle on which a surface electrode has been positioned laterally to increase the recording area. The action potentials of two muscle fibers belonging to the same motor unit can thus be recorded. The time interval (latency) between the two potentials is constant in normal muscle and is called jitter (mean difference between consecutive interpotential intervals).

Jitter variability indicates the presence of an abnormality in neuromuscular transmission (myasthenia) resulting from impulse blockage at the neuromuscular junction.

Electromyography of an individual muscle fiber can also be used to:

- determine the mean density of the motor unit fibers (average number of muscle fibers per motor unit in the recording area)
- evaluate the number of motor units in a muscle.

Surface electromyography

Recording of the potential differences between the electrodes located linearly on the surface of a muscle with the onset of action potentials of different motor units.

During the maximal voluntary contraction of a muscle (force increasing linearly from 0 to 100%), based on the onset of different action potentials that identify different motor units, it is possible to assess the phenomenon of motor unit recruitment and, more precisely, the type of motor units:

- always active
- recruited at low contraction levels
- recruited at high contraction levels.

By extrapolating each motor unit potential from the overall signal recorded on the skin, it is possible to calculate the motor unit conduction velocity. During a contraction sustained over time, this can be maintained only for a certain period, after which there is a decrease in force (mechanical fatigue). The point of decline in force is preceded, among other things, by a reduction in the motor unit conduction velocity, which is related to the prevalence of type II (fast) fibers over the type I (slow) fibers. Surface electromyography can indicate the composition of muscle fibers during endurance effort.

In general, surface electromyography provides information on:

- moment, duration and extent of the activation of one or more muscles during movement
- overall activity of a muscle or muscle group
- anatomy and geometry of superficial motor units.

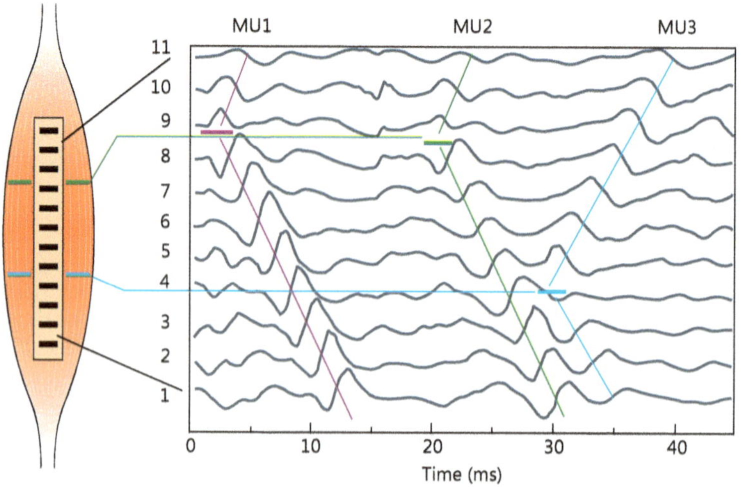

This image shows 11 recordings obtained from a linear series of 12 electrodes placed at a distance of 5 mm from each other on the surface of the biceps brachii during a low-level contraction. The traces show three different action potentials attributable to three different motor units (MU).

Muscles most frequently subjected to electromyography

Head and neck
- Frontal
- Masseter
- Orbicularis oculi
- Orbicularis oris
- Sternocleidomastoid
- Temporal

Intrinsic muscles of the vertebral column
- C5-C6
- C6-C7
- C7-T1
- L2-L3
- L3-L4
- L4-L5
- L5-L1

Shoulder and trunk
- Deltoid
- Serratus anterior
- Latissimus dorsi
- Pectoralis major
- Rhomboid major
- Teres major
- Infraspinatus
- Supraspinatus
- Trapezius

Arm
- Abductor pollicis longus
- Biceps brachii
- Brachialis
- Brachioradialis
- Extensor pollicis brevis
- Extensor digitorum
- Extensor indicis
- Extensor carpi radialis brevis
- Extensor carpi radialis longus
- Extensor carpi ulnaris
- Flexor digitorum profundus
- Pronator quadratus
- Flexor carpi radialis
- Flexor digitorum superficialis
- Flexor carpi ulnaris
- Pronator teres
- Supinator
- Triceps brachii

Hand
- Abductor pollicis brevis
- Adductor pollicis longus
- Abductor digiti minimi
- Flexor pollicis brevis
- First dorsal interosseous

Pelvis
- Gluteus maximus
- Gluteus medius

Thigh
- Biceps femoris
- Rectus femoris
- Sartorius
- Vastus lateralis
- Vastus medialis

Leg
- Extensor digitorum longus
- Gastrocnemius
- Peroneus longus
- Soleus
- Tibialis anterior

Foot
- Abductor digiti minimi
- Abductor hallucis
- Extensor digitorum brevis

Study of the motor nerve conduction velocity

Definition: recording of the electrical response of a muscle (muscular action potential) to stimulation of its motor nerve fibers in two or more points along their course.

Two or more stimulation electrodes are used, each at a different point of the nerve, and a recording electrode in the innervated muscle (surface electrode).

Motor conduction velocity: relationship between the distance (s) between two stimulation sites and the difference between the two corresponding muscular action potentials, given by the difference ($\Delta t_1 - \Delta t_2$) be-

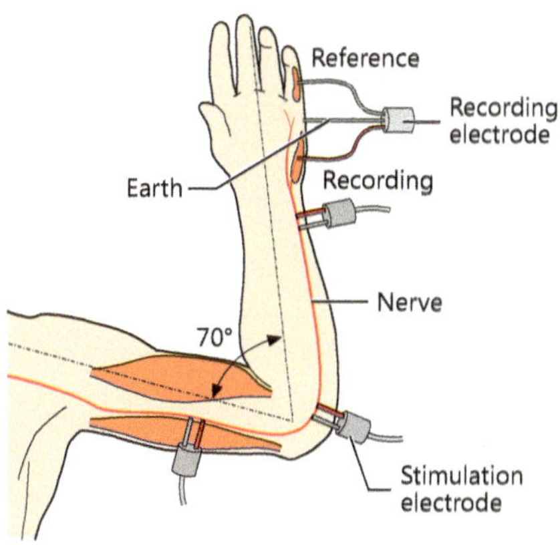

Recording of the electrical response of a muscle to stimulation of the motor fibers.

tween the proximal interval (latency) (Δt_1) and the distal interval (latency) (Δt_2) of the action potential (the value obtained is compared with the normal reference values stable for the majority of nerves tested).

Amplitude of the action potential

The amplitude of the muscular action potential is measured by applying the recording electrode (surface electrode) over the muscle and stimulating (through stimulation electrodes) the motor fibers of the nerve at different frequencies or in different locations.

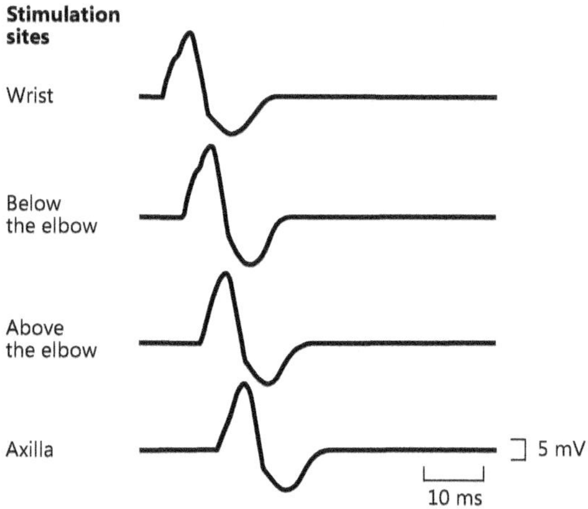

This image shows the action potential of an abductor digiti minimi recorded after high-frequency stimulation of the ulnar nerve in different locations.

More commonly studied nerves

- Accessory nerve
- Axillary nerve
- Lateral cutaneous nerve of the thigh
- Facial nerve
- Femoral nerve
- Median nerve
- Musculocutaneous nerve
- Fibular (or peroneal) nerve
- Plantar nerve
- Radial nerve
- Suprascapular nerve
- Sural nerve
- Tibial nerve
- Ulnar nerve

Models to study movement

In the past hundred years, many researchers have contributed to models to study movement derived mainly from analyses of neuropsychology. The most important schools that have dealt with movement are, in chronological order:

- behavioral school
- cognitive school
- ecological school.

None of these models can be considered outdated. The applications of each of these schools, in both sports and rehabilitation medicine, are sometimes alternative or complementary depending on the subjects, the type of exercise and/or pathology to be treated.

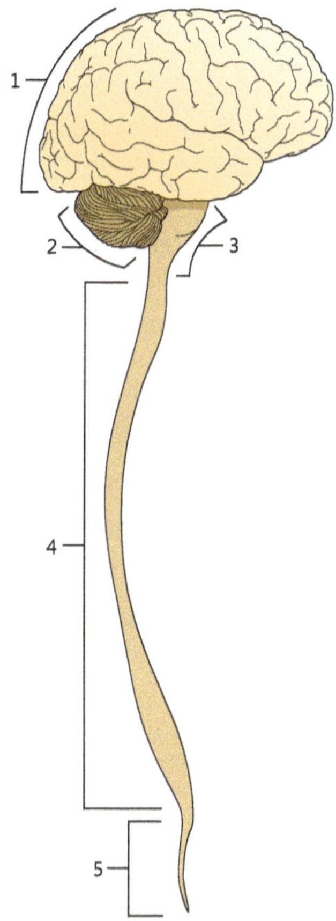

General lateral view of the central nervous system. **1**, Brain; **2**, cerebellum; **3**, brainstem; **4**, spinal cord; **5**, filum terminale.

Behavioral model

It has been developed and disseminated in the first fifty years of the 20th century.
Main proponents:

- in USA: E.L. Thorndike, J.B. Watson, C. Hull, E.C. Tolman, B.F. Skinner
- in Russia: I.P. Pavlov.

Theories and methods

It answers the question: what?
Since the neurophysiological and emotional phenomena underlying autonomous movement or in response to environmental stimuli that can determine or favor it are not objectively verifiable, it is possible to verify or induce an action only through what is visible or comparable. In fact, the behavioral school does not deal with the modalities in which a movement can be performed.

Examples

- Pavlov's "conditioned movements": after switched on a light bulb, a dog was usually given a steak. The repetition of these two modalities induced the animal to always expect a steak after switched on the light bulb, so it reacted with salivary hypersecretion even if after the light stimulus the food did not appear.
- Mutilations to experimental animals in parts of the central nervous system (CNS) to verify correspondences between the site of injury and peripheral damage.
- Thorndike and Skinner's programs related to the theory of "positive and negative reinforcement", which are followed by different behaviors by subjects to whom they are applied (operant conditioning). Operant conditioning differs from Pavlov's "classical conditioning," in which the organism's action is a response to a stimulus, in that it represents "an operation that the organism performs on the environment in view of a purpose... it can be regarded as

a form of behavioral therapy where the therapist rewards or reinforces with his/her attitude certain speech or actions of the patient that are in line with the desired behavior" [1].

Cognitive model

It emerged in the 1960s largely replacing the behavioral model.
It has its origins in cognitive psychology and neuropsychophysiology studies.
Main proponents:

- in Russia: P.K. Anochin, N.A. Bernstein, A.R. Luria
- in USA: J.A. Adams, F. Bartlett, S.W. Keele, S. Miller, U. Neisser, etc.
- in Switzerland: J. Piaget.

Theories and methods

It answers the question: how?
For cognitivists, it is important to research and evaluate, in a straightforward manner, what underlies the movement, that is, "what are the processes that the nervous system implements to carry it out and which of these processes need to be strengthened to achieve the best results". Therefore, cognitive functions are important: memory, language, attention, perception, space-time orientation, reaction times, motor skills, etc. These functions can interact in the environment using information received from sensitive and sensory structures, such as: vision, hearing, touch, proprioceptive receptors, etc. The result is, for the athlete, an optimal use of his/her motor skills and, for the disabled person, a better reorganization of his/her impaired motor skills.

Examples

- In rehabilitation, an example of the use of cognitive theories is "the cognitive therapeutic exercise" by the Italian C. Perfetti.
- In sport, the best-known example involves teams of experts associated with large teams whose aim is to sharpen neurosensory skills, with particular regard to vision, to make gestures and actions more effective in a specific sport and/or in a particular role the athlete plays in that sport.

The phases of the movement are divided into:

- perceptive (or afferent synthesis)
- organizational
- execution.

The *perceptive phase* is divided into two stages:

- perception of the stimulus
- identification of the stimulus.

A stimulus can be internal, for example, when a thought activates a decision. Examples of external stimuli, whose response can still make use of internal data contained in the individual's memory, are:

- the sound produced by the racket hitting the ball alerts the tennis player to the imminent arrival of the opponent's response

[1] Galimberti U. *Dizionario di Psicologia.* Utet ed.; 2006.

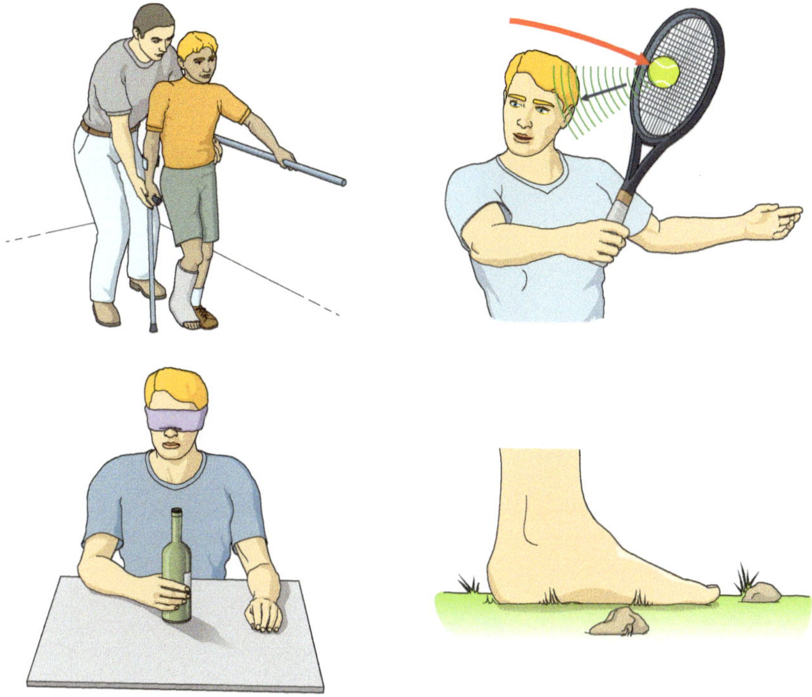

Perception of the stimulus.

- the carrier of a lower limb injury often also acoustically evidences an "escape limp" by showing a faster and acoustically sharper half-step than that of the healthy limb
- manipulating an object in the dark still allows to perceive its shape, consistency and weight
- by placing the feet on a ground, information is obtained regarding the friction that characterizes it: soft, firm, hard, slippery, etc.

In this way the stimulus is first perceived, then identified.
It should be noted that the speed of perception and identification depends on:
- filtering of stimuli (attentiveness)
- identification of the most important information (ability to choose).

The *organizational phase* is divided into two stages:
- choice of the motor response
- programming of the response.

The choice answers the question, "what to do?"

Examples

- In volleyball and basketball, the choice can be between passing the ball to a teammate or shooting towards the goal.

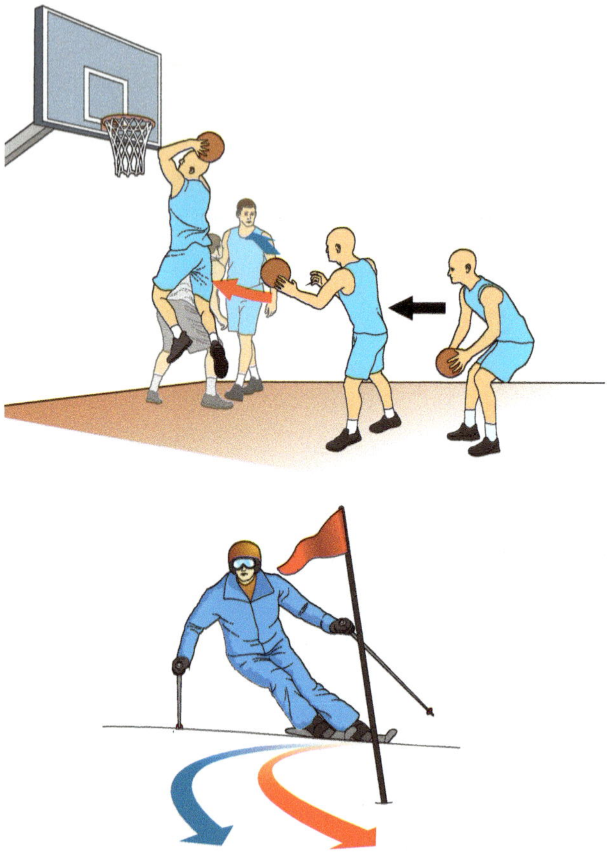

Choice of motor response.

- In skiing, the decision can be to make a wide or narrow turn or to stop.
- In contact sports (boxing, karate, fencing, etc.) the choice can be to attack, retreat or defend.

The programming answers the questions, “how and when to do?”

Examples

- In basketball, it is decided when and how to pass or shoot to the basket.
- In contrast sports, it is chosen when and how to stop, hit or retreat.

The *execution phase* represents the realization of the motor act.

Reaction time and movement time

Reaction time (RT): represents the time interval between the moment the stimulus is presented to the subject and the start of the movement. A premotor or cognitive reaction time (PRT) and a motor reaction time (MRT) can be distinguished.

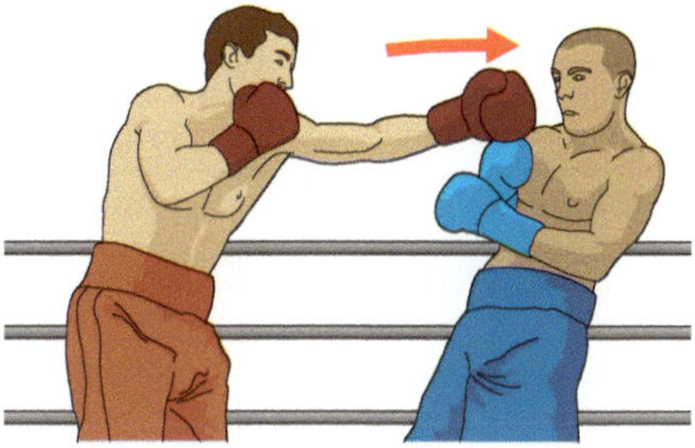

MT (movement time) very short.

Movement time (TM): is the interval time between the beginning and the end of the movement.

Total time (TT): is the time required to execute the response to a stimulus. It is given by the sum of RT + TM.
During PRT, nothing is still happening at the muscle level.
The MRT is signaled by the EMG detected at the level of the muscles responsible for executing the response. It indicates the start of neuromuscular activity that is not yet visually evident as movement. It is, in fact, the tension due to anticipatory (feedforward) muscle actions.

In many sports, and in particular motor situations, such as in contract sports and penalty kicks, there are TMs so fast that the RTs are too long to be able to respond with the same speed. So almost always the response relies on chance.

In rehabilitation, speed turns less importance even if the final and possible goal is still to improve it. It should be kept in mind that, in the case of peripheral injuries not caused by CNS damage, the most frequent impediment is related to pain and, if the injured site is in the lower limbs, also to the fear of falling. In damage caused by CNS injuries, however, the entire movement system is unstructured.
The latter condition is far more serious. The most classic example is hemiplegia (paralysis of half of the body) where, due to the destructuring of the CNS and PNS (peripheral nervous system), there are at least five penalizing conditions, namely:

- total or partial deficit on the affected side
- postural tone abnormality on the affected side
- central loss of general movement patterns
- psychological deficits related to the patient's new situation
- slowing down or/and abnormal responses of RT, PRT, MRT, MT.

The task of the rehabilitation team will be to:

- adapt to the patient's RTs and MTs
- avoid the acceleration of his/her time
- promote a recovery that aims at a gradual autonomy through voluntary and conscious movement patterns that, before the injury, were mainly automatic and unconscious.

Movement realization according to the cognitive school

PHASES of the movement	**TIMES** of the movement	**ANATOMICAL SITES** of origin of movement
Perceptive phase **1** Perception of the stimulus ↓ **2** Identification of the stimulus ↓	**Total time (TT)** *Reaction time* (RT) Cognitive or premotor reaction time (PRT) Motor reaction time (MRT) detectable at EMG ↓	**Sensitive** *Central sites*: occipital cortex, temporal cortex, parietal cortex (areas 3-1-2...), limbic system (mental impulses) *Intermediate central site*: thalamus *Peripheral sites*: receptor structures of eyes (70-80%), ears, skin, muscles, tendons, joints...
Organizational phase **3** Choice of the answer ⇅ **4** Programming of the answer	*Movement time* (MT)	**Organizational** *Central sites*: – premotor cerebral cortex (area 6) – cerebellum – extrapyramidal systems – hippocampus, mammillothalamic tract and opposite hemisphere (for the evocation of data from motor experiences) *Peripheral sites*: the same as those indicated above
Execution phase **5** Execution of the answer		**Motor** *Central sites*: – motor cerebral cortex (area 4) – cerebellum (only through the cerebral cortex) – extrapyramidal systems – medulla oblongata – pons – spinal cord *Peripheral sites*: – peripheral axon – motor plate – muscle fiber

Note - From the "ontogenetic" point of view, it should be remembered that the prefrontal regions mature late: from 4 to 7 years. "Phylogenetically" these regions have a strong development in humans: they are more than a quarter of the brain.

Ecological school

It emerged in the 1970s.
Main supporters:
- J. Gibson, M. Turvey, P. Kugler, J.A.S. Kelso and, for Italy, L. Grimaldi.

Theories and methods

Main observations of the ecological school:
- the CNS has too many tasks to deal in detail with all aspects of movement. Its main function is to deal with thinking, that is, with ideas, theories, programs
- the memory (computer hardware) of the CNS is too limited to intervene in both individual muscles and individual movements. Just think of how many muscles are part of our locomotor system and all the possible variations during their use
- the CNS uses the reflex to perform the movements, and the stretch threshold of the muscle is independent of the central commands that go to the motor neurons α and γ
- there is an equilibrium point (EP) in the various muscle groups that depends on the joint excursion achieved during movement and the degree of tension present at the level of the muscles
- there are various activation thresholds in the muscle, which should be viewed as a spring. A first stretch may simply deform the muscle without it reacting. A second elongation may cause the typical "spindle reflex," which is a phasic contraction of short duration. Further stretching causes more resistance called the tonic stretch reflex
- from the idea that the brain does not know the muscles but the movements, it has passed to the hypothesis that the brain does not know the movements but the objectives to be achieved, therefore, it must be assumed that the neural architecture of the CNS possesses, especially at the spinal level, all the details of knowledge useful for carrying out the different muscle kinetics
- cognitive afferences of the cognitivists and behaviorists should be interpreted not as fundamental factors of movement, but only as elements that facilitate it.

Postural control

There are two main models to refer to when discussing postural control: the feedback model, which implies the activation of strategies when moving away from an ideally correct posture, and the feedforward model, which instead predicts that voluntary movements that determine an alteration of the ideal posture are anticipated, in turn, by postural adjustments that compensate for these deviations [1].

The feedback model is fundamentally based on two theories.

According to the first, postural control would be fundamentally conditioned by a single predominant variable (such as the position of the center of mass, or the orientation of the longitudinal axis of the body); if this predominant variable deviates from what is preprogrammed in terms of position in space, the motor centers are activated, which in turn compensate for the deviation with a motor response.

The other theory hypothesizes instead that posture is somehow determined and conditioned by a series of reflex activities and by an innumerable series of interactions between these reflexes (vestibular, visual, somatosensory in origin): this reflex activity may have convergent components to the determination of the posture itself or divergent components.

The postural system normally functions as a functional unit, with a main characterization for the associated control of the head and trunk. However, under certain conditions, the system clearly dissociates into subsystems the control of these two segments, and it now also seems to be well established that the two body antimeres may have separate control as a function of lateralized sensory input.

A similar situation seems to be established in the cat for the anterior part of the body compared to the posterior.

These data are difficult to explain within the framework of the hypothesis of control over a single predominant variable; instead, it is possible to hypothesize that a complex system of reflex activities independently controls different portions of the body.

A similar functional organization is present in quadrupeds at the level of the locomotor system, where the pectoral (shoulder) girdle and the pelvic girdle have autonomous control mechanisms, even with respect to the most distal control of the four limbs: thus, an extremely complex system is configured, capable of responding in a decidedly timely and precise manner at the segmental level.

This organized model ensures, on the one hand, the optimization of the response to destabilizing stimuli with respect to ideal postural alignment and simultaneously their self-amplification: in fact, it has been suggested that a control system consisting of semiautonomous subsystems better adapts to the complex of environmental conditions and stimulations [2].

Control optimization would then be ensured by a model that can be functionally considered an outgrowth of feedback or feedforward systems: the central nervous system would be able to control instantly with a response that is not pre-established, but rather correlated and parameterized to the destabilizing stimulus in place: learning would then guarantee, for a portion of the repeated responses, the anticipatory capacity in counteracting a destabilizing stimulus when it has already been experienced and known.

It is reasonably to say that good postural alignment can reduce incongruous overloads on the joint support surfaces and periarticular soft tissues, thus preventing natural responses to misalignment, such as increased stiffness and decreased muscle strength.

In addition, there is no incontrovertible speculative certainty that an imperfect muscular alignment can be the cause of some symptomatology: a much-discussed topic in recent years is, for example, the relationship between malocclusion and postural problems; some authors have demonstrated their coexistence, while in many clinical studies there is no proven correlation [3].

More generally, generic associations between postural attitudes of non-adjacent segments of the body (cervical spine/anterior cruciate ligament) have been demonstrated, and some studies based on mathematical examples have highlighted the possibility that alterations in the position of one segment may cause similar problems for an adjacent segment [4].
Another topic with a strong epidemiological impact is certainly low back pain: even for this pathological condition, there are conflicting results regarding the search for an incontrovertible relationship between symptomatology and posture alteration.
Although there is a plausible relationship between the position of the head of the femur, pelvic tilt and decreased lumbar lordosis, there are strong doubts as to whether the alteration of these relationships is a causal factor for low back pain. Finally, more certainty seems to be in studies on the lower limb between static tibial alignment and patellofemoral pain syndrome or excessive pronation of the subtalar joint and between some foot pathologies (cavus and/or planus) and pathologies due to overload of the lower limb.
Thus, it cannot be certain about the causal factors of postural defect (asymptomatic deviation, only morphological, from ideal postural alignment) and even less of the postural dysfunction (which may be consequent to a prolonged state of postural defect, characterized by the presence of structural alterations and pain): although without any certainty, it is not possible to exclude that, in some subjects, asymmetries between body segments may be identified as the main causes of symptomatology.

[1] Deliagina T, Zelenin P, Beloozerova I, et al. Nervous mechanisms controlling body posture. Physiol Behav 2007; 92(1-2): 148-54.
[2] Gelfand IM, Zetlin ML. On the mathematical modeling of mechanisms of the central nervous system. In: Gelfand IM, Fomin SV, Zetlin ML, eds. Models of the structural and functional organization of certain biological systems. Cambridge (MA): MIT Press; 1971: 2-23.
[3] Ben-Bassat Y, Yitschaky M, Kaplan L, Brin I. Occlusal patterns in patients with idiopathic scoliosis. Am J Orthod Dentofacial Orthop 2006; 130(5): 629-33.
[4] Berthonnaud E, Dimnet J, Roussouly P, Labelle H. Analysis of the sagittal balance of the spine and pelvis using shape and orientation parameters. J Spinal Disord Tech 2005; 18(1): 40-7.

Biomechanics

Definition: science that applies the laws of mechanics to living organisms.

It is subdivided into:
- kinematics
- statics
- kinetics.

Kinematics and kinetics are components of dynamics.

Physical quantities of mechanics

Type	Symbol	Unit of measure
Fundamental		
– length	L o S (space)	meter (m)
– mass	M	kilogram (kg)
– time	T	second (s)
Derived (examples)		
– velocity	V	m/s
– acceleration	a	m/s^2
– force	F	Newton (N)
– pressure	p	N/m^2
– energy	E	Joule (J)
– momentum	Q	m × v
– power	P	Watt (W)

In addition to the fundamental and derived quantities, there are scalar quantities, whose value is expressed by a number that represents its measurement (examples include: mass, time, volume, surface, energy, temperature, power), and vector quantities, which are represented by a vector (examples include: force, velocity, acceleration, weight).

Vectors

Characteristics:
- direction (expresses the orientation in space)
- sense (expresses the origin and end of the line and is indicated by an arrow)
- modulus (amplitude, measure, value or intensity) (expresses the value with respect to the reference unit of measure)
- point of application (when the vector is applied to a body).

Vectors are indicated by a letter in bold or with an arrow above it, for example:

$$\mathbf{F} \text{ o } \vec{F}$$

Note: the vector quantities must be highlighted when a number is not sufficient to express its characteristics.

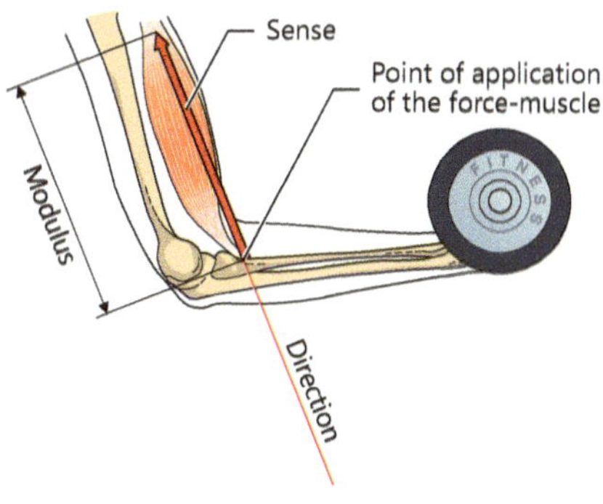

Example of vector quantity: internal force. |—| = reference segment = 1 mm = 1 kg modulus = 35 mm = 35 kg = scalar quantity (of the modulus).

Physical reference system: the human body

Internal forces – exerted by bodies forming part of the system (the point of application of the vector is that of the force-muscle).

External forces – exerted by bodies not forming part of the system (the point of application of the vector can be an object such as a balloon).

Representation of movement

Space – real path traveled by a body (wavy line, ~): scalar quantity measured in meters.

Displacement – theoretical path (straight line, –): vector quantity that unites two different positions in the body.

Kinematics

Definition: study of the trajectories of movement independent of the forces applied (causes).

Quantities of kinematics

- Position (vector quantity between the reference point or position of the observer and the point considered)
- Space (scalar quantity) and displacement (vector quantity)
- Time (scalar quantity)
- Velocity (scalar quantity)
- Acceleration (scalar quantity).

Types of movement

- Translational motion – all the points of a body travel the same distance in the same sense at the same time (they all have the same displacement vector)

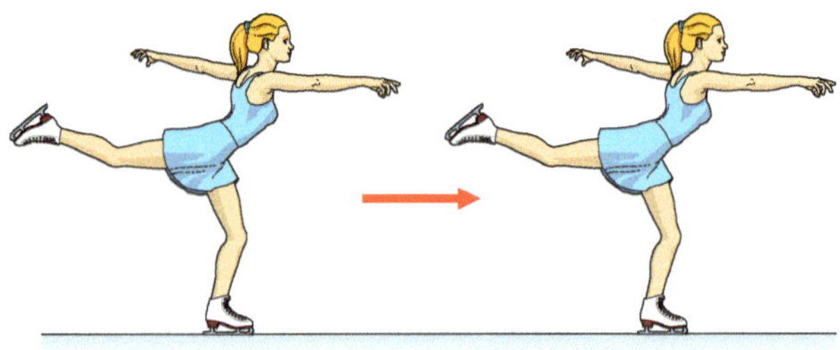

- Angular motion (rotational or circular motion) – all the points of a body travel at the same angle in the same sense at the same time

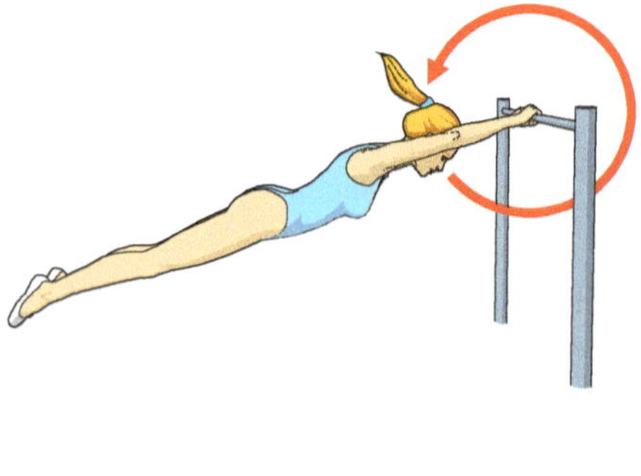

- Mixed or compound motion (natural human motion) – predominantly characterized by a combination of translational and rotatory motions, except for some short periods in which it is only translational or rotatory.

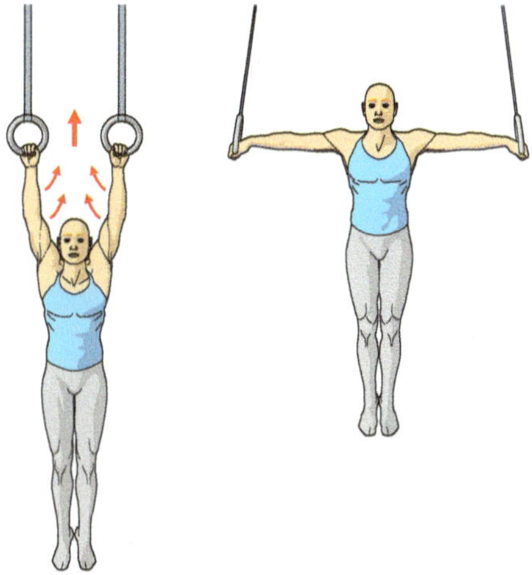

Human motion is rarely constant in velocity or acceleration and has complex trajectories, so it is also necessary to refer to the movements identified by the type of velocity:
- uniform motion
- varied motion

and by the type of trajectory:
- rectilinear motion
- curvilinear motion.

Reference system

It is represented by cartesian coordinates – a system formed by three straight lines perpendicular to each other:
- vertical axis (y-axis)
- horizontal axis (x-axis)
- axis orthogonal to the xy plane (z-axis).

With reference to the human body, its **center of gravity** (center of mass), located between the second and third lumbar vertebra (L2-L3) and the first sacral vertebra (S1) can be made to coincide with the origin of the cartesian axis system (0), the **vertical** or **longitudinal axis**, that crosses the body's center of gravity from top to bottom with the y-axis; the **frontal** or **transverse axis**, that crosses the body's center of gravity horizontally from left to right, with the x-axis; and the **sagittal** or **anteroposterior axis**, that crosses the body's center of gravity from back to front, with the z-axis.

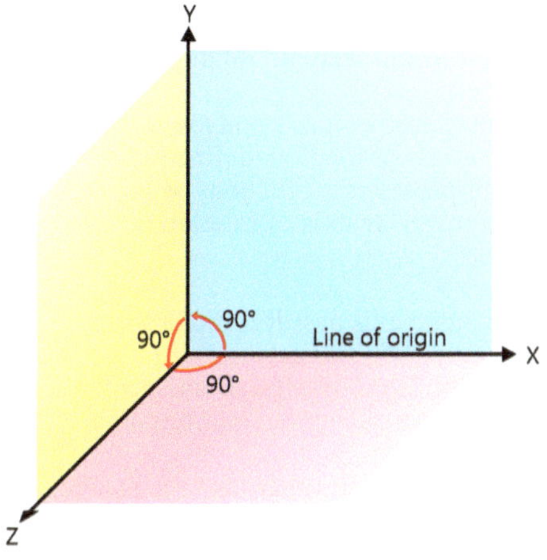

Cartesian coordinates.

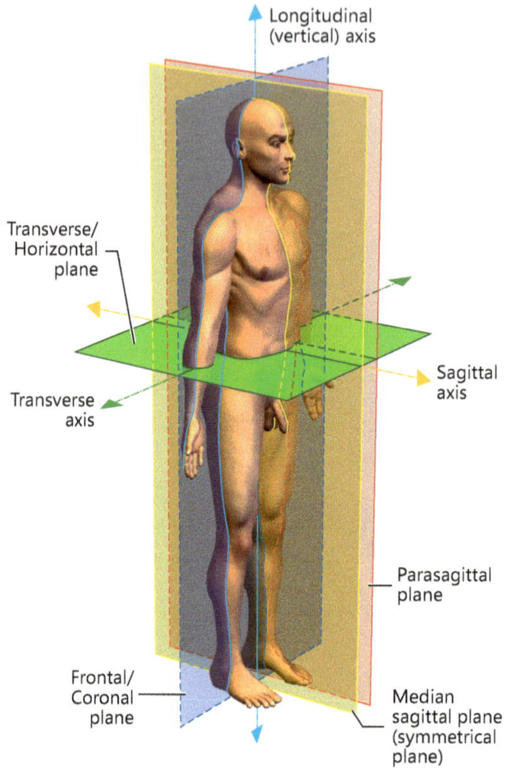

Body planes.

These **axes of movement** allow the three fundamental body planes to be defined:

- **transverse**
  - plane in which the sagittal and frontal axes intersect perpendicularly
  - divides the body in two asymmetrical halves: superior and inferior
- **sagittal**
  - plane in which the sagittal and longitudinal axes intersect perpendicularly
  - divides the body in two symmetrical halves: right and left
- **frontal**
  - plane in which the longitudinal and frontal axes intersect perpendicularly
  - divides the body in two asymmetrical halves: anterior and posterior.

Considering the anatomical reference position (upright position with upper limbs relaxed alongside the trunk and palms facing forward):

- all displacements of a body segment on the transverse plane occur around the **vertical** or **longitudinal axis** of rotation (defined by the intersection of the frontal and sagittal planes)
- all displacements of a body segment on the sagittal plane occur around a **frontal** or **transverse axis** of rotation (defined by the intersection of the frontal and transverse planes)
- all displacements of a body segment on the frontal plane occur around a **sagittal** or **anteroposterior axis** of rotation (defined by the intersection of the sagittal and transverse planes).

The rotation axis passes through the center of rotation of each joint.

In addition to the sagittal, frontal and transverse planes, that divide the body in two halves, infinite sagittal, frontal and transverse planes pass parallel to each other.

Each sagittal plane other than the median sagittal plane has two surfaces:

- medial or internal (facing the median plane)
- lateral or external (opposite to the medial surface)

Each frontal plane has two surfaces:

- anterior (ventral; volar or palmar at the level of the hands; volar or plantar at the level of the feet)
- posterior (dorsal)

Each transverse plane has two surfaces:

- superior (cephalic, cranial or rostral)
- inferior (caudal).

The terms proximal and distal indicate a lesser or greater distance, respectively, from the median sagittal plane (symmetrical plane).

Simple motions

It is only possible to describe and understand complex or compound motions if the different types of simple motions are known. Each motion is characterized by its trajectory, defined by the different spatial positions of a body due to its displacement, and by its velocity.

Most important simple motions

- Rectilinear:
  - uniform
  - uniformly accelerated or decelerated
- Parabolic
- Circular (rotatory or angular)
- Uniform circular
- Harmonic
- Various:
  - circular
  - curvilinear
  - rectilinear.

Uniform rectilinear motion

Characteristics:

- translational motion with rectilinear trajectory
- the body travels through the same spaces at the same time
- constant velocity.

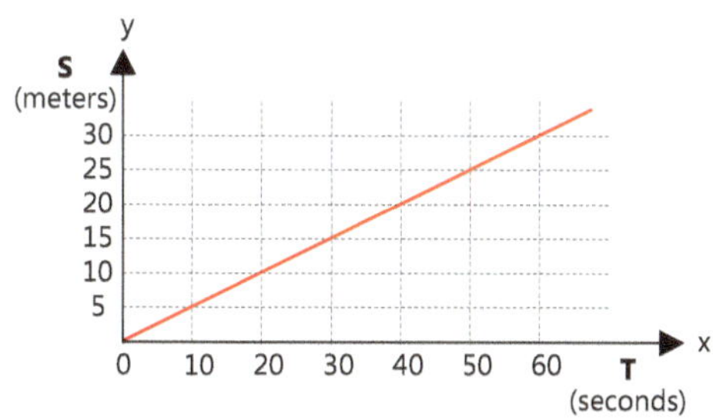

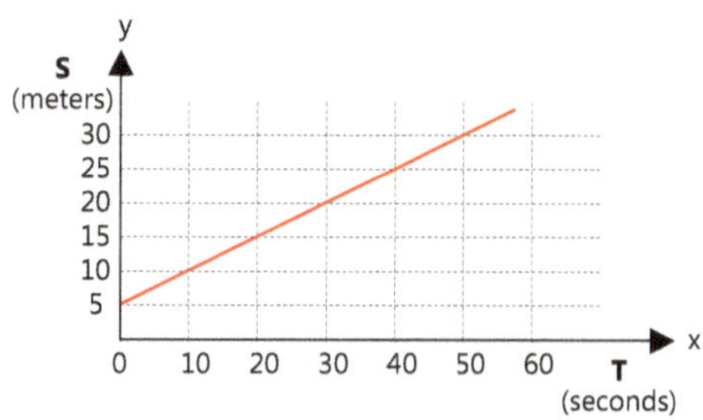

T (time) – x-axis
S (space) – y-axis

The space traveled between two points (S_1 and S_2) is $\Delta S = S_2 - S_1$
The time taken is $T_2 - T_1$
The relation $S_2 - S_1/T_2 - T_1$
is constant.

The mean velocity is
$V_m = S_2 - S_1/T_2 - T_1$

In the graph above, the origin of the movement examined occurs when this begins (S = 0, i.e., the position of the body = 0).
Below, the movement is examined when the position of the body has already traveled 5 m.

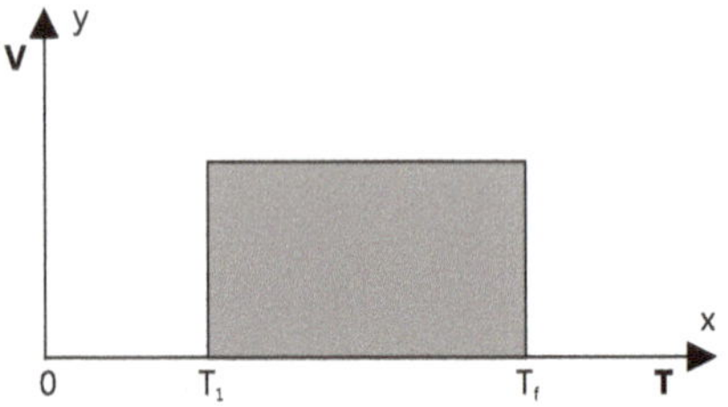

Graph representing the constant velocity characteristic of the uniform rectilinear motion. V = velocity; T = time; T_1 = time at which the initial observation occurs; T_f = time at which the final observation occurs.

T (time) – x-axis
V (velocity) – y-axis
The space traveled is $S - S_0$ (observation of the motion starts after the body has traveled the distance $S - S_0) = \Delta S$

Position S_0 corresponds to the initial time or instant T_1 (time at which the initial observation occurs), equal to 0, whereas position S corresponds to the final time or instant T_f (time at which the final observation occurs), equal to T.

The area of the rectangle gives the space traveled:

$\Delta S = V \times T$

The instantaneous velocity is $V_{inst} = \Delta S/T$, also constant as V_m

Uniformly accelerated or decelerated rectilinear motion

Characteristics:
- the body travels through the same spaces at ever increasing velocity (accelerated motion-positive velocity) or ever decreasing velocity (decelerated motion-negative velocity), or gradually greater or lesser spaces due to the effect of a constant increase or decrease in velocity, thus
  - the velocity is variable
  - the acceleration is constant.

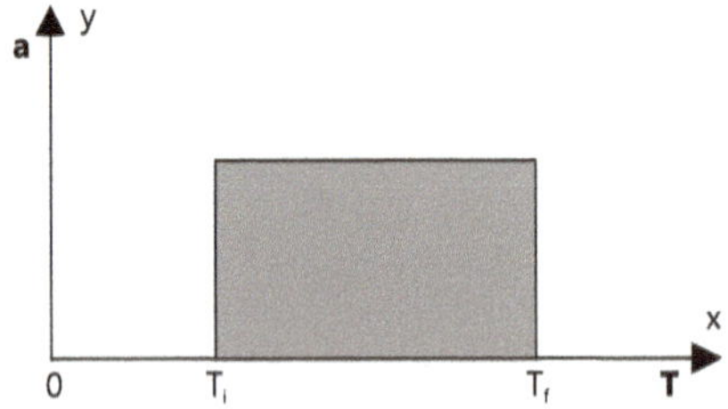

Graph representing the constant acceleration:

$$a = \frac{V_f - V_i}{T_f - T_i} = \text{constant.}$$

V_i = initial velocity; V_f = final velocity;
T_i = initial time; T_f = final time.

a (acceleration) – y-axis
T (time) – x-axis

$a = V/T \rightarrow V/T = (V_f - V_i)/(T_f - T_i) \rightarrow$
$a = (V_f - V_i)/(T_f - T_i) \rightarrow (V_f - V_i) =$
$a \times (T_f - T_i) \rightarrow V_f = V_i + a \times (T_f - T_i)$

If $T_i = 0$ and $T_f = T$, $V_i = V_0$ and $V_f = V$

you will have $V = V_0 + a \times T$

Positive velocity – The area of the triangle corresponds to the space traveled.

> If $V_i = 0$ ($V_f - V_i = V_f = V$) you will have ΔS (area of the triangle) = $(V \times T)/2 \rightarrow (aT \times T)/2 \rightarrow aT^2/2$

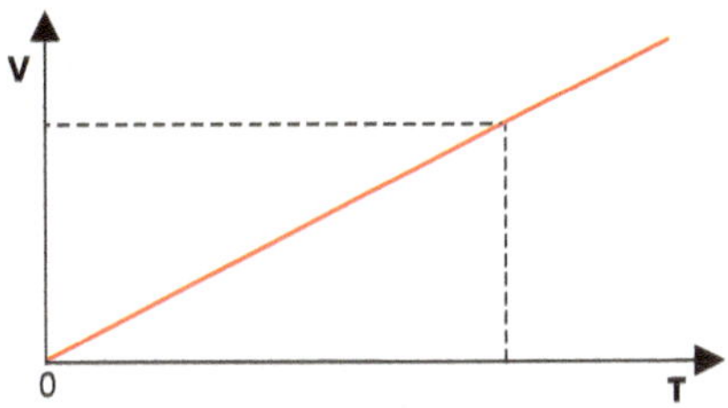

Representation of the space traveled by a body with uniformly accelerated motion (UAM) with initial velocity $V_0 = 0$.

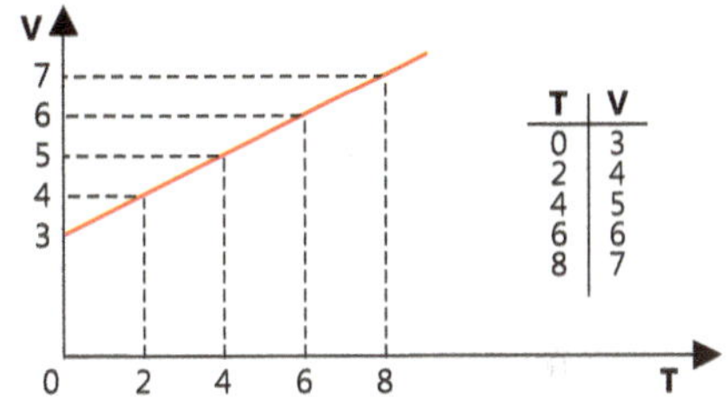

T	V
0	3
2	4
4	5
6	6
8	7

Representation of the space traveled by a body with uniformly accelerated motion with initial velocity other than 0. This graph and the previous graph show that the relationship between the variation in velocity and the interval of time is constant. This graph indicates such relationship alongside it.

Negative velocity – The area of the triangle corresponds to the space traveled.

> If $V_i \# 0$ you will have ΔS (area of the triangle) = $(V + V_0) \times T/2 = (V_0 + aT + V_0) \times T/2 = V_0 \times T + 1/2\, a\, T^2$

Graph representing negative acceleration. The body is proceeding at a velocity of 40 m/s when it starts to decelerate and stops after 18 seconds. The space traveled is represented by the area under the triangle:

$$\frac{40 \cdot 18}{2} = 360$$

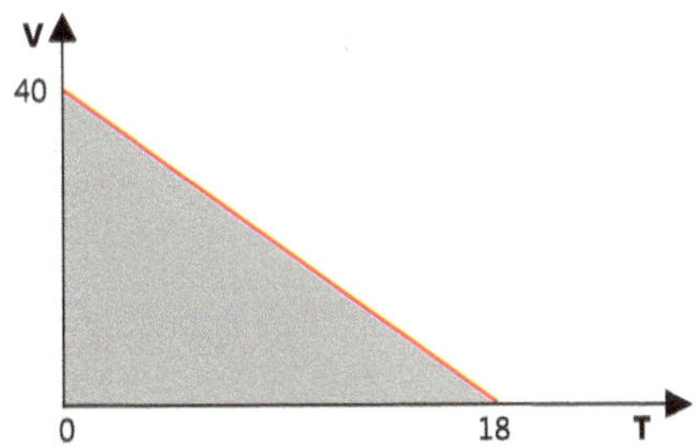

Space-time diagrams

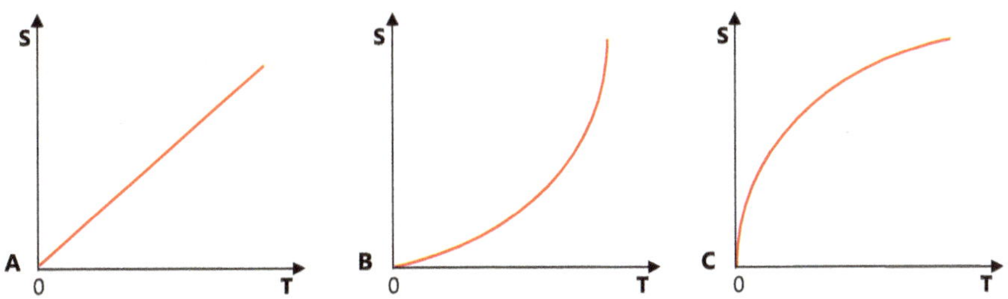

Space-time graphs. **A**, Uniform rectilinear motion (URM): the velocity is constant, there is no acceleration. **B**, Uniformly accelerated rectilinear motion (UARM): the velocity increases, the "positive" acceleration is constant. **C**, Uniformly accelerated rectilinear motion (UARM): the velocity decreases, the "negative" acceleration (deceleration) is constant.

The importance of uniformly accelerated rectilinear motion is related to the action of the force of gravity, which causes constant accelerations of body movements.

In the presence of gravity, acceleration (a) is constant and is represented by g (acceleration of gravity = 9.81 m/s^2).

In the absence of friction, if we want to know the time taken by a body falling from a certain height (flight time), we need to use the formula $\Delta S = aT^2/2$ (see section "Uniformly accelerated or decelerated rectilinear motion", page 50).

$\Delta S = aT^2/2 \rightarrow \Delta S = gT^2/2 \rightarrow T^2 = 2\Delta S/g$

The mean velocity will be: $V_{med} = \Delta S/T$

The final velocity will be: $V_{fin} = aT$

Parabolic motion

It is a motion composed of:
- uniform rectilinear motion
- uniformly accelerated rectilinear motion

that occurs along orthogonal directions.

Half-parabola or simple parabola – The simplest of the parabolic movements is that in which the direction in the initial phase is almost horizontal, with slight deviations and prevalence of uniform rectilinear motion, while in the intermediate and terminal phases there is an accentuation of the deviations from the horizontal line with prevalence of uniformly accelerated rectilinear motion (example: a stone thrown forward). This is represented by a line (with a descending arc) whose direction derives from the composition of the two motions.

> 0 is the origin of the launch point, the x-axis shows the horizontal distance (ΔS horizontal), the y-axis shows the vertical distance (ΔS vertical).
>
> ΔS horizontal (uniform rectilinear motion) = $V \times T$
>
> ΔS vertical = $-gT^2/2$ (the acceleration has a negative sign because the value of the quadrant where the half-parabola occurs is negative; in fact, gravity causes a downward acceleration)
>
> If height h (ΔS vertical) is known, we can obtain the fall time T_c from $T^2 = 2\Delta S/g$: $T^2 = 2h/g$

Complete parabola – It is a complex motion that often occurs in human motions. It is represented by a complete arc whose point of origin (origin of the flight) can be at the same height as the point of arrival (example: high jump) or at a greater height (release height, detachment or projection) (example: throwing an object). The release angle is the angle formed by the body or object with the horizontal (ground) to perform the required action. The theoretical release angle that allows the maximum horizontal distance to be obtained is 45°.

Representation of a simple parabolic motion. There is no "angle" of detachment, i.e., the throw (or flight) is horizontal, as in the case of a bullet, a javelin, or a body thrown after a run-up or push from an elevated position and forward. Note that the horizontal spaces occupied in the graph by the uniform rectilinear motion are always equal (constant velocity), whereas the vertical spaces emphasize the increase in velocity, therefore, the presence of a uniformly accelerated motion. On the right, the "dots" give us an idea of the non-uniform increase in vertical velocity (for equal horizontal spaces). The space traveled from the moment of launch to the arrival of the body on the ground (25.5 m) is represented horizontally, whereas the space traveled in flight (50 m) is shown vertically.

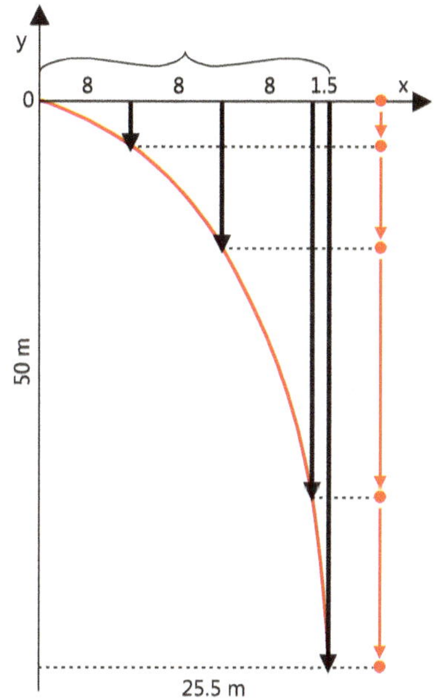

Characteristics:

- trajectory, defined by the points of displacement of the body's center of gravity
- projection velocity (of running, pushing, throwing, also defined as power), divided into two components – horizontal velocity and vertical velocity
- range (space traveled), which is proportional to the square of the velocity and is dependent on the horizontal velocity and the flight time, which in turn depends on the vertical velocity
- the ideal release angle can be defined with analytical methods that require the use of trigonometry, or with the evolutive method, which proposes to verify the so-called current interval, i.e., the interval within which the angles that offer the best result to each athlete can be determined
- the projection velocity is divided into a horizontal and a vertical component. The intensity (or modulus) of each individual component depends on the release angle.

For a release angle of 45°, the height reached is greater than for a release angle of 25°. In the latter case, however, the horizontal distance is greater.

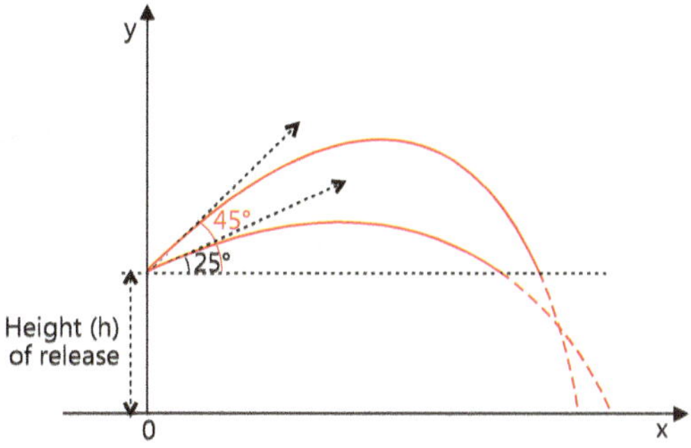

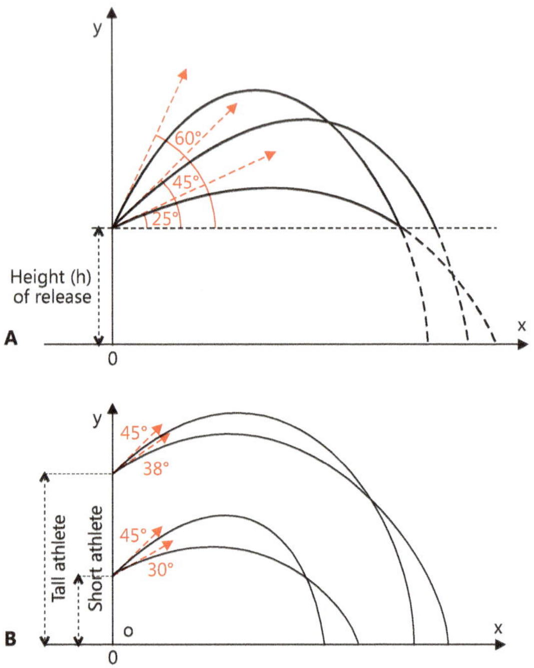

A, As can be seen from the figure, while a release angle > 45° is always disadvantageous, an angle < 45° is, on the other hand, advantageous. **B**, Since an athlete of short stature is closer to having no height difference than a tall athlete, the former will throw, for example, with an angle = 42° and the latter with an angle = 40°.

The parabola is formed by two phases: ascending and descending. Knowing the initial horizontal velocity (V_{0x}), the initial vertical velocity (V_{0y}) and the release angle, the parabolic motion can be described through the positions assumed by the body – horizontal and vertical – second by second.

In fact: $x = V_{0x} \times T$

$y = V_{0y} \times T - gT^2/2$ (the displacement depending on negative acceleration, ΔS vertical $= - gT^2/2$, must be subtracted to calculate the vertical position)

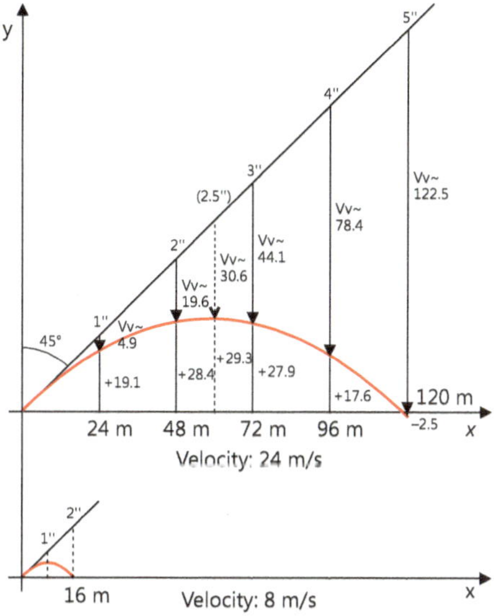

Complete parabolic motion (with release angle of 45°). At a velocity of 8 m/s, a small parabola is obtained with a flight time of less than 2 s (horizontal space traveled = 16 m). At a velocity of 24 m/s, a large parabola is obtained with a flight time of around 5 s (horizontal space traveled = ~ 120 m).

Circular motion (rotational or angular motion)

Characteristics:

- all points on a body move around a rotation axis describing a circular trajectory (complete motion) or an arc of a circle (incomplete motion)
- the center of rotation can be internal or external.

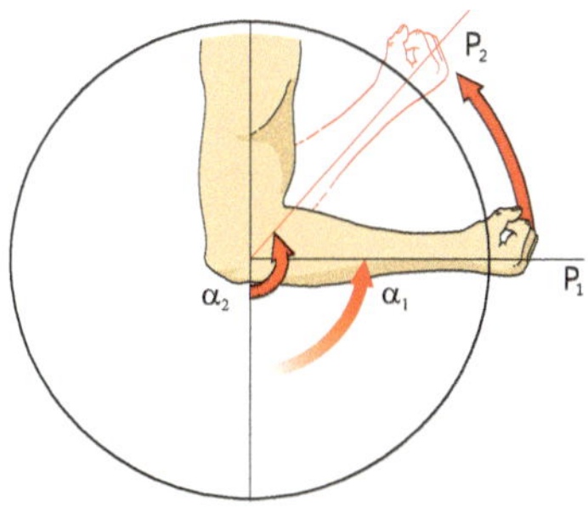

Angular excursion of the forearm on the arm, i.e., "flexion of the elbow". The forearm moves with a uniform circular motion (UCM). The trajectory traveled by the body under observation is given by the difference between the total angle (a_2) from the reference position (vertical forearm) to the arrival position (P_2) and the angle (a_1) from the reference position to that of the beginning of the observation (P_1).

Uniform circular motion

The circular trajectory is traveled with a velocity constant in modulus (but not in direction, which varies continuously). There are two types of velocity:

- angular (ω) – the relationship between the angle (measured in radians) described as the radius for a section of circumference (arc of circumference) and time taken by the body to travel it (measured in seconds)
- tangential (u) (peripheral, linear or centripetal) – the relationship between the section of circumference (arc) and the time taken by the body to travel it.

A radian is defined as the relationship between the arc of circumference and the radius (rad = l/r). When the arc of circumference is equal to the radius (l = r), α is equal to 1 rad (1° corresponds to 0.01745 rad).

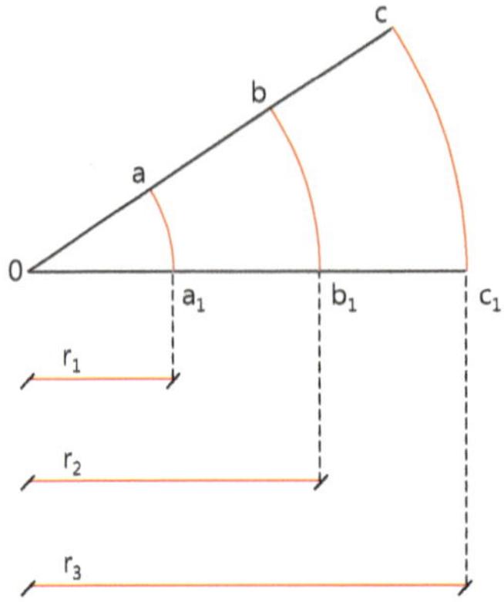

Exemplification of the increase in peripheral velocity compared to the increase in radius. The bodies a, b, c, which travel the trajectories a-a_1, b-b_1 and c-c_1 respectively in a uniform circular motion whose center of rotation is at 0; the bodies move with gradually increasing peripheral velocity ($u_c > u_b > u_a$) since their radii are different ($r_3 > r_2 > r_1$).

Angular velocity:

$\omega_{med} = (\alpha_2 - \alpha_1)/(T_2 - T_1) = \Delta\alpha/\Delta T$

where ω_{med} = average velocity, α_1 = angle traveled in time T_1, α_2 = angle traveled in time T_2

Peripheral velocity: $u = \Delta l/\Delta T$

Since $\Delta\alpha$ (angle measured in radians) is equal to $\Delta l/r$ (where Δl is the arc of circumference traveled in time ΔT), $\omega = \Delta l/r/\Delta T = u/r$; from $\omega = u/r$ we obtain $u = \omega r$, therefore the tangential velocity is the product of the angular velocity and the radius (thus, with constant angular velocity, there will be an increase in the peripheral velocity with the increase in radius).

To define uniform circular motion, in addition to the angular and tangential velocity, it is necessary to know the distance from the rotation axis and the centripetal acceleration (**a**C). In uniform circular motion, unlike uniform rectilinear motion, there is a continuous change in vectoral direction, due to the presence of vector distances of the same length tangent to the circular trajectory. These variations in direction of the trajectory change the velocity. Acceleration therefore occurs, which is precisely **a**C, directed towards the center of rotation, which prevents the body from continuing along the tangent by inertia. Since **V** : r = a : **V** (the scalar velocity is proportional to the radius, as well as the acceleration is proportional to the scalar velocity)

$$\mathbf{a}C = \mathbf{V}^2/r$$

Other parameters are the period (measured in seconds), i.e., the time taken by the body to travel the entire circumference, and the frequency (measured in Hertz), i.e., the number of laps traveled in one second, which is the inverse of the period.

Harmonic motion

It is a motion characterized by oscillations produced by elastic forces whose intensity is proportional to the displacement of the body from the position of equilibrium or rest.

Varied circular motion

In uniform circular motion, the peripheral velocity (u) in modulus is constant, but not in varied motion. It is therefore necessary to find out its average value (u_{med}).

Varied curvilinear motion

It is the most general motion possible, characterized by a body subjected to forces that make it perform varied and partial circular movements.

Varied rectilinear motion

It is a rectilinear motion with variable acceleration.

Statics

Definition: field of mechanics that deals with the equilibrium conditions of bodies and the forces that affect them.

Forces

The force (derived physical quantity) acts on a body causing an effect, which can be:
- static (the body remains in the state in which it is, or is deformed)
- dynamic (variation in the state of rest or motion of the body).

The first type of effect is studied by statics, the latter by dynamics.

In human motions, the two most frequent types of force are the **muscular force** and the **force of gravity**.

The unit of measure for forces is the Newton (N), defined as the force that, applied to a mass of 1 kg, causes its acceleration of 1 m/s^2 (1 N = 0.1 kg).

Forces are applied vectors. In addition to having direction, sense and intensity, they are characterized by a straight line (or point) of application. When this varies, different effects can be produced.

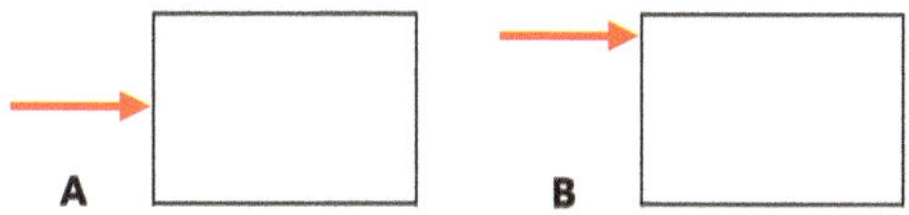

Two forces of equal modulus produce, in **A**, the translation of the body, and in **B**, the rotation.

Composition of the forces

Definition: search for the resultant force (**R**) of different forces acting simultaneously on a body. The latter are coplanar when they act on the same plane, concurrent when they converge on the same point, colinear when they act on the same line.

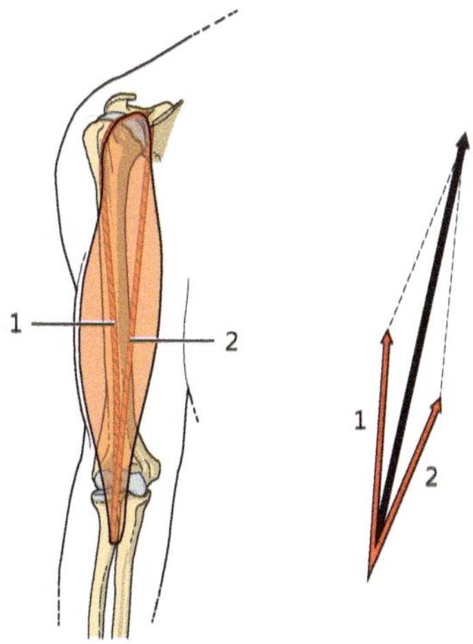

Biceps brachii (frontal projection). **1**, Long head of the muscle; **2**, short head of the muscle. With the construction of the parallelogram of the forces, we obtain the resultant of the action of the two heads.

Composition of more than two concurrent forces

To obtain **R**, the **polygon of forces** is used, uniting a first vector (any) with a second, this to a third and so on up to the last vector; the line that joins the origin of the first vector with the end of the last constitutes **R** in both sense and modulus.

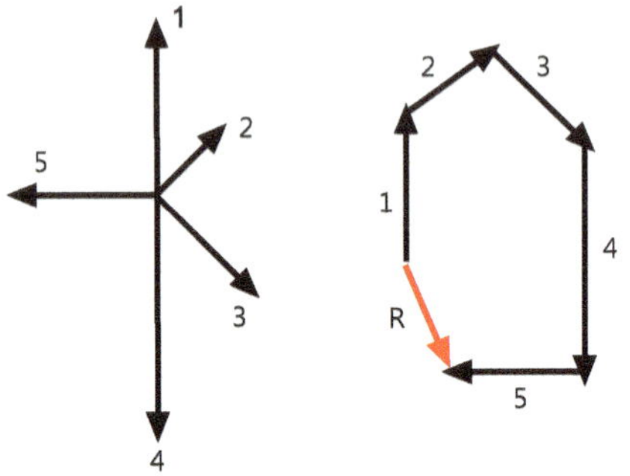

Graphic example of the resultant of more than three concurrent forces with different directions and senses.

Calculating the modulus of **R** *in the case of non-colinear forces*

The cosine rule applies.

For the cosine theorem

$c = \sqrt{a^2 + b^2 - 2ab\cos\theta}$.

Since $\theta = 180 - \varphi$,
$\cos\theta = \cos(180 - \varphi) = \cos\varphi$,

therefore, c is equal to

$\sqrt{a^2 + b^2 - 2ab\cos\varphi}$

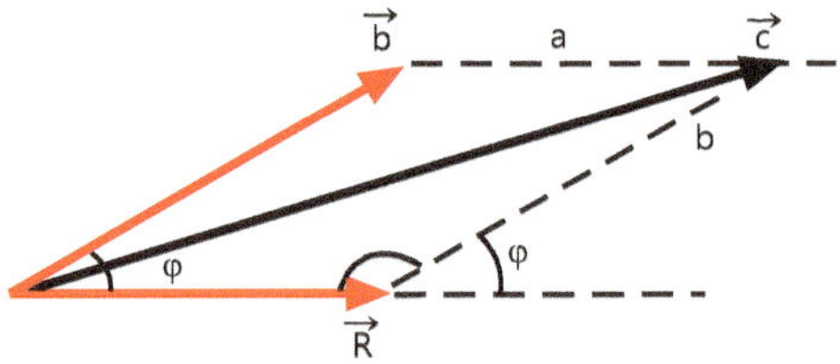

Illustration of the cosine rule.

Calculating the modulus of **R** *in the case of perpendicular forces*

The Pythagorean theorem applies, **R** represented by the hypotenuse.

$$R = \sqrt{AO^2 + OB^2}$$

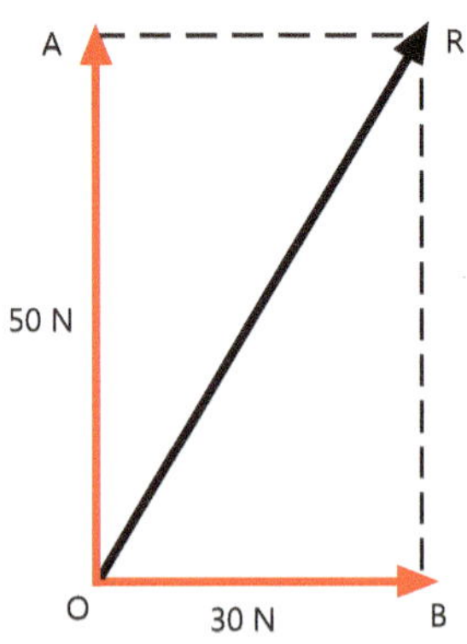

Search for the value of the resultant (R) when the two forces have an angle of 90° between them.

The smaller the angle between the two forces, the larger **R** is, and vice versa.

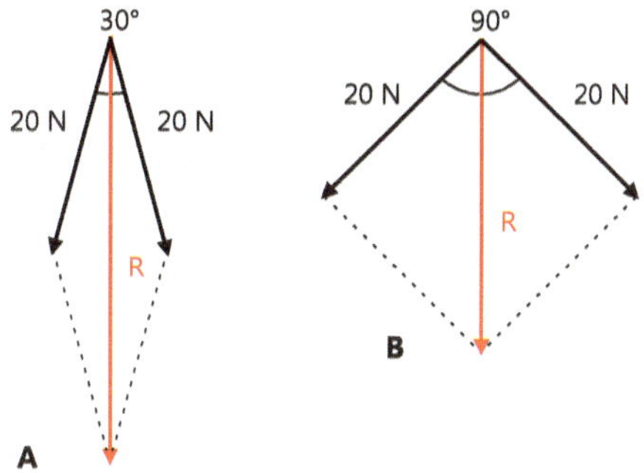

A, Two forces of 20 N, each acting on the same point with an interposed angle of 30°. The resultant will be 40 N. **B**, Two forces of 20 N, each acting on the same point with an interposed angle of 90°. The resultant will be ~29 N.

Concurrent non-coplanar forces

R is given by the diagonal of the solid that is formed by these forces.

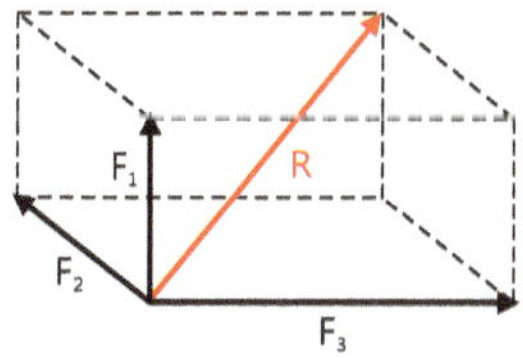

Resultant of three concurrent non-coplanar forces.

Coplanar forces with different points of application

This is the case of the biceps brachialis and brachialis, which are synergic with each other (they perform the same function), but with different points of application of their forces; the property of rigid bodies is exploited (the assumption is that the bodies on which the forces act are undeformable) to slide the force vectors until they cross, making it possible to determine **R**.

Parallel forces with the same sense (concordant) or opposite sense (discordant)

- In the first case, two other forces are applied to the two original forces directed along the joining line, equal and opposite and with the same modulus. Thus two concurrent **R** are obtained, which are projected until they cross; through the point of intersection we obtain the **R** of the two original forces, which is found within these and is the sum of the two original forces
- In the second case, after having applied the same procedure, **R** is found outside the greater force and is the difference between the greater force and the lesser force.

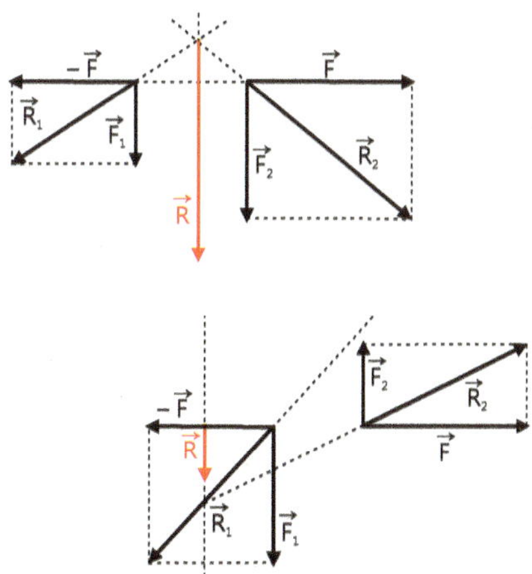

Determination of the line of application (resultant) in the presence of concordant (above) and discordant (below) parallel forces.

Pair of forces

It consists of two parallel forces, with opposite sense and equal modulus, whose **R** is equal to 0 (being the difference between the two forces equal to zero).
The pair of forces produces a rotational effect on the body.

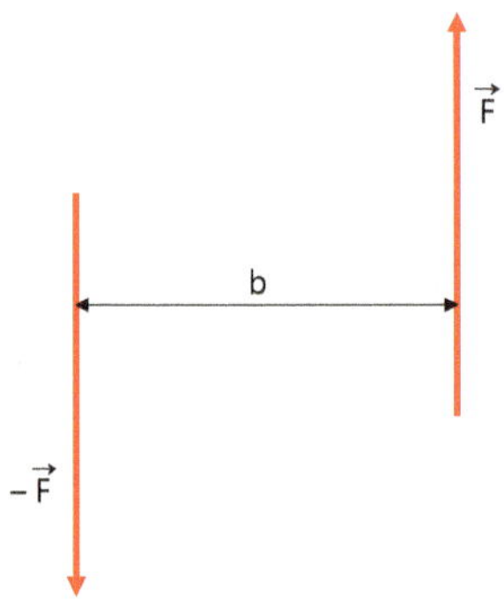

Pair of forces.

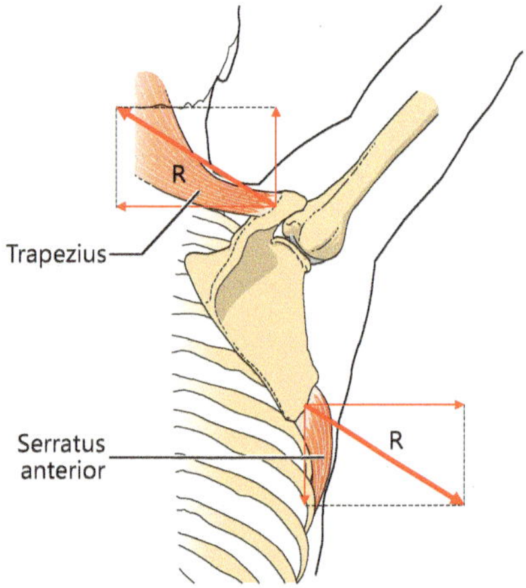

Anatomical example of a pair of forces: descending part of the trapezius and serratus anterior.

Moment of a pair of forces

Definition: product of the modulus of the force and the distance between the two forces (measured in N × m).

If two pairs of forces have the same moment of force, the effect on the body will be the same.

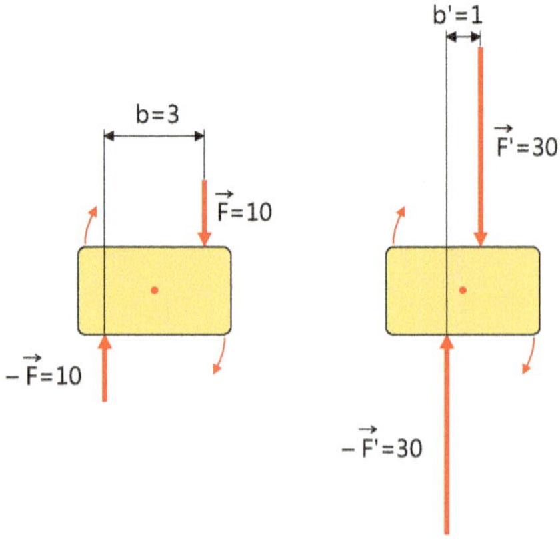

On the left, a pair of forces with a motion equal to the pair of forces on the right: the body rotates in the same way.

2

Decomposition of the forces

Definition: from a resultant (**R**), the forces that have determined it must be sought.

It is the opposite of composition. However, it is necessary to know the direction of the forces whose composition gives **R**. The same **R** can have variable components.

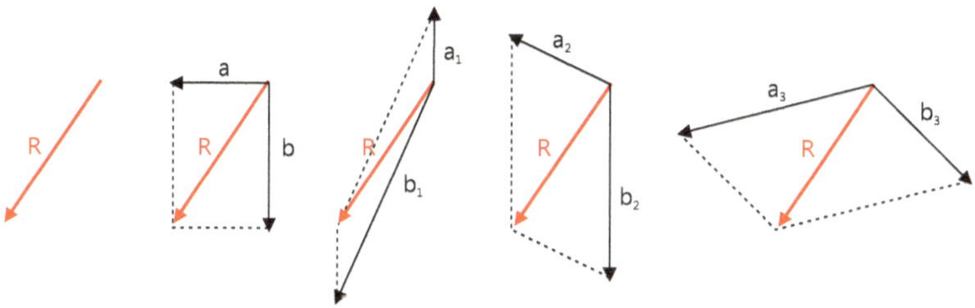

Variable components of a same resultant.

Decomposition of the muscular force

The **R** of a muscle (i.e., the force on which the movement produced by a muscle depends) has a direction that corresponds to the average line of direction of the muscle fibers from the origin to the insertion. During contraction, which causes the movement of the mobile bone segment (where the muscle fibers are inserted) compared to the fixed bone segment (where the muscle fibers originate), the direction of the muscle fibers continuously changes and, therefore, the direction of **R**. This can be broken down into two forces:

- rotational (angular or motor)
- longitudinal (stabilizing).

The rotational force is the only effective force for the purposes of movement, whereas the longitudinal force (so defined because it is directed along the bone axis) has mainly stabilizing effects (sometimes also coaptation or dislocation). The predominance of the rotatory force compared to the longitudinal force depends on the angle between the insertion of the muscle and the mobile bone segment.

A typical example is the flexion of the forearm (mobile segment) on the arm (fixed segment) performed by the biceps brachii. The angle between **R** and the axis of the forearm, on

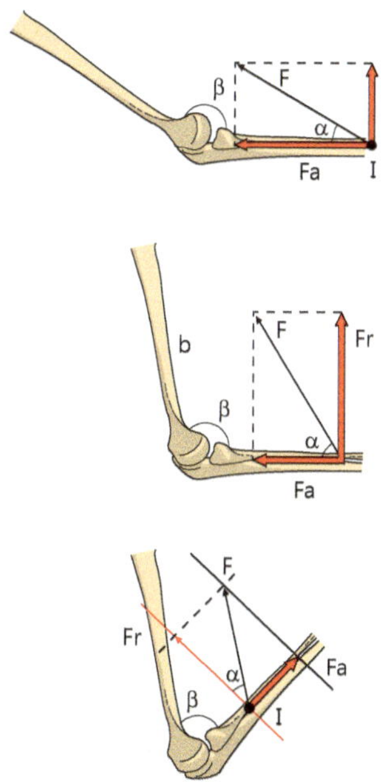

Relationship between angle "α" and angle "β". Angle α, angle between the resultant vector force of the muscle (F) and the axis of the forearm; angle β, angle between the axis of the forearm and the axis of the arm; F, resultant vector force of the muscle; Fr, rotational component vector force; Fa, axial component vector force.

which the prevalence of the rotational force with respect to the longitudinal force depends, in turn depends on the angle between the arm and the forearm.

During flexion of the forearm on the arm, the rotational force has maximum intensity and maximum prevalence in relation to the longitudinal force when the movement occurs from a flexion position of the forearm equal to 90°.

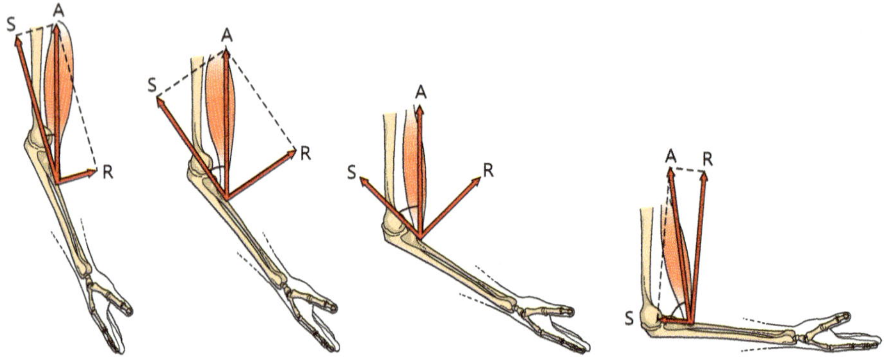

Angle = 15°
S = 95.6 N
R = 25.9 N

Angle = 30°
S = 86.6 N
R = 50 N

Angle = 45°
S = 70.7 N
R = 70.7 N

Angle = 75°
S = 25.9 N
R = 96.6 N

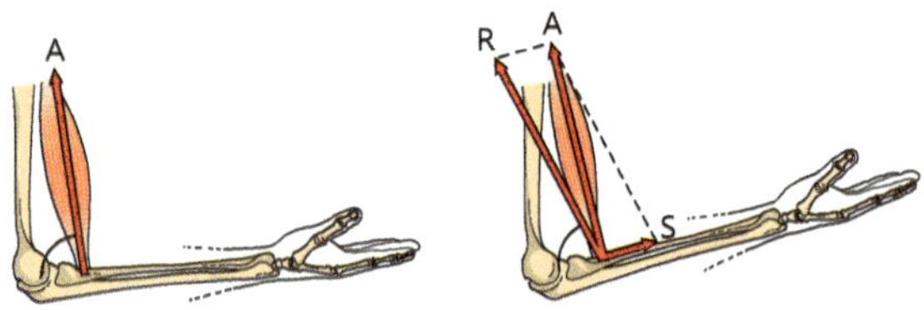

Angle = 90°
S = 0
R = A = 100 N

Angle = 120°
S = 50 N
R = 86.6 N

Angle of insertion of the muscle. **A**, Resultant force of the muscle; **R**, rotational component; **S**, stabilizing or axial component. For angles of insertion near 90°, the force exerted by the muscle becomes more efficient, simultaneously with the reduction of the axial component (**S**) and the increase in the rotational component. For practical reasons, we refer to a total force of 100 N.

Decomposition of a force into two parallel forces

It is necessary to know the point of application of each component force; the component force with the greater modulus will be the one closest to **R**:

- **R** within the component forces
- **R** outside the component forces.

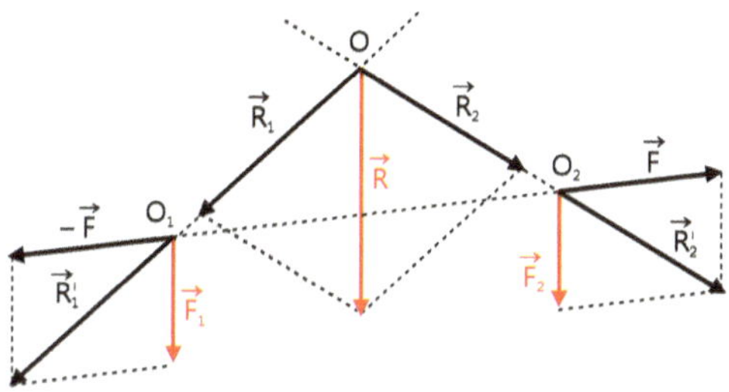

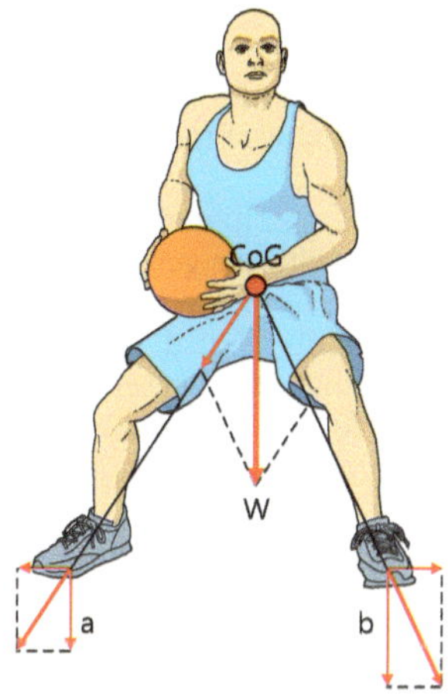

Decomposition of a force (R) into two forces (F_1, F_2) parallel to it. The force is within the two points of application of its components (R_1, R_2). Given R, O, O_1 and O_2:

- OO_1 and OO_2 unite
- R is decomposed and $\vec{R}_1$ and $\vec{R}_2$ are found
- $\vec{R}_1$ and $\vec{R}_2$ in $\vec{R}'_1$ and $\vec{R}'_2$ are reported
- any two forces are considered $-\vec{F}$ and $\vec{F}$ (which being directed along the same line, balance each other)
- they are subtracted from a $\vec{R}'_1$ and $\vec{R}'_2$, and finally $\vec{F}_1$ and $\vec{F}_2$ are found.

Similarly, we proceed to the next figure in the case where the extension of R is external to the segment O_1 O_2.

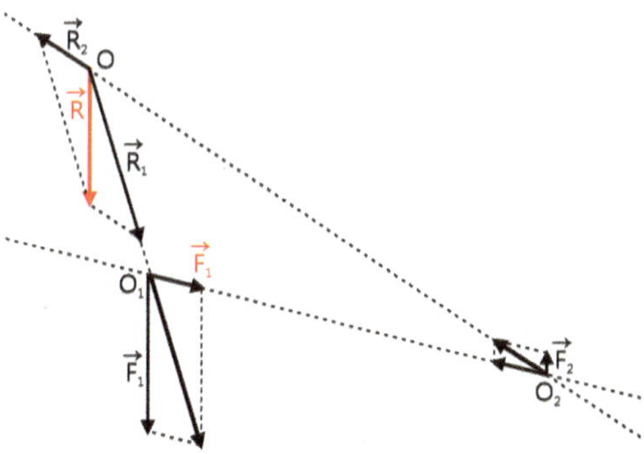

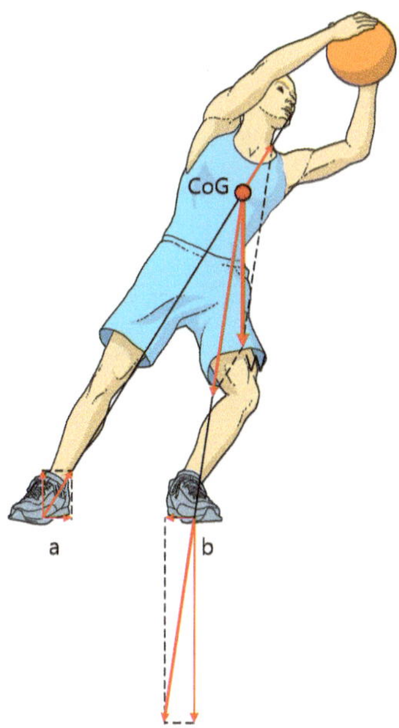

Decomposition of a force (R) into two forces (F_1, F_2) parallel to it. The force has points of application of its components (R_1, R_2) on the outside and on one side only.

Center of gravity (or center of mass)

Definition: point of a body on which the resultant (**R**) of the forces of gravity acts (representing the weight of the entire body).

If the mass is distributed symmetrically and is homogeneous, the center of gravity (CoG) will coincide with the geometric center.

If the mass is distributed asymmetrically with respect to the horizontal plane (as occurs in the human body), the center of gravity will be located on the line that unites the center of gravity of the two body parts (superior and inferior) divided by the horizontal plane. The localization point will be proportionally closer to the center of gravity than the heaviest part.

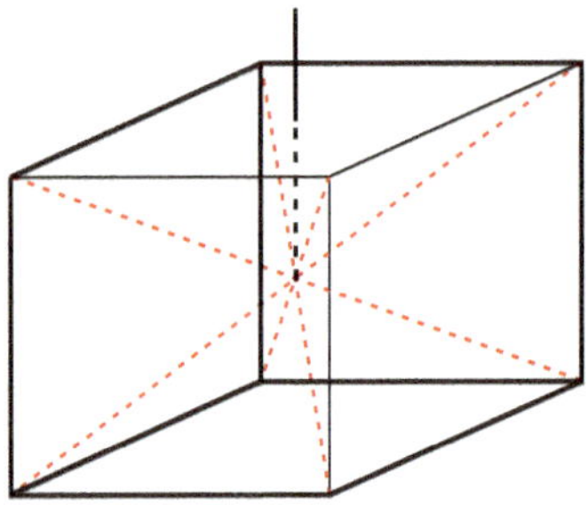

Determination of the center of gravity of a body of homogeneous shape and mass (density): the diagonals that join the four upper vertices of the cube with the four lower vertices all intersect the CoG. By hanging the cube from this point, it will remain perfectly balanced.

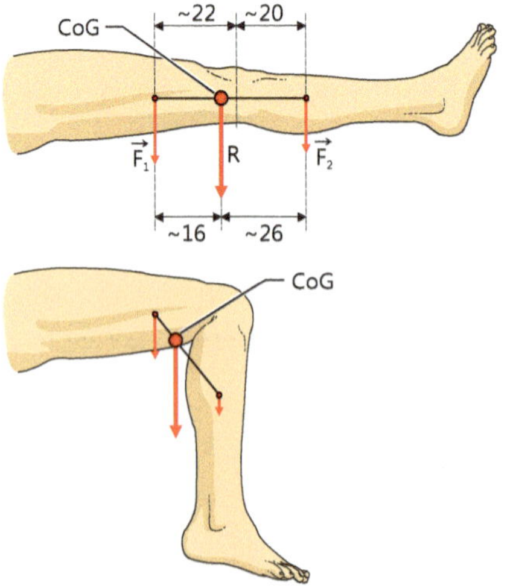

Position of the CoG in the lower limb when extended (above) and flexed (below).

The center of gravity of the human body is located between the second lumbar vertebra (L2) and the first sacral vertebra (S1), in front of the vertebral column and around 56% of the total height of the individual from the ground. It is generally lower in women and higher in children.
The position of the center of gravity is modified by various static and dynamic postures.

The center of gravity of a limb is located in a point of the line that joins the centers of gravity of the two parts of the limb (arm and forearm in the upper limb, and leg and thigh in the lower limb). The location of this point can be determined by making use of the composition of parallel forces having the same sense.

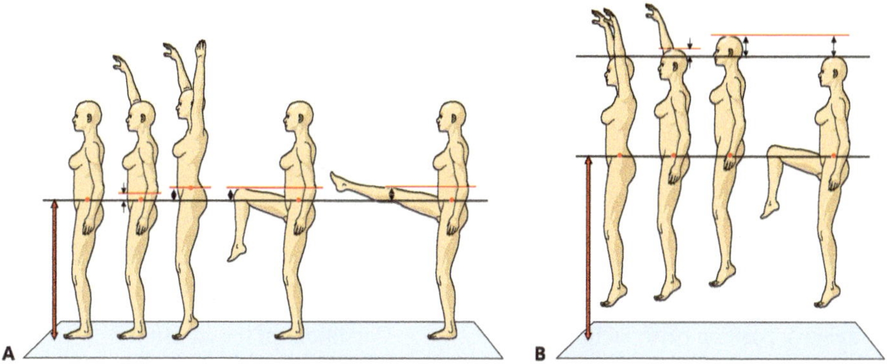

In figure **A**, where all persons have their feet (or one foot) in contact with the ground, a height of approximately 100 cm of the CoG from the ground is assumed for the first person (in normal upright position) which rises from 4 to 10 cm in the other assumed positions.
In figure **B**, where all persons perform an upward jump, the CoG always remains at the same height with respect to the ground, for example, 160 cm (but the position of the CoG with respect to the body varies). From the figures it can be understood that, for example, to reach a high ball with the hand it is better to jump with one upper limb raised and one upper limb along the flank, to touch a ball with the head it is better to jump with both upper limbs along the flanks and to overcome an obstacle during a run it is useful, after overcoming it, to keep high the leg that has passed second and raise the arms to facilitate faster contact with the ground of the first lower limb.

The weight of different body segments (trunk, upper limb, arm, forearm, hand, lower limb, thigh, leg and foot) and the distance of their center of gravity from the respective joints has been determined.

In image **A**, the red dots indicate the centers of gravity of various body segments and the numbers represent the percentage distance from the respective joints; in image **B**, the percentage weight of the various body segments is shown.

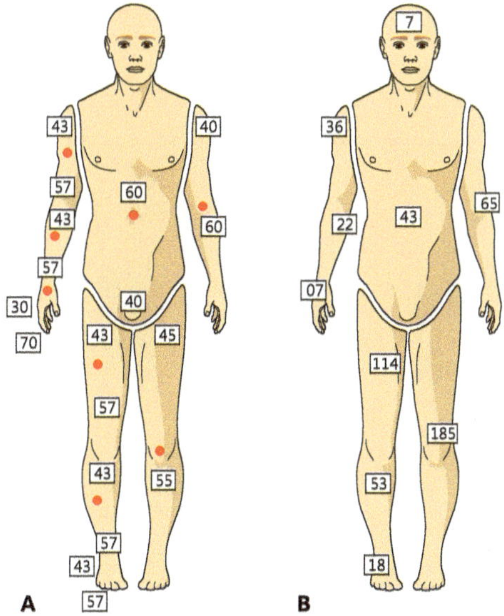

Position of the CoG in various body segments (on the left) and percentage weight of each body segment referred to 100 (on the right).

Balance

There are two types of balance:
- static (maintaining a static position)
- dynamic (stability of all the parts that carry out a movement).

Factors that influence the stability of a body

Main	Secondary
• Height of the center of gravity • Width and shape of the support base • Relative position between line of gravity and support base • Momentum of the body	• Orientation of the support base with respect to the line of force • Conditions of the constraint • Orientation of the gaze • Physical and emotional state

Height of the center of gravity

A body is much more stable when the height of the center of gravity is lower compared to the height of the body (the human body, for example, is more stable when the lower limbs are flexed and, during walking, when both limbs are in contact with the ground; in this phase, in fact, the body's center of gravity is found to be lower compared to the height of the single-leg stance or swing phase).

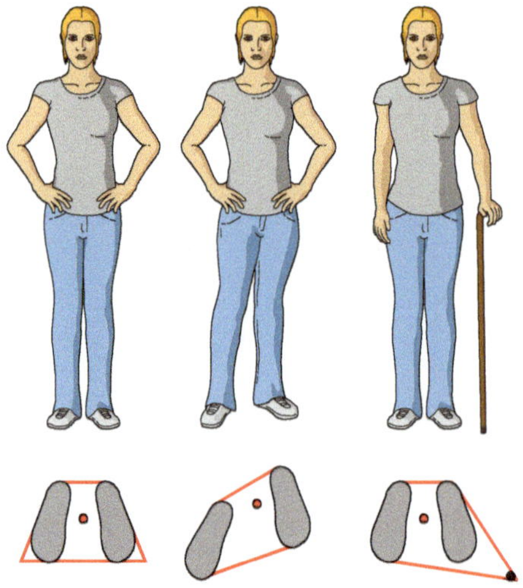

The width of the body's support surface is determined by the position of the feet. The further the feet are apart, the greater the support surface; the aid of a stick causes widening of the support surface (right).

Width and shape of the support base

- The support base of an individual in the upright position is given by a polygon (trapezium) whose sides are formed by the lateral profile of the feet and the two bases (major and minor) by lines that join, respectively, the anterior and posterior parts of the feet:
  - moving the feet apart produces greater stability (if these, however, are moved beyond the width of the pelvis, a lateral force that facilitates sliding of the feet is added to the vertical force on the ground)
  - bringing the feet together produces lesser stability.
- Assistive devices can help to widen the support base or to discharge the body weight onto more points, decreasing it on the lower limbs.

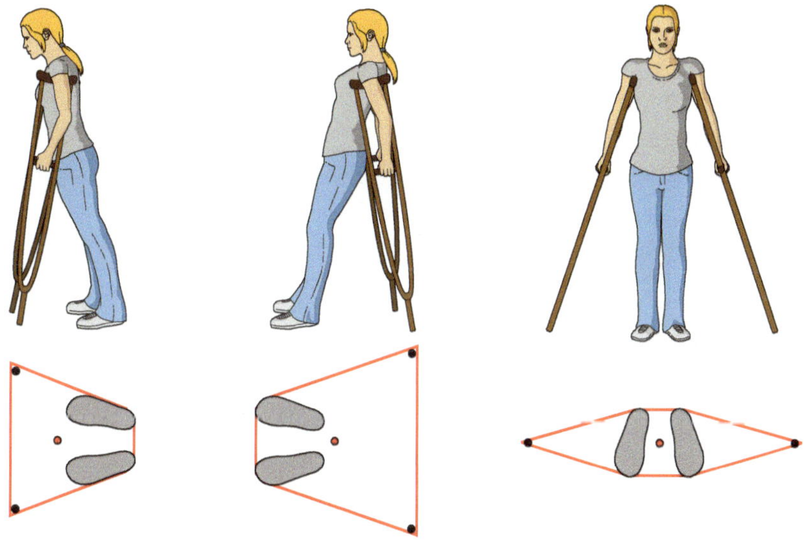

The different support position of the assistive devices on the ground (for example, crutches) allows a greater stability during walking. The figure shows that the subject has a greater stability in the anteroposterior direction in the first two cases, whereas it is more stable in the lateral direction in the third case.

Relative position between line of gravity and support base

- The line of gravity is the vertical on which the force of gravity acts (it can be identified by tracing the vertical from the center of gravity to the support base):
  - the more this line falls within the support polygon, the greater the stability
  - the closer this line gets to the edges of the support polygon, the lesser the stability
- Through displacements of the trunk and the pelvis, the line of gravity is maintained inside the support polygon (forward flexion of the trunk when rising from a seated position, backward displacement of the pelvis when picking up an object from the floor, contralateral movement of the trunk when carrying a load on one side of the body).

Momentum of the body

- It is the product of mass and velocity ($M \times V$)
- Greater stability (greater impact resistance) corresponds to a greater momentum (greater body mass at the same velocity of movement or greater velocity for the same mass).

Orientation of the support base with respect to the line of force

The upright position with feet parallel is less stable than the position with one foot in front of the other. The impact of a ball caught or a body to be opposed, the need to move an object or to punch, or to maintain balance while standing on a bus, are all actions facilitated by orienting the support base in the direction of the force.

Conditions of the constraint

- A body is said to be constrained when the presence of other bodies prevents its displacement
- The are two types of constraint:
  - body suspended at a point (stability is greater when the center of gravity is located below the constraint)
  - body resting on a smooth surface.

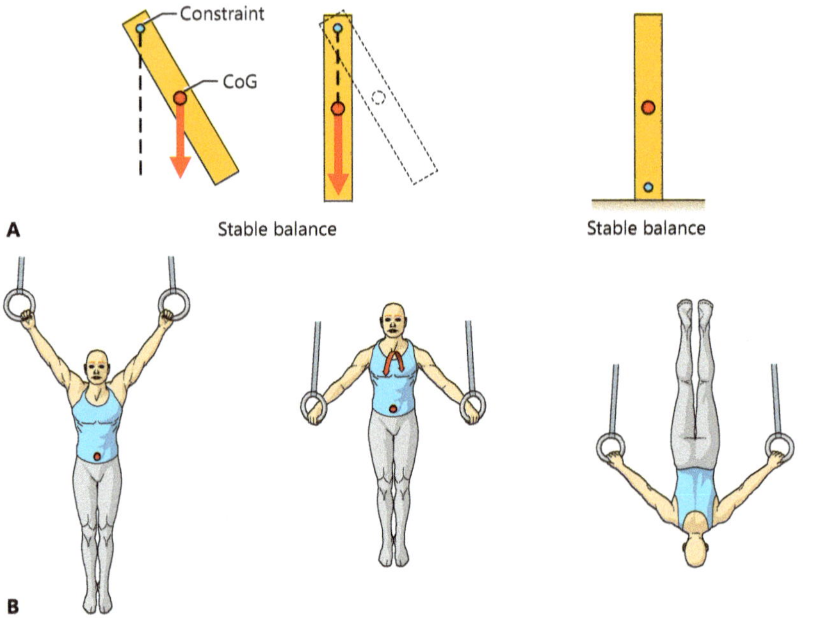

Displacement of the center of gravity and stability conditions in a constrained body. **A**, Schematic representation showing that the position of the constraint modifies a body's state of stability. **B**, The athlete on the left is in suspension, therefore, in a situation of stability; in the center, in a position "resting on the rings", the athlete is in a state of instability; on the right, the athlete performs a forward movement due to the unstable position.

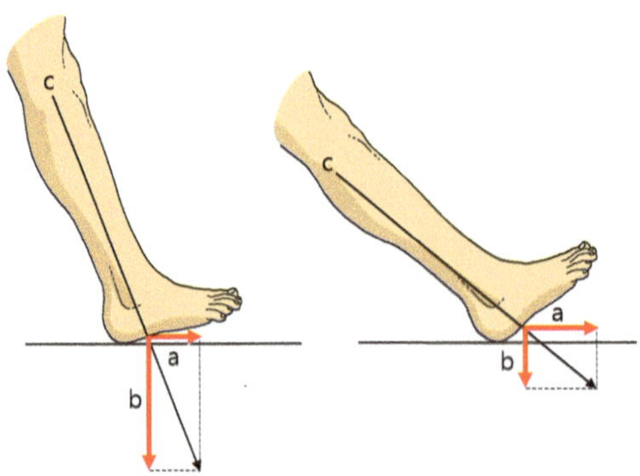

Constraint due to the ground: the body (foot) is supported by the ground. On the left, force "a" (destabilizing) is minimal compared to force "b" (stabilizing). On the right, force "a" prevails over force "b". In this case, the balance will be more unstable. "c" is the axis of the leg with respect to the ground.

Orientation of the gaze

The stability of the body improves when the gaze is oriented towards a fixed point as compared to when it is oriented downward, upward or towards mobile points.

Physical and emotional state

Negative influence of psycho-emotional disorders during the execution of movements that require balance.

Balance conditions

The balance of a body is divided into:

- stable (small movements of the body due to the raising of the center of gravity or displacement of the line of gravity towards the periphery of the support polygon do not cause the body to lose balance, which automatically returns to the previous condition)
- unstable (small movements of the body that make the body's stability precarious)
- indifferent (any displacement on the same type of constraint does not influence balance).

Lever

Components	In the human body
• Rigid segment	• Body segment on which the muscle is applied
• f: fulcrum (or axis)	• Joint (pivot or axis around which the body segment rotates)
• P: power (or motor force)	• Axis of the muscle
• R: resistance (or resistant force)	• Weight of the body segment on which the muscle is applied

The vector P has a sense opposite to the vector R. The latter has its point of application in the center of gravity of the body segment.

Power arm (Pa) – distance of f from P
Resistance arm (Ra) – distance of f from R
Moment of P (mP) – Pa × modulus of P
Moment of R (mR) – Ra × modulus of R
When mP = mR, the lever is in balance

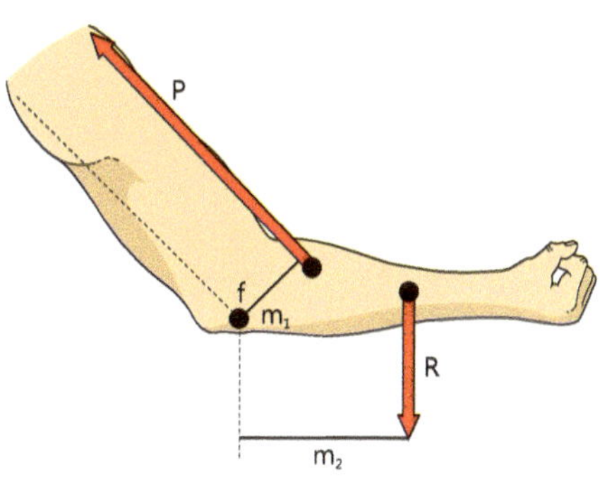

Balance conditions of a muscle lever (biceps brachii). P, power; R, resistance; m_1, power arm; m_2, resistance arm. In the example, if P = 20 N, m_1 = 5 cm, R = 10 N, m_2 = 10 cm, it follows that: $m_1P = m_2R = 100$ Ncm, i.e., in this case, the forearm and arm remain in the position they are in: they are in balance. It will therefore be necessary to apply a fraction of N to P if you want to allow the flexion movement of the forearm on the arm.
Note: the power arm (Pa) and the resistance arm (Ra) change with the angle because they are originated from distances in a perpendicular direction.

Types of lever

- f between P and R – interfulcrum (class 1) – neutral lever (i.e., advantageous or disadvantageous if Pa > Ra or vice versa)
- R between f and P – interresistant (class 2) – advantageous lever (Pa > Ra)
- P between f and R – interpotent (class 3) – disadvantageous lever (Pa < Ra).

The advantage of a lever is due to the fact that if Pa > Ra, the muscle will need less force to carry out the movement. Human muscular levers are largely disadvantageous (i.e., with P between f and R), but the mechanical advantage of a muscle also depends on the other factors:

- angle of insertion
- diameter and arrangement of the fibers
- pre-stretch
- capacity and velocity of contraction.

The brachioradialis, being an advantageous lever, can exert a lesser force to perform flexion of the forearm compared to the brachialis, which is a disadvantageous lever.
However, the brachialis forms (with the forearm flexed 90° on the arm) an angle of insertion > 60°, with prevalence of the rotational force over the axial force, whereas the angle of insertion of the brachioradialis is 20-25°, with prevalence of the axial force over the rotational force.

According to the angle of insertion, the muscles are divided into:

- spurt muscles – with the insertion close to the center of rotation and, therefore, with a rotational force prevalent over the axial force (for example, the brachialis)
- shunt muscles – with the insertion far from the center of rotation and, therefore, with an axial force prevalent over the rotational force (for example, the brachioradialis).

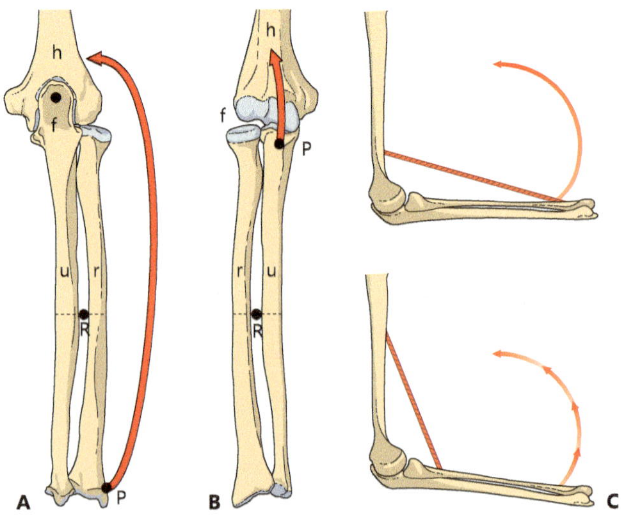

Elbow joint: shunt and spurt muscles. **A**, Posterior view; **B**, anterior view; **C**, lateral view, h, humerus; u, ulna; r, radius; f, fulcrum; P, power (localization); R, resistance (localization).

Examples of muscular levers

Muscle(s)	Action	Type of lever	Insertion	Fulcrum	Resistance
Splenius capitis and splenius cervicis and semispinalis capitis and semispinalis cervicis	Extension of the head	Class 1	Cranial base	Atlanto-occipital joint	Weight of the head
Triceps brachii	Extension of the elbow	Class 1	Olecranon of the ulna	Elbow joint	Center of gravity of the forearm
Triceps surae	Upright position on the forefoot	Class 1 Class 2	Calcaneus Calcaneus	Ankle joint Metatarsophalangeal joints	Reaction of the ground on the metatarsal heads in response to body weight
Brachioradialis	Flexion of the elbow	Class 2	Distal epiphysis of the radius	Elbow joint	Center of gravity of the forearm
Masseter	Elevation of the mandible (closure of the mouth)	Class 2	Angle of the mandible	Temporomandibular joint	Center of gravity of the mandible (last molar tooth)
Brachialis	Flexion of the elbow	Class 3	Tuberosity of the ulna	Elbow joint	Center of gravity of the forearm
Biceps brachii	Flexion of the elbow	Class 3	Tuberosity of the radius	Elbow joint	Center of gravity of the forearm
Quadriceps femoris	Extension of the knee	Class 3	Tuberosity of the tibia	Knee joint	Center of gravity of the leg and foot
Deltoid	Movements of the shoulder	Class 3	Deltoid tuberosity of the humerus	Glenohumeral (or shoulder) joint	Center of gravity of the upper limb

Pulley

Definition: machine through which the line of action of a force is modified without changing its modulus.

In the human body, pulleys are applied to internal forces (muscles) and are fixed.

Muscle(s)	Pulley	Advantage
Quadriceps femoris	Patella	Greater angle of insertion of the tendon with increase in the rotational force
Sartorius	Medial condyle of the femur	The insertion tendon, sliding behind the condyle, improves the action of the internal rotation of the leg
Fibularis longus and fibularis brevis	Malleolus of the fibula	The insertion tendons of the two muscles, sliding behind the malleolus, improve the flexion and, especially, the pronation of the foot
Biceps brachii (long head)	Bicipital groove of the humerus	The sliding of the tendon in this groove favors the abduction of the shoulder above 90° (mainly isometric)

Wheel

It is a class 2 lever (R between f and P).

The force can be applied to the outside of the wheel or on the wheel axle. The greater the diameter of the wheel, the greater the force obtained (rotational force or effect).

An example of force applied to the outside of the wheel is that exerted on the steering wheel by a hand (the wheel being a class 2 lever, the force exerted is on the steering wheel, the fulcrum is the center of the rotation axis and the resistance is located near the fulcrum, on the surface of the axle). The rotational force is equal to the force exerted by the radius. If the force exerted by the other hand is added to the steering wheel (thus applying one force upwards and the other downwards), a pair of forces is obtained.
The pair of forces produces a rotational effect.

Examples of pairs of forces in the human body

- Rotation of the scapula produced by the serratus anterior and by the descending part of the trapezius
- Rotation of the head produced by the splenius capitis (ipsilateral) and by the sternocleidomastoid (contralateral)
- Rotation of the trunk produced by the transversospinales muscles (semispinalis, multifidus and rotatores muscles), with action on the vertebral column, and by the external oblique and internal oblique and iliocostalis, with action on the thorax.

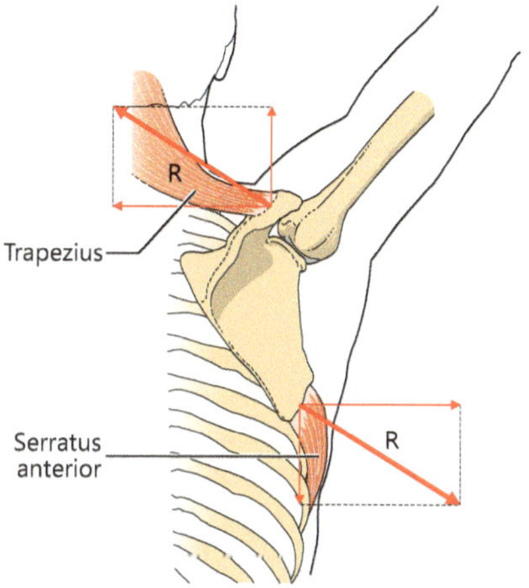

Anatomical example of a pair of forces: descending part of the trapezius and serratus anterior.

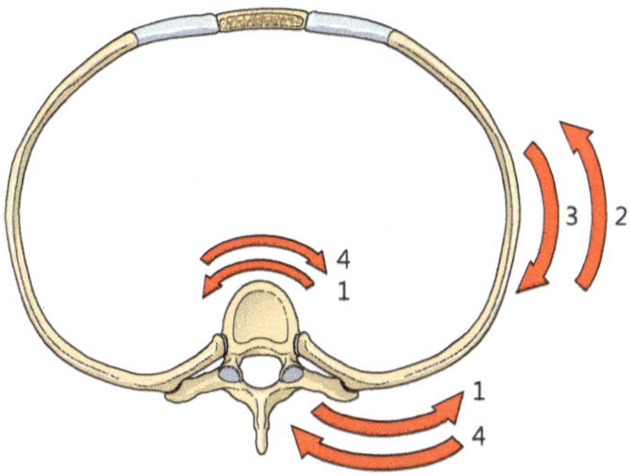

Thoracic cage as seen from above: muscle actions in pairs of forces. **1**, Multifidus, semispinalis, rotatores muscles. **2**, External oblique. **3**, Internal oblique. **4**, Iliocostalis. Action: rotation of the thorax.

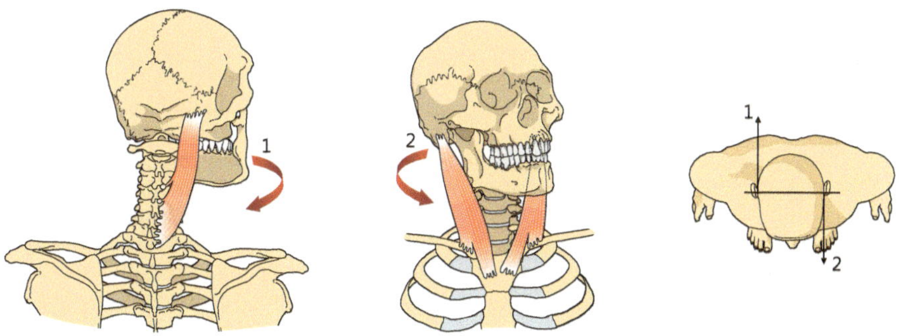

Pair of forces. **1**, Splenius capitis: rotates ipsilaterally. **2**, Sternocleidomastoid: rotates contralaterally. Action: rotation of the head.

Kinetics

Definition: field of mechanics that studies the movement of bodies in relation to the forces that determine it.

The way in which forces influence the movement are described by Newton's three laws:

- law of inertia (first law of motion)
- law of acceleration (second law of motion)
- law of action and reaction (third law of motion).

Inertia

A body maintains its state of rest or uniform rectilinear motion as long as no external forces act on it.

Muscular forces are the most common example of forces that can change the state of a body. If a ball is rolled along the ground, an object is thrown upward or in water, these would continue to move if the friction on the ground, the resistance of the air and the force of gravity in space, the resistance of the liquid, the force of gravity and Archimedes buoyant force in water did not act.

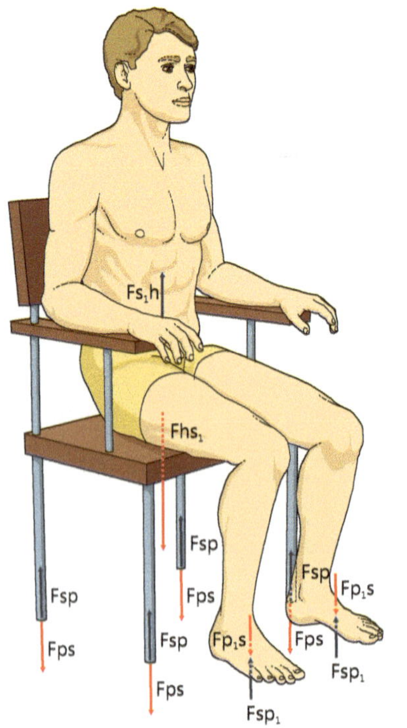

Forces of action and reaction in a sitting position. p, chair leg; s, floor; h, man; s_1, chair; p_1, foot.

Acceleration

When a force acts on a punctual body, the body undergoes acceleration that has the same direction and the same sense as the acting force and is proportional to it.

$F = ma$ or $\mathbf{F} = m\mathbf{a}$ (in vector form)

The proportionality constant m is the mass of the body, therefore, the force is proportional to acceleration, or, with the same force, acceleration is inversely proportional to the mass. It follows that if the mass of a ball to which a thrust (force) is applied is greater than the mass of another ball to which the same thrust is applied, with the same friction, there will be a reduction in acceleration, i.e., in velocity and space traveled by the ball.

Properties of the mass of a body:

- invariable in space and time
- additive (the mass of two bodies m_1 and m_2 is equal to $m_1 + m_2$).

Action and reaction

When a body exerts an action on another body, the latter exerts on the former a reaction force of equal intensity, in the opposite direction and sense, and applied to the same line.

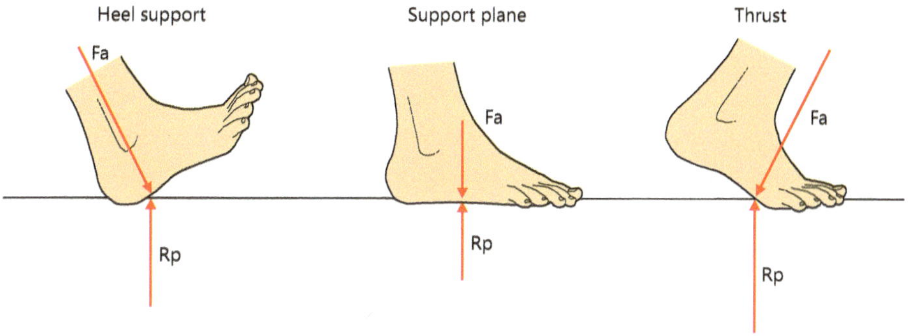

Fa, axial force of the foot; Rp, perpendicular reaction of the floor.

An individual sitting on a chair receives a response force from the chair; if the feet are not resting on the floor, the floor responds to the weight of the chair and the person with a force equal to one fourth of the weight to which it is subjected, exerted on each of the four chair legs (Fsp).

When the feet are resting on the ground, a part of the body weight is discharged directly on the floor, so that the force of the person exerted on the chair (Fhs_1) is less than the body weight. Two new forces have been created: the force exerted by the foot on the floor (Fp_1s) and the response force exerted by the floor on the foot (Fsp_1).

In the upright position, there is a reaction of the ground that is of greater or lesser intensity in relation to the muscular forces exerted by the lower limbs.

During walking, different forces are produced by variable angles of the axis of the lower limb. The reaction of the ground will be of greater intensity during the thrust phase, decreasing in the initial support phase and becoming lesser in the full support phase. While the axial force of the foot (Fa) is oriented along the longitudinal axis of the body segment (leg), the reaction of the floor (Rs) is always perpendicular to the plane.

Applications of the second law of motion

According to the law of acceleration, the force can be considered constant (even if in reality it is not) when its variation is slow. A constant force determines a constant acceleration (the mass of the body in turn being constant).

In translational motion (all the points of a body travel the same distance in the same sense at the same time), the three formulas of the law of acceleration apply:

$F = ma \rightarrow a = F/m \rightarrow m = F/a$

Acceleration is directly proportional to the force and inversely proportional to the mass of the body. Therefore, the mass hinders the acceleration and, for this reason, it is called inertial.

Translational motion refers to a punctual body with a mass of m. However, when considering an extended body, which can be rigid or not, other physical quantities must be used. If it is assumed that the body is rigid, the motion that characterizes it will not be translational,

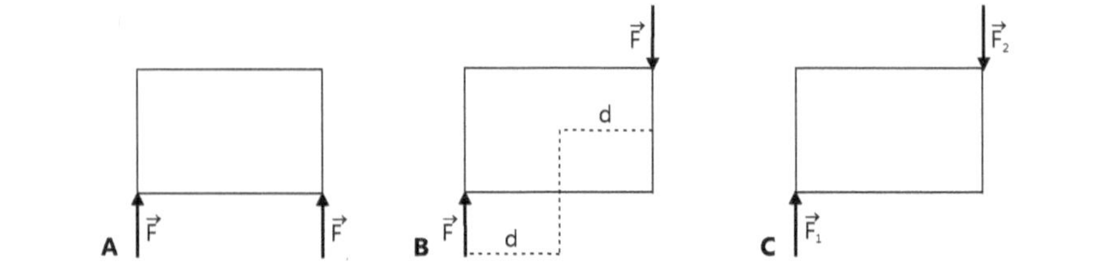

Motions due to the forces applied: **A**, translational motion; **B**, rotational motion; **C**, rototranslational motion.

but rototranslational (natural human motion), which is characterized by a rotational (angular) motion around the center of mass or center of gravity (all points of a body travel at the same angle in the same sense at the same time), whereas it moves as if the body were punctual (translational motion).

The second law of motion applies to the movement of the center of mass (translational motion): $\mathbf{R} = m\mathbf{a}_{cm}$, where R is the vector sum of all forces applied to the body, m is the mass of the body and $\mathbf{a}_{cm}$ is the acceleration of the center of mass.

In the motion around the center of mass (rotational motion), instead of the resultant of the forces (R), the resultant of the moments is introduced; instead of mass (m), the moment of inertia (measured in kg × m² and dependent not only on m, but also on how m is distributed around the center of gravity); instead of linear acceleration ($\mathbf{a}_{cm}$), the angular acceleration ($a_\omega = \Delta\omega/\Delta T$, measured in rad/s²; see section "Uniform circular motion", page 55).

If we consider a rigid body on which two forces are applied, the following three cases can be considered for the purposes of motion:

- translation – the two forces:
  - are equal
  - have the same sense
  - are applied to the edge of a side of the rigid body
  - $F_1 + F_2 = ma \rightarrow a = 2F/m$
- rotation – the two forces:
  - are equal
  - have opposite sense
  - are applied to the opposite edges of the two opposite sides of the rigid body
  - $a_\omega = M/I = 2Fr/I$ (where M is the moment of the pair of forces and I is the moment of inertia)
- rototranslation – the two forces:
  - have opposite sense
  - are applied to the opposite edges of the two opposite sides of the rigid body
  - have different modulus.

Constant and impulsive forces

The impulse (I) of a constant force is equal to $F \times \Delta T$ (where ΔT is the time for which the force is maintained) and is measured in N × s. In a force/time diagram, it takes the appearance of a rectangle.

Since $F = ma \rightarrow F = m \times \Delta V/\Delta T$ we get $I = F \times \Delta T \rightarrow I = m \times \Delta V \rightarrow I = mV_2 - mV_1$

Impulsive forces are defined as those that appear suddenly and last for a very short time (ΔT).

Knowing the mass and velocity (V_2, supposing $V_1 = 0$) we can calculate the impulse, and knowing the impact time (ΔT) we can calculate the force through the formula: $F = I/\Delta T$.

The force obtained is an average force and not a real force (the latter is variable and, in this case, the impulse is obtained by calculating the area in the force/time diagram through the sum of many small impulses $\delta I = F\ (\delta T)$, i.e., a force which corresponds to the same area and the same impulse and that produces the same dynamic effects. The smaller ΔT is, the greater this force is.

Theorem of momentum conservation

When two bodies of masses m and M, with velocity v_1 and V_2 collide with each other, there is always:

$mv_1 + MV_1 = mv_2 + MV_2$

where 1 and 2 indicate the values before and after the impact.

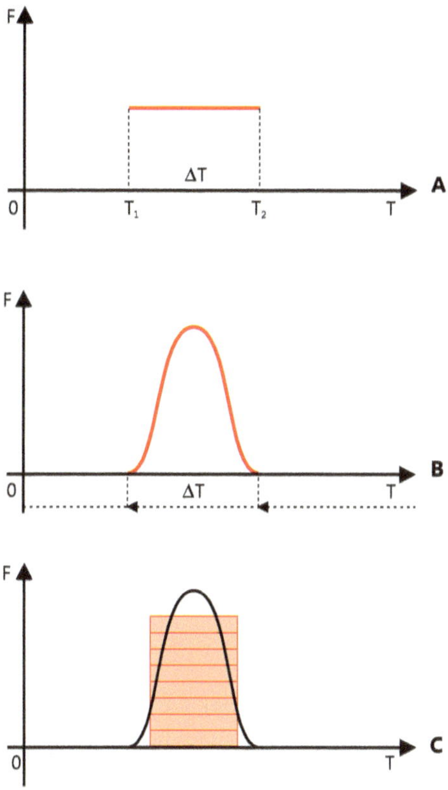

A, Constant force impulse. **B**, Impulsive forces. **C**, Average force: area identification, impulse and dynamic effects.

Work and kinetic energy

Work

Definition: physical quantity dependent on the relationship between the force and the displacement

$L = F \times \Delta x$

where Δx = displacement from the point of application of F.

L is measured in Joules (1 Joule = 1 N × 1 m): a force of 1 Newton does the work of 1 Joule if its point of application shifts 1 m in the direction of the force sense. Since 1 N = 0.1 kg, if a weight of 0.1 kg is lifted by 1 m, the work done will be equivalent to 1 Joule.

Kinetic energy theorem

From the uniformly accelerated rectilinear motion:

$\Delta s = AT^2/2 \rightarrow AT_2^2/2 - AT_1^2/2$

and from the second law of motion

$F = ma$

$L = F \times \Delta x \rightarrow ma^2T_2^2/2 - ma^2T_1^2/2 \rightarrow mV_2^2/2 - mV_1^2/2$

The quantity $mV^2/2$ is called kinetic energy (or kinetic movement) and is indicated using E_k, so:

$L = \Delta E_k$

Force, displacement and velocity are related to each other without the mediation of time.

Different direction between force and displacement

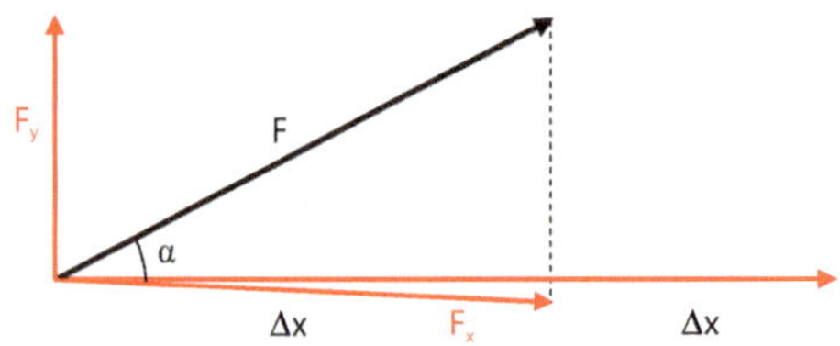

The forces perpendicular to the displacement cause a curvature of the trajectory but do not modify its velocity (see section "Uniform circular motion", page 55). In this case:

$L = F \times \Delta x \cos\alpha$.

Variable forces acting along a trajectory curve

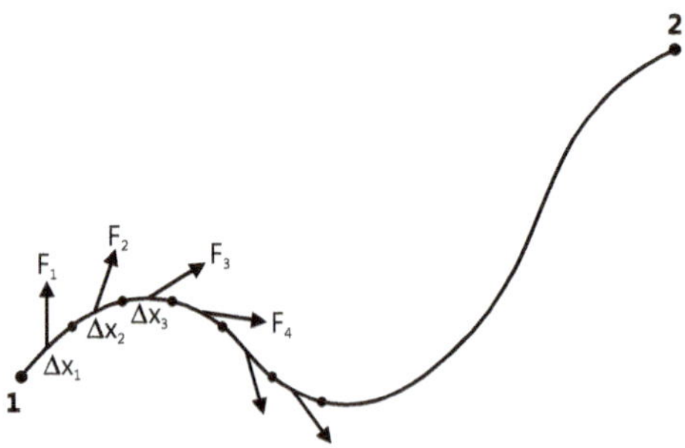

The trajectory must be divided into such small elements:

$L = F_1 \times \Delta x_1 \cos\alpha_1 + F_2 \times \Delta x_2 \cos\alpha_2 + ...$

When more forces act on a body, it is necessary to calculate the resulting work of all the forces acting on it. All this work is positive when the force acts in the sense of the displacement and negative in the opposite case. If the force is perpendicular to the displacement: $L = 0$ and $Fx = 0$.

Unit of measurement of energy

In addition to the Joule (defined by the International System of Units), the erg and the calorie are used:

1 erg = 10^{-5} Joule

1 cal = 4180 Joule (energy required to raise the temperature of one gram of water by 1 °C).

Energy in biological processes

The energy of the human body, whose origin is at the biochemical level, is dissipated by the body for its own functions, at rest and in motion, producing heat and work. The muscular effort can be assessed by calculating the consumption of oxygen in the unit of time, and converting it to J/s or cal/min.

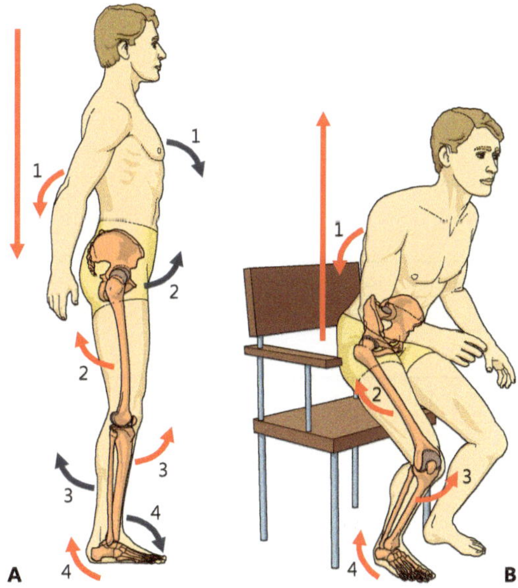

Positive and negative work. **A**, Upright position. In *red*, the muscular forces that oppose gravity and produce "negative work" (1, extensors of the vertebral column; 2, hip extensors; 3, knee extensors; 4, plantar flexors of the foot). In *black*, the gravitational forces (1, flexors of the trunk and vertebral column; 2, hip flexors; 3, knee flexors; 4, dorsal flexors of the foot). **Note**: the body goes in the direction of gravity. **B**, Act of raising oneself from a sitting position, i.e., "positive work". In *red*, the muscular forces are moving in the direction of the body that is rising from the chair (they are the same ones that, on the left, work eccentrically, here concentrically). **Note**: the body goes in the opposite direction to gravity. The trunk leans forward to bring the line of gravity into the support polygon of the feet. Moreover, the pre-lengthening, in particular of the extensors of the vertebral column (1) and hip extensors (2) facilitates their subsequent "concentric" work.

The human body uses energy when the body's center of gravity is raised (positive work with increase in potential energy), but dissipates energy even when this is lowered (to slow down the descent, i.e., the spontaneous process of acquiring kinetic energy deriving from the transformation of potential energy previously acquired). In the second case, the work done by weight is not exploited and it is not possible to accumulate the energy that this movement produces.

Power

Definition: relationship between a variation of energy (ΔE) or work (ΔW) and the time interval in which this occurs (ΔT).

$P = \Delta E$ (o ΔW)/ΔT

P is linked to the speed with which a phenomenon occurs, being greater the smaller ΔT is.

The unit of measurement of P is the Watt (1 W= 1 J/1 s, or J/s), but all the calculations referring to variations in energy over time (independently of various types of measurement unit used) are attributable to P.

Basal metabolism (basal metabolic power)

The quantity of energy dissipated at rest by the human body for maintaining all the biochemical processes, respiratory and cardiac activities, smooth muscle activity of the organs and vessels, body temperature and muscle tone (all these activities are defined as basal metabolism) is 1.2 W/kg of body weight in men and 1.1 W/kg in women (P/m, measured in W/kg, expresses the power per unit of mass).

Physical activity

The percentage efficiency (E%) is defined as the relationship between the actual mechanical work done (ΔW) and the difference between the energy expended at the metabolic level and basal energy ($\Delta E - \Delta Eb$) × 100:

$$E\% = \Delta W/(\Delta E - \Delta Eb) \times 100$$

Power per unit of mass in relation to daily physical activities		**Percentage efficiency in relation to physical activities**	
Activity	*P/m (W/kg)*	*Activity*	*E%*
Sleeping	1.1	Shoveling	3
Lying	1.2	Weight-lifting	9
Sitting	1.5	Turning a wheel	13
Standing	2.6	Climbing a ladder	19
Walking	4.3	Climbing stairs	23
Cycling	7.6	Cycling	25
Swimming	11	Walking uphill (slope of 5%)	30
Skiing	15		
Running	18		

Angular momentum

In rotational (or angular) motion, all the points of a body move along concentric circumferences whose centers are on the same axis, known as rotation axis. The linear velocity is different for each point, while the angular velocity is the same:

$$\omega = \Delta\alpha/\Delta T.$$

If we consider two particles of mass m_1 and m_2 at a distance of r_1 and r_2, respectively, from a fixed rotation axis (rigid body), the velocity of the first particle (tangential velocity; see section "Uniform circular motion", page 55) will be $V_1 = \omega r_1$ and the velocity of the second particle will be $V_2 = \omega r_2$.
The kinetic energy of the due particles is given by:

$$E_k = m_1V_1^2/2 = m_1r_1^2\omega^2/2$$

$$E_k = m_2V_2^2/2 = m_2r_2^2\omega^2/2$$

The kinetic energy of the system is equal to the sum of the kinetic energy of the constituents:

$E_k = E_{k1} + E_{K2} = \omega^2 (m_1 r_1^2 + m_2 r_2^2)/2$

The physical quantity $m_1 r_1^2 + m_2 r_2^2$ is called the moment of inertia (energy of rotation or rotational inertia) and is indicated with I and measured in kg · m². The mass distribution of the system with respect to the rotation axis depends on I.

By substituting $m_1 r_1^2 + m_2 r_2^2$ with I, we get:

$E_k = \omega^2 I/2$

The kinetic energy of a rotating particle system is equal to half the product of the moment of inertia and the square of the angular velocity.

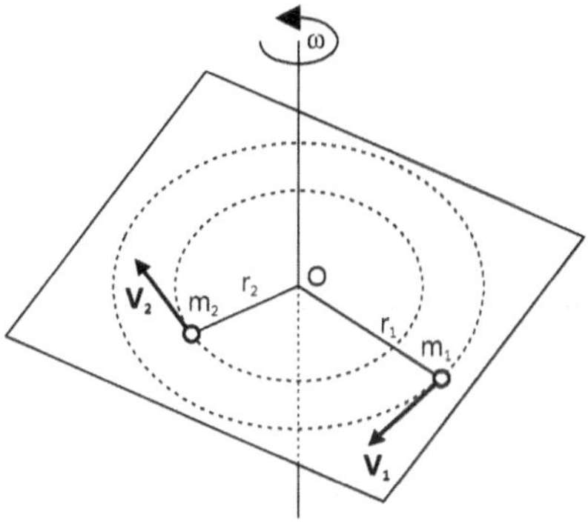

Kinetic energy of a rigid body that rotates around an axis.

If we consider a rotating body (around a fixed axis) on which forces act and we indicate with M the algebraic sum of the moments, at the instant T1, the body will have an angular velocity ω_1 and a kinetic energy E_{k1} and, at the instant T2, an angular velocity ω_2 and a kinetic energy E_{k2}, so we will have:

$E_{k2} - E_{k1} = \omega_2^2 I/2 - \omega_1^2 I/2$

For the kinetic energy theorem:

$\Delta E_k = mV_2^2/2 - mV_1^2/2$

and thus:

$mV_2^2/2 - mV_1^2/2 = \omega_2^2 I/2 - \omega_1^2 I/2$

$mV_2 - mV_1 = \omega_2 I - \omega_1 I$

$maT_2 - maT_1 = \omega_2 I - \omega_1 I$

$F\Delta T = I\omega - I\omega_1$

$M\Delta T = I\omega - I\omega_1$

The physical quantity defined by the product of angular velocity and the moment of inertia is called the angular momentum ($L = I\omega$).

Since $I\omega_2 - I\omega_1 = L_2 - L_1 = \Delta L \rightarrow M\Delta T = \Delta L$ (fundamental law of dynamics for a rigid body in rotation: the algebraic sum of the moment of external forces is equal to the variation of the angular momentum in time).

The sum of the moments of the internal forces is equal to 0.

Conservation of the angular momentum

If we assume $M\Delta T = 0$, then $\Delta L = 0$ and therefore constant.

This is the law of conservation of the angular momentum: the angular momentum of a system for which the moment of the forces is equal to 0 remains constant.

M is equal to 0 when a body is subject only to the weight force and the rotation axis is the one passing through the center of gravity.

When a body rotates around an axis, the internal forces, whose sum of movements is equal to 0, cannot modify the angular momentum (and therefore the movement of the center of gravity), but they can vary the distance between the parts (r) and therefore the moment of inertia ($m_1r_1^2 + m_2r_2^2$). In the case of variation of I by the internal forces, there will be a corresponding opposite variation of ω to keep the angular momentum unchanged.

Conservation of energy and energy efficiency

Energy is a quantity that is quantitatively conserved while changing its form.

Law of the conservation of energy: the variation in total energy of a physical system is equal to the balance between input energy (E_{in}) and output energy (E_{out}).

By indicating the (internal) energy contained in the system with ΔE_{in}, we can say that E_{in} + $E_{in} - E_{out}$ = constant.

An energy transformation can be assessed in terms of energy efficiency (transformation efficiency). If E_{in} is input energy, E_{out} is output energy in the desired form, and E_{lost} is energy lost during the process (for example, in the form of heat), the percentage efficiency η will be:

$$\eta\% = E_{out}/E_{in} \times 100 = (E_{in} - E_{lost})/E_{in} \times 100 = 100 \times (1 - E_{lost}/E_{in})$$

Potential energy

There are forces whose work done to achieve a displacement between two points (A and B) depends only on the initial point (A), not on the final point (B) nor the path followed. These forces are represented by:
- weight force
- elastic force
- electric force.

Frictional forces, muscular action forces and forces that induce permanent deformation of a body do not have this property.

Potential (or positional) energy U is expressed by the relation

$$U_A - U_B = L_{A\rightarrow B}$$

where $U_A - U_B$ is the work done to go from A to B.

In a system in which conservative forces (fc; forces that conserve energy) and non-conservative forces (fnc; forces that dissipate energy) act, L (from A to B) will be equal to $L_{fc} + L_{fnc}$.

For the kinetic energy theorem, $\Delta E_k = L$, so:

$$(E_{kB} - E_{kA}) = L_{A\rightarrow B} = U_A - U_B + L_{fnc\,A\rightarrow B}$$

$$(E_{kB} - E_{kA}) + (U_B - U_A) = L_{fnc\,A\rightarrow B}$$

$$(E_{kB} + U_B) - (E_{kA} + U_A) = L_{fnc\,A\rightarrow B}$$

The quantity $E_k + U$ (kinetic energy + potential energy) is called mechanical energy.

In any system, the variation of mechanical energy is equal to the work of non-conservative forces (mechanical energy is transformed into heat).

In the absence of non-conservative forces ($L_{fnc} = 0$), $E_{kB} + U_B = E_{kA} + U_A$ (the mechanical energy of the system is conserved). Since the non-conservative forces always do negative work, the mechanical energy decreases (in the presence of non-conservative forces), while kinetic energy and potential energy are transformed from one into the other (for example, when a body slides along an inclined plane, its potential energy decreases and its kinetic energy increases; however, the mechanical energy does not remain constant, but decreases due to the negative work done by frictional forces, being converted into heat).

In the case of weight force, potential energy at a generic point A is: $U_A = mgh_A$, where h is height with respect to a generic reference level (with positive values above the reference level and negative values below it).

Frictional forces

Definition: forces that hinder the motion between two bodies or between a body and the medium in which the body is located.
There are three types of friction:
- sliding (when two solids slide against each other)
- rolling
- drag.

Sliding friction

Sliding frictional forces (F_a):
- are formed by contact between two solids, hindering the sliding
- work in pairs (third law of motion)
- their energy depends on the microroughness of the surfaces (it therefore depends on the state of the surfaces and not on their extension)
- are proportional to the component of the force applied perpendicularly to the contact surface
- are greater under static conditions than under dynamic conditions (from 0 to 3-4 times).

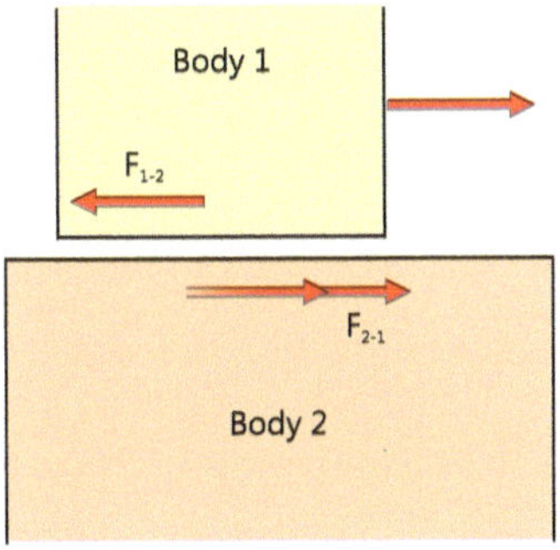

Sliding friction.

Under static conditions:

$F_a < \mu_s \times F_n$, where μ_s is the static friction coefficient and F_n is the component of the force applied perpendicularly to the contact surface (under this condition, F_a is variable, adapting to the value of the force applied, because vice versa would move the body instead of opposing its motion).

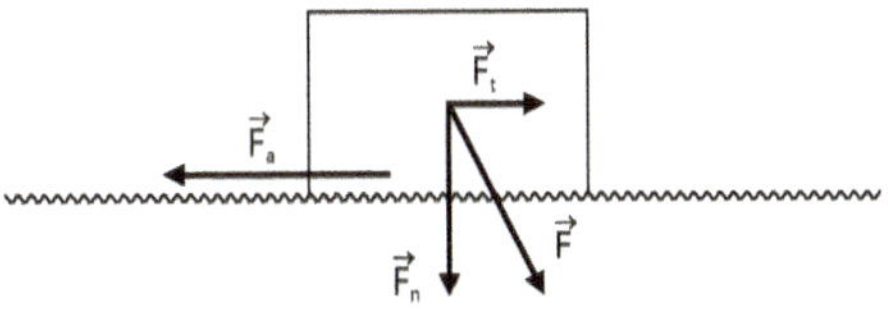

Under dynamic conditions:

$F_a = \mu_d \times F_n$, where μ_d is the coefficient of dynamic friction.

The frictional forces are responsible for movement.
When walking, an oblique force (F_{pu}) with respect to the vertical is exerted on the floor and its components are F_t (parallel to the plane) and F_n (perpendicular to the plane).
If α is the angle formed by F_{pu} with the vertical, then:

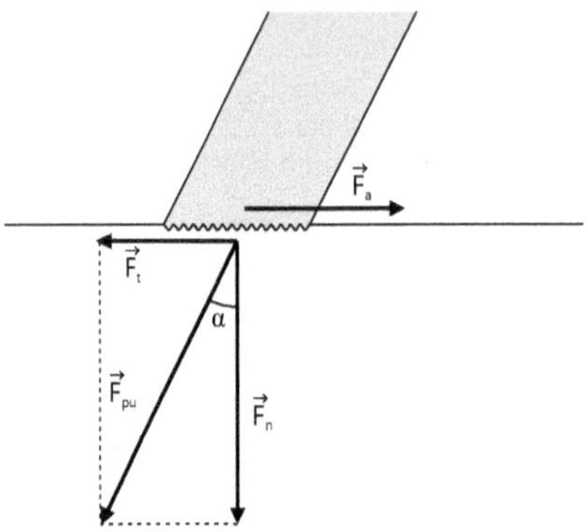

$F_n = F_{pu} \times \cos\alpha$
$F_t = F_{pu} \times \mathrm{sen}\alpha$

The floor responds to F_n with an elastic force due to its deformation, while the response to F_t is the static friction (F_a) that pushes the body forwards (by reaction to F_t). Increasing the angle α with respect to the vertical (i.e., the obliqueness), increases F_t (increasing acceleration), but decreases F_n and F_a proportionally, which allows movement, so the increase in α can only occur to a certain extent.

$F_a = F_t = F_n \times \mathrm{tg}\alpha$

For $F_a < \mu_s \times F_n$, it follows that $F_a = F_n \times \mathrm{tg}\alpha \leq F_n \times \mu_s$

When $\mathrm{tg}\alpha = \mu_s$, there is a maximum forward thrust of F_a (which, however, corresponds to a sliding condition). The optimal condition is instead: $F_a = \mu_s \times F_n$ (maximum thrust on the floor and high friction coefficient).

Rolling friction

It occurs when two bodies, at least one of which is circular, rotate with respect to one another.

The rolling frictional force (F_a) depends on:

- deformability characteristics of the bodies in contact
- weight force
- radius of curvature

and is equal to $\mu_v \times F_n/r$, where μ_v is the coefficient of rolling friction (measured in millimeters) and r is the radius (also measured in millimeters).

Drag (viscous resistance)

When a body is immersed in a fluid (liquid or gas) it undergoes a force that opposes its movement.

This depends on:

- transverse section of the body
- shape of the body
- velocity of the body.

When a body is falling in a fluid, as the velocity increases (due to the effect of gravity), the viscous frictional force also increases, until, at a certain point, the velocity stops. This velocity value, known as limited velocity, is reached when $F_p = F_a$.

The limited velocity depends on the dimensions of the body (F_a increases quadratically by increasing the surface of the body, whereas F_p increases cubically by increasing the volume of the body). F_a also depends on the shape of the body (with the same transverse section and velocity of the body), influencing the establishment of a laminar or turbulent regime in the fluid.
The viscous frictional force always causes a negative work in the presence of motion, with decrease in the mechanical energy and reduction in range, force of impact and velocity.

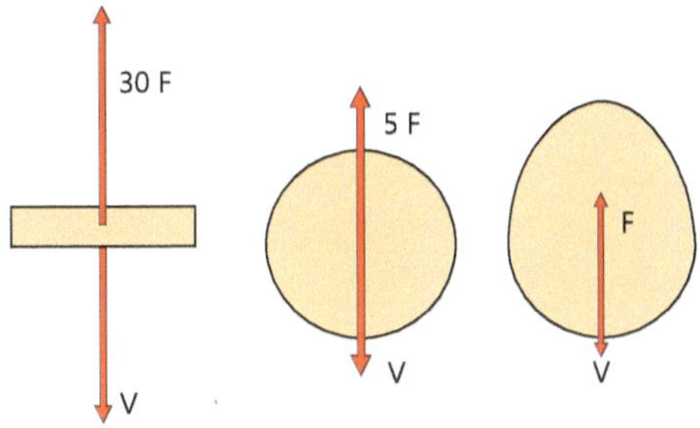

Different aerodynamics of the bodies. Three bodies with the same transverse section moving at the same velocity have, depending on their shape, frictional forces up to thirty times greater.

Examples of limited velocity in free fall as a function of the body size

Body in free fall	Limited velocity (m/s)
Lead ball weighing 10 g	40
Raindrop	7
Man in free-fall	60
Ping pong ball	8
Plastic microbead (1 μm)	10^{-4}
Parachute	6
Grain of dust	$2 \cdot 10^{-2}$

Aerodynamics and sport

The transverse section of the body, in the case of athletes such as cyclists or speed skiers, can be reduced with flexion of the trunk and head.
Divers perform an aerodynamic shape through an appropriate profile, swimmers do it by maintaining optimal directions that facilitate laminar flow. In fact, a poorly aligned arrangement in the water can lead to the formation of vortices.

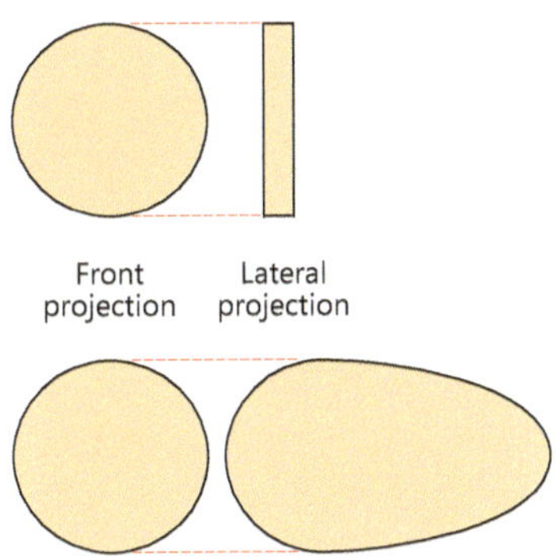

Different projections of solid bodies: depending on their arrangement in a fluid, the opposite resistance will be different.

The same can occur in throwing, particularly in discus, or ski jumping. In these cases, both the launch angle of the discus and the take-off angle of the jumper are important, but also the mode chosen to overcome resistance.
In ski jumping, in addition to the angle, it is the position of the skier with respect to the skis that makes the flight aerodynamic.

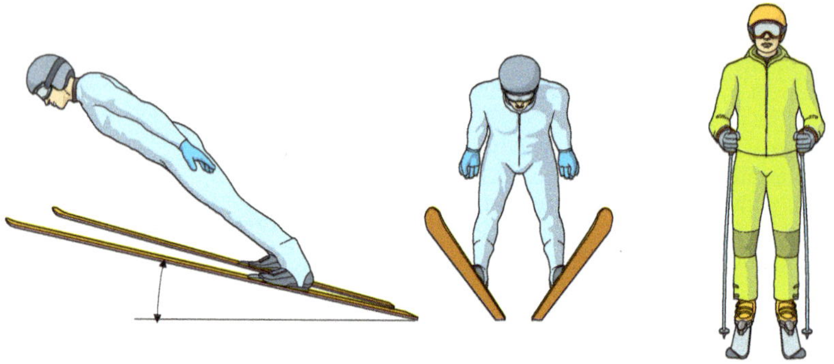

Differet projections of presentation of a skier. On the left and in the center, the frictional forces decrease, whereas on the right they increase.

In the case of discus throw, it is the rotation of the object during flight that stabilizes the trajectory, thus avoiding the formation of vortices.
In fact, for reasons related to the vectoral nature of angular momentum, the rotation axis of a body in motion tends to retain the same direction and this stabilizes its motion.
This principle underlies the choice of rotating the objects during the launching process (jugglers, discus and weight throwers).
Another interesting case is the Magnus effect, related to the decrease in air pressure (and therefore of its own resistance) when its velocity increases.

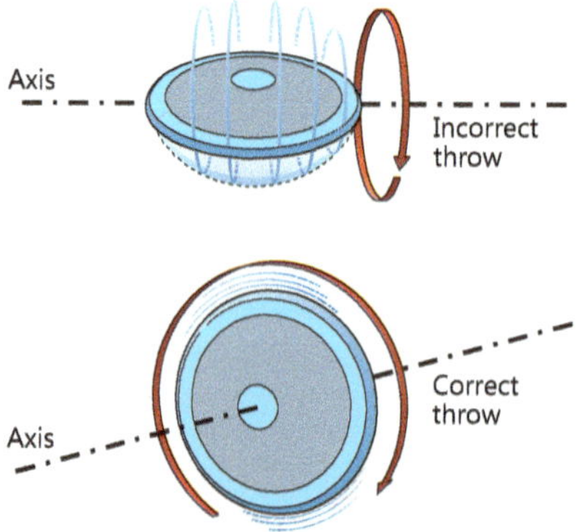

When throwing the discus, the rotation of the object during flight stabilizes the trajectory, avoiding the formation of vortices.

This phenomenon, applied to a ball thrown in the air, can give three different responses. First, if the ball is thrown into the air, it will head towards the areas of lower pressure. If the ball rotates around itself while in flight, there will be a rototranslational motion which, as such, is faster:

- if the ball is driven clockwise, the laminar air flows accompanying the rotation, such as the resistance to motion, are divided into higher flows that, by pushing in the opposite direction, move more slowly due to the effect of the increase in pressure and lower flows that, by reducing pressure, increase in velocity. The result of these actions leads the ball to favor a downward trajectory.
- The opposite occurs when the rotation of the ball is counterclockwise. Therefore, there is an upward trajectory.

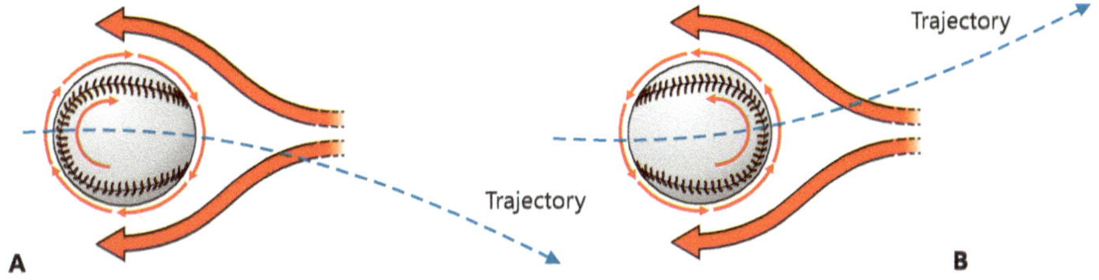

A, The ball pushed downward rotates in a clockwise direction for the observer. The air that opposes the movement is the one that "flows" over the ball, whereas the air underneath, flowing in the same direction is faster. This is the reason why the downward motion of the ball is favored. **B**, In the second case, the counterclockwise rotation favors upward motion.

In any case, the ball that has undergone a rotation, with the same thrust applied, will go higher or lower, respectively, than a ball that has not undergone a rotation and, moreover, the type of rotation will favor the curve that you want to impose on the ball.
Naturally, the larger the ball and the greater its velocity, the more resistance it will encounter in the air.

Cranium

Viscerocranium (facial skeleton)

1 Nasal bone
2 Lacrimal bone
3 Ethmoid
4 Zygomatic bone
5 Maxilla
6 Mandible

The vomer, inferior nasal concha (turbinate) and palatine bone (not visible in lateral projection of the cranium) are added to those mentioned above.

Neurocranium

7 Occipital bone
8 Parietal bone
9 Temporal bone
10 Sphenoid
11 Frontal bone

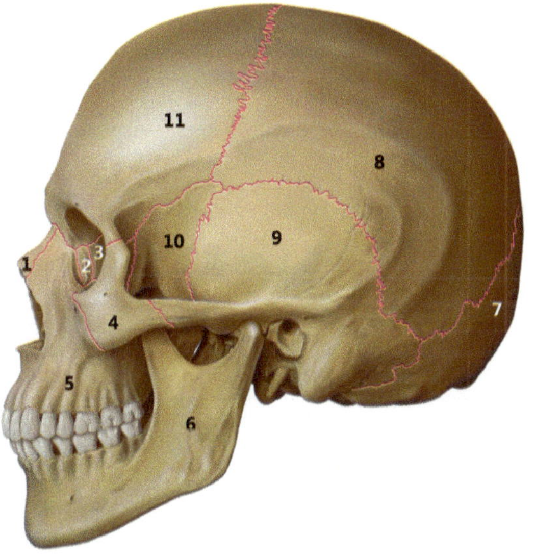

Cranial bones.

Cranial sutures

- Sagittal (between the parietal bones)
- Lambdoid (between the occipital bone and the parietal bones)
- Coronal (between the frontal bone and the parietal bones).

Meninges

- Dura mater (it lines the internal surface of the cranium):
  - outer layer (periosteal)
  - inner layer
  - reflections of the dura mater:
    - falx cerebri (between the cerebral hemispheres)
    - falx cerebelli (between the cerebellar hemispheres)
    - tentorium cerebelli (between the occipital lobes and the cerebellum)
- Leptomeninx (internally to the dura mater, it lines the gyri and sulci of the brain):
  - outer layer (arachnoid mater)
  - inner layer (pia mater)
  - subarachnoid space between the two layers (containing the cerebrospinal fluid)

The falces and tentorium constitute an important longitudinal and transverse support system, respectively.

Cranium mobility

- The cranium is not a rigid but an elastic structure
- Each cranial bone is characterized by a specific movement, the frequency of which is 10 to 14 times per minute
- The direction of these movements depends on the characteristics of the sutures, which perform unloading functions.

Cranial osteopathy exploits cranial mobility.

The cranial dura mater attaches to the borders of the foramen magnum, where it continues with the spinal dura mater, which in turn attaches to the vertebral bodies of C1 and C2 and the anterior surface of S2. This is why the mobilization of the cranium is always associated with the mobility of the sacrum and vice versa.

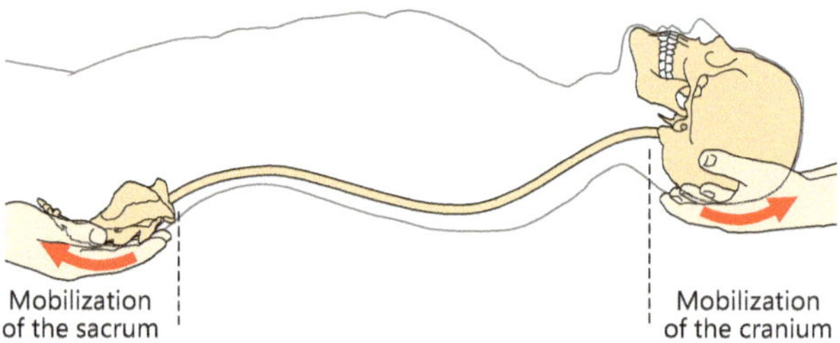

Mobilization of the sacrum and cranium.

Mandible

- Ramus:
  - coronoid process (insertion of the temporalis)
  - head
  - pterygoid fovea (insertion of the lateral pterygoid)
  - articular surface (cylindrical shape with biconvex curvature – axis directed posteromedially)
- Body:
  - alveolar processes (with alveolar yokes for tooth roots)
  - inferior border
  - digastric fossa (on the internal surface, insertion of the digastric)
- Angle:
  - width (140° in the infant, 120° in active mastication, > 120° in the edentulous)
  - masseteric tuberosity (on the external surface, insertion of the masseter)
  - pterygoid tuberosity (on the internal surface, insertion of the medial pterygoid).

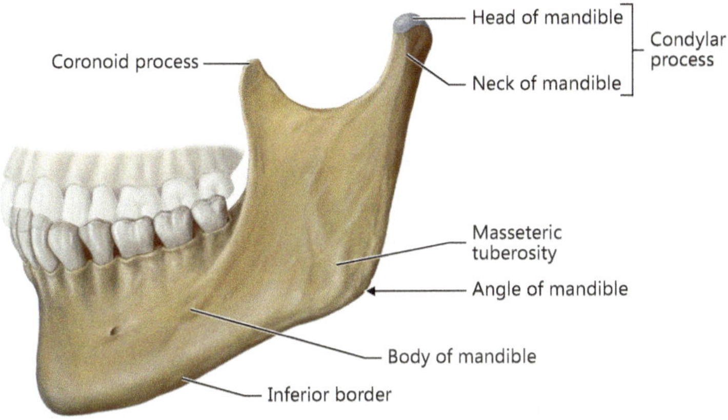

Mandible.

Articular surface of the temporal bone

Mandibular fossa:
- concave
- delimited anteriorly by the articular tubercle
- extracapsular posteriorly and forms the lateral wall of the external acoustic meatus
- it is two to three times wider than the head of the mandible.

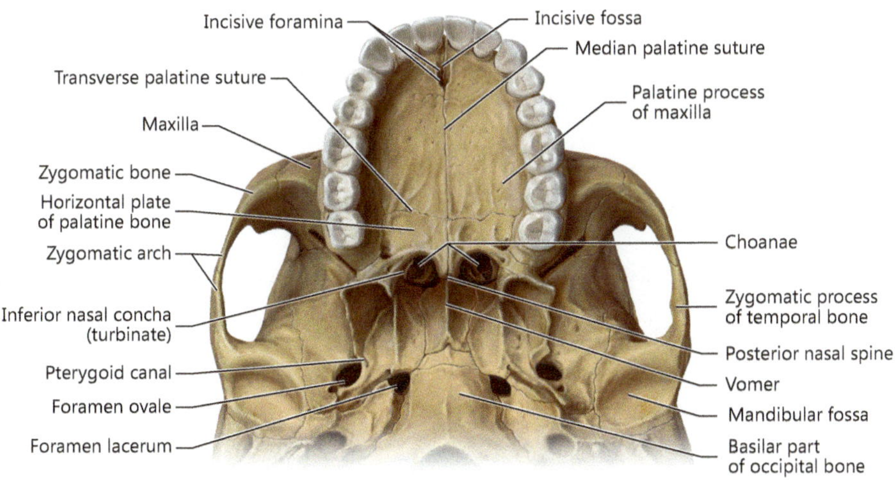

Detail of the external surface of the cranial base.

Temporomandibular joint

Articular surfaces

The articular surfaces are the heads of the mandible and mandibular fossae of the two temporal bones; a fibrocartilagenous disc interposes between the discordant articular surfaces, dividing the articular cavity into lower and upper parts.

Type

Bicondylar, synovial joint [due to the presence of a disc between the articular convexities of the mandible and the concavities (fossae) of the temporal bones].

Articular disc

- Elliptical shape
- Attached to the inner layer of the capsule
- An anterosuperior surface convex posteriorly (posterior part of disc), corresponding to the articular fossa, and concave anteriorly (anterior part of disc) attached to the articular tubercle
- A posteroinferior surface concave in relation to the anterior part of the condyle.

Joint capsule

- Encloses the articular tubercle but not the posterior part of the fossa
- Its flaccidity allows wide extension movements.

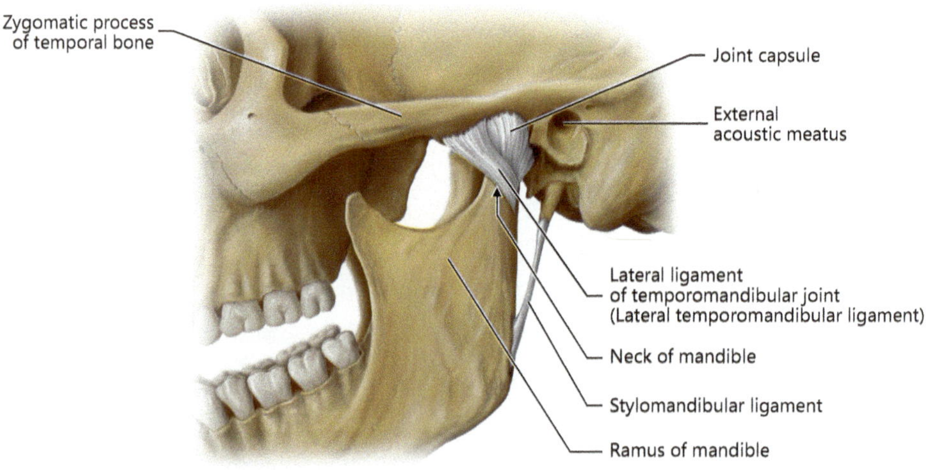

Temporomandibular joint in lateral projection. The mandible is firmly attached to the temporal bone by several remote ligaments.

Ligaments

- Temporomandibular
- Sphenomandibular
- Stylomandibular.

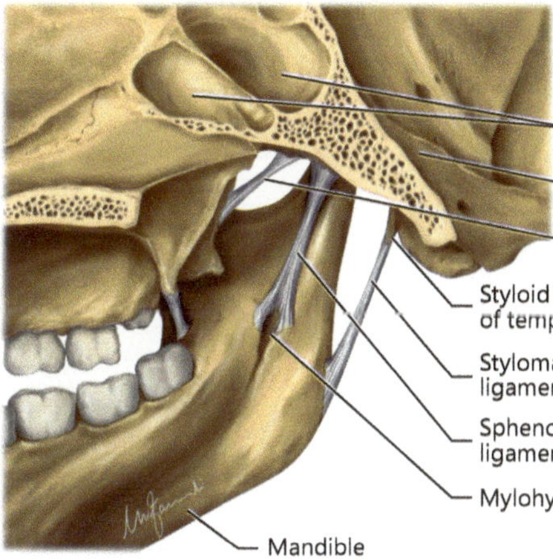

Temporomandibular joint seen in lateral projection of the internal side. Several remote ligaments reinforce the joint medially.

Mandibular movement

Elevation of the mandible	→	The mouth closes
Depression (descent) of the mandible	→	The mouth opens
Protrusion of the mandible (anterior protrusion)	→	Anterior movement (gliding) of the mandible
Retrusion (retraction) of the mandible	→	Posterior movement (gliding) of the mandible
Lateral deviation of the mandible	→	Lateral movements (lateromedial translation of the mandible)

Temporomandibular joint movements

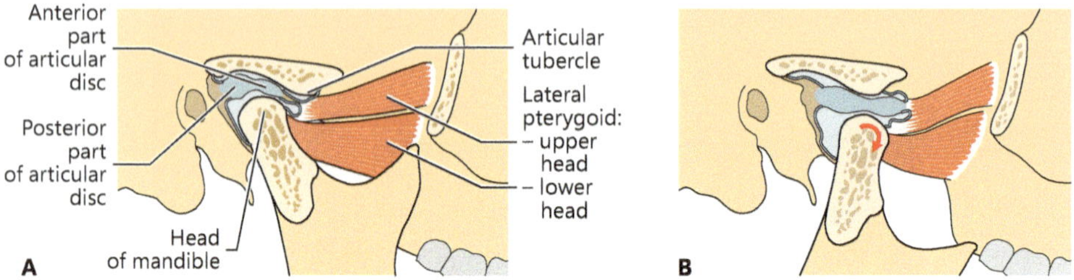

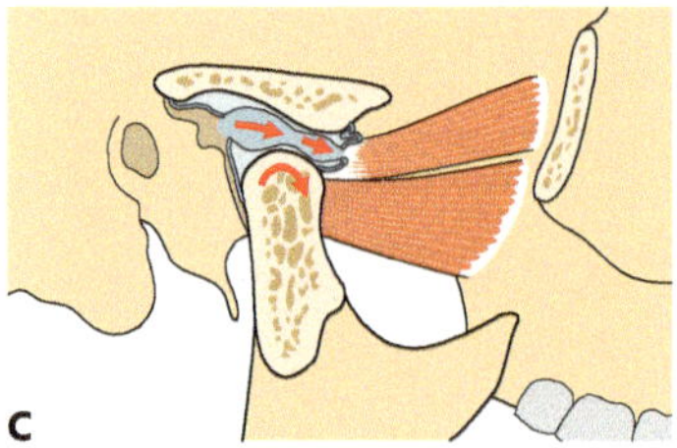

Position of the temporomandibular joint. **A**, Mouth closed; **B**, mouth open; **C**, with maximal mouth opening.

- Combined movements of both articulations
- Symmetrical mouth opening and closing movements
- Asymmetrical masticatory movements.

Rest position of the temporomandibular joint: in this position, the action potential of the mandibular muscles is minimal and there is no occlusion between the dental arches. The head and neck are in anatomical position. From the resting position, the mandible rises, lowers, protrudes and deviates laterally, first to one side and then to the other.

Mouth opening (depression of the mandible): the opening of the mouth is a combination of circumduction and rotation movements:

- the disc in the upper articular cavity is moved forward, towards the temporal bone;
- the condyle moves in the gap delimiting the anterior and posterior parts of the disc and drags the disc with it in anteroinferior direction;
- the posterior part of the disc is stretched by the condyle movements, while the anterior part is stretched contraction of the lateral pterygoid;
- during maximal mouth opening, the condyle is rotated out of the mandibular fossa and rests on the anterior part of the disc at the level of the articular tubercle.

Deviation of the mandible from the midline should not occur during active mouth opening. In fact, the mandible moves along a straight line during normal opening:

- a deviation to the left, with a "C"-shaped curve, indicates temporomandibular joint hypomobility on the convex or closed side of the curve, or a joint hypomobility on the concave or open side of the curve
- an "S"-shaped deviation may indicate muscular disequilibrium or dislocation of the condyle.

Functional mobility is determined by inserting two or three fingers between the upper and lower central incisors, which corresponds to a distance of 35-40 mm. Variations in the opening of the mouth can be measured with a ruler, using the upper and lower central incisors as a reference.

Mouth closing (dental arch occlusion): elevation of the mandible until the dental arches are completely occluded:

- the condyle and the posterior part of the disc are in the anterior mandibular fossa.

Protrusion of the mandible: forward gliding of the mandible. The movement should be sufficient to allow the protrusion of the lower dental arch with respect to the upper dental arch. It is possible to measure with a ruler the distance between the upper and lower central incisors. Normal protrusion from the rest position varies from 3 to 7 mm.

Retrusion of the mandible: movement opposite to the previous one. The protrusion and retrusion movements of the mandible are circumduction movements that occur mainly in the upper articular cavity.

Lateral movement of the mandible: this can occur only when the mandible is slightly lowered and has an amplitude of 2-3 cm, of which only 0.5 cm in the posterior direction.

Deviation of the mandible to one side and to the other: these are combined movements of laterality that occur during mastication. In this phase a distinction should be made between:

- balance side, characterized by:
  - lateral deviation of the mandible
  - inferior displacement of the mandibular condyle
  - modest protrusion of the mandible
- side in action, characterized by:
  - stabilization by the masticatory muscles
  - masticatory pressure
  - minimum amplitude of combined movements of:
    - rotation around a vertical axis
    - modest lateral translation.

The distance between two specific points can be measured, one at the level of the upper teeth and the other at the level of the lower teeth, for example, the space between the central incisors. Normal joint mobility is between 5 and 12 mm.

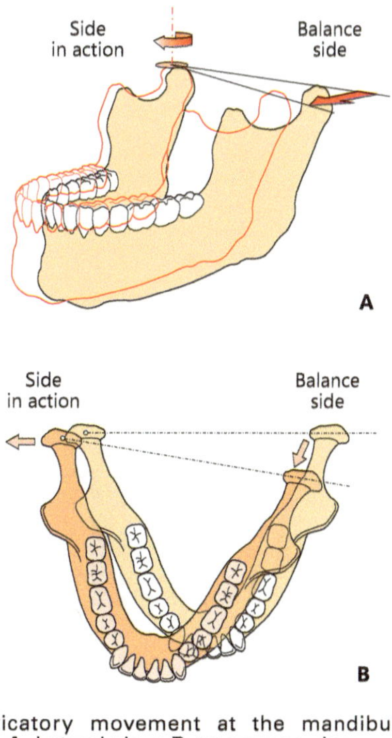

Masticatory movement at the mandibular joint. **A**, Lateral view; **B**, transverse view.

Masticatory muscles

Muscle	Action	Origin	Insertion	Innervation
Temporalis	Elevation of the mandible; deviation of the mandible to one side and to the other; retrusion of the mandible mediated by the action of the posterior fascicles	Temporal fossa; deep surface of the temporal fascia	Coronoid process of the mandible; anterior margin of the ramus of the mandible as far as the last molars	Trigeminal nerve [V]
Masseter	Vigorous elevation of the mandible; modest deviation of the mandible to one side and to the other; protrusion and retrusion of the mandible; due to the oblique orientation of its fibers it can move the mandible in inferoposterior direction	*Superficial part*: zygomatic process of the maxilla; anterior two-thirds of the zygomatic arch *Intermediate part*: medial surface of the anterior two-thirds of the zygomatic arch; inferior margin of the posterior third of the ramus of the mandible *Deep part*: deep surface of the zygomatic arch	*Superficial part*: angle and lower half of the lateral surface of the ramus of the mandible *Intermediate part*: central part of the ramus of the mandible *Deep part*: superior part of the ramus of the mandible; coronoid process of the mandible	Trigeminal nerve [V]
Medial pterygoid	Elevation of the mandible: protrusion of the mandible (with protrusion of the lateral pterygoid); lateral deviation of the mandible; during mastication it stabilizes the side that is in action	Medial plate of the pterygoid process; pyramidal process of the palatine bone; maxillary tuberosity	Posteroinferior part of the medial surfaces of the ramus and angle of the mandible	Trigeminal nerve [V]

(*continued*)

Masticatory muscles *(continued)*

Muscle	Action	Origin	Insertion	Innervation
Lateral pterygoid	Protrusion of the mandible (with protrusion of the medial pterygoid); depression of the mandible; control of the posterior movement of the articular disc of the temporomandibular joint and of the mandibular condyle when the mouth closes; deviation of the mandible to one side and to the other; during mastication it stabilizes the side in action	*Upper head*: lower part and lateral surface of the greater wing of the sphenoid *Lower head*: lateral plate of the pterygoid process	Pterygoid fossa on the internal surface of the neck of the mandible; joint capsule and disc of the temporomandibular joint	Trigeminal nerve [V]

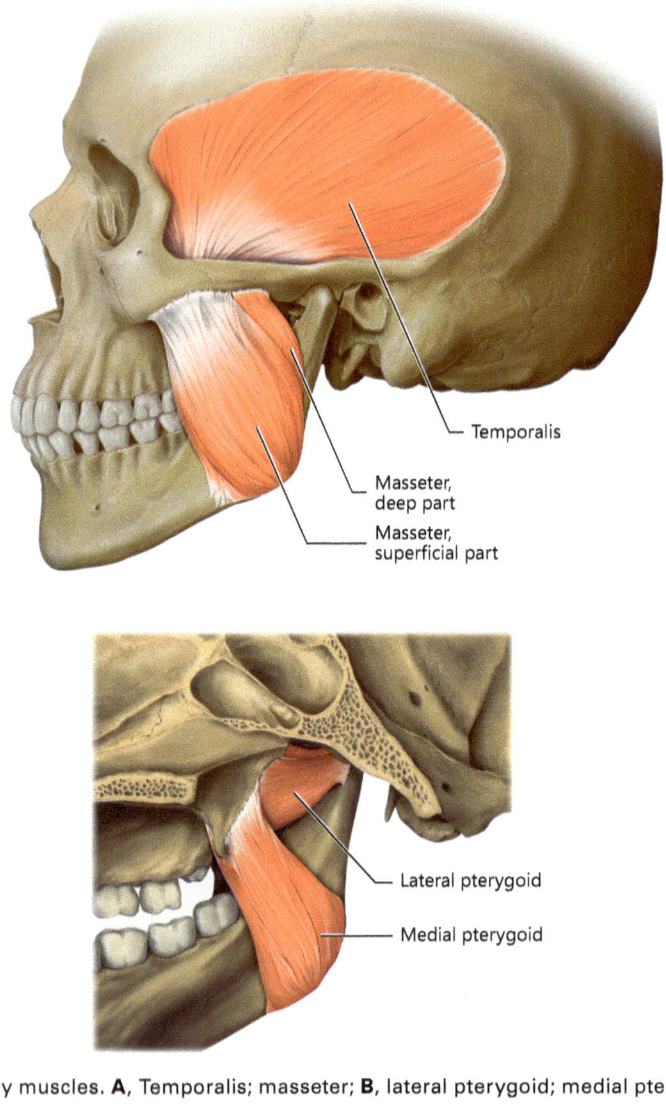

Masticatory muscles. **A**, Temporalis; masseter; **B**, lateral pterygoid; medial pterygoid.

Examination of the masticatory muscles

The masticatory muscles are innervated by the V cranial nerve (trigeminal nerve, through the mandibular nerve).

Movements evaluated:
- elevation and retrusion of the mandible
- depression of the mandible
- protrusion of the mandible
- lateral deviation of the mandible.

Elevation and retrusion of the mandible

Muscles	Temporalis, masseter, medial pterygoid
Movement	Mouth closing with tight occlusion of the teeth
Palpation	Contraction force and bellies of the temporalis and masseter: • the temporalis is palpated above the zygomatic arch • the masseter is palpated above the angle of the mandible

Depression of the mandible

Muscles	Lateral pterygoid (as well as the mylohyoid, digastric and suprahyoid muscles described in Chapter 4 "Neck and cervical column")
Movement	Mouth opening with complete depression of the mandible (the lateral pterygoid is active during the entire range of movement, while the digastric is active only during the phase of full descent or forced descend of the mandible)
Palpation	The anterior part of the digastric is palpated below the mandible

Protrusion of the mandible

Muscles	Medial pterygoid, lateral pterygoid
Movement	Protrusion of the mandible with mouth partially open

Lateral deviation of the mandible

Muscles	Temporalis, medial pterygoid, lateral pterygoid, masseter
Movement	Deviation of the mandible to one side and to the other with the mouth slightly open

Mandible-cervical column as a functional unit

The mandible and the cervical column, as well as the other cranial bones, the hyoid bone and the pectoral girdle form a functional unit.
This means that functional changes in one of these parts will affect the others.

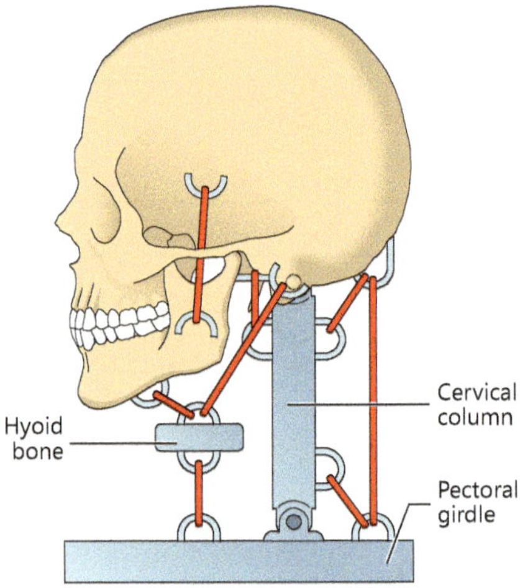

Mandible-cervical column as a functional unit.

Example: flexion of the cervical column moves the mandible forward, while its extension moves the mandible backward. Changes in the posture of the cervical column consequently alter the closing of the mouth. In case of forward flexion there is, for example, an alteration of the bite after retraction of the mandible by the infrahyoid muscles.

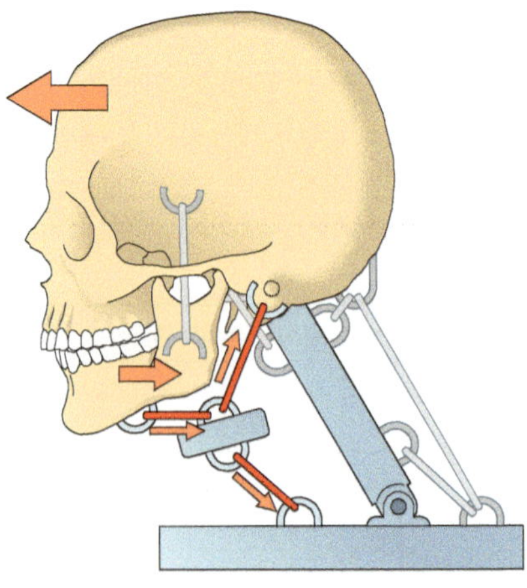

Change in the position of the cervical column and its consequences on the bite.

Muscles of facial expression

Also called cutaneous muscles, they insert, with at least one of the two heads, in the deep surface of the skin and are determinant in the facial expression.

Muscle	Action	Origin	Insertion	Innervation
Epicranius				
Frontal (procerus included)	Moves the scalp forward; wrinkles the forehead	Anterior margin of the epicranial aponeurosis	Deep surface of the skin corresponding to the eyebrow, the glabella and the upper part of the dorsum of the nose	Facial nerve [VII]
Occipital	Moves the scalp backward	Posterior margin of the epicranial aponeurosis	Lateral two-thirds of the superior nuchal line; mastoid process	Facial nerve [VII]
Epicranial aponeurosis (galea aponeurotica – origin of the frontal, occipital and anterosuperior auricular muscles)				
Extrinsic auricular muscles				
Auricularis anterosuperior	Moves the auricle forward and upward	Lateral margin of the epicranial aponeurosis	Lateral surface of the auricle corresponding to the helix, the spine of the helix and the anterosuperior part of the convexity of the concha of the auricle	Facial nerve [VII]
Auricularis posterior	Moves the auricle backward	Lateral margin of the epicranial aponeurosis and mastoid process	Medial surface of the auricle, at the level of the eminentia conchae of the auricle	Facial nerve [VII]

(continued)

3

Muscles of facial expression *(continued)*

Muscle	Action	Origin	Insertion	Innervation
Palpebral muscles				
Orbicularis oculi	Closes the palpebral fissure; draws tears towards the internal angle of the eye; dilates the lacrimal sac; facilitates the outflow of tears	*Orbital part*: upper margin of the medial palpebral ligament; medial third of the supraorbital margin	Lower margin of the palpebral ligament; medial third of the infraorbital margin; lacrimal sac	Facial nerve [VII]
		Palpebral part: medial palpebral ligament	Lateral palpebral ligament	
		Deep or lacrimal part: posterior lacrimal crest	Converge towards the palpebral part of the muscle	
Corrugator supercilii	Medial descent of the eyebrow skin	Medial end of the superciliary arch	Skin of the eyebrow in correspondence of the supraorbital notch/foramen	Facial nerve [VII]
Muscles of the nose				
Nasalis	Compression of the lateral wall of the nose, restricting the nares (nostrils) and nasal vestibule	Alveolar yokes of the upper incisors and canines; incisive fossa	*Transverse part*: nasal dosum *Alar part*: skin of the posterior end of the mobile part of the nasal septum and of the nares (nostrils)	Facial nerve [VII]
Dilator of nares	Moves the ala of the nose laterally, dilating the nares and vestibule	Lateral margin of the piriform opening	Skin of the lower margin of the ala of the nose	Facial nerve [VII]

(continued)

Muscles of facial expression (*continued*)

Muscle	Action	Origin	Insertion	Innervation
Muscles of the lips				
Zygomaticus	Moves the labial commissure upward and backward	Lateral surface of the zygomatic bone	Deep surface of the skin and mucosa of the labial commissure	Facial nerve [VII]
Levator labii superioris (quadratus labii superioris)	Raising of the upper lip and dilation of the nares	*Zygomatic part*: lateral surface of the zygomatic bone	Skin of the upper lip	Facial nerve [VII]
		Infraorbital part: infraorbital margin	Skin of the upper lip	
		Angular part: frontal process of the maxilla; nasal bone	Skin of the ala of the nose and of the upper lip	
Levator anguli oris (caninus)	Raising of the labial commissure in the medial part	Canine fossa of the maxilla	Skin and mucosa of the labial commissure	Facial nerve [VII]
Buccinator	Retraction of the labial commissure and adheres the cheeks and lips to the dental arches	External surface of the upper alveolar process; maxillary tuberosity; pterygoid hamulus; pterygomandibular raphe; external surface of the lower alveolar process at the level of the molars	Deep surface of the lip and mucosa of the labial commissure	Facial nerve [VII]

(*continued*)

3

Muscles of facial expression *(continued)*

Muscle	Action	Origin	Insertion	Innervation
Muscles of the lips				
Risorius	Retraction of the labial commissure	Parotid fascia	Deep surface of the skin of the labial commissure	Facial nerve [VII]
Depressor anguli oris (triangularis labiorum)	Lowering of the labial commissure	External surface of the body of the mandible, close to the base	Skin of the labial commissure; confluence at the orbicularis muscle at the level of the upper lip	Facial nerve [VII]
Depressor labii inferioris (quadratus labii inferioris)	Moves the lower lip downward and outward, inverting it	External surface of the body of the mandible	Deep surface of the skin and mucosa of the lower lip	Facial nerve [VII]
Mentalis	Raising and corrugation of the skin of the chin	Alveolar yoke of the lower medial incisor	Skin of the chin	Facial nerve [VII]
Incisivus labii superioris and incisivus labii inferioris	Move the labial commissure medially (upward and downward, respectively)	Alveolar yokes of the upper and lower lateral incisors	Skin of the chin	Facial nerve [VII]

(continued)

Muscles of facial expression (*continued*)

Muscle	Action	Origin	Insertion	Innervation
Muscles of the lips				
Orbicularis oris (including the depressor septi nasi)	Sphincter of the oral opening: pushes the lips forward	*External part*: fascicles coming from the caninus, buccinator, triangularis and incisivus muscles; these fascicles form two half-rings with center in correspondence of the commissure and extremity on the midline	Deep surface of the skin of the lips near the midline and of the skin lining the posterior contour of the nares and the posterior part of the membranous septum (depressor septi nasi)	Facial nerve [VII]
		Internal part: ring close to the free margin of the lips	Deep surface of the skin and mucosa of the lips	

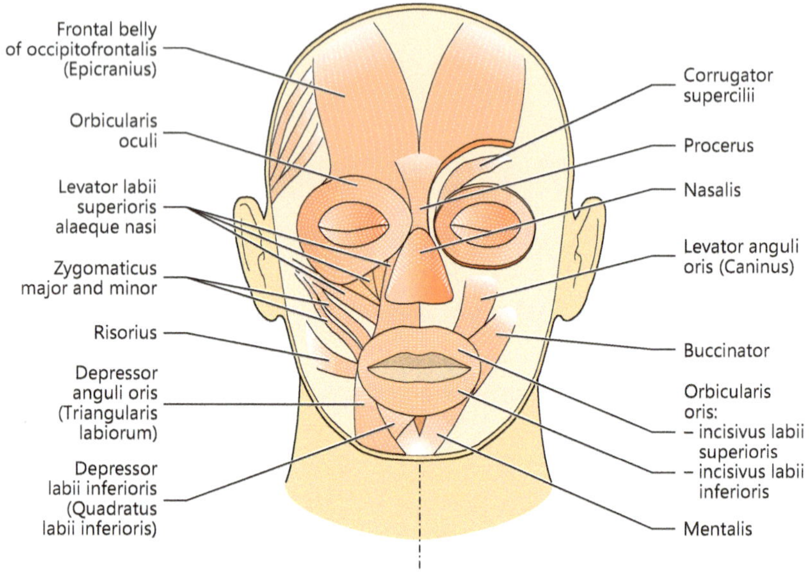

Muscles of facial expression.

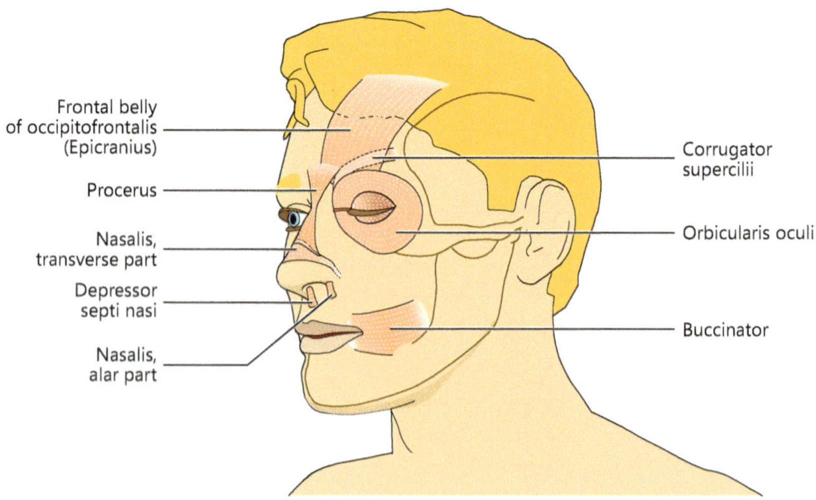

Muscles of facial expression.

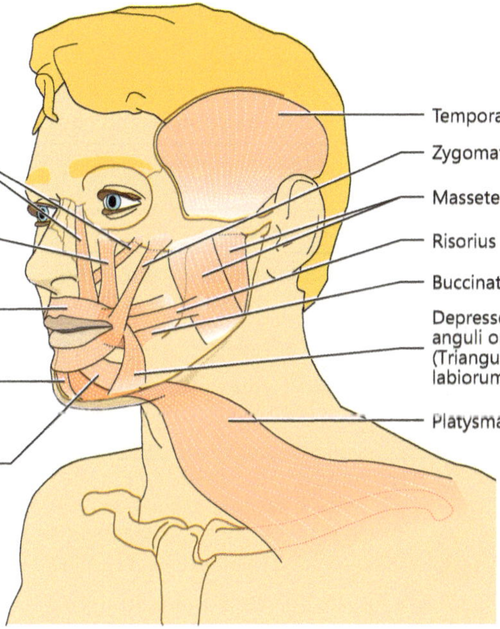

Muscles of facial expression.

Examination of the muscles of facial expression

The muscles of facial expression are innervated by the VII cranial nerve (facial nerve). The evaluation of their functions includes facial expression and control of the muscles of the eyebrows, eyelids, nose and mouth.

Movements evaluated:

- Eyebrows:
  - elevation
  - adduction
  - depression of medial angles
- Eyelids:
  - closing
- Nose:
  - dilation of nares (nostrils)
  - constriction of nares (nostrils)
- Mouth:
  - occlusion and protrusion of the lips
  - compression of cheecks against teeth
  - elevation, retraction and depression of the angle of the mouth
  - elevation of the upper lip
  - elevation and protrusion of the lower lip.

Elevation of eyebrows

Muscle	Epicranial (occipitofrontal)
Movement	Elevation of eyebrows; the action of the muscle causes the appearance of transverse wrinkles on the forehead and an expression of surprise

Adduction of eyebrows

Muscle	Corrugator supercilii
Movement	Closeness of the medial extremities of the eyebrows; the action of the muscle causes the appearance of vertical wrinkles between the eyebrows and a threatening expression

Depression of the medial angles of the eyebrows

Muscle	Procerus
Movement	Depression of the medial angles of the eyebrows and elevation of the skin of the nose; the action of the muscle causes the appearance of transverse wrinkles on the dorsum of the nose; it can also corrugate the skin on the dorsum of the nose, as in the expression of disgust

Closing of eyelids

Muscle	Orbicularis oculi
Movement	Tight closure of the eyelids; the action of this muscle stretches the skin of the forehead, temples and cheeks in a medial direction, towards the nose

Dilation of nares (nostrils)

Muscles	Nasalis (alar part) and depressor septi nasi
Movement	Dilation or enlargement of the nares (nostrils); in order to speed up the movement, a deep breath may be taken

Constriction of nares (nostrils)

Muscle	Nasalis (transverse part)
Movement	Constriction of the nares (nostrils)

Closing and protrusion of lips

Muscle	Orbicularis oris
Movement	Closing and protrusion of the lips, as in whistling, wrinkling the lips at the same time

Compression of the cheeks against the teeth

Muscle	Buccinator
Movement	Compression of the cheeks against the teeth, as when blowing into a wind instrument; during the movement it is possible to palpate the buccinator at the level of the cheek

Elevation of the angle of the mouth

Muscle	Levator anguli oris (caninus)
Movement	Elevation of the angle of the mouth or labial commissure; the action of the muscle accentuates the nasolabial sulcus

Elevation and retraction of the angle of the mouth

Muscle	Zygomaticus
Movement	The angle of the mouth is drawn upward and laterally; the action of the muscle gives the face a smiling expression; palpation of the muscle is possible above and lateral to the angle of the mouth

Retraction of the angle of the mouth

Muscle	Risorius
Movement	Retraction or displacement of the angle of the mouth in the posterior direction; the action of the muscle causes a grimace of the face

Depression of the angle of the mouth and of the lower lip

Muscles	Platysma (for its action, origin and insertion see Chapter 4 "Neck and cervical column"), depressor anguli oris (triangularis labiorum), depressor labii inferioris (quadratus labii inferioris)
Movement	Lowering of the lower lip and angles of the mouth by stretching the skin between the chin and clavicle, as if to loosen the pressure produced by a shirt collar that is too tight

Elevation of the upper lip

Muscles	Levator labii superioris (quadratus labii superioris) and zygomaticus
Movement	Elevation and protrusion of the upper lip (lip eversion), as if to show the upper incisors and gums

Elevation and protrusion of the lower lip

Muscle	Mentalis
Movement	Elevation of the skin of the chin and protrusion of the lower lip; the action of the muscle determines grumpy facial expression

Extraocular muscles

Muscle	Action	Origin	Insertion	Innervation
Levator palpebrae superioris	Raising of the upper eyelid	Inferior surface of the lesser wing of the sphenoid, above and in front of the optic canal	Skin of the upper eyelid; anterior surface of the superior tarsus; upper conjunctival fornix; zygomatic bone tubercle; superior surface of the orbital septum	Oculomotor nerve [III]
Superior rectus	Elevation of the abducted eye	Common tendinous ring (anulus of Zinn) (fibrous ring that surrounds the superior, medial and inferior margins of the optic canal)	Superior part of the sclera, posteriorly to the cornea	Oculomotor nerve [III]
Inferior rectus	Lowering of the abducted eye	Common tendinous ring (anulus of Zinn)	Inferior part of the sclera, posteriorly to the cornea	Oculomotor nerve [III]
Superior oblique	Lowering of the adducted eye	Body of the sphenoid, above and medial to the optic canal; tendinous insertion of the superior rectus	The tendon passes through the trochlea (circular fibrocartilaginous formation that inserts into the fossa of the frontal bone) and then passes posteriorly, laterally and downward to insert into the sclera, posterior to the equatorial zone, in the superolateral part of the eyeball	Trochlear nerve [IV]
Inferior oblique	Elevation of the adducted eye	Orbital surface of the maxilla, lateral to the nasolacrimal sulcus	Lateral part of the sclera, posterior to the equatorial zone of the eyeball	Oculomotor nerve [III]
Lateral rectus	Abduction of the eye	Common tendinous ring (anulus of Zinn); orbital surface of the greater wing of the sphenoid	Lateral part of the sclera, posterior to the corneoscleral junction	Abducens nerve [VI]
Medial rectus	Adduction of the eye	Common tendinous ring (anulus of Zinn)	Medial part of the sclera, posterior to the corneoscleral junction	Oculomotor nerve [III]

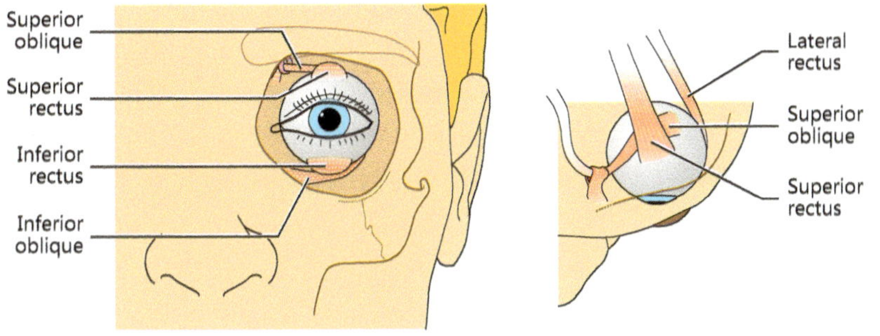

Frontal and superior aspects of the left eye.

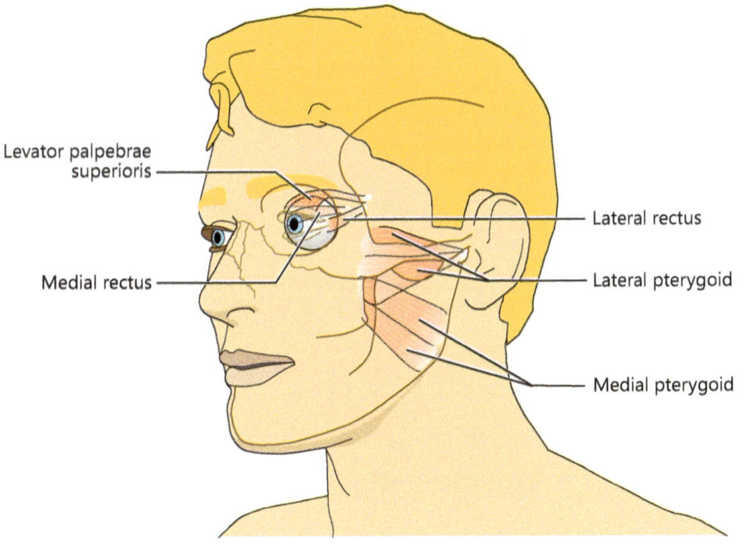

Lateral aspect of the left eye.

3

Examination of the extraocular muscles

The extraocular muscles are innervated by the III, IV and VI cranial nerves (the oculomotor, trochlear and abducens nerves). Their functions are to open the eyes (levator palpebrae superioris) and to control movements (six extraocular muscles).

Movements evaluated:

- elevation of the upper eyelid
- elevation, abduction, lowering and adduction of the eye.

Elevation of the upper eyelid

Muscle	Levator palpebrae superioris
Movement	Elevation of the eyelids (ptosis is the clinical term for the inability to perform this movement)

Eye movements

Muscles	Superior rectus, inferior rectus, superior oblique, inferior oblique, lateral rectus, medial rectus
Movement	Each extraocular muscle can be examined when it is in its most efficient position, which is reached when the muscle is at a right angle to the axis of eye movement: – start with a forward-directed gaze – then move the gaze to other direction

Diplopia (double vision) should be investigated during the examination of each extraocular muscle. The examination can focus on only one eye. However, it is preferable to examine concurrently the muscles of both eyes by observing their simultaneous movements.
Possible muscular combinations are:

- right superior rectus and left inferior oblique
- left superior oblique and right inferior rectus
- right superior oblique and left inferior rectus
- left superior rectus and right inferior oblique
- left medial rectus and right lateral rectus
- right medial rectus and left lateral rectus.

It should be noted whether the movement is normal (i.e., regular for its full amplitude) or abnormal.

Superior rectus

Movement	Upward and outward gaze; thus any deficits in eye elevation can be observed

Inferior rectus

Movement	Downward and outward gaze; thus any deficits in the descent of the eyes can be observed

Superior oblique

Movement	Downward and inward gaze; thus any deficits in the descent of the eyes can be observed

Inferior oblique

Movement	Upward and inward gaze; thus any deficits in eye elevation can be observed

Lateral rectus

Movement	Outward gaze (abduction); thus any deficits in eye abduction can be observed

Medial rectus

Movement	Inward gaze (adduction); thus any deficits in eye adduction can be observed

Movements of the head

For the examination of the movements of the head, see Chapter 4 “Neck and cervical column”.

Palpation of the head

External occipital protuberance

Prominence in the center of the occipital region.

Superior nuchal line

It extends on both sides of the external occipital protuberance. It has the shape of a ridge with slightly arched course and inferior convexity. The following muscles originate in this line:

- trapezius
- sternocleidomastoid.

(For the action, origin, insertion and innervation of the trapezius and sternocleidomastoid, see Chapter 7 "Shoulder and pectoral girdle" and Chapter 4 "Neck and cervical column", respectively).

Mastoid process

Prominence at the extremity of the superior nuchal line and immediately behind the ear. The sternocleidomastoid inserts into the mastoid process.

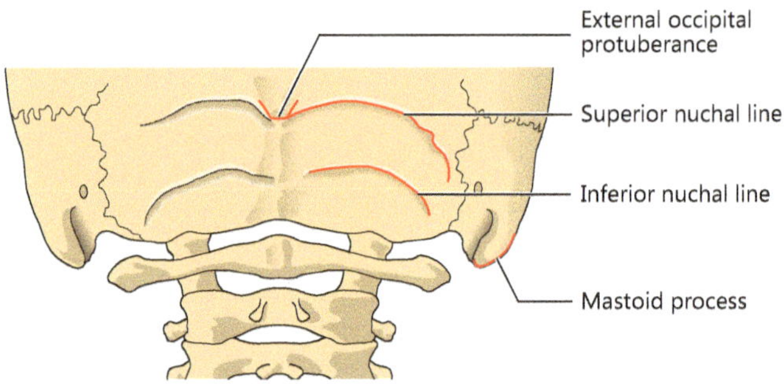

Palpation of the cranium: bony structures.

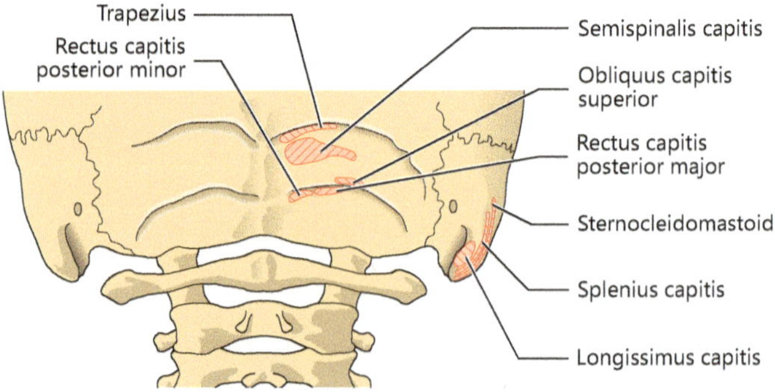

Palpation of the cranium: muscle origins.

(For the action, origin, insertion and innervation of the semispinalis capitis and the longissimus capitis, see Chapter 5 "Vertebral column and movements of the trunk").

Inferior nuchal line

It passes about two fingers below the superior nuchal line. In this line originate, in a mediolateral direction, the muscles:
- semispinalis capitis
- rectus capitis posterior minor
- rectus capitus posterior major
- obliquus capitis superior
- longissimus capitis
- splenius capitis.

(For the action, origin, insertion and innervation of the rectus capitis posterior minor, rectus capitis posterior major, obliquus capitis superior and splenius capitis, see Chapter 4 "Neck and cervical column").

Head of the mandible

The head of the mandible is anterior to the external acoustic meatus and moves forward when the mouth is opened.

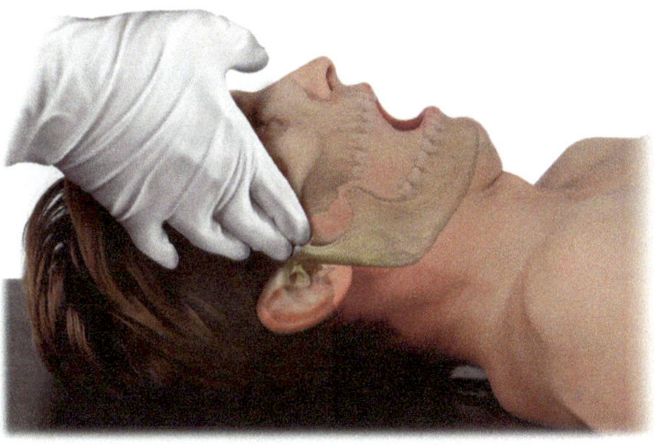

Palpation of the head of the mandible.

Coronoid process

When the mouth is closed, the coronoid process is positioned behind the zygomatic arch, and cannot be palpated; when the mouth is opened, it moves forward under the zygomatic arch, allowing palpation. The temporalis inserts on the coronoid process.

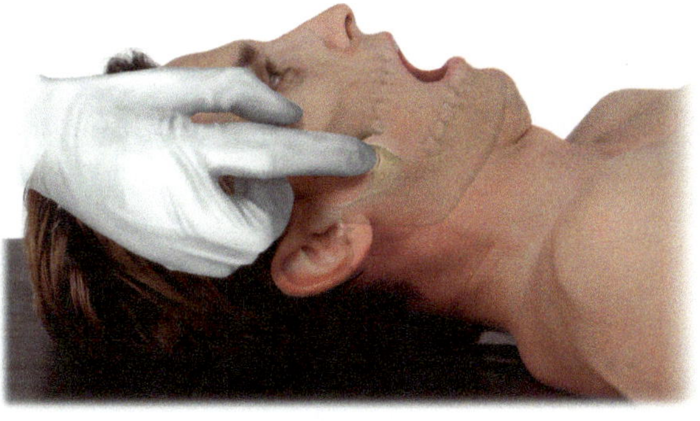

Palpation of the coronoid process.

Masseteric tuberosity

Palpation is easier when the mouth is closed.

Masticatory muscles

- Temporalis: When the mouth is open, it is palpated in its insertion, in the coronoid process of the mandible; when the mouth is closed, it is palpated in its origin, in the temporal fossa.

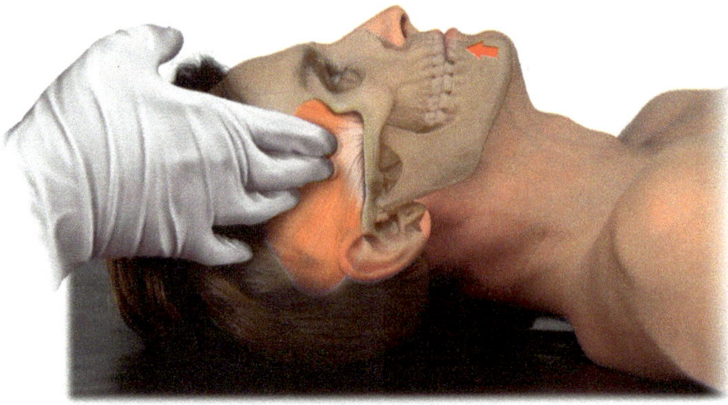

Palpation of the temporalis.

- Masseter: A thick, rectangular muscular mass, palpated at the level of the angle of the mandible when the mouth is opened, even partially; it becomes a muscular protuberance when the mouth is closed.

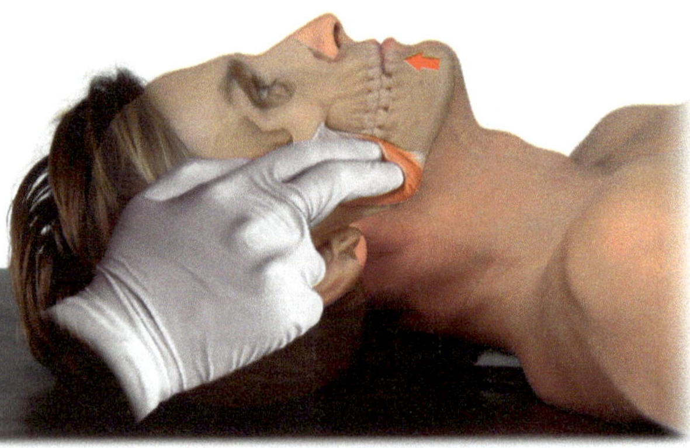

Palpation of the masseter.

• Medial pterygoid: When the mouth is closed, it can be palpated at the level of its insertion on the inner surface of the ramus of the mandible.

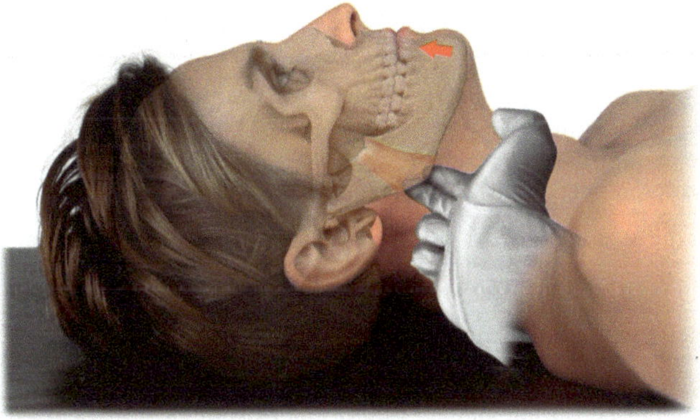

Palpation of the medial pterygoid.

• Lateral pterygoid: Can only be palpated from the oral cavity, proceeding from the last upper molar in the direction of the neck of the mandible, while the patient opens and closes the mouth; muscle contraction is evaluated during mouth opening.

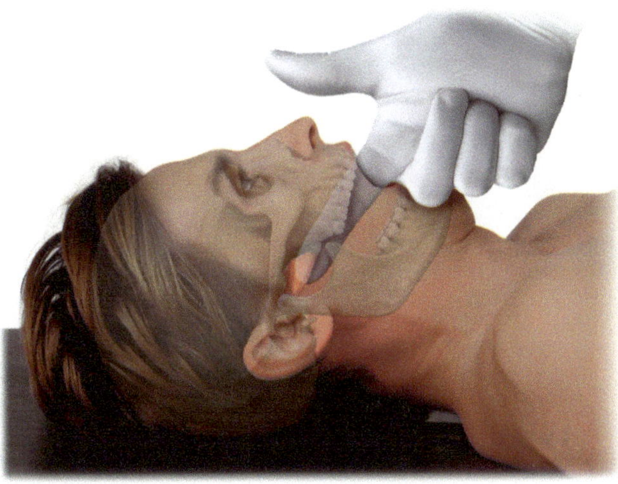

Palpation of the lateral pterygoid.

Anatomical landmarks on the surface of the head and neck

1	Jugular (suprasternal) notch: a rounded depression on the upper margin of the sternum, between the medial ends of the clavicles
2	Thyroid cartilage: most prominent cartilage of the larynx, located at the level of the fourth and fifth cervical vertebrae; subcutaneous prominence (laryngeal prominence)
3	Hyoid bone: a U-shaped submandibular bone lying above the thyroid cartilage at the level of the third cervical vertebra; its body can be palpated along the midline under the chin, at the angle formed by the floor of the oral cavity and the anterior part of the neck
4	Angle of the mandible: the angle located medially and distal to the ear lobe
5	Angle of the mouth: the angle formed laterally by the upper and lower lips
6	Nasolabial sulcus: skin furrow between the ala of the nose and the lip
7	Temporomandibular joint: can be palpated anteriorly to the tragus of the external ear during mouth opening and closing
8	Mastoid process: a bony prominence of the cranium located behind the ear
9	Acromion: lateral projection of the spine of the scapula at the apex of the shoulder

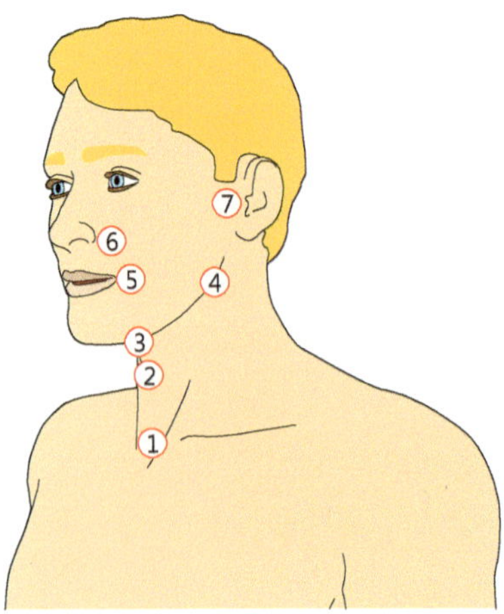

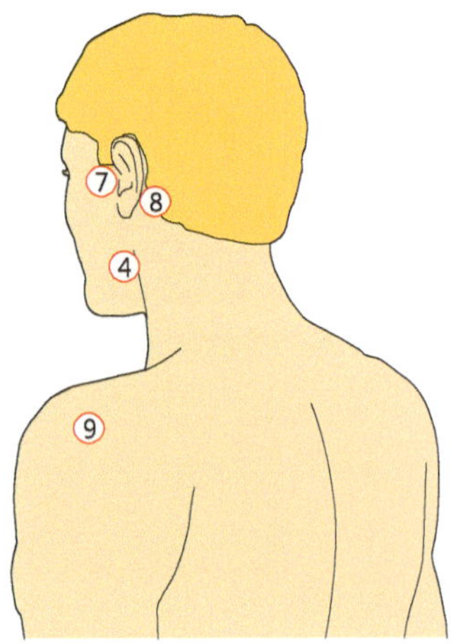

Upper cervical column

1st cervical vertebra (atlas)

Two joined lateral masses:
- anterior to the anterior arch (on which the anterior tubercle can be seen)
- posterior to the posterior arch (on which the posterior tubercle can be seen).

Articular surfaces:
- superior (joint with the occipital bone)
- inferior (joint with the 2nd cervical vertebra)
- medial (facet for dens – joint with the dens of the axis or odontoid process).

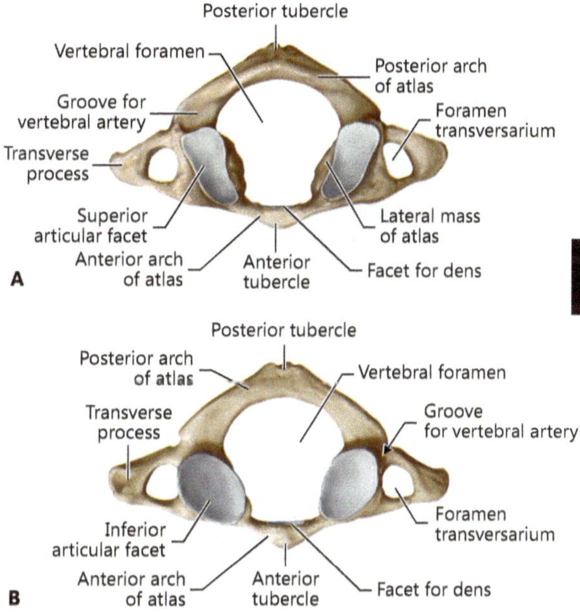

Atlas. **A**, View from above; **B**, view from below.

2nd cervical vertebra (axis)

- Dens of the axis originating from the vertebral body
- Bifid spinous process
- Foramen transversarium for the passage of the vertebral artery.

Articular surfaces:
- anterior articular facet of the dens (joint with the atlas)
- posterior articular facet of the dens (where the transverse ligament of the atlas is attached)
- superior articular facets (joint with the masses of the atlas)
- inferior articular facets (joint with C3).

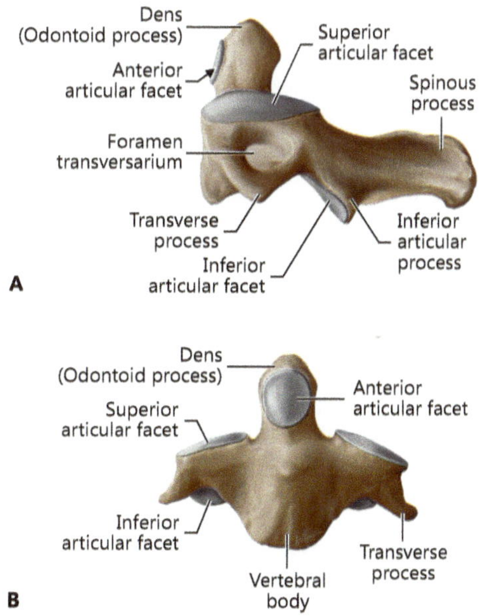

Axis. **A**, Sagittal view; **B**, frontal view.

Atlanto-occipital joint

Articular surfaces:
- occipital condyles – ellipsoidal shape, convex surface
- superior articular facets of the atlas – oval shape, concave surface (medial to anterior orientation).

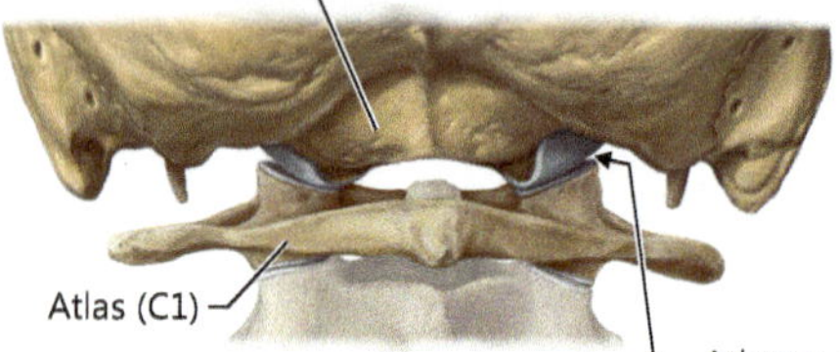

Atlanto-occipital joint.

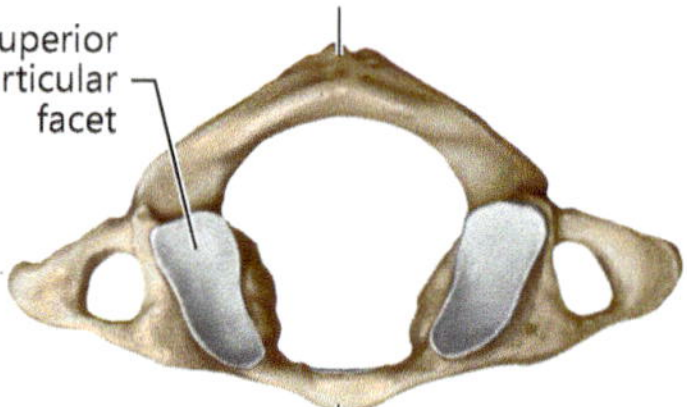

Superior articular facets of the atlas.

Median atlantoaxial joint

Articular surfaces:
- facet for dens – slightly concave surface
- anterior articular facet of the dens – oval shape, convex surface.

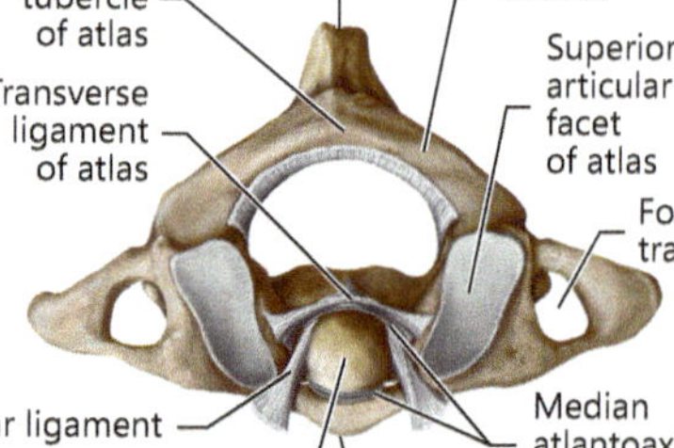

Medial atlantoaxial joint.

Lateral atlantoaxial joints

- Inferior articular facets of the atlas – flat or slightly convex surface
- Superior articular facets of the axis, convex surface (posterior to lateral orientation).

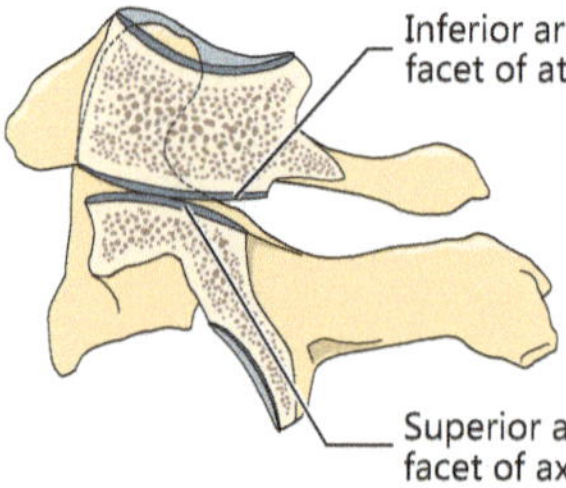

Left lateral atlantoaxial joint.

Ligaments of the upper cervical column

Anterior ligaments

Anterior atlanto-occipital membrane	Between the superior border of the anterior arch of the atlas and anterior border of the foramen magnum (some fiber bundles are fixed to the transverse process of the atlas; two layers, one deeper in contact with the atlanto-occipital joint capsule, the other closer to the surface corresponding to the anterior longitudinal ligament).
Anterior atlantoaxial ligament	Between the anterior parts of the atlas and axis.
Anterior longitudinal ligament	Covers the anterior surface of the vertebral bodies from the axis to the superior part of the sacrum.

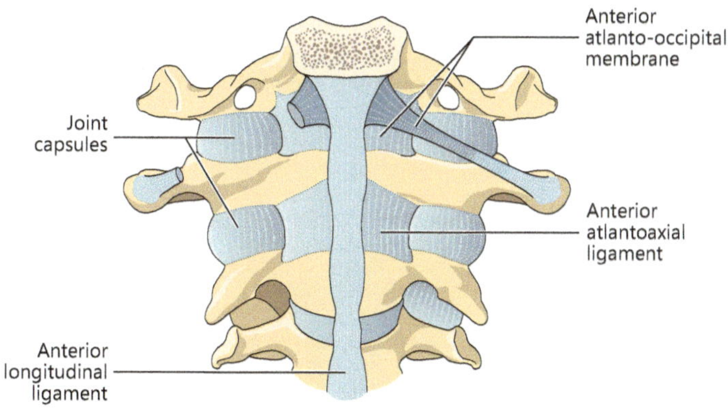

Anterior ligaments of the upper cervical column.

Posterior ligaments (from surface to depth)

Ligamentum nuchae	Between the external occipital protuberance and C7, where it continues with the spinal ligament, it is anchored to the spinous processes of the cervical vertebrae and joins the interspinous ligament.
Posterior atlanto-occipital membrane	Between the superior border of the posterior arch of the atlas and the posterior border of the foramen magnum.
Posterior atlantoaxial ligament	Between the posterior parts of the atlas and axis.

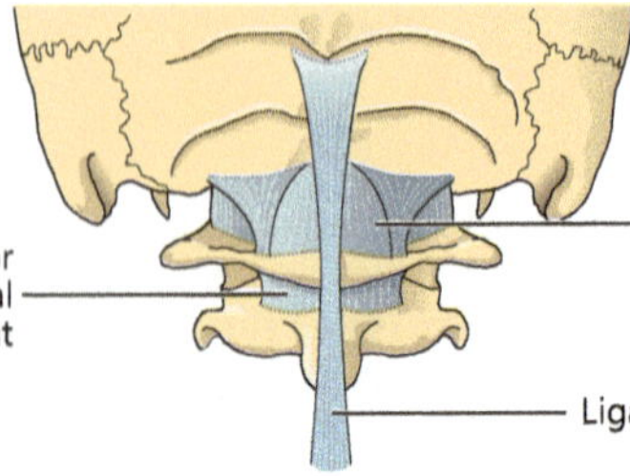

Posterior ligaments of the upper cervical column.

After removal of the vertebral arches

Superficial plane

Tectorial membrane	Between the clivus of the occipital bone and posterior surface of the body of the axis.
Posterior longitudinal ligament	Covers the posterior surface of the vertebral bodies from the occipital bone to the sacrum.

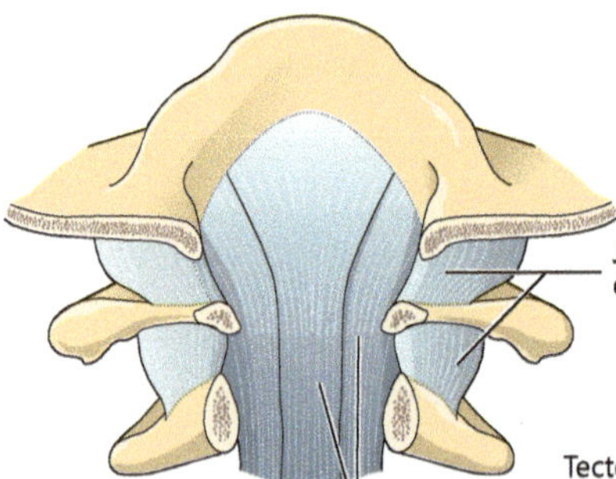

Posterior ligaments of the upper cervical column after removal of the vertebral arches. Superficial plane.

Intermediate plane

Cruciate ligament:

• Transverse ligament of the atlas	Between the medial surfaces of the lateral masses of the atlas and the posterior articular facet of the dens (transverse part of the cruciate ligament).
• Transverse occipital and transverse axial ligaments	Between the body of the axis and the border of the foramen magnum (longitudinal part of the cruciate ligament).

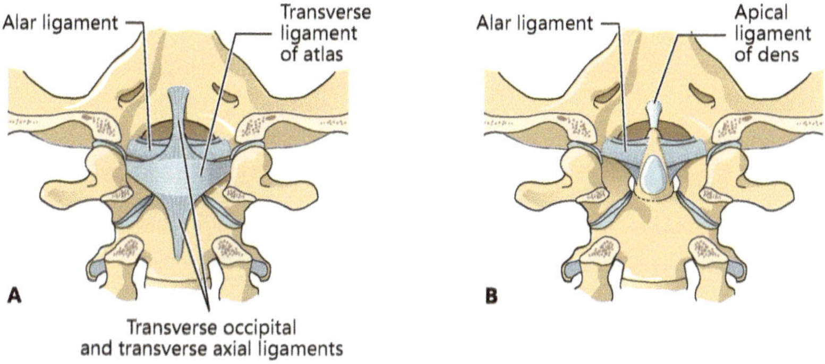

Posterior ligaments of the upper cervical column after removal of the vertebral arches. **A**, Intermediate plane; **B**, deep plane.

Deep plane

Apical ligament of the dens	Between the apex of the dens of the axis and central part of the border of the foramen magnum.
Alar ligaments	Between the dorsolateral surface of the apex of the dens and the anteromedial border of the occipital condyles (the posterior fascicles are inserted in the lateral masses of the atlas).

Functions of the ligaments of the upper cervical column

The ligaments of the upper cervical column, in addition to providing support, limit flexion-extension and rotation movements.

Limitation of flexion

- Posterior ligaments arranged longitudinally (ligamentum nuchae, posterior longitudinal ligament, tectorial membrane, posterior atlanto-occipital membrane, posterior atlantoaxial ligament)
- Cruciate ligament (transverse occipital and transverse axial ligaments).

Limitation of extension

Anterior ligaments (anterior atlantoaxial ligaments, anterior atlanto-occipital membrane, anterior longitudinal ligament).

Limitation of rotation

Contralateral part of the posterior atlanto-occipital membrane, the tectorial membrane and the alar ligaments.

Movements of the upper cervical column

The joints between the occipital bone, the atlas and the axis constitute a functional unit.

Flexion

Atlanto-occipital joint

The occipital condyles slide on the superior articular facets of the atlas moving in posterior direction, increasing the distance between the occipital bone and the posterior arch of the atlas.

Altogether the entire cervical column flexes 40°.

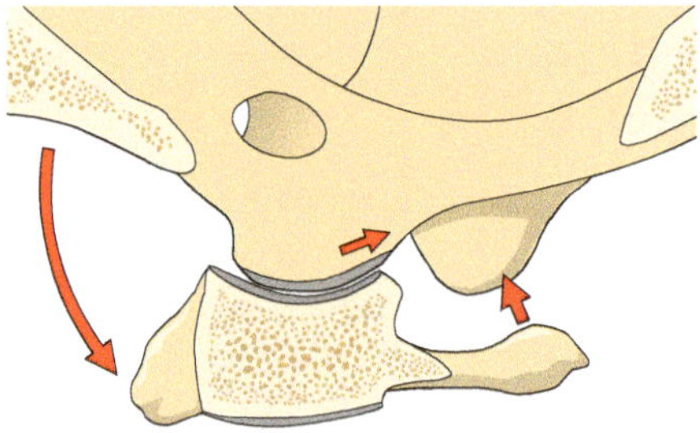

Flexion of the atlanto-occipital joint.

Atlantoaxial joints

- The inferior articular facets of the atlas slide backward and upward
- The fossa of the dens moves downward and away from the dens
- It increases the distance between the posterior arch of the atlas and the spinous process of C2.

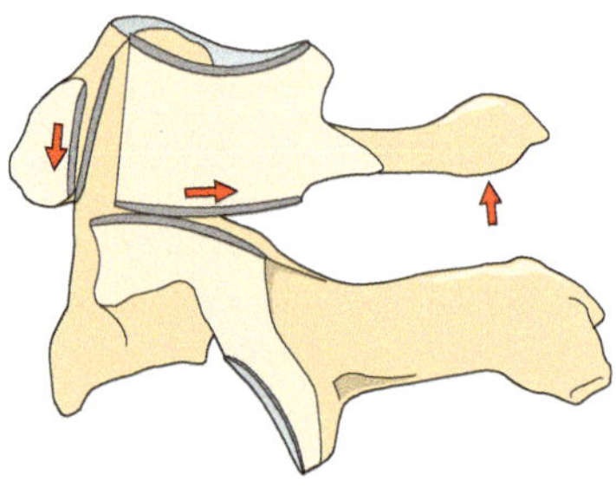

Flexion of the atlanto-axial joints.

Extension

Atlanto-occipital joint

- The occipital condyles move in anterior direction
- Approach between the occipital bone and the posterior arch of the atlas.

Altogether the entire cervical column extends 45°.

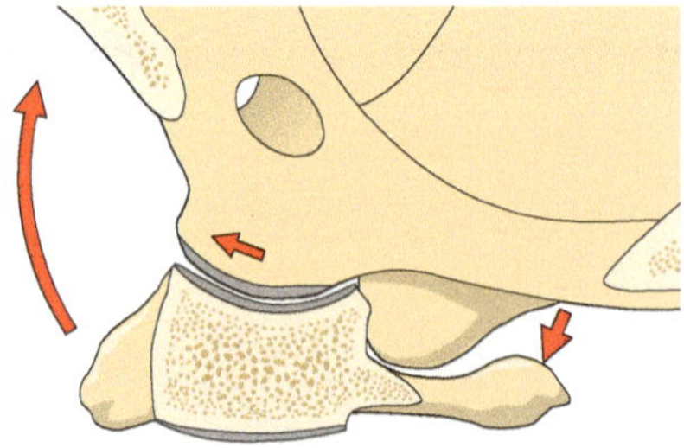

Extension of the atlanto-occipital joint.

Atlantoaxial joints

- The inferior articular facets of the atlas slide forward and upward
- The fossa of the dens moves upward, anteriorly approaching the dens and posteriorly moving away from it.

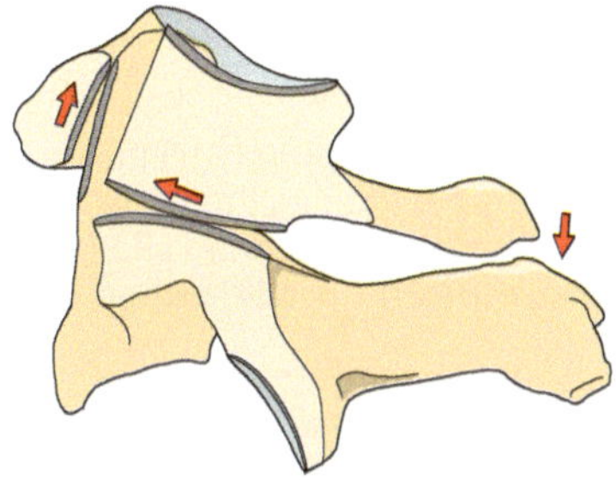

Extension of the atlantoaxial joints.

The amplitude of the flexion-extension of the upper cervical column is around 30° and is greater in flexion than extension.

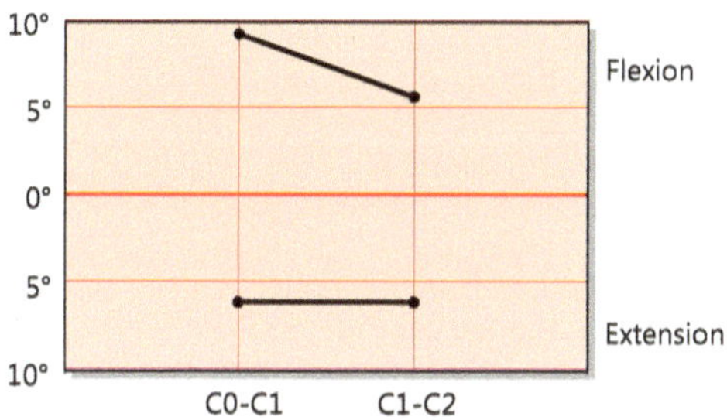

Diagram of the extent of flexion and extension movements between the occiput and C1 (C0-C1) and C1 and C2 (C1-C2).

Lateral inclination

Atlanto-occipital joint

Modest movements of the occipital condyles in the lateral and medial direction (not exceeding 3-5° in one direction or the other direction).

Atlantoaxial joints

The movements of the dens of the axis in lateral direction are so modest that cannot be measured and are accompanied by rotation.

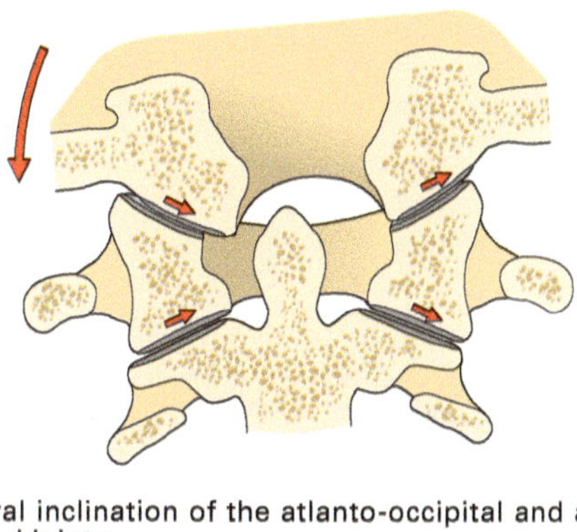

Lateral inclination of the atlanto-occipital and atlantoaxial joints.

Rotation

Atlanto-occipital joint

- The occipital bone rotates around the atlas with forward sliding of the contralateral condyle and backward sliding of the ipsilateral condyle upon rotation
- The contralateral alar ligament is tensed and exerts traction on the corresponding condyle by bringing it towards the dens of the axis causing a slight contralateral inclination
- The amplitude of movement is 5°.

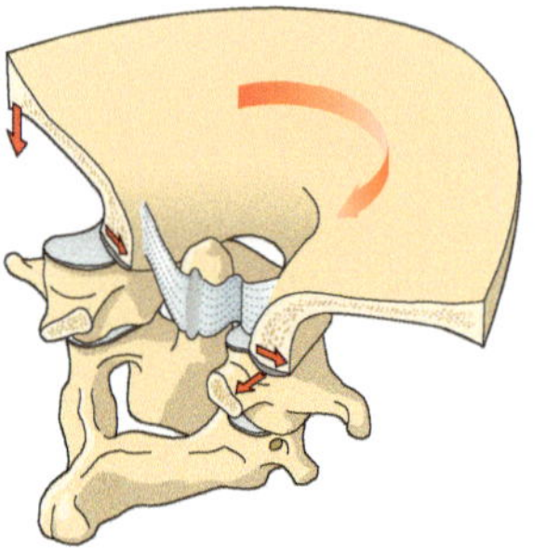

Rotation combined with lateral inclination of the atlanto-occipital joint.

Atlantoaxial joints

- The osteofibrous ring, formed by the transverse ligament of the atlas, in which the dens of the axis is enclosed, rotates around the dens
- The lateral mass of the atlas ipsilateral to the rotation moves posteriorly and in opposite direction (anteriorly) with respect to the contralateral
- Starting from 20° of rotation, there is a lowering of the atlas towards the axis caused by the convexity of the articular surfaces
- The amplitude of movement reaches 40°.

Real rotation is considered to occur with the mutually supporting occiput and atlas rotating around the dens of the axis.

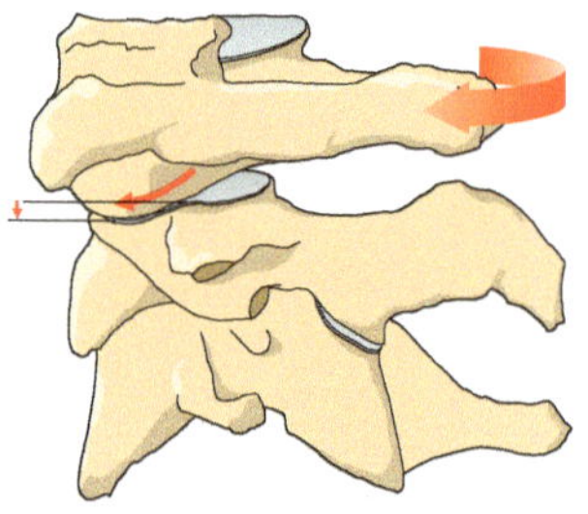

Rotation of the atlantoaxial joints.

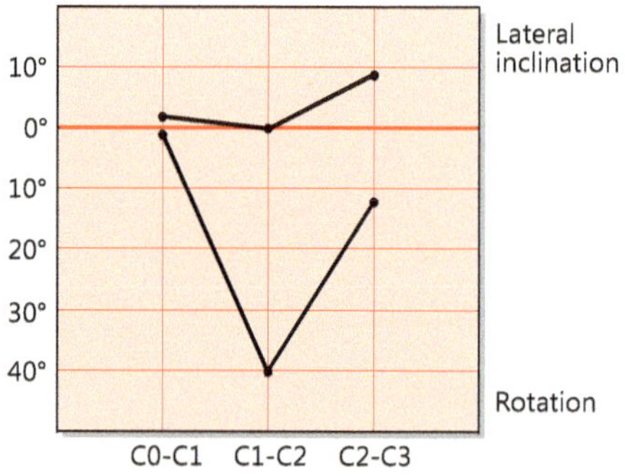

Diagram of the extent of lateral inclination and rotation movements between the occiput and C1 (C0-C1), C1 and C2 (C1-C2), C2 and C3 (C2-C3).

To evaluate the degree of rotation of the upper cervical column, the lower cervical column should be brought to maximum lateral inclination; to evaluate the degree of lateral inclination of the upper cervical column, the lower cervical column should be brought to maximum rotation.

Lower cervical column

3rd, 4th, 5th, 6th and 7th cervical vertebrae

Vertebral body

On both lateral borders, it is characterized by an upwardly directed projection, called the uncus of the body (or uncinate process), which articulates through a fissure with the latero-inferior border of the overlying vertebra (uncovertebral joint). This type of joint favors the mobility of the disc but impedes its protrusion, which could damage the spinal artery and nerve that pass close to the uncovertebral joint.

Transverse process

- Foramen transversarium (where the vertebral artery and vein pass)
- Anterior and posterior tubercles
- Groove for the spinal nerve.

Spinous process

Short, bifid and orientated downward, except for C7, which is long and often with a nearly horizontal course (vertebra prominens).

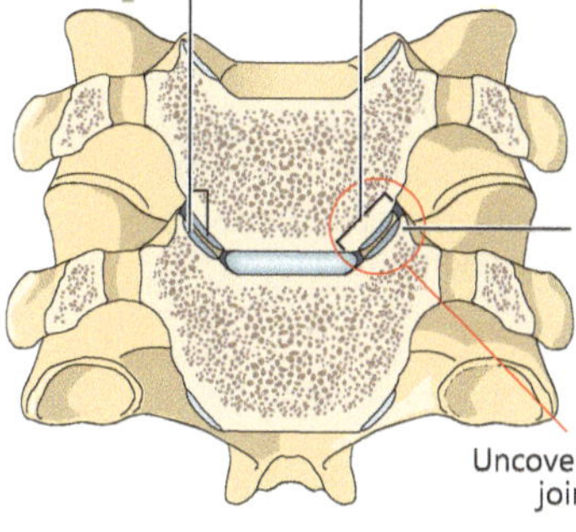

Cervical vertebra: frontal view.

Articular processes

Superior and inferior articular facets – circular shape and flat surface, with a 45° orientation in relation to the transverse plane (this angle is progressively reduced towards C7, reaching 10° at this level).

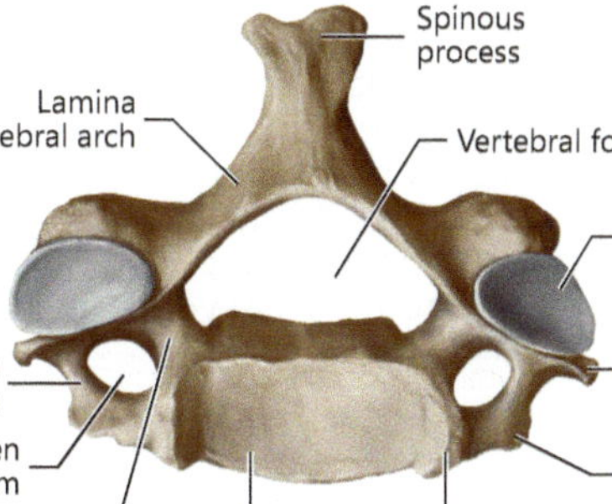

Cervical vertebra: view from above.

Ligaments of the lower cervical column

- Anterior longitudinal ligament
- Posterior longitudinal ligament
- Interspinous ligaments
- Intertransverse ligaments
- Supraspinous ligament
- Ligamenta flava.

(For their characteristics and functions, see Chapter 5 "Vertebral column and movements of the trunk").

Movements of the lower cervical column

Flexion

- The articular facets move away from each other and the articular space widens with the formation of an open angle posteriorly
- When the range of motion is maximum, there is a distance of only two fingers between the chin (with the mouth closed) and the sternum.

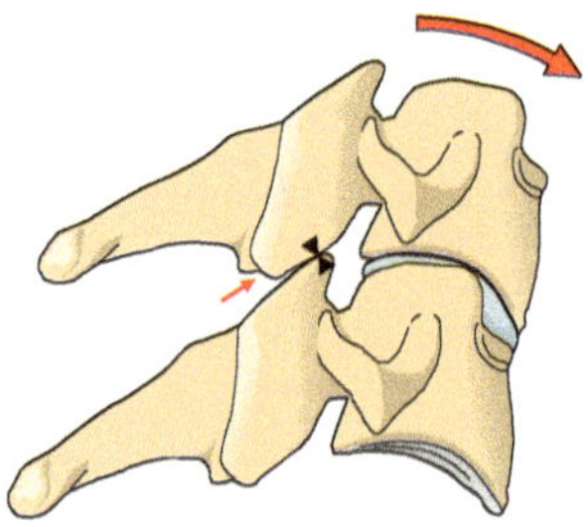

Flexion of the lower cervical column.

Extension

- The articular facets slide one over the other by moving upward and forward
- The anterior capsuloligamentous structures inhibit the movement, which is also impeded by the contact between the spinous processes and the posterior parts of the articular facets
- When the range of motion is maximum, the nasofrontal line is localized on a plane forming an angle of 30° in relation to the transverse plane.

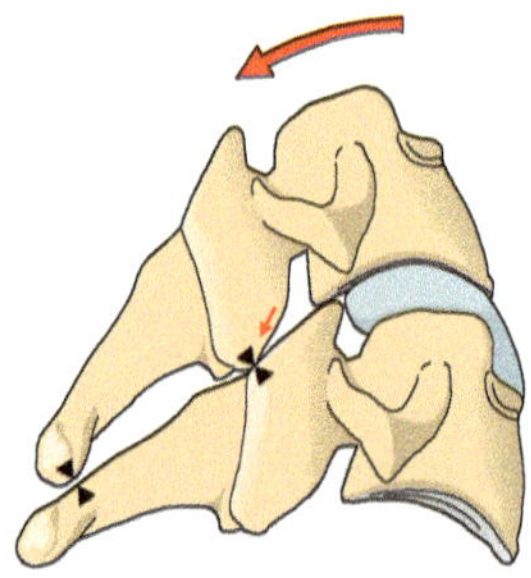

Extension of the lower cervical column.

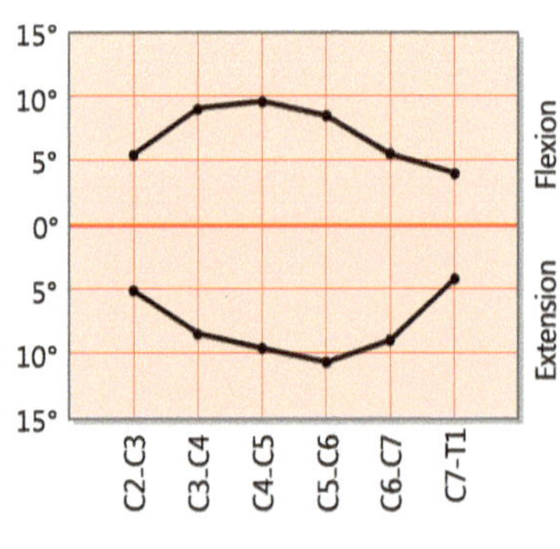

Diagram of the extent of flexion and extension movements between C2 and C3 (C2-C3), C3 and C4 (C3-C4), C4 and C5 (C4-C5), C5 and C6 (C5-C6), C6 and C7 (C6-C7), C7 and T1 (C7-T1).

Lateral inclination

- The movement is hindered by the orientation of the articular processes and by the presence of the semilunar processes, accompanied by an ipsilateral rotation whose amplitude varies from segment to segment (5° between C2 and C3 and even less between C7 and T1)
- The maximum amplitude of movement is 50°.

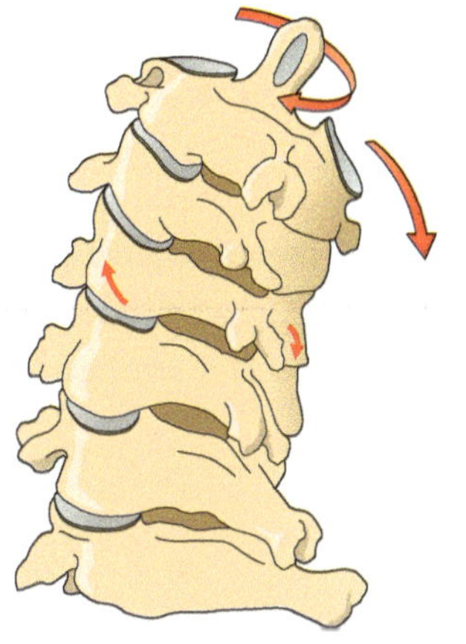

Combination of lateral inclination and consensual rotation movements of the lower cervical column.

Rotation

- The movement is accompanied by the ipsilateral inclination of the superior vertebra
- The orientation of the articular facets of the most cranial vertebra is such that an angle of 40-50° is formed between the vertical axis and the rotation axis, enabling a greater lateral inclination in relation to the more caudal vertebrae (between C7 and T1 the lateral inclination is only 10°)
- The amplitude of rotation is greater in flexion than in extension
- The maximum amplitude of movement is 40°.

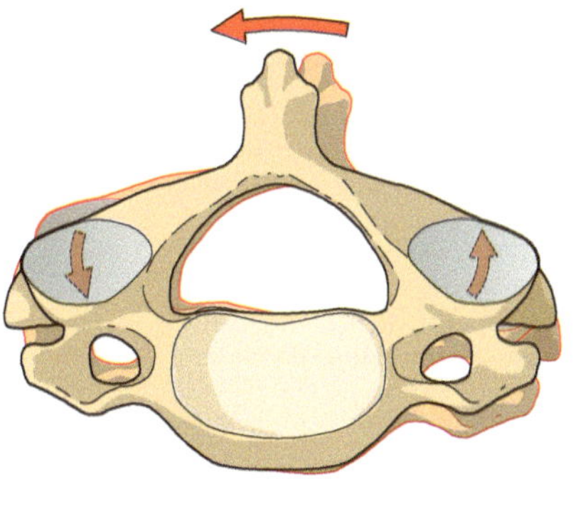

Rotation of the lower cervical column.

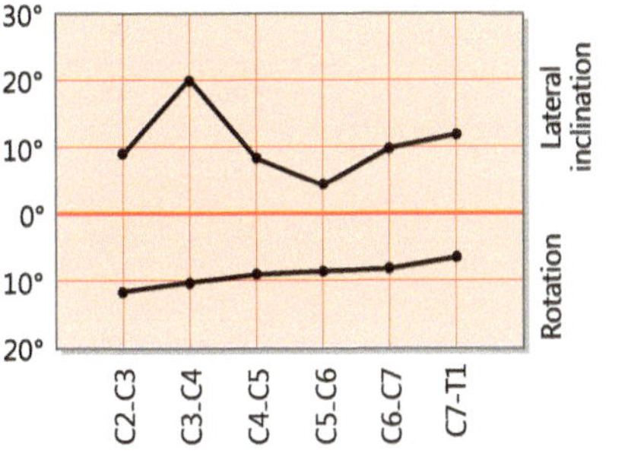

Diagram of the extent of lateral inclination and rotation movements between C2 and C3 (C2-C3), C3 and C4 (C3-C4), C4 and C5 (C4-C5), C5 and C6 (C5-C6), C6 and C7 (C6-C7), C7 and T1 (C7-T1).

Radiology of the cervical column

Anteroposterior projection

- The dens and the spinous process of the axis are arranged on the median line
- The occipital condyles and the lateral masses of the atlas are parallel and symmetrical
- The transverse processes of the atlas have the same length and are at equal distance from the occipital bone
- The line that passes through the inferior boundaries of the occipital condyles (intercondylar line) is parallel to the line that passes through the inferior borders of the lateral masses of the atlas (line of the atlas)
- The distance between the atlas and axis is 3 mm
- The inferior and superior limitings of the vertebral bodies are parallel
- The spinous processes are aligned along the central axis
- The pedicles of the vertebral arches are aligned and arranged symmetrically at an equal distance from the midline
- The distance between the pedicles is 24-33 mm.

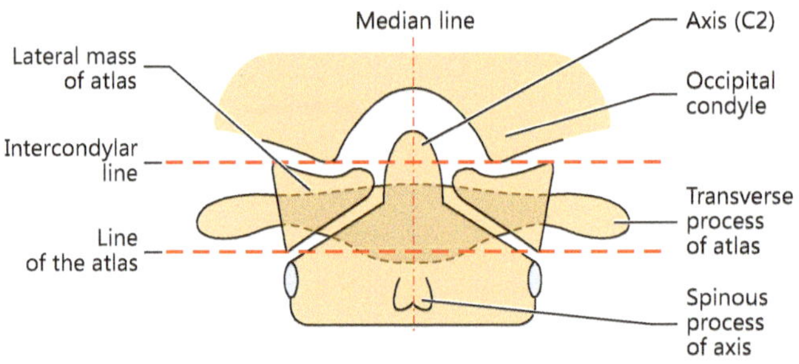

Anteroposterior projection of the upper cervical column.

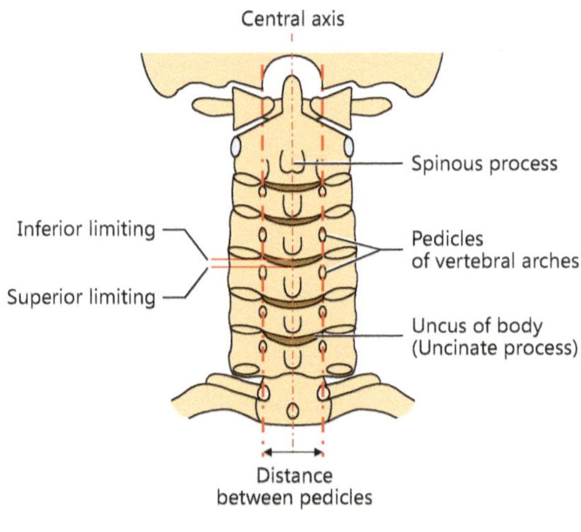

Anteroposterior projection of the lower cervical column.

Lateral projection

- The anterior limiting of the vertebral bodies, the posterior limiting of the vertebral bodies and the line that passes through the vertebral arches form parallel arches
- The distance between the latter two lines is 15-20 mm
- The horizontal line that passes through the atlas and the line between the inferior border of the vertebral arch and the spinous process of the axis are parallel.

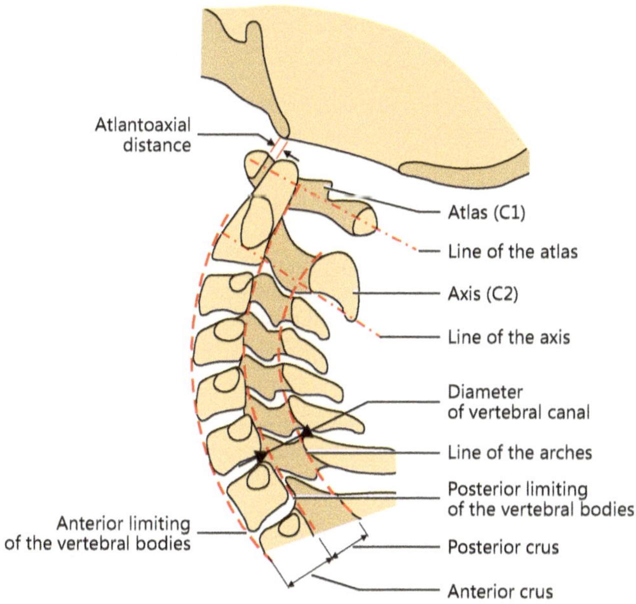

Lateral projection of the cervical column.

Assessment of neck joint mobility

It is possible to obtain a linear measurement of cervical column movements. The test is performed in a seated position, with the trunk supported by the back of the seat and the head and neck in the anatomical position.

Flexion of the neck

- The neck should be flexed to the limit of movement allowed
- The distance between the tip of the chin and the jugular (suprasternal) notch is measured
- Under normal conditions, it should be possible to touch the thorax with the chin.

Extension of the neck

- The same landmarks used to measure the flexion of the neck are utilized
- One measurement is taken in the anatomical position, the other in the extension position
- The difference between these two measurements indicates the amplitude of the extension of the neck.

Lateral inclination of the neck

- The neck should be tilted laterally (without rotating it) to the limit of movement allowed
- The distance between the mastoid process and the acromion is measured
- One measurement is taken in the anatomical position, the other at the limit of lateral inclination.

Rotation of the neck

- Rotation of the head (without flexing or extending it) to the limit of movement allowed
- The distance between the tip of the chin and the acromion is measured
- One measurement is taken in the anatomical position, the other at the limit of rotation.

The examination of the head and neck movements is contraindicated in some circumstances, for example, in the case vertebral artery disease. This artery passes through the foramina transversaria of the cervical vertebrae and, after exiting the foramen transversarium of the atlas, it proceeds along the sulcus on the posterior surface of the lateral mass of the atlas. Some movements of the neck reduce the lumen of the artery, decreasing the bloody supply, but the appearance of disorders only occurs in the case of alterations in the elasticity of the vessel.

> The lower cervical column is functionally connected to the upper thoracic column. From a functional perspective, the movements of the cervical column terminate at T5.

> Reduced mobility of one or more functional spinal units (FSU) can cause excessive mobility of nearby FSU, at which level inclination or sliding may occur.

Variation in blood supply from the vertebral artery during movements of the neck

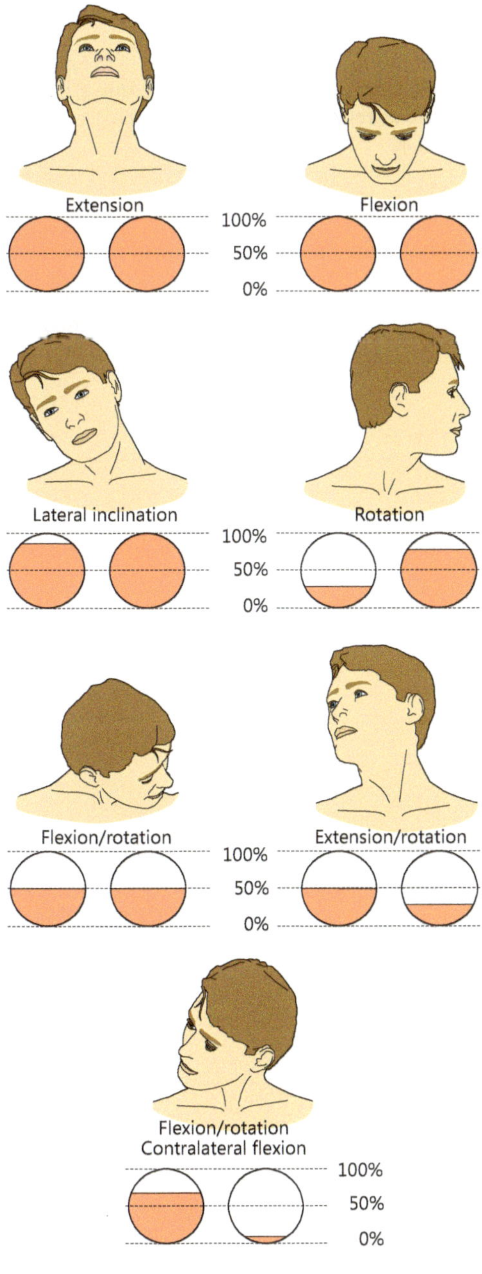

Functional applications of neck mobility

- Neck mobility is necessary for the function of the sense organs located in the head and for expression of non-verbal communication, such as indicating agreement or disagreement
- The flexion, extension, lateral inclination and rotation of the neck are particularly important because they allow the interaction with the environment through the sense of sight
- The importance of the close relationship between vision and neck movements is clear from various daily activities
- In case of reduced eye mobility, a greater range of motion of the cervical column is required, or the position of the head during sight accommodation may be affected by the reduction in the visual field
- For most activities of daily living, a complete range of motion along all planes is not required
- Close to maximum mobility may be necessary for certain activities, such as looking over one's shoulder when driving a car (which involves lateral inclination and rotation), painting a ceiling in a room, placing an object on a high shelf, looking at the stars (which involves extension).

Muscles of the neck

The muscles of the head and neck help to maintain the head's posture, the position of the head for sight accommodation and nutrition. It also contributes to the movements of breathing and coughing.

Extensor muscles of the head and neck

- Muscles with extensor capacity:
  - descending part of the trapezius
  - sternocleidomastoid
  - levator scapulae
- Extensor muscles proper:
  - rectus capitis posterior minor
  - rectus capitis posterior major
  - splenius cervicis
  - splenius capitis
  - obliquus capitis superior
  - obliquus capitis inferior
- Common extensor muscles:
  - iliocostalis cervicis
  - longissimus capitis
  - longissimus cervicis
  - spinalis capitis
  - spinalis cervicis
  - semispinalis capitis
  - semispinalis cervicis
  - cervical intertransversarii
  - interspinales cervicis
  - transversospinales of the neck:
    - rotatores
    - multifidus
    - semispinalis capitis
    - semispinalis cervicis.

(For the action, origin, insertion and innervation of the common extensor muscles of the head and neck, see Chapter 5 "Vertebral column and movements of the trunk").

(For the action, origin, insertion and innervations of the levator scapulae, see Chapter 7 "Shoulder and pectoral girdle").

4

Extensor muscles of the head and neck

Muscle	Action	Origin	Insertion	Innervation
Descending part of trapezius	Extension of the head and neck	Medial third of the superior nuchal line; external occipital protuberance; ligamentum nuchae	Posterior border of the lateral third of the clavicle	Spinal root of the accessory nerve [XI] and branches of the cervical plexus [C3, C4]
Splenius capitis	Extension of the neck; ipsilateral rotation of the neck	Inferior half of the ligamentum nuchae; spinous processes of C7 and T1 to T4 and corresponding supraspinous ligaments	Mastoid process of the temporal bone; occipital bone below the lateral third of the superior nuchal line	Posterior rami of the cervical nerves [C2-C4]
Splenius cervicis	Extension of the neck; ipsilateral rotation of the neck	Spinous processes from T3 to T6	Posterior tubercles of the transverse processes of the three superior cervical vertebrae	Posterior rami of the cervical nerves [C2-C4]
Rectus capitis posterior major	Extension of the head; ipsilateral rotation of the head	Spinous process of the axis	Lateral part of the inferior nuchal line and immediately underlying osseous area	Posterior rami of the first cervical nerve [C1]
Rectus capitis posterior minor	Extension of the head	Posterior tubercle of the atlas	Medial part of the inferior nuchal line and osseous area between this and the foramen magnum	Posterior rami of the first cervical nerve [C1]
Obliquus capitis inferior	Ipsilateral rotation of the head	Lateral surface of the spinous process and adjacent superior surface of the lamina of the axis	Inferior and posterior surfaces of the transverse process of the atlas	Posterior rami of the first cervical nerve [C1]
Obliquus capitis superior	Extension and ipsilateral inclination of the head	Superior surface of the transverse process of the atlas	Occipital bone between the superior and inferior nuchal lines, laterally to the semispinalis capitis	Posterior rami of the first cervical nerve [C1]
Sternocleido-mastoid	Extension of the neck; flexion of the neck; contralateral rotation of the neck; ipsilateral inclination of the neck	*Sternal head*: superior surface of the manubrium of the sternum *Clavicular head*: superior surface of the medial third of the clavicle	Lateral surface of the mastoid process; lateral half of the superior nuchal line	Spinal root of the accessory nerve [XI] and branches of the cervical plexus (C2, C3 and sometimes C4)

Functional aspects of the extensor muscles of the head and neck

Muscles with extensor capacity

- The trapezius is an extensor and contracts bilaterally through the superior and middle fascicles (descending and transverse parts), maintaining as a fixed point its insertion on the clavicle and on the spine of the scapula
- The sternocleidomastoid extends the head; it contracts bilaterally when the insertion at the mastoid level is located posteriorly to the origin on the clavicle and on the sternum, rather than anteriorly to it
- The levator scapulae muscle extends the neck and contracts bilaterally with fixed point on the scapula; during unilateral contraction, with fixed point on the scapula, it tilts and rotates the neck ipsilaterally.

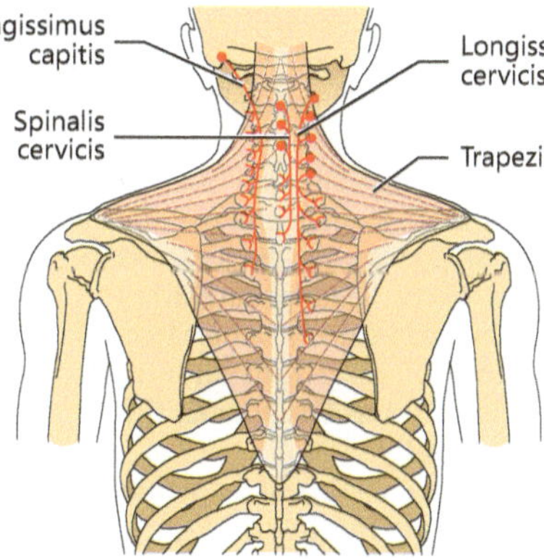

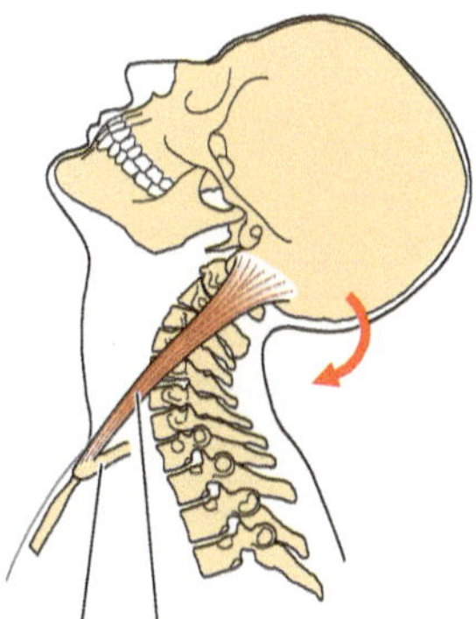

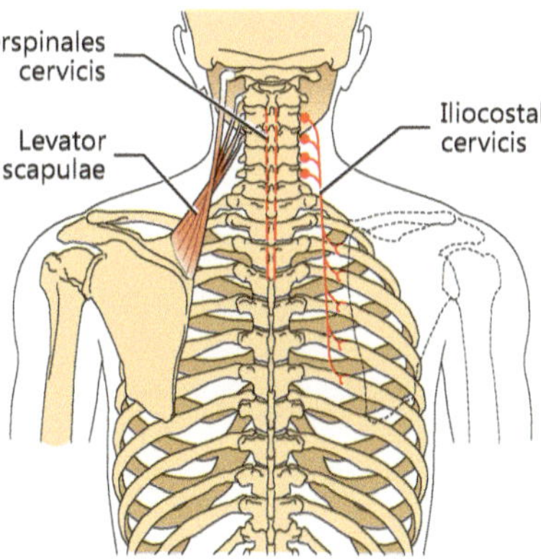

Extensor muscles proper of the head and neck

- They are only found in this region
- The rectus capitis posterior minor, rectus capitis posterior major, obliquus capitis inferior and obliquus capitis superior extend the head by bilateral contraction
- The unilateral contraction of these muscles tilts the head laterally
- The rectus capitis posterior major and rectus capitis posterior minor (which replace the interspinales between the occiput and the atlas and the atlas and the axis), and the obliquus capitis inferior rotate the head ipsilaterally
- The obliquus capitis superior (which replaces the intertransverse muscle between C2 and C1) rotates the head contralaterally
- The splenius capitis and splenius cervicis extend the head and neck by contracting bilaterally, whereas their unilateral contraction rotates the head and neck ipsilaterally.

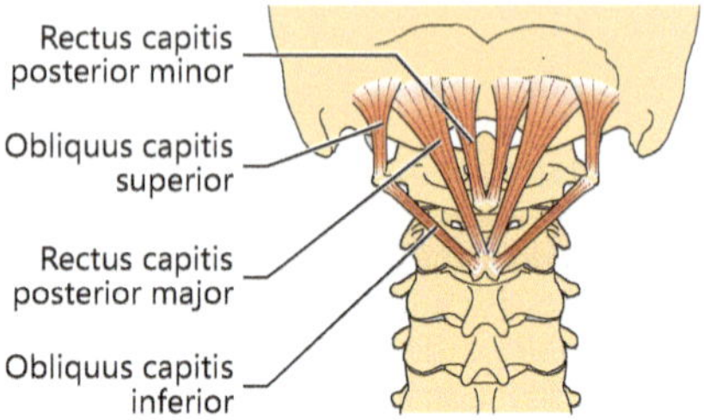

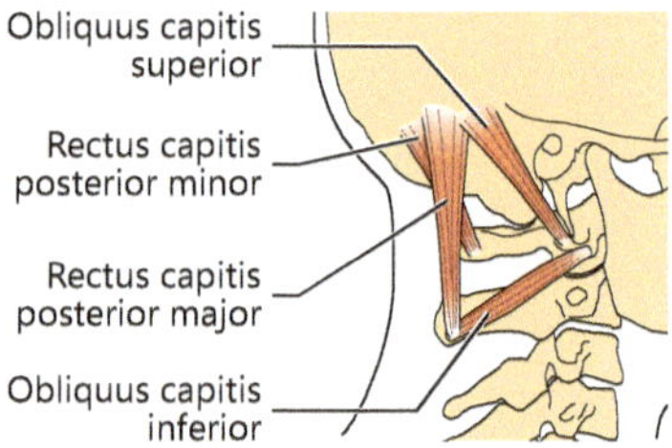

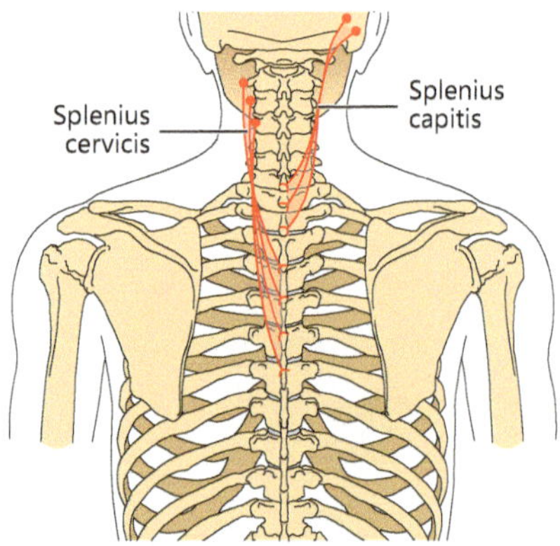

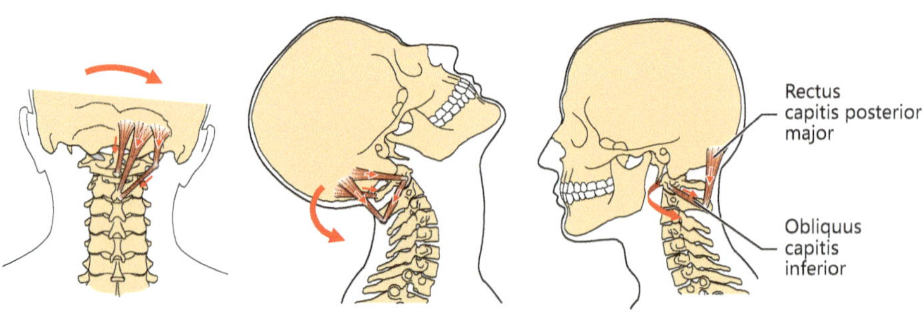

Common extensor muscles of the head and neck

- They are also found throughout the vertebral column
- They are extensors when contracted bilaterally
- Their unilateral contraction contributes to the lateral inclination of the head and neck, except for the transversospinal complex of the neck and the longissimus capitis (the former rotates the head and neck contralaterally, while the latter rotates the head and neck ipsilaterally).

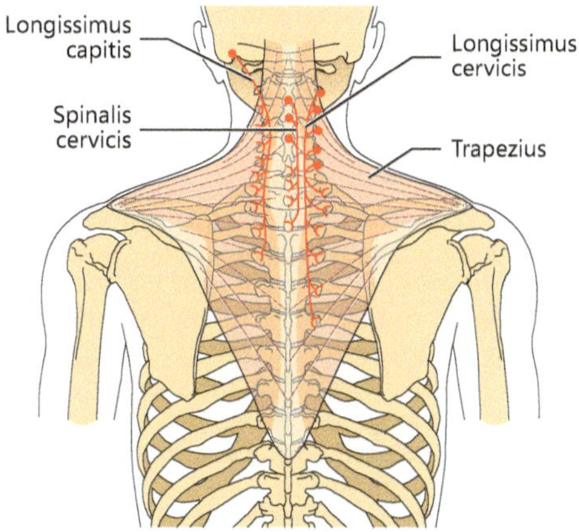

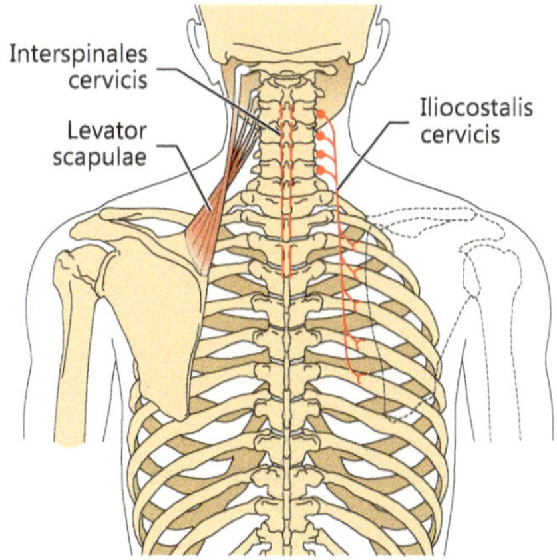

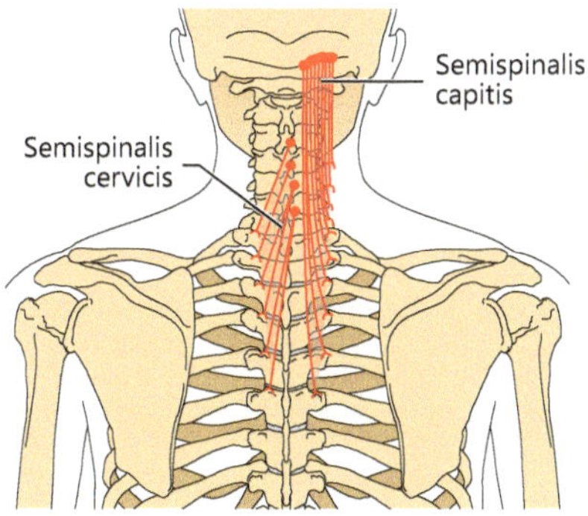

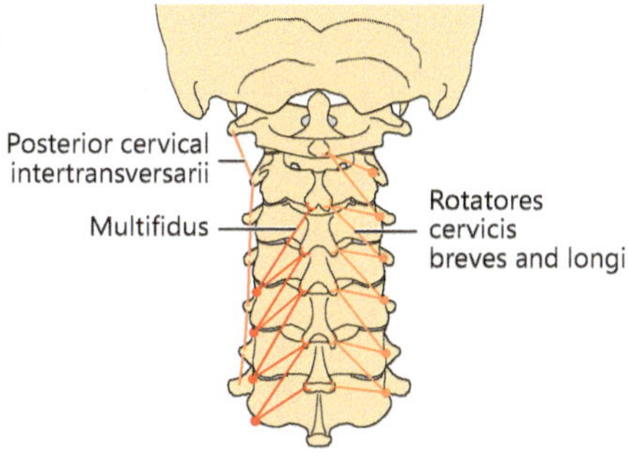

4

Functional applications of the extensor muscles of the head and neck

- Their bilateral contraction causes the extension of the neck by eliminating the actions of lateral inclination and rotation which occur in unilateral contraction
- They contract in cases of forced extension once the joint excursion movement is completed or when the extension is executed against resistance
  - the actions performed with the upper limbs above the head require contraction of these muscles due to the amplitude of the joint movement, as happens, for example, when taking a book from a high shelf
  - other activities that require contraction of these muscles due to the amplitude of joint excursion are, for example, drinking from a glass or looking down a bowling lane when throwing the ball with the hand
- They contract and work against resistance when the head is lifted from a support surface in the prone position and control the flexion of the neck when the head is lowered back to the support surface
- They contract during activities in which the head is inclined forward, such as reading and writing
- The activity of these muscles ceases when the neck is completely flexed and when the position of the head is maintained by the tension of the ligamentum nuchae.

Flexor muscles of the head and neck

- Suprahyoid muscles:
  - digastric
  - stylohyoid
  - mylohyoid
  - geniohyoid
- Infrahyoid muscles:
  - sternohyoid
  - sternothyroid
  - thyrohyoid
  - omohyoid
- Prevertebral muscles:
  - longus capitis
  - longus colli (longus cervicis)
  - rectus capitis anterior
  - rectus capitis lateralis
- Scalene muscles (anterior, middle and posterior)
- Sternocleidomastoid.

Flexor muscles of the head and neck

Muscle	Action	Origin	Insertion	Innervation
Suprahyoid muscles				
Digastric	Depression of the mandible; elevation of the hyoid bone (deglutition, mastication)	*Posterior belly*: mastoid process of the temporal bone *Anterior belly*: digastric fossa on the base of the mandible close to the midline	The direction of the muscle changes after it passes through a fibrous ring fixed to the hyoid bone	Facial nerve [VII] (posterior belly) and mylohyoid nerve (anterior belly)
Stylohyoid	Elevation and retrusion of the hyoid bone (deglutition)	Posterior surface of the styloid process of the temporal bone	Junction between the body and the greater horn of the hyoid bone	Facial nerve [VII]
Mylohyoid	Elevation of the floor of the mouth (deglutition); elevation of the hyoid bone; depression of the mandible	Mylohyoid line of the mandible	Body of the hyoid bone; medial fibrous raphe of the mandibular symphysis to the hyoid bone	Mylohyoid nerve (branch of the mandibular nerve, V_3 or Vc)
Geniohyoid	Elevation and protrusion of the hyoid bone; depression of the mandible	Inferior mental spine on the posterior surface of the mandibular symphysis	Anterior surface of the body of the hyoid bone	First cervical nerve [C1] through the hypoglossal nerve [XII]
Infrahyoid muscles				
Sternohyoid	Depression of the hyoid bone	Posterior surface of the medial end of the clavicle; posterior sternoclavicular ligament; superior and posterior surface of the manubrium of the sternum	Inferior surface of the body of the hyoid bone	Ansa cervicalis (branches of C1, C2 and C3)

(continued)

4

Flexor muscles of the head and neck (*continued*)

Muscle	Action	Origin	Insertion	Innervation
Sterno-thyroid	Depression of the larynx	Posterior surface of the manubrium of the sternum below the origin of the sternohyoid and border of the first costal cartilage	Oblique line on the lamina of the thyroid cartilage	Ansa cervicalis (branches of C1, C2 and C3)
Thyrohyoid	Depression of the hyoid bone; elevation of the larynx	Oblique line on the lamina of the thyroid cartilage	Inferior border of the greater horn and the adjacent part of the body of the hyoid bone	Thyrohyoid branch of the first cervical nerve [C1] that branches off through the hypoglossal nerve [XII]
Omohyoid	Depression of the hyoid bone	Superior border of the scapula adjacent to the scapular notch; superior transverse scapular ligament	A band of the deep cervical fascia holds the intermediate portion of the muscle inferiorly, in the direction of the clavicle and the first rib, changing direction at this level; inferior border of the body of the hyoid bone	Ansa cervicalis (branch of C1, superior root, for the superior belly; branches of C1, C2 and C3, for the inferior belly)
Prevertebral muscles				
Longus capitis	Flexion of the head	Anterior tubercles of the transverse processes from C3 to C6	Inferior surface of the basilar part of the occipital bone	Anterior rami of the cervical nerves [C1-C3]
Longus colli (Longus cervicis)	Flexion of the neck; contralateral rotation of the neck (inferior oblique fibers); lateral inclination of the neck (oblique fibers)	*Inferior (oblique) lateral part*: anterior surface of the vertebral bodies from T1 to T3 *Superior (oblique) lateral part*: anterior tubercles of the transverse processes from C3 to C5 *(Vertical) medial part*: anterior surface of the vertebral bodies from T1 to T3 and from C5 to C7	*Inferior (oblique) lateral part*: anterior tubercles of the transverse processes of C5 and C6 *Superior (oblique) lateral part:* anterolateral surface of the anterior tubercle of the atlas *(Vertical) medial part*: anterior surface of the vertebral bodies from C2 to C4	Anterior rami of the cervical nerves [C2-C6]

(*continued*)

Flexor muscles of the head and neck (*continued*)

Muscle	Action	Origin	Insertion	Innervation
Rectus capitis anterior	Flexion of the head	Anterior surface of the lateral mass of the atlas; root of the transverse process of the atlas	Inferior surface of the basilar part of the occipital bone, anterior to the occipital condyle	Anterior rami of the cervical nerves [C1, C2]
Rectus capitis lateralis	Ipsilateral inclination of the head	Superior surface of the transverse process of the atlas	Inferior surface of the jugular process of the occipital bone	Anterior rami of the cervical nerves [C1, C2]
Scalene muscles				
Scalenus anterior	Flexion of the neck and its ipsilateral inclination; contralateral rotation of the neck	Anterior tubercles of the transverse processes from C3 to C6	Tubercle of the scalene muscle on the internal border of the 1st rib and ridge on the superior surface of the rib anterior to the groove for the subclavian artery	Anterior rami of the cervical nerves [C4-C6]
Scalenus medius	Ipsilateral inclination of the neck	Transverse process of the axis; anterior surface of the posterior tubercles of the transverse processes from C3 to C7	Superior surface of the 1st rib between the costal tubercle and the groove for the subclavian artery	Anterior rami of the cervical nerves [C3-C8]
Scalenus posterior	Ipsilateral inclination of the neck	Posterior tubercles of the transverse processes from C4 to C6	Lateral surface of the 2nd rib	Anterior rami of the cervical nerves [C6-C8]
Sterno-cleido-mastoid	Extension of the neck; flexion of the neck; contralateral rotation of the neck; ipsilateral inclination of the neck	*Sternal head*: superior surface of the manubrium of the sternum *Clavicular head*: superior surface of the medial third of the clavicle	Lateral surface of the mastoid process; lateral half of the superior nuchal line	Spinal root of the accessory nerve [XI] and branches of the cervical plexus (C2, C3 and sometimes C4)

Functional aspects of the flexor muscles of the head and neck

- Flexion of the head and neck requires less muscular strength than extension due to the tendency of the head to fall forward
- The suprahyoid muscles flex the head and neck with a fixed point (origin) on the hyoid bone and insertion on the mandible and other bones of the cranium
- The infrahyoid muscles flex the head and neck with a fixed point (origin) on the bones and cartilages of the neck and trunk, and insertions on the hyoid bone
- Flexion of the head and neck by the suprahyoid and infrahyoid muscles is only possible with the mouth closed (thanks to the action of the masticatory muscles which act as fixator muscles)
- The prevertebral muscles (longus capitis, longus colli, rectus capitis anterior, rectus capitis lateralis) flex the head and neck by contracting bilaterally; when they contract unilaterally, all four muscles tilt the neck ipsilaterally; additionally, the longus capitis and rectus capitis anterior rotate the head contralaterally and ipsilaterally, respectively
- The scalene muscles are primarily inspiratory muscles; by contracting bilaterally and acting synergistically they flex the head; when they instead contract unilaterally, they tilt the head laterally
- The sternocleidomastoid is a secondary inspiratory muscle; the rectus capitis anterior and rectus capitis lateralis contract and bring the mastoid insertion of the muscle anteriorly to the clavicular and sternal origin, thus allowing for them to have a flexor action on the head and neck.

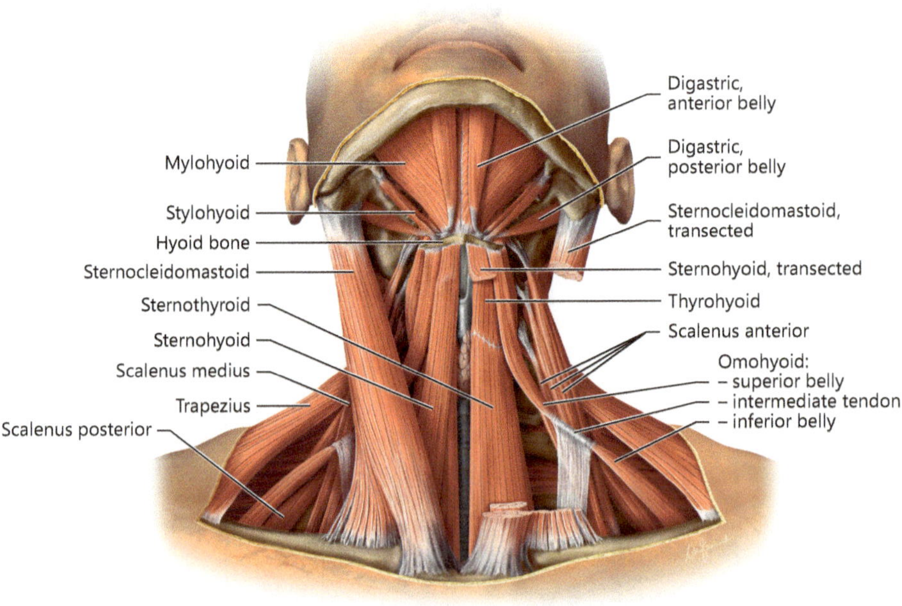

View of the anterior muscles of the neck. The left sternocleidomastoid and sternohyoid have been transected and removed.

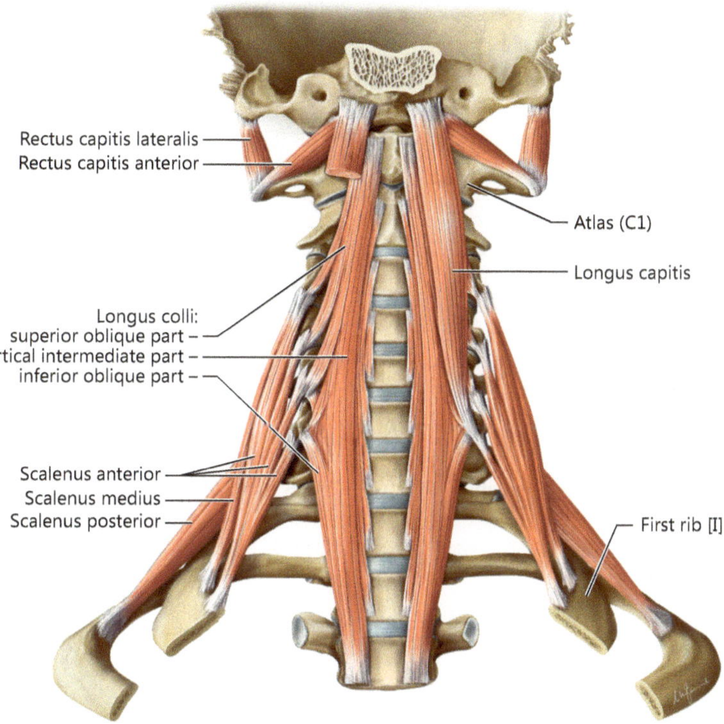

Preparation of the prevertebral muscles viewed from the front. These are long muscles that are adjacent to the ventrolateral surface of the vertebral column, covered by the deep cervical fascia; the anterior, middle and posterior scalene muscles are at the side of the prevertebral muscles. The prevertebral muscles extend between the cranial base and the cervical column, while the scalene muscles extend from the vertebral column to the upper part of the thorax.

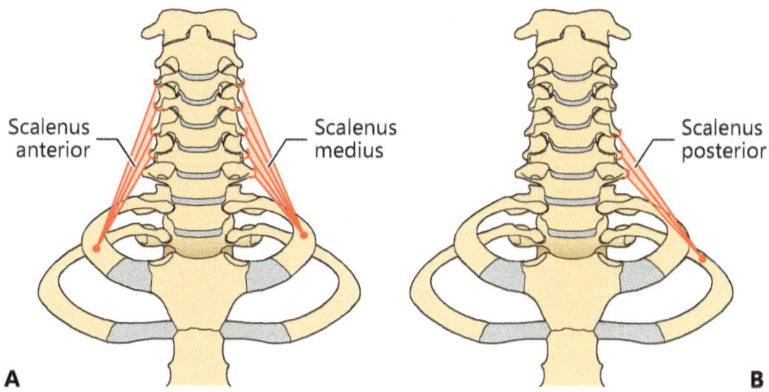

Scalene muscles. **A**, Scalenus anterior, scalenus medius; **B**, scalenus posterior.

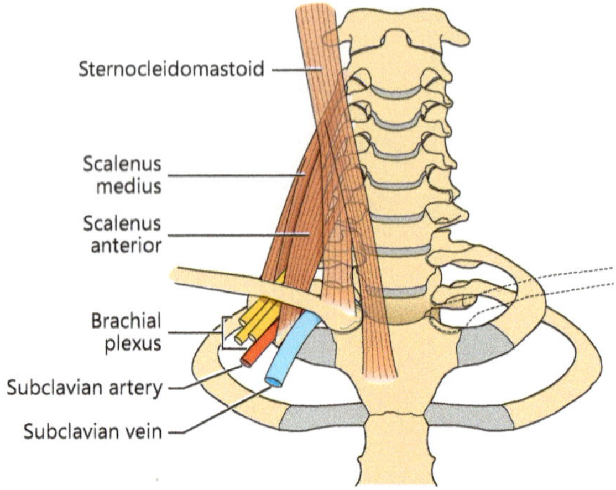

Interscalene triangle.

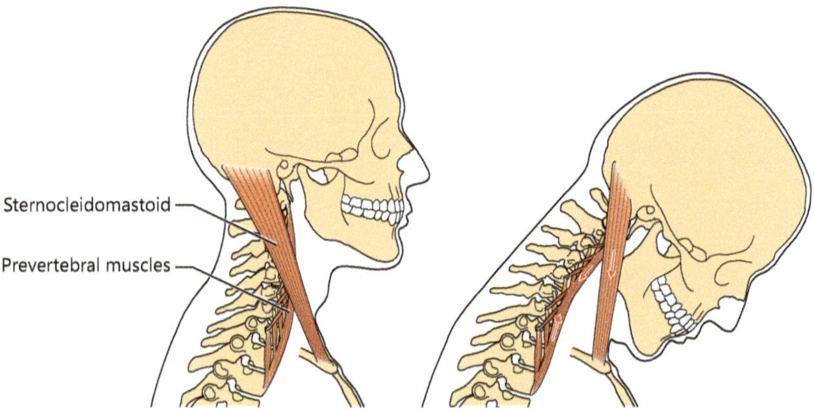

Action of the sternocleidomastoid. Anterior stabilization.

Functional applications of the flexor muscles of the head and neck

- They contract when the movement occurs against resistance, which can be represented by the weight of the head itself
- They flex the head and neck and maintain this position when the head is raised from a supporting surface in a supine position, such as, for example, when getting up from a bed

- They control the extension of the neck when the head lowers back towards the supporting surface, as occurs when you stretch out in a supine position
- In the upright position the flexor muscles of the head and neck contract only with complete, forced flexion
  - this combined action of the flexor muscles occurs, for example, when, looking down, you loosen or fasten the first button of your shirt, or when you fasten a necklace around your neck
- When you eat, the bilateral contraction of the sternocleidomastoid muscles brings the head forward and helps the longus colli to flex the cervical column
- Electromyographic studies have shown a moderate bilateral activity of the longus colli and sternocleidomastoid in maintaining the head's forward position.

Hyoid bone

It is located just below the mandible and has the following characteristics:
- body with four appendices – greater and lesser horns
- the suprahyoid and infrahyoid muscles attach there.

The suprahyoid and infrahyoid muscles may be considered as a muscular sling with the hyoid bone as its pivot. Deglutition, mastication and speech are the main functions of the suprahyoid and infrahyoid muscles, which are accomplished by acting on the hyoid bone, the mandible and the thyroid cartilage. These muscles can also flex the cervical column when the masseter and temporalis contract to close the mandible, thus ensuring a correct closure of the mouth while the masticatory muscles stabilize the temporomandibular joint.

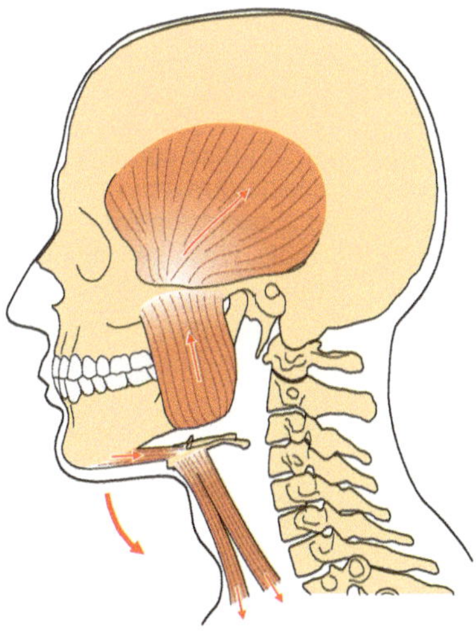

Flexion of the cervical column caused by the suprahyoid and infrahyoid muscles during the closure of the mouth.

Lateral inclination of the head and neck

It is produced by the unilateral contraction of the muscles:
- levator scapulae (with a fixed point on the scapula)
- rectus capitis posterior minor
- rectus capitis posterior major
- obliquus capitis superior
- obliquus capitis inferior
- iliocostalis cervicis
- longissimus cervicis
- spinalis capitis
- spinalis cervicis
- semispinalis capitis
- semispinalis cervicis
- intertransversarii cervicis
- interspinales cervicis
- longus capitis
- longus colli (longus cervicis)
- rectus capitis anterior
- rectus capitis lateralis
- scalene muscles.

Functional applications

- The unilateral contraction of the extensor muscles and many flexor muscles of the head and neck tilt the head and neck laterally to the same side
- From a functional perspective, these muscles contract ipsilaterally to:
  - tilt the cervical column laterally
  - position and control the inclination of the head so as to allow a proper view of objects placed on different planes
  - regulate the position of the head and facilitate corporal realignment in the upright position starting from a decubitus or upside-down position
  - maintain the position of the head in the transition from the lateral decubitus position to the seated position, such as, for example, when getting out of bed.

Rotation of the head and neck

Ipsilateral rotation

It is produced by the unilateral contraction of the muscles:

- rectus capitis posterior minor
- rectus capitis posterior major
- obliquus capitis inferior
- splenius capitis
- splenius cervicis
- longissimus capitis
- levator scapulae
- rectus capitis lateralis.

The most powerful ipsilateral rotator muscles are the splenius capitis and splenius cervicis.

Contralateral rotation

It is produced by the unilateral contraction of the muscles:

- obliquus capitis superior
- semispinalis cervicis
- semispinalis capitis
- multifidus cervicis
- rotatores cervicis
- descending part of the trapezius
- sternocleidomastoid
- longus capitis.

The most powerful contralateral rotator muscle is the sternocleidomastoid.

Functional applications

- The primary function of the rotator muscles of the head and neck consists of rotating the head and neck to look from one side to the other, for example, when you look over your shoulder when backing up your car or when you hit the ball after having followed its trajectory while playing tennis
- In the rolling motion from the supine position to the lateral decubitus or prone position, the movement of the trunk may begin with the rotation of the head and neck in the desired direction
- The rotator muscles of the head and neck contract when you express refusal with your head
- Even activities such as combing hair, which require hand movement behind the head, can produce a rotation of the cervical column and head.

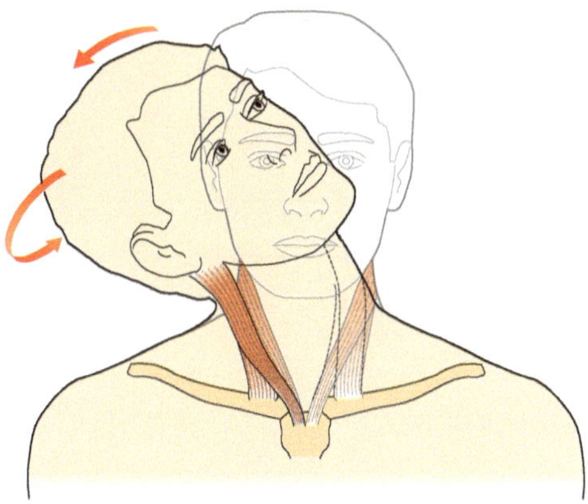

Action of the sternocleidomastoid: ipsilateral inclination, contralateral rotation.

Assessment of head and neck muscle strength

Extensor muscles of the head and neck

Muscles	Rectus capitis posterior (major and minor), obliquus capitis (inferior and superior), splenius capitis, splenius cervicis, semispinalis capitis, semispinalis cervicis, longissimus capitis, longissimus cervicis, spinalis capitis, spinalis cervicis, iliocostalis cervicis
Movement	Extension and rotation (and lateral flexion) of the head from the prone position
Palpation	In the paravertebral region 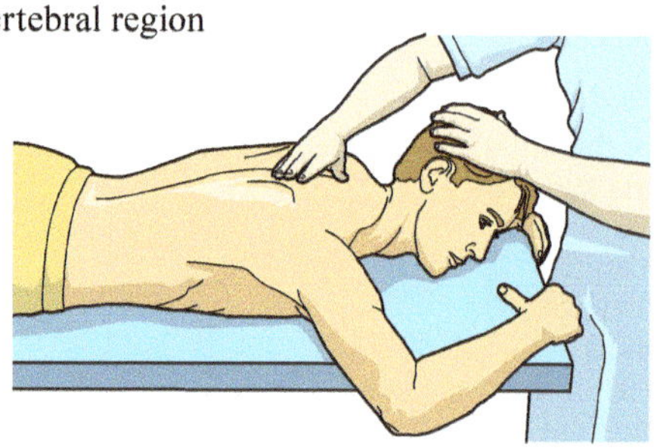
Resistance to movement	It is applied to the head in front of the occipital bone
Note: these muscles are examined in an antigravity position.	

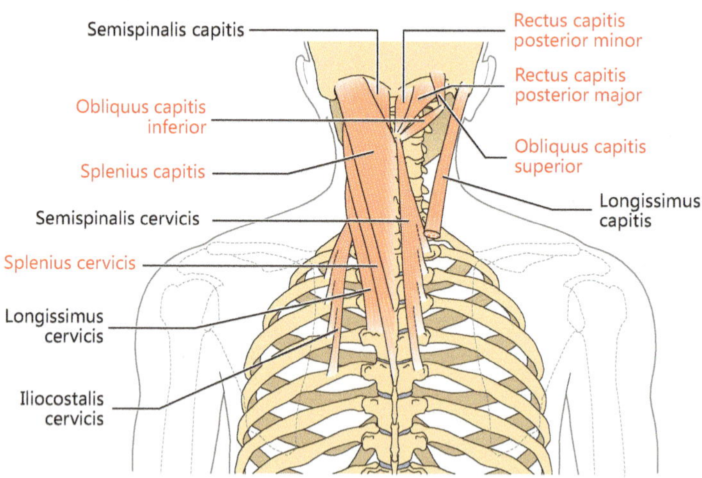

Main extensor muscles of the head and neck: the extensor muscles proper of the head and neck are shown in red.

Flexor muscles of the head and neck

Muscles	Rectus capitis anterior, longus capitis, longus colli, scalenus anterior, sternocleidomastoid (accessory muscles: scalenus medius, scalenus posterior, suprahyoid muscles, infrahyoid muscles and rectus capitis lateralis)
Movement	Flexion of the head and neck only in part (degree 2) or for the entire range of motion (degree 3) from the supine position, with the chin down and the arms extended backwards 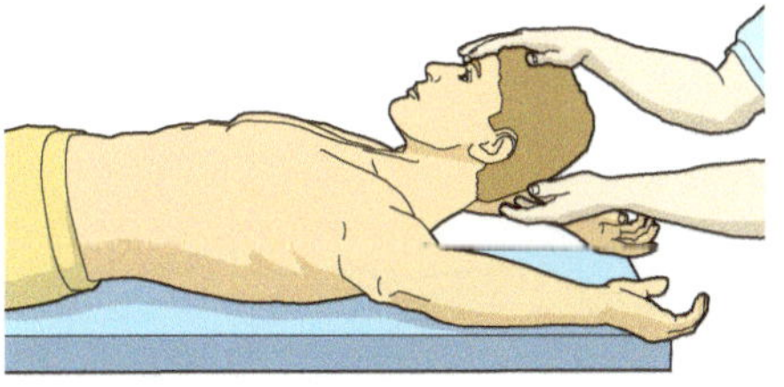
Palpation	The longus capitis, longus colli and rectus capitis anterior are too deep to be palpated; the sternocleidomastoid can be palpated proximal to the clavicle or sternum and more easily during the isolated examination of the muscle with head rotation; the scalenus anterior can be palpated above the clavicle and behind the sternocleidomastoid
Resistance to movement	It is applied to the forehead

Note: these muscles are examined in an antigravity position (first all muscles and then only the sternocleidomastoid).

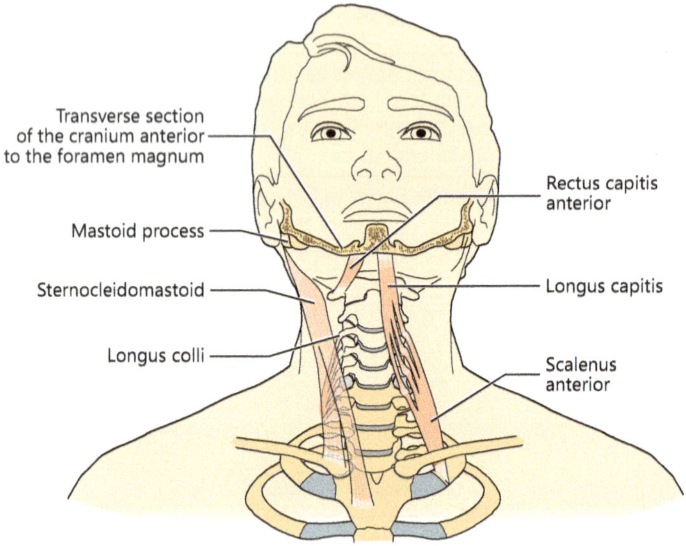

Main flexor muscles of the head and neck.

Sternocleidomastoid (anterolateral flexion of the neck)

Muscle	Sternocleidomastoid
Movement	Anterolateral flexion of the neck with ipsilateral inclination and contralateral rotation from the supine position; the muscles are evaluated separately 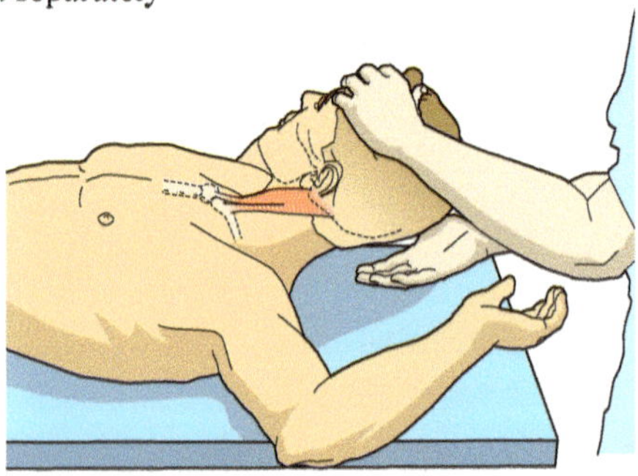
Palpation	Oblique margin of the muscle, direct to the mastoid process, to the sternum and to the clavicle
Resistance to movement	It is applied to the temporal region of the head

Infrahyoid muscles

The main function of these muscles is to lower the hyoid bone during deglutition and speech.

Muscles	Sternohyoid, thyrohyoid, omohyoid, sternothyroid
Movement	Lowering the root of the tongue with consequent descent of the hyoid bone (hyoglossus muscle), as in deglutition
Palpation	Contraction of the infrahyoid muscles inferior to the hyoid bone

Genioglossus (protrusion of the tongue)

The genioglossus is innervated by the XII cranial nerve (hypoglossal nerve).

With the mouth open and the tongue on the floor of the oral cavity, a tongue depressor is placed on the midline of the chin to provide a reference point for the midline of the tongue. The tongue should protrude to that the tip touches the tongue depressor. Any lateral deviation of the line formed by the lingual septum and the edge of the tongue depressor must be observed. During the movement of the tongue, the geniohyoid moves the hyoid bone forward and upward and this movement can be detected by palpation.

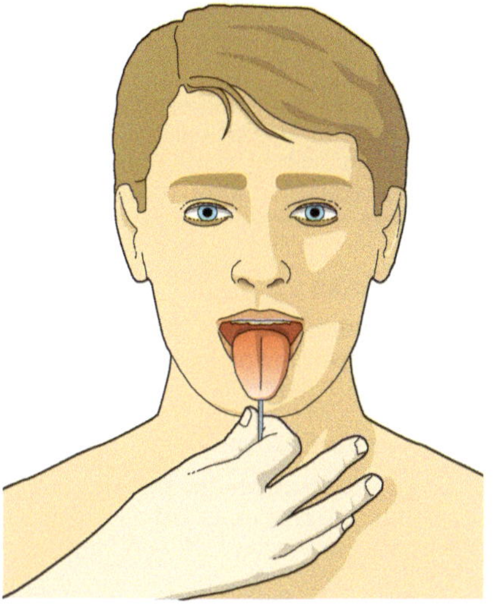

Palpation of the cervical column

Transverse process of C1

Immediately below the mastoid process and posterior to the ramus of the mandible, it can be palpated at depth, being the point of insertion and origin of many muscles.

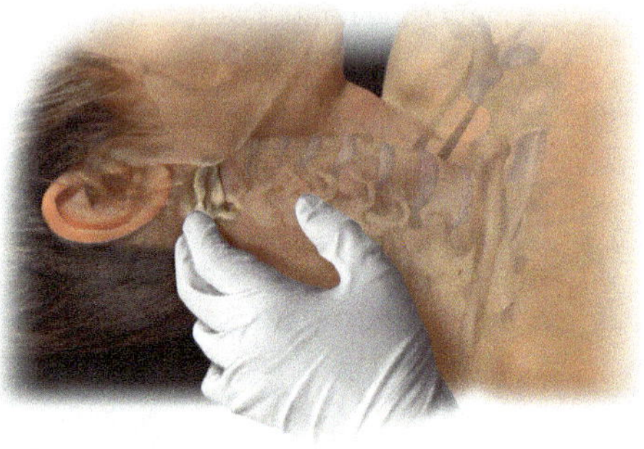

If there is a defective posture in rotation, the transverse process of C1 is more evident and posterior when the head is rotated to one side, more anteromedial and displaced behind the ramus of the mandible when the head is rotated in the opposite direction.

Spinous processes

The spinous process of the atlas can be felt immediately below the cranium moving downward from the external occipital protuberance; the spinous process of C7 (vertebra prominens) is also easily felt.

Ligamentum nuchae

It can be palpated between the spinous processes of the cervical vertebrae, more easily when in tension, during flexion of the cervical column.

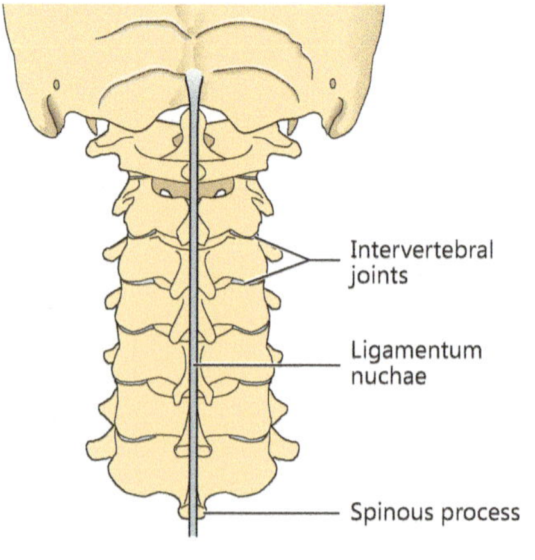

Intervertebral joints

The joints between the cervical vertebrae can be felt by placing two fingers next to the respective spinous processes.

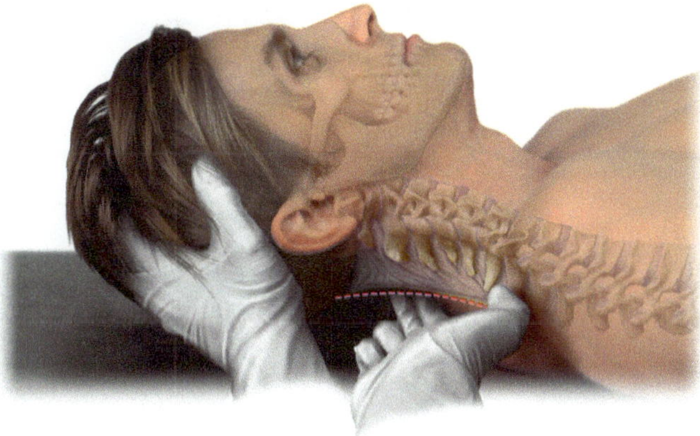

Hyoid bone

It can be palpated just immediately below the mandible, feeling its concave arch shape and the greater horns. It is mobile on both sides.

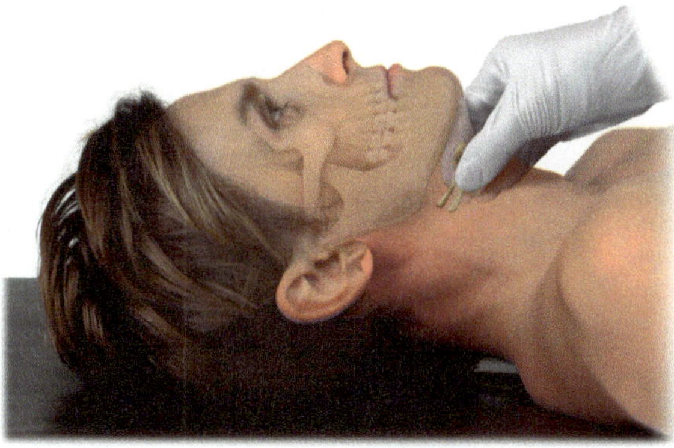

Carotid artery

The carotid pulse can be felt at the anterior border of the sternocleidomastoid, around the midpoint of the muscle belly.

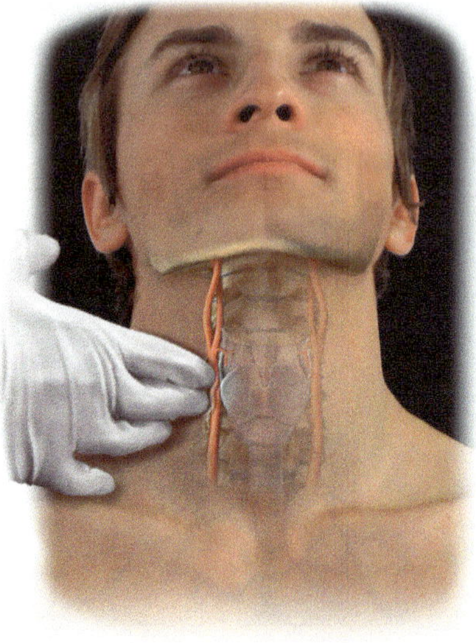

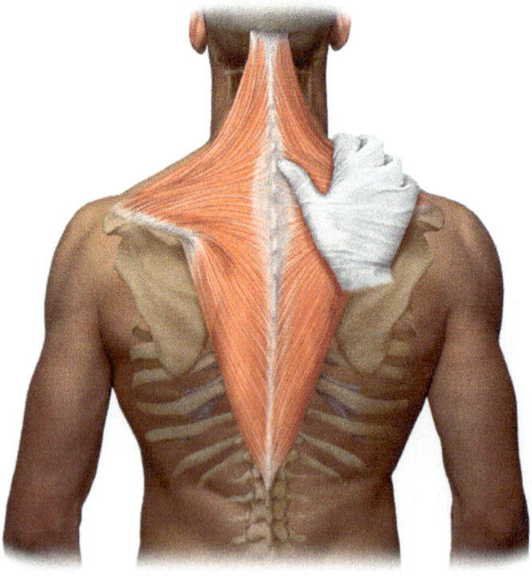

Trapezius

Laterally to the external occipital protuberance, the ligamentum nuchae and the spinous processes from T1 to T12, it extends to the lateral third of the clavicle, the acromion and the spine of the scapula.

Levator scapulae

It can be identified only at the point of insertion on the superior angle of the scapula.

Splenius capitis

Despite being largely covered by the trapezius, it can be identified in depth, extending between the mastoid process and the superior nuchal line and the spinous processes from C3 to T3.

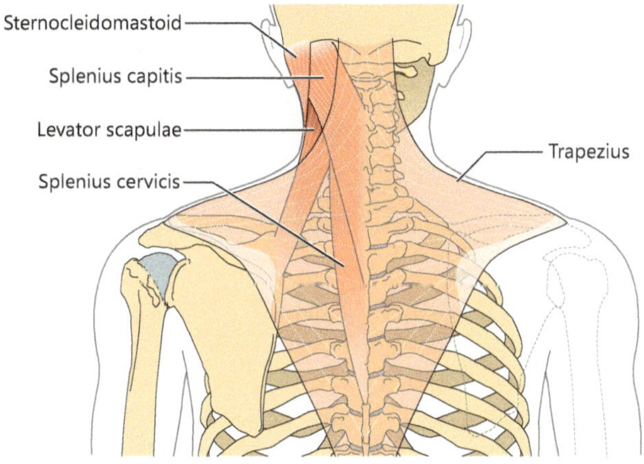

Sternocleidomastoid

Its oblique margin is palpable between the mastoid process and the sternum and clavicle. Between the sternal origin, just medial to the sternoclavicular joint, and the clavicular origin, along the middle third of the bone, a small indentation can be detected.

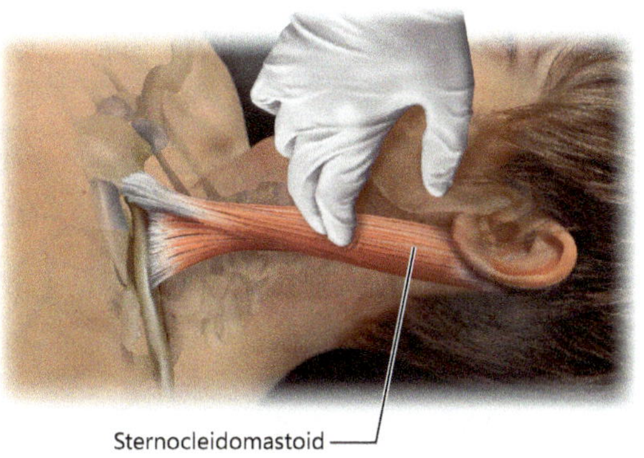

Scalene muscles

The origin of the anterior and middle scalene muscles, at the transverse processes of C3 and C7, can be palpated in depth along the sides of the trachea, while the muscles are contracted, such as during the lateral inclination of the neck. The insertion on the 1st rib can be palpat-

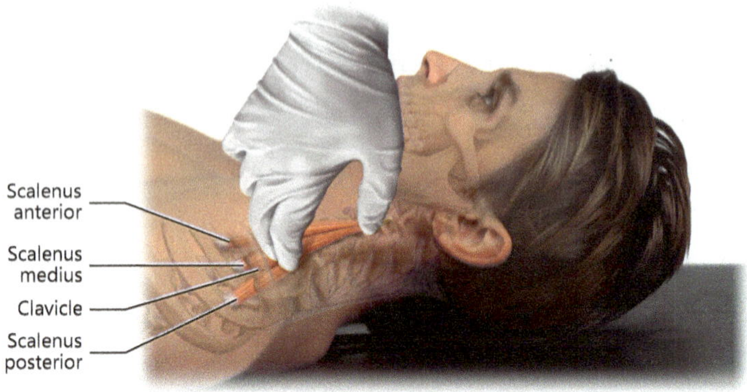

ed posteriorly to the clavicle and the sternocleidomastoid. The scalenus posterior passes in front of the anterior border of the trapezius, of which it is partially covered.

Digastric

It can be palpated at the mastoid process, in front of the sternocleidomastoid, while the mouth is open. Then proceed along the internal surface of the mandible in the direction of the symphysis.

Mylohyoid

With the mouth open, it can be palpated from the mandibular symphysis, in a posterior direction, along the floor of the oral cavity.

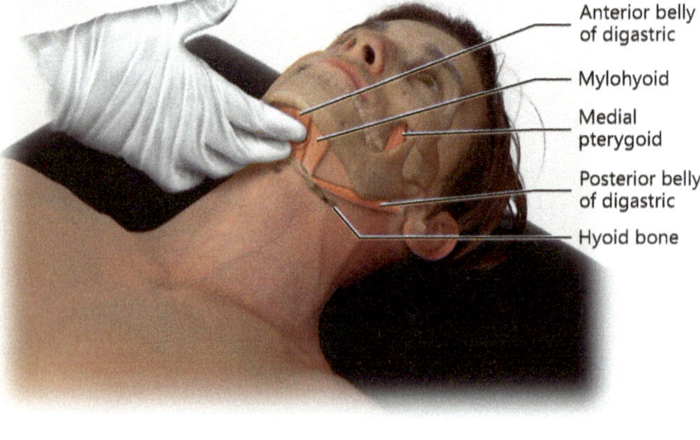

Anatomical landmarks on the surface of the head and neck

(See Chapter 3 “Head”).

Vertebral column

Functions

- Protecting the spinal cord
- Supporting the head, trunk and upper limbs (two thirds of body weight)
- Cushioning (stress transfer, in particular to the pelvis and the upper limbs)
- Adaptation of the trunk to the approaching movements of the body segmants.

Morphology

On the sagittal plane → 4 curvatures:
- 2 with posterior concavity (lordosis)
- 2 with posterior convexity (kyphosis).

Cervical lordosis: 7 cervical vertebrae: 35° angle: mobile

Thoracic kyphosis: 12 thoracic vertebrae: 35° angle: mobile

Lumbar lordosis: 5 lumbar vertebrae: 40° angle: mobile

Sacral kyphosis: 5 sacral vertebrae and 3-4 coccygeal vertebrae: almost immobile

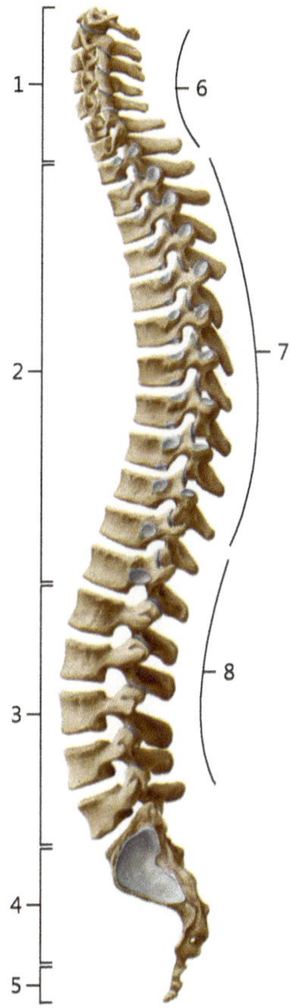

Vertebral column, left lateral view. **1.** Cervical vertebrae; **2.** thoracic vertebrae; **3.** lumbar vertebrae; **4.** sacrum; **5.** coccyx; **6.** cervical lordosis; **7.** thoracic kyphosis; **8.** lumbar lordosis.

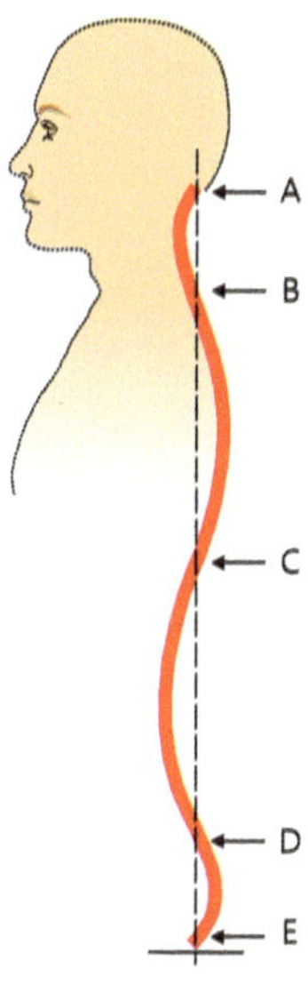

Curvature of the vertebral column (computer analysis)

In orthostatism, the axis of gravity crosses the column, perpendicular to the surface, at:
- the anterior tubercle of the 1st cervical vertebra (**A**)
- 6th cervical vertebra (**B**)
- 9th thoracic vertebra (**C**)
- 3rd sacral vertebra (**D**)
- end of the coccyx (**E**).

The column's resistance to vertical pressure → directly proportional to the square of the number of mobile curves (i.e., 3^2) + 1 = 10, thus ten times superior to that of a column without curvatures, i.e., straight.

Angles: cervical (35°), thoracic (35°) and lumbar (40°)

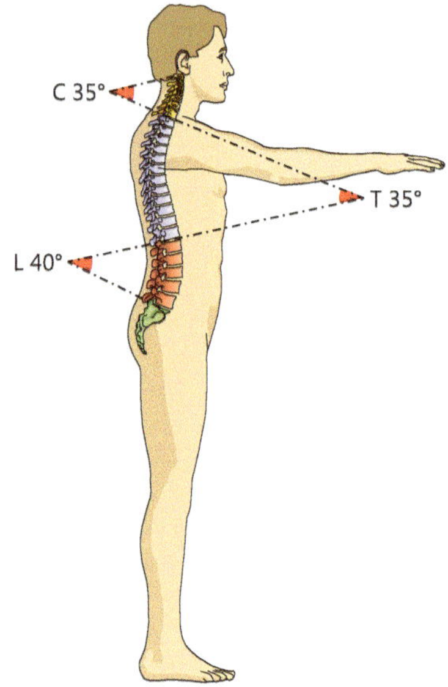

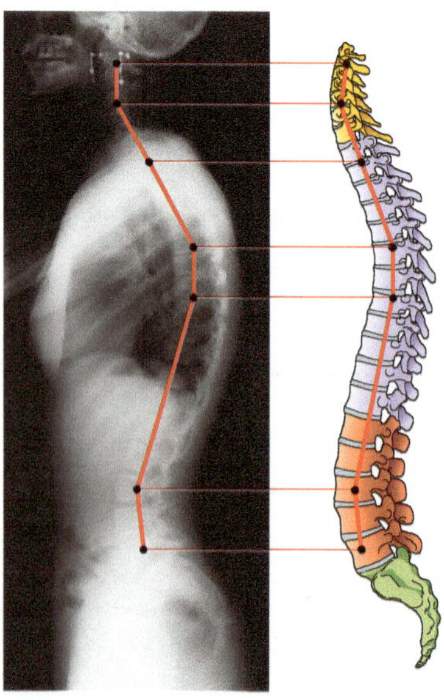

Delmas index:

$$\frac{h \times 100}{l}$$

where h = body height (measured on an X-ray in the upright position from the first cervical vertebra to the base of the sacrum) and l = length of the column ("straightened", that is, the sum of the measurements of the various segments of the column carried out on an X-ray of the column).

94-96 = normal
< 94 = accentuated curvatures (dynamic subject)
> 96 = attenuated curvatures (static subject)

Development of the vertebral column

Age	Development
Embryo and fetus	Single curve of posterior convexity (total kyphosis)
At birth	Thoracic kyphosis (will reach its definitive shape during puberty)
Infant 6-7 weeks old	Initial formation of the cervical lordosis (when the infant begins to lift the head while trying to move from the prone position)
Between 3-6 months of age	Completion of the cervical lordosis
Child 3 years old	Formation of lumbar lordosis (with the acquisition of the upright position, the reduction of the stretch of the hip flexor muscles determines, with each extension of the hip, an inclination of the pelvis – anteversion – which is reflected in the lumbar column causing lordosis).

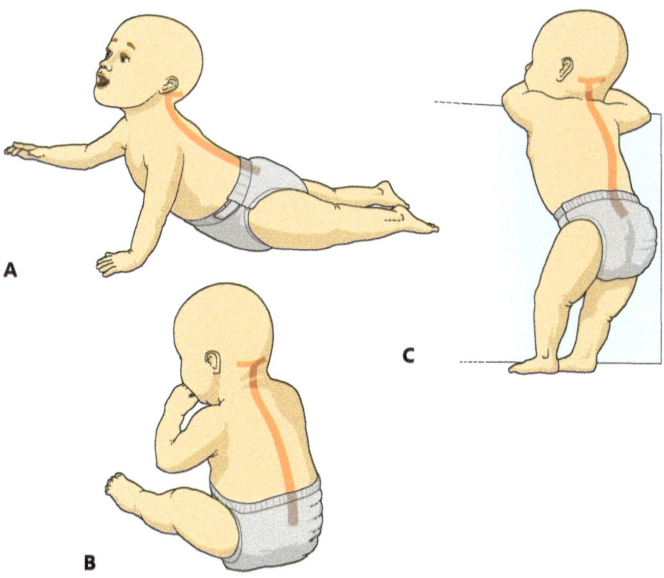

Development of physiological curvatures of the vertebral column in early years of life. **A.** At around 6 months there is an almost complete cervical lordosis. After a sitting position (**B**), during which there is an evident cervical lordosis and a wide thoracolumbar convexity, we have the upright position (**C**). Here the lumbar lordosis begins to form, which will be complete by the age of 8 years.

Structure of the vertebrae

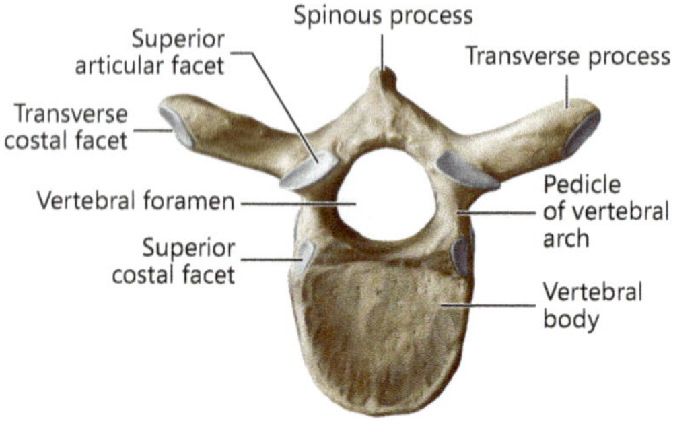

Sixth thoracic vertebra, view from above.

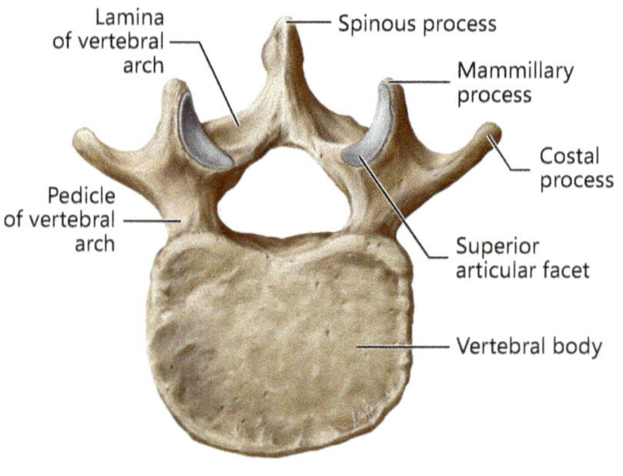

Third lumbar vertebra, view from above.

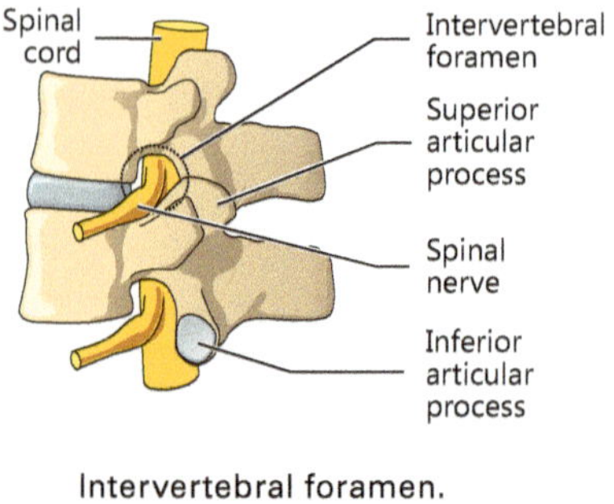

Intervertebral foramen.

Vertebral body: spongy bone tissue bounded externally by compact bone tissue.

Vertebral arch: originates in the posterior part of the vertebral body and is formed from two symmetrical halves fused to each other delimiting the **vertebral foramen**, together with the body. The overlapping vertebral foramina form the vertebral canal, which houses the spinal cord.
Anterior part of the vertebral arch: **pedicles**.
Posterior part of the vertebral arch: **laminae**.

Vertebral joints: each of the two pedicles is characterized by a **superior** and an **inferior articular process**.

Transverse and spinous processes: the transverse process project to the sides of the pedicles. Posteriorly to these, the two laminae of the arch join posteriorly and medially at the spinous process. The transverse processes of the thoracic vertebrae articulate with the ribs. The transverse processes of the lumbar vertebrae are characterized by the accessory, mammillary and costal processes. Numerous muscles originate from and insert on the spinous and transverse processes.

Intervertebral foramen: each pedicle has two notches, one superior and one inferior. The superior and inferior notches of two contiguous vertebrae delimit the intervertebral foramen, which gives passage to the spinal nerve.

Thoracic vertebrae

The thoracic vertebrae articulate with the ribs through:

- articular demifacets (facets in certain cases) present on the vertebral bodies (joint with the head of the ribs)
- articular facets, known as costal facets, present on the transverse processes (joints with the tubercle of the rib or costotransverse joints).

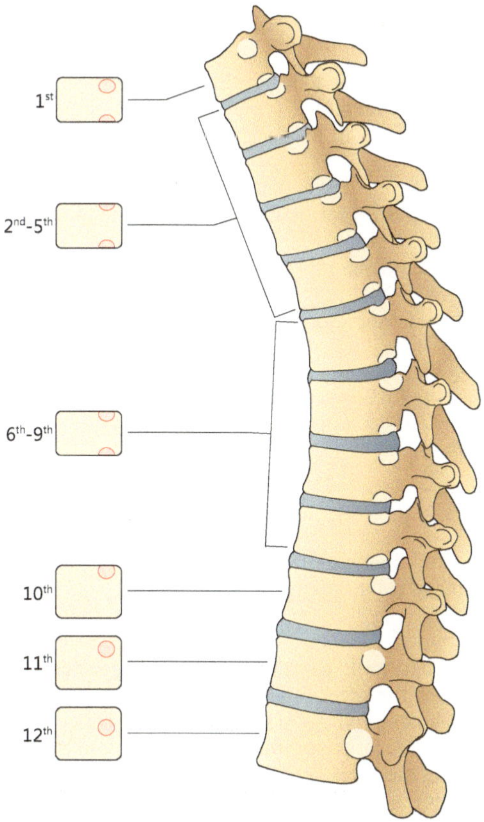

Thoracic vertebrae	Distinctive features
1st	• Superior facet • Inferior demifacet • Costal facet with flat surface (gliding of the rib)
2nd-5th	• Superior demifacet • Inferior demifacet • Costal facet with hollow surface (rotation of the rib)
6th-9th	• Superior demifacet • Inferior demifacet • Costal facet with flat surface (gliding of the rib, 6th, 9th)
10th	• Superior demifacet • Costal facet with flat surface
11th	• Superior facet • Costal facet with flat surface
12th	• Intermediate facet • Costal facet with flat surface

The mobility of the ribs (rotation or gliding) is conditioned by the shape of the surface of the articular facet.

Cervical vertebrae

- The transverse processes of the cervical vertebrae are characterized by the transverse foramina, through which the vertebral arteries pass
- Pointed tuberosities, called the uncinate processes, are created on the superior endplate of the vertebral bodies in the first year of life. Between the upper inner part of the uncinate processes and the lateroinferior border of the body of the overlapping vertebra, fissures that increase disc mobility (uncovertebral joints) open up before the tenth year of life.
- Meniscal structures located at the ends, superior and inferior, of the articular facets increase joint amplitude
- 1st cervical vertebra (atlas):
  - wide vertebral foramen
  - vertebral body replaced by an anterior arch with an anterior tubercle
  - large posterior arch with a smaller posterior tubercle
  - in the posterior arch, behind and inferiomedially to the foramen transversarium, is the groove for the vertebral artery
  - five articular facets: two concave superior facets that articulate with the occipital bone, two flat inferior facets that articulate with the 2nd cervical vertebra and one facet (facet for dens) that articulates with the dens of the axis
  - the atlanto-occipital joint is a condyle with movements of flexion-extension and lateral inclination (limited)
  - the intervertebral disc is not present between the 1st and 2nd cervical vertebrae
- 2nd cervical vertebra (axis):
  - the dens of the axis articulates with the atlas
  - the atlantoaxial joint is a pivot joint with only movements of rotation (the head and the atlas are integral to each other during rotation, with a fixed point represented by the axis).

Lumbar vertebrae

- 2nd and 3rd lumbar vertebrae – greater sagittal diameter
- 4th lumbar vertebra – capable of supporting greater weight
- 5th lumbar vertebra:
  - greater transverse diameter
  - the intervertebral disc that separates it from the 1st sacral vertebra has a greater height and presents a greater asymmetry between the anterior and posterior height
  - wide posteroinferior articular facets articulated with the sacrum
  - iliolumbar ligaments between transverse processes and iliac crest
  - greater mobility, limited by the joints with the sacrum and by the iliolumbar ligaments.

Articular facets of the vertebral processes

The orientation of the articular facets of the vertebral processes varies in the cervical, thoracic and lumbar regions of the vertebral column, conditioning the mobility of the different segments of the vertebral column.

Articular facets	Inclination with respect to the sagittal plane	Inclination with respect to the horizontal plane
Cervical	45°	Backward open arch (almost coinciding with the frontal plane)
Thoracic	60°	Forward open arch (20° per side)
Lumbar	90°	Backward open arch (45° per side)

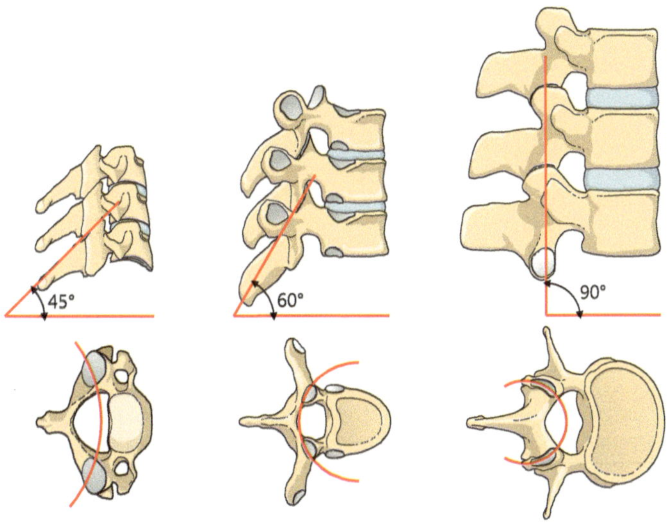

Angular difference between the epiphysial joints of the cervical, thoracic and lumbar regions.

How to unload the joints of the vertebral arches
Since the traction exerted is perpendicular to the articular surface, it should be directed towards the superior articular processes and towards the underlying vertebrae:
- downwards and forwards in the cervical column
- downwards, forwards and medially in the thoracic column
- forwards and laterally in the lumbar column.

Vertebral resistance to pressure

Resistance elements:

- compact bone tissue of the vertebral body, situated externally
- direction of the trabeculae (horizontal, oblique, vertical) of spongy bone of the vertebral body, situated internally.

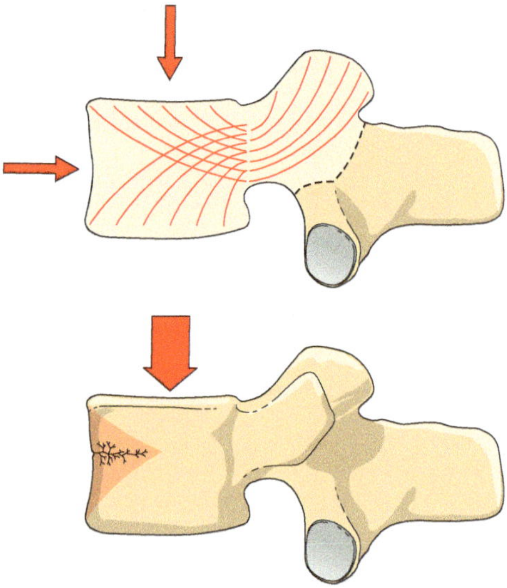

The image shows a triangular-shaped area of least resistance, with the base corresponding to the anterior surface of the vertebral body. At this stage there is a lack of fan-shaped oblique trabeculae which are directed backwards towards the arch from the superior and inferior parts of the vertebral body.

The anterior part of the vertebral body is therefore more subjected to crushing or fracture due to compression forces.

Joints of the vertebral column

- Joints of the vertebral bodies (anterior): main function of support
- joints of the vertebral arch (posterior and apophysial): main function of movement.

Joints of the vertebral bodies

Composition	Type	Characteristics
Intervertebral disc and inferior and superior surfaces of the vertebral bodies	Cartilaginous synarthrosis (synchondrosis)	Is the most mobile of the synarthroses. This mobility is due to the structure of each disc, to the overall number of discs and to their height

5

Intervertebral discs

There are 23 intervertebral discs, which are missing between the occipital bone and atlas and between the atlas and the axis. Together, they account for approximately one quarter of the column height.
The intervertebral disc consists of:

- anulus fibrosus
- nucleus pulposus.

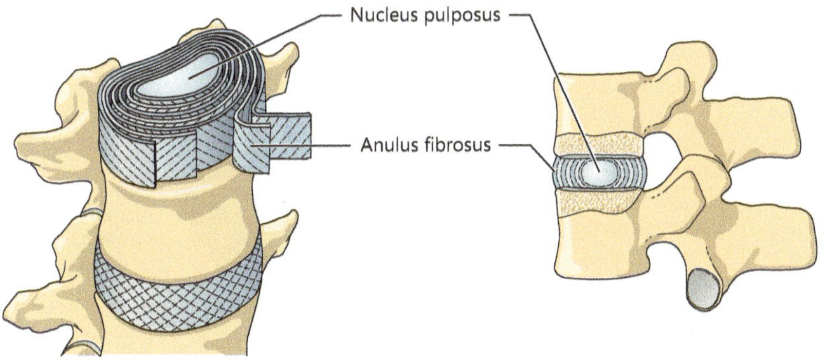

Shape of intervertebral discs

Cervical and lumbar segments of the column	Thoracic segment of the column
Greater anterior height of the intervertebral disc	Greater posterior height of the intervertebral disc

Since the vertebral bodies have similar dimensions, with the exception of the thoracic discs which are slightly wedge-shaped, with a greater posterior height, the physiological curvature of the vertebral column largely depends on the shape of the discs and not that of the vertebral bodies.

The height of the intervertebral discs is lower at the cervical level, medium at the thoracic level and higher at the lumbar level.

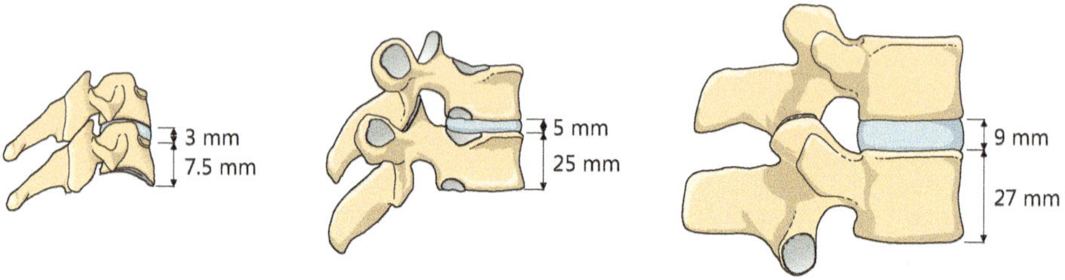

The different heights of the intervertebral discs compared to the height of the vertebral bodies. **A.** Cervical vertebrae; **B.** thoracic vertebrae; **C.** lumbar vertebrae.

Since the higher the ratio between the height of the disc and the height of the vertebral body, the higher the mobility, the most mobile portion of the vertebral column is the cervical, followed by the lumbar and thoracic.

Anulus fibrosus

Composition:

- collagen fibers distributed from the inside out in several layers
- a moderate amount of elastic fibers.

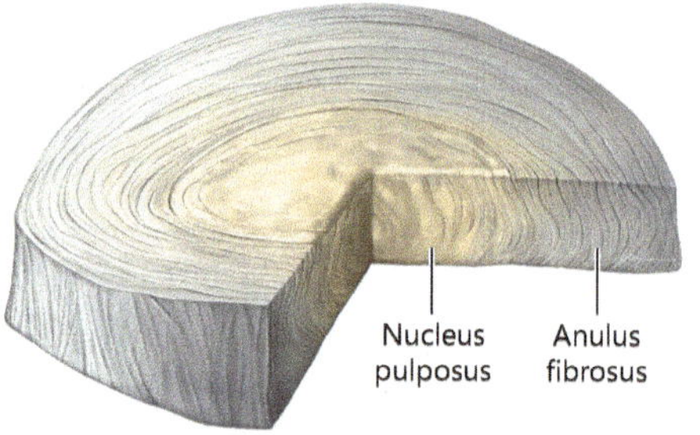

Characteristics:

- the fibers present varying degrees of obliquity in each layer
- the fibers of one layer form an angle of 90° with those of the adjacent layers
- the fibers in the outer layers are almost vertical
- the obliquity of the fibers increases from the outer layers to the inner layers
- the fibers on the innermost layer are almost horizontal.

Properties:

- the orientation of the fibers allows some of them to stretch, limiting certain movements, and others to relax, allowing other movements
- under normal load, and at rest, all of the fibers are stretched.

Nucleus pulposus

Is the center of the intervertebral disc.

Composition:

- network of elastic fibers of connective tissue
- Mucopolysaccharides capable of retaining water (colloidal gel consisting of 80% water).

Characteristics:

- the amount of water decreases with age and so does the number of elastic fibers and the amount of mucopolysaccharides. The reduced joint mobility of the vertebral column that occurs in older people depends on this
- hydroelastic shock absorber (supports 75% of the load, whereas the other 25% is borne by the anulus fibrosus)
- the displacements of the nucleus pulposus caused by the load tense or relax the fibers of the anulus fibrosus.

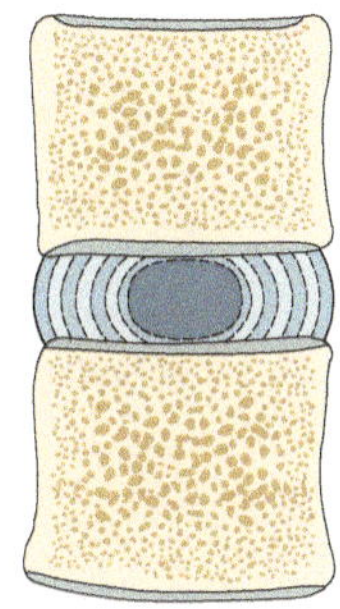

The nucleus pulposus, being incompressible (Pascal's law), maintains the distance between the vertebral bodies, and its deformation is responsible for the varying kinetics of the annulus fibrosus.

The mucopolysaccharides and the other components of the nucleus pulposus (proteins, sodium, calcium) exert a significant influence on the elasticity and hydration of the intervertebral disc and are responsible for the osmotic pressure that opposes the orthostatic pressure exerted on the intervertebral disc.
The incompressibility allows it to protect the distance between the vertebral bodies.
The deformability allows it to press the anulus fibrosus due to its variable kinetics.
In addition:

- in young people, the anulus fibrosus has many elastic fibers, which enable a wide range of motion
- after 40-45 years, due to the increase in the fibrotic component and the decrease in mucopolysaccharides, there is a lower absorption of fluids and lower joint mobility of the vertebral column.

The alternation of loading and unloading is very important in the treatment of disc-related pathologies because it allows an even distribution of nutritive substances throughout the disc.

Interdiscal pressure

The balance between hydration and dehydration by the intervertebral disc is established at a threshold level of orthostatic pressure in the disc, equal to approximately 800 N, which represents the intradiscal pressure.
The various positions modify the intradiscal pressure. For example, at the 3rd lumbar vertebra, this is equal to:

- 250 N in a supine position
- 350 N in lateral decubitus
- 1000 N in upright position
- 1400 N in a seated position

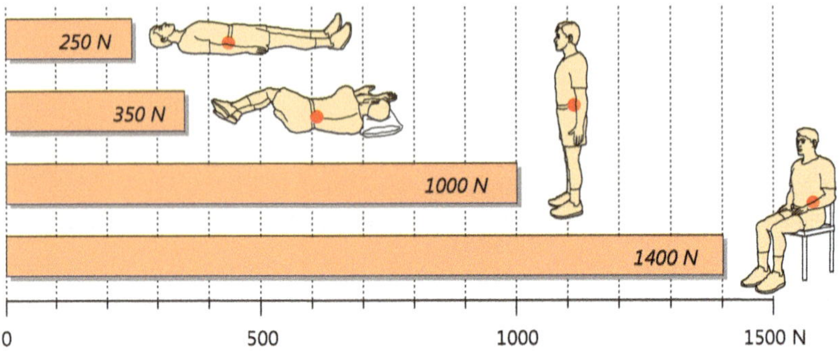

Increase in intradiscal pressure → **dehydration**
Reduction in intradiscal pressure → **hydration**

Body posture and movements during the day (loading position) determine dehydration with an increase in intradiscal pressure, while the opposite occurs during sleep (unloading position), with fluid recovery and reduction of intradiscal pressure.
The **traction** exerted on the intervertebral space facilitates hydration of the disc, which is thus relieved.

Variations in intradiscal pressure during lifting and carrying weights

Example:
- 20° forward flexion of the trunk with the back straight → if a load is carried in this position, this leads to a three to fourfold increase in intradiscal pressure
- 20° forward flexion of the trunk with the back curved → if a load is carried in this position, this leads to a seven to eightfold increase in intradiscal pressure.

For this reason, the starting position to be assumed when lifting and carrying weights must respect the physiological curvature of the column, otherwise the column is not be able to support the maximum tolerable load.

Modifications of the intervertebral disc during movement

For example, forward flexion of the trunk:
- the vertebral body leans forwards
- the intersomatic space assumes a wedge shape
- the anterior collagen fibers of the anulus fibrosus are compressed
- the posterior collagen fibers of the anulus fibrosus are stretched
- the nucleus pulposus slides backwards, dragging the elastic fibers of the anulus fibrosus
- the posterior space between the vertebral bodies increases
- the posterior collagen fibers of the anulus fibrosus reach the limit of extensibility

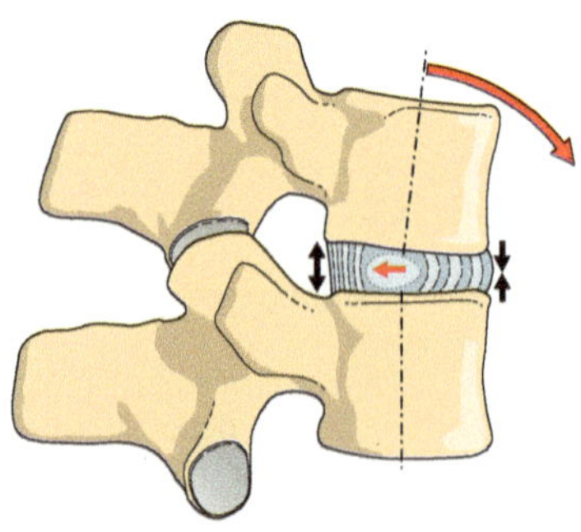

Behavior of the intervertebral disc during flexion.

- the tension of the fibers in the anulus fibrosus, in addition to holding the vertebra together, limits movement.

Axes of movement of the intervertebral disc

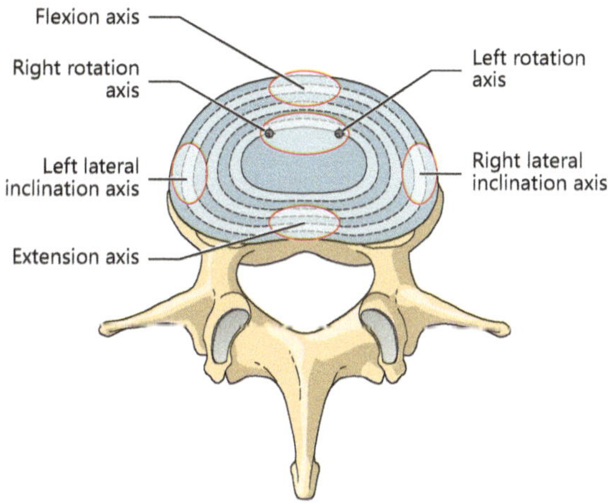

The axes of movement depend on the adaptive capacity of the nucleus pulposus. They cannot be accurately predetermined.

Alterations in the intervertebral disc

Protrusion

Definition	Intervertebral disc progress over the posterior border of the vertebral bodies.
Etiopathogenesis	Degeneration of the collagen fiber bundles of the anulus fibrosus (due to overload). Formation of fissures in the layers of collagen fibers of the anulus fibrosus. Dislocation of the nucleus pulposus that seeps into the fissures formed by moving the intact fiber layers (due to an asymmetric load).

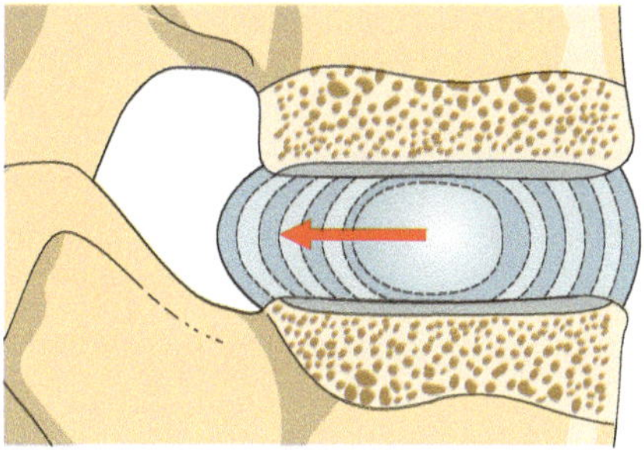

Herniation

Definition	Displacement of the nucleus pulposus in the direction of the spinal canal or spinal nerve.
Etiopathogenesis	Degenerative formation of fissures in all the layers of collagen fibers of the anulus fibrosus.

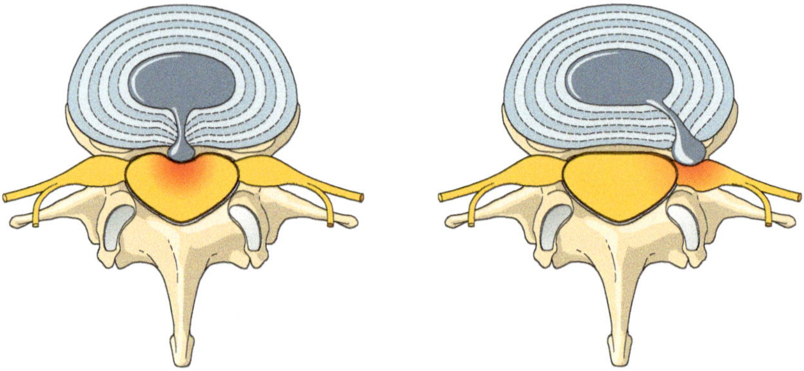

Degeneration of the intervertebral disc

- Alterations of the lines of fluid diffusion in the disc with reduction of hydration
- Loss of uniform load distribution and capacity to adapt to varying stresses
- Reduction of the space between the vertebral bodies
- Increased stress on the joints of the vertebral arch
- Origin of the spurs (osteophytes) from the borders of the vertebral bodies.

According to the severity of the disc displacement, hernias can also be classified into:
- contained subligamentous hernias
- protruding subligamentous hernias
- extruded hernia (*in situ*)
- extruded hernia (migrated).

Joints of the vertebral arch

Articular facets of the superior and inferior processes (for their orientation, see page 165). Each joint has an articular cartilage, fibrous capsule, synovial membrane and synovial fluid.

> Between the superior and inferior articular processes of a vertebra, there is an area of predominantly compacted bone tissue with limited presence of spongy bone tissue. A break in this area, known as the pars interarticularis, can cause vertebral gliding.

Ligaments of the vertebral column

Interspinous ligament	Between two adjacent spinous processes.
Supraspinous ligament	Between the apices of the spinous processes. It extends from the 7th cervical vertebra to the sacrum, whereas it is replaced by the ligamentum nuchae in the cervical segment.
Ligamentum flavum	Between the laminae of two adjacent vertebrae. The characteristic yellow color, from which the name derives, is due to the almost exclusive presence of elastic fibers. It favors the recovery of the upright position of the trunk from the flexed position.

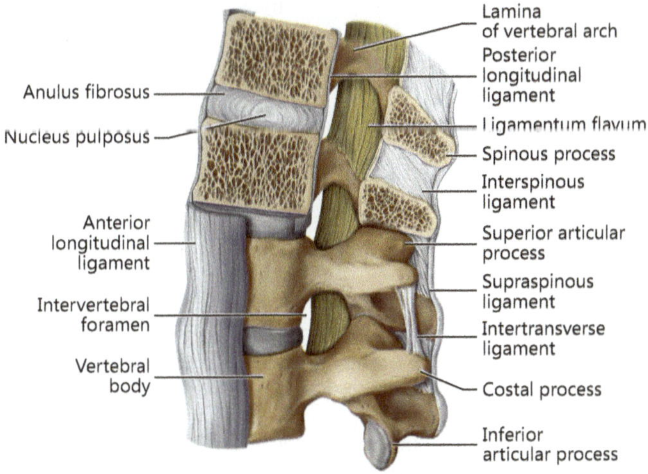

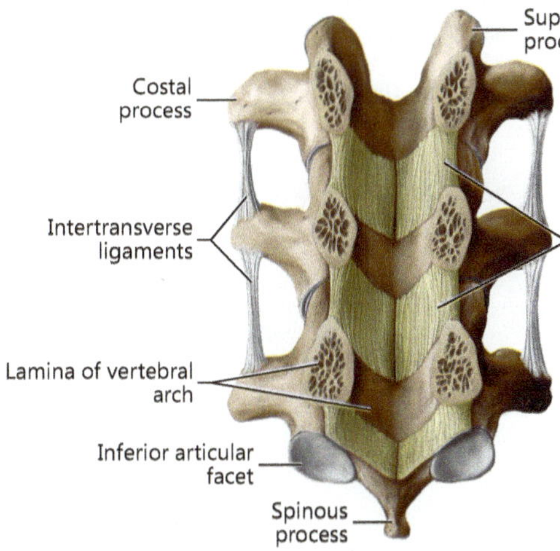

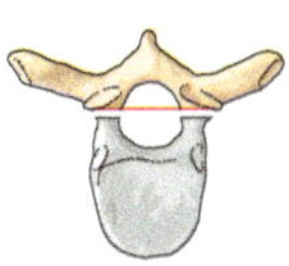

When these ligaments are tensed, their restraining action favors the resistance of the nucleus pulposus to vertical pressure.

Posterior longitudinal ligament

It extends from the 2nd cervical vertebra to the sacrum, becoming narrower during its course. It attaches to the intervertebral discs posteriorly, whereas at the level of the vertebral bodies it only attaches to the superior and inferior borders. It limits the flexion of the vertebral column. Together with the anulus fibrosus, it counteracts the diastasis of the nucleus pulposus.

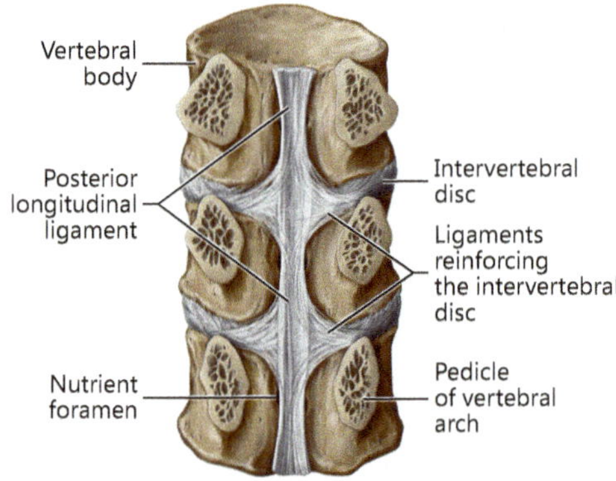

Anterior longitudinal ligament

It extends from the anterior tubercle of the 1st cervical vertebra to the sacrum, widening along its course. It adheres to the anterior surface of the vertebral bodies, leaving the superior and inferior borders free and adhering only partially to the intervertebral discs. It limits the extension of the vertebral column. Together with the anulus fibrosus, it counteracts the diastasis of the nucleus pulposus.

Intertransverse ligament

Between the transverse processes.

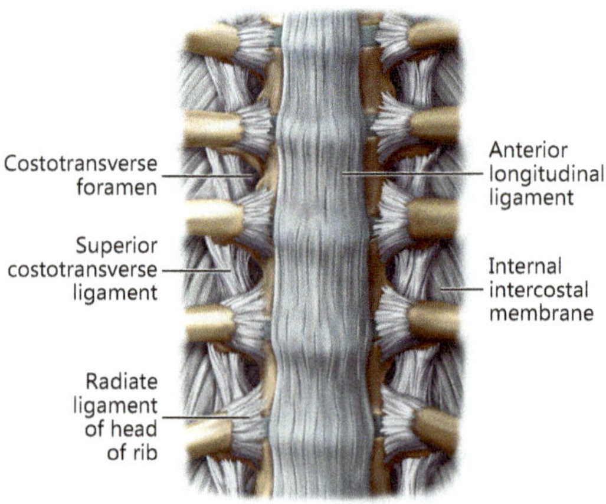

Functional spinal unit

(Functional spinal unit, FSU, or "motion segment").

Definition: space formed by two adjacent vertebrae including the soft tissues interposed between the vertebrae with the exclusion of the muscles. The two rib heads (left and right) and their ligaments are also included in the FSU at the level of the thoracic column. (As far as the others are concerned, the intersegmental muscles are also part of the FSU).

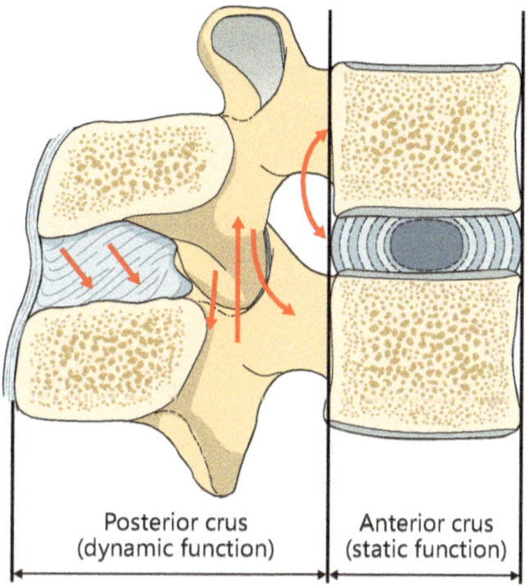

Unit of motion

The unit of motion corresponds to the FSU.

In the space between the two vertebrae, there are:
- the joints of the vertebral arch (in addition to the joint capsules there is also the ligamentum flava)
- the spinal canal and the intervertebral foramen (with the spinal nerves, the meningeal branches and vessels)
- the intervertebral disc (in addition to the cartilaginous surfaces of the vertebral bodies, with the borders of the vertebral endplates, the nucleus pulposus and the anulus fibrosus, there are also the anterior and posterior longitudinal ligaments).

It also includes the spaces between the vertebral arches, the spinous processes and overlying transverse processes, with all ligaments and muscles included in these spaces.

The structures of the unit of motion are anatomically and functionally coordinated. An injury to one of its components also affects the other structures.

The unit of motion can be divided into two parts:
- anterior crus (vertebral body and intervertebral disc), with support function (absorbs axial compressive forces, such as the body load, which are discharged through the column of the vertebral bodies and then transmitted)
- posterior crus (joints of the vertebral arch), with movement direction function (allowing or blocking the movements permitted by the shape of the joints of the vertebral arch and limited by the ligamentous structures, the position of the joints and the anulus fibrosus).

Movements of the vertebral column

All types of movements are possible (joint structure with three degrees of freedom):
- flexion-extension
- lateral inclination
- rotation.

The sliding of the vertebral bodies on the discs in the three spatial planes can be added to these movements. For this reason, six degrees of freedom can be attributed to the vertebral column.
The mobile part of the column is the sum of 24 vertebrae, including:
- 25 anterior intervertebral joints (the atlanto-occipital and atlantoaxial joints and 23 discs)
- 46 (23 × 2) posterior vertebral (or interapophysial) joints.

Axes of rotation

The vertebral column can move around three axes of rotation:
- longitudinal (or vertical)
- sagittal (or lateral)
- frontal (or transverse).

Movements can also be carried out by a single vertebra, with respect to the overlying or underlying vertebrae, or by a single segment of the column.
The center of longitudinal rotation is located:
- on the spinous processes at the level of the lumbar vertebrae (helical traction on the disc)
- at the center of the intervertebral disc in the thoracic vertebrae (torsion of the disc on itself).

The center of rotation and the axis of rotation move from vertebra to vertebra and even within the same FSU, as a result of the vertebral translations allowed by the discs and by the various directions of the facets of the posterior vertebral joints.
In turn, the movements of the column change the center of rotation. When a vertebra or FSU has reached the maximum range of motion, the center of rotation moves above or below it, depending on the direction of motion and the position of the first center of rotation from which the motion originated. In fact, in vertebral kinetics, partial movements of all the other FSU in the direction of the movement take place simultaneously with the movement of a single FSU. For example, during flexion of the column, the movement starts from the head, if the different FSU are progressively mobilized in craniocaudal direction, but also at the lumbar level, if the different FSU are progressively mobilized in caudocranial direction.

Flexion-extension of the vertebral column

Plane of movement → Sagittal
Axis of rotation → Transverse

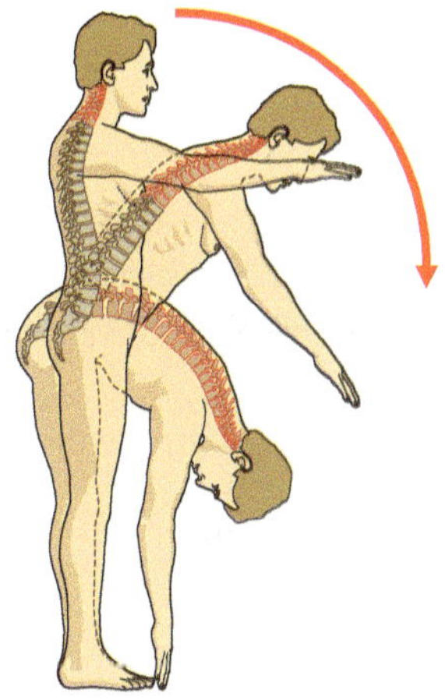

Flexion:
- cervical 40°
- thoracic 40°
- lumbar 60°

Lumbopelvic rhythm
Lumbar flexion is accompanied by the movement of the pelvis around the bicondylar (or coxofemoral) axis, which extends the range of motion; otherwise, it would not exceed half of the indicated values.

5

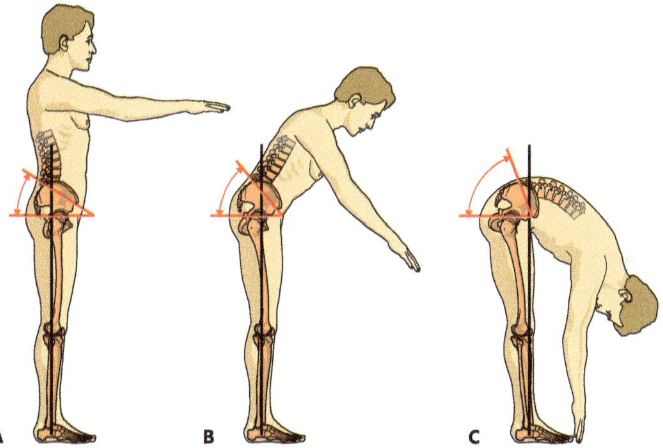

Lumbopelvic rhythm in the anterior flexion of the trunk. **A.** Upright position: normal lumbar lordosis; **B.** beginning of the flexion: flattening of the lumbar lordosis and beginning of anteversion of the pelvis; **C.** end of the flexion: moderate inversion of the lumbar lordosis and wide anteversion of the pelvis that, for reasons of balance, moves posteriorly.

Lumbar flexion:
- 70% at L5-S1 level
- 20% at L4-L5 level
- 10% at L1-L2/L2-L3/L3-L4 level

Flexion of the trunk
(thoracolumbar) 100°

Extension:
- cervical 45°
- thoracic 15°
- lumbar 30°

Extension of the trunk
(thoracolumbar) 45°

In a normal subject there is a total flexion-extension of the vertebral column equal to 230° (total flexion of 140° + total extension of 90°); this value can reach 250° in a flexible subject.

Formations limiting flexion of the vertebral column:
- posterior longitudinal ligament
- ligamenta flava
- interspinous ligaments
- supraspinous ligaments
- intertransverse ligaments
- ligamentum nuchae
- superior fascicle of the lumbosacral ligament
- joint capsules of the posterior joints of the column
- anterior obstruction of the disc
- posterior traction of the anulus fibrosus
- extensor muscles of the trunk.

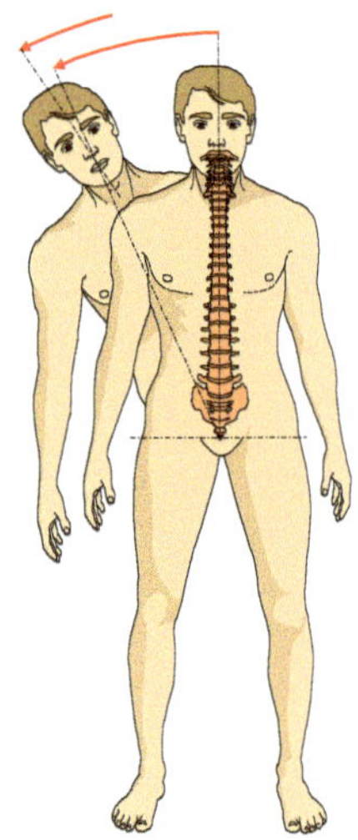

Formations limiting extension of the vertebral column:
- anterior longitudinal ligament
- compaction of the posterior articular facets and the spinous processes
- anterior traction of the anulus fibrosus
- posterior obstruction of the disc
- flexor muscles of the trunk.

Lateral inclination of the vertebral column

Plane of movement → Frontal
Axis of rotation → Sagittal

Lateral inclination:
• cervical 40°
• thoracic 25°
• lumbar 15°
Lateral inclination of the trunk (thoracolumbar) 40°

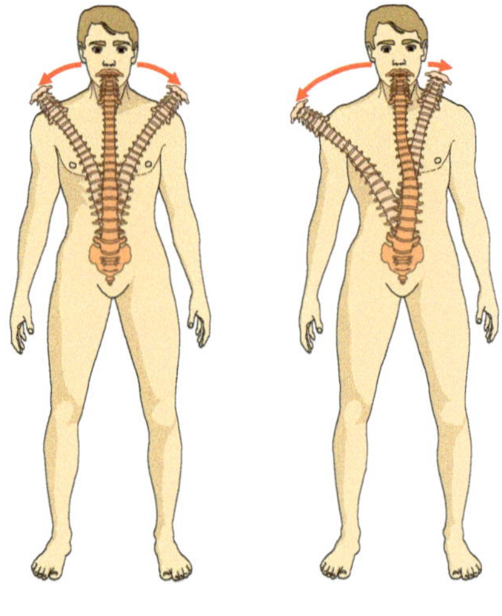

The lateral inclination of the vertebral column displays the same amplitude in both sides. The presence of scoliosis can limit the inclination in one or both sides to a considerable extent.

Physiological rotation of the vertebrae
The lateral inclination of the column results in a physiological rotation of the vertebrae that, while expanding the radius of the arc of a circle produced by the lateral inclination of the column, limits the movement.

Formations limiting the lateral inclination of the vertebral column:
- physiological rotation of the vertebral bodies
- tension of the intertransverse and flava contralateral ligaments and interspinous ligaments
- joint capsules of the posterior joints of the contralateral vertebral column
- tension of the contralateral lumbosacral ligament
- contralateral tension of the anulus fibrosus
- obstruction of the disc ipsilaterally.

Rotation of the vertebral column

Plane of movement → Transverse
Axis of rotation → Longitudinal

Rotation:
- cervical 50°
- thoracic 35°
- lumbar 5°

Rotation of the trunk (thoracolumbar) 40°

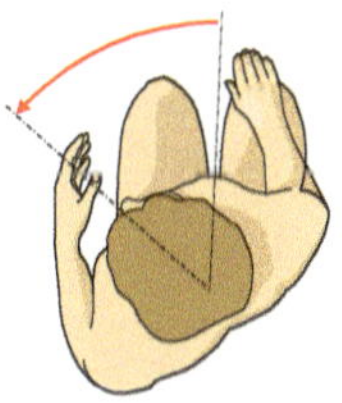

Formations limiting the rotation of the vertebral column:
- traction on the intervertebral discs or variations in their thickness that are determined during movement
- muscular, ligamentous, bone and articular structures opposing the movement in the various degrees of rotation
- the iliolumbar ligament.

Mobility of the different segments of the vertebral column

Cervical column	175° (flexion, extension, lateral inclination and rotation have approximately the same range of motion, between 40° to 50°; maximum rotation at C1-C2 level; maximum flexion-extension at C6-T1 level)
Thoracic column	115° (the most limited movement is extension)
Lumbar column	110° (flexion-extension range of motion is 90°, greater than that of the thoracic column, lateral inclination range of motion is 15° and rotation range of motion is 5°; greater mobility at the T11-L1-L2 and L4-L5-S1 levels)

Muscles of the vertebral column

- They act in a global and non-metameric manner, with a mainly postural significance
- The movements produced have characteristics of elementary reflexes (antigravity), i.e., not voluntary and not very conscious
- Their function is mainly controlled by the brainstem and the spinal cord.

Muscular layers:
- superficial
- intermediate
- deep: I, II, III.

Extrinsic muscles: they do not insert on the vertebral column but can indirectly determine movements
- Serratus anterior, pectoralis minor and pectoralis major
  - act on the thoracic cage
- Internal oblique, external oblique, rectus abdominis and transversus abdominis
  - act on the thoracic cage and the pelvis
- Gluteus maximus, gluteus medius, gluteus minimus, tensor fasciae latae, adductor longus, adductor brevis and adductor magnus
  - act on the pelvis.

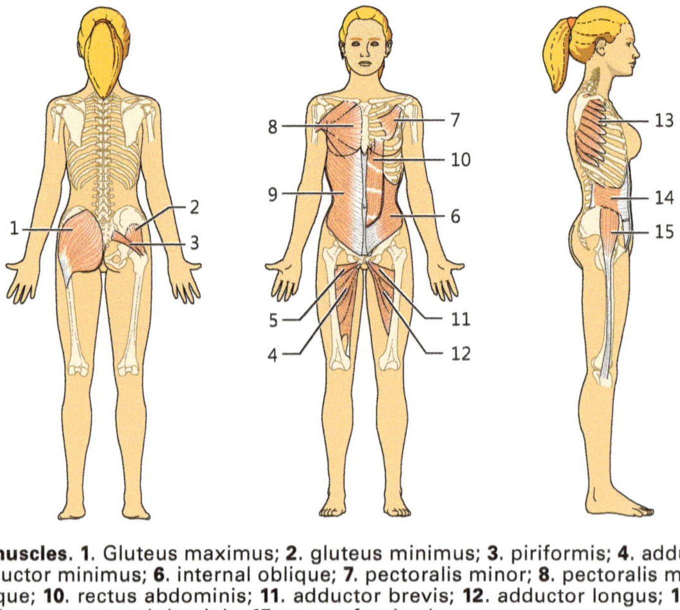

Extrinsic muscles. **1**. Gluteus maximus; **2**. gluteus minimus; **3**. piriformis; **4**. adductor magnus; **5**. adductor minimus; **6**. internal oblique; **7**. pectoralis minor; **8**. pectoralis major; **9**. external oblique; **10**. rectus abdominis; **11**. adductor brevis; **12**. adductor longus; **13**. serratus anterior; **14**. transversus abdominis; **15**. tensor fasciae latae.

(See Chapters 6 "Thorax and thoracic column" and 10 "Hip and pelvis" for the origin, insertion and action of these muscles, with the exception of those of the abdomen referred to in section "Muscles of the abdomen", page 187).

Intrinsic muscles: they are inserted or originate on the vertebral column
- Flat muscles:
  - trapezius and latissimus dorsi (superficial layer), rhomboids and serratus posterior superior and inferior muscles (intermediate layer), quadratus lumborum and iliopsoas (deep layer) muscles

- Long muscles, they are divided based on the orientation of the fibers into:
  - longitudinal system (all paravertebral muscles, with the exception of the iliocostalis and the transverse spinous muscle complex)
    - spinalis (capitis, colli and thoracis – medially in the deep layer I)
    - longissimus (capitis, colli and thoracis – in intermediate position, between the medial and lateral, in the deep I layer)
    - intertransversarii (cervicis and lumborum – deep layer III)
    - interspinales (cervicis, thoracis and lumborum – deep layer III)
  - oblique system
    - iliocostalis (cervicis and lumborum – laterally in the deep layer I)
    - transverse spinous muscle complex
      - semispinalis (capitis, cervicis and thoracis – superficially in the deep layer II)
      - multifidus (thoracis and cervicis – in intermediate position, between the superficial and deep, in the deep layer II)
      - rotatores (breves and longi – in deep position in the deep layer II).

5

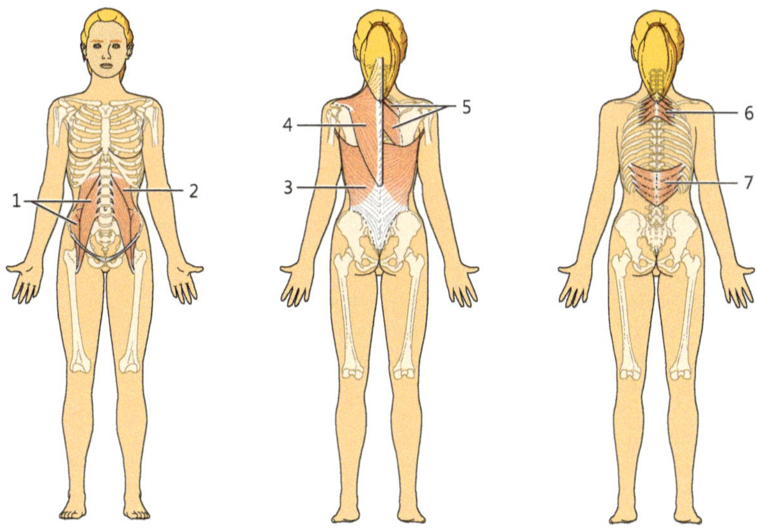

Flat intrinsic muscles. **1.** Iliopsoas; **2.** quadratus lumborum; **3.** latissimus dorsi; **4.** trapezius; **5.** rhomboids; **6.** serratus posterior superior; **7.** serratus posterior inferior.

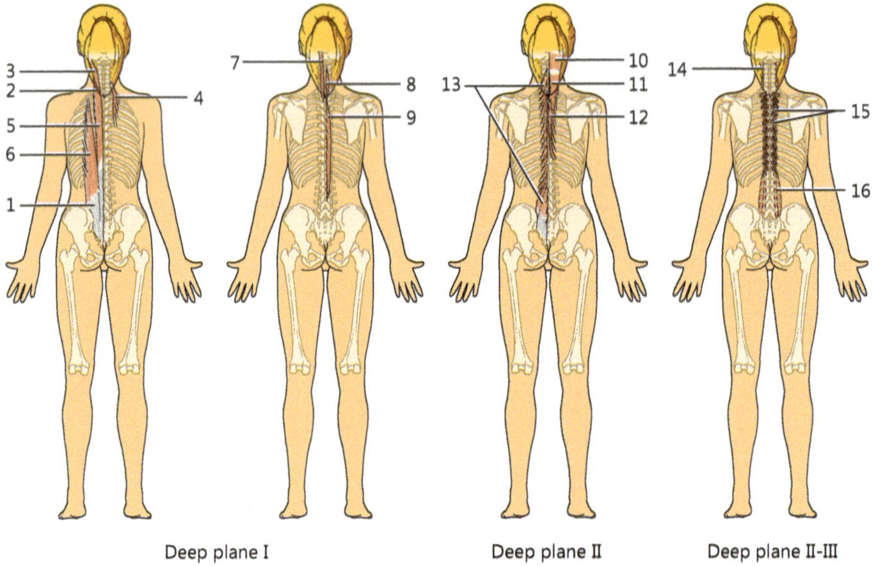

Long intrinsic muscles. **1**. Iliocostalis lumborum, lumbar part; **2**. longissimus cervicis; **3**. longissimus capitis; **4**. iliocostalis cervicis; **5**. longissimus thoracis; **6**. iliocostalis lumborum, thoracic part; **7**. spinalis capitis; **8**. spinalis cervicis; **9**. spinalis thoracis; **10**. semispinalis capitis; **11**. semispinalis cervicis; **12**. semispinalis thoracis; **13**. multifidus; **14**. cervical intertransversarii; **15**. rotatores; **16**. lumbar intertransversarii. **Note**: the interspinales are not represented, for which see the figures on page 186.

Long intrinsic muscles of the vertebral column

Also called paravertebral muscles, they constitute the erector spinae.
The erector spinae is located on both sides of the vertebral column and is made up of three main columns of muscle tissue (from lateral to medial: iliocostalis, longissimus and spinalis) with common origin in:

- the posterior surfaces of the sacrum and the iliac crest
- the sacrotuberous and dorsal sacroiliac ligaments
- the spinous processes and their corresponding supraspinous ligaments from L1 to L5 and from T11 and T12.

The three columns also originate from other bony structures. They are located at different levels of the lumbar region and each column is composed of three parts extending from six to ten vertebral metomeres.

Long intrinsic muscles of the vertebral column

Muscle	Action	Origin	Insertion	Innervation
Iliocostalis				
• cervicis	Extension of the neck; lateral inclination of the neck (ipsilateral)	Costal angles from the first six ribs	Posterior tubercles of the transverse processes from C4 to C6	Posterior rami of the spinal nerves (from C1 to L5)
• lumborum				
– thoracic part	Extension of the trunk; lateral inclination of the trunk (ipsilateral)	External surface of the ribs from the sixth or seventh to the twelfth	Superior border of the costal angles from the first to the sixth or seventh ribs; posterior surface of the transverse process of C7	
– lumbar part	Extension of the trunk; lateral inclination of the trunk (ipsilateral)	Iliac tuberosity, outer lip of the iliac crest, posterior layer of the thoracolumbar fascia	Last eight ribs, near the costal angle	
Longissimus				
– capitis	Extension of the head and neck and lateral inclination of the neck (ipsilateral)	Transverse processes from T1 a T5; articular processes from C3 or C4 to C7	Mastoid process of the temporal bone	Posterior rami of the spinal nerves (from C1 to L5)
– cervicis	Extension and lateral inclination of the neck (ipsilateral)	Transverse processes from T1 to T5 or T6	Posterior tubercles of the transverse processes from C2 to C6	
– thoracis	Extension of the trunk and lateral inclination of the back (ipsilateral)	Spinous processes from L3 to L5 and dorsal surface of the sacrum; posterior layer of the thoracolumbar fascia	Apex of the transverse processes from T1 to T12 and external surface of the ribs, between the tubercles and costal angles, excluding the first; costal and accessory processes from L1 to L5	

(continued)

Long intrinsic muscles of the vertebral column (*continued*)

Muscle	Action	Origin	Insertion	Innervation
Spinalis				
– capitis	Extension of the head and neck	Spinous processes of C6, C7, T1 and T2	Squamous part of the occipital bone between the superior and inferior nuchal lines, merging with the semispinalis capitis	Posterior rami of the spinal nerves (from C1 to T12)
– cervicis	Extension and lateral inclination of the neck	Spinous processes of C6, C7, T1 and T2	Spinous processes from C1 or C2 to C3 or C4	
– thoracis	Extension and lateral inclination of the trunk	Spinous processes of T10, T11, T12, L1 and L2	Spinous processes from T1 to T8	
Transversospinales				
Semispinalis				
– capitis	Extension of the head; contralateral rotation of the head	Apices of the transverse processes of C7 and from T1 to T7; articular processes from C4 to C7	Medial part of the region between the superior and inferior nuchal lines of the occipital bone	Posterior rami of the spinal nerves (from C1 to L5)
– cervicis	Extension of the neck; contralateral rotation of the neck	Transverse processes from T1 to T6	Spinous processes from C1 or C2 to C5	
– thoracis	Extension of the trunk; contralateral rotation of the trunk	Transverse processes from T6 to T10	Spinous processes of C6 and C7 and from T1 to T4	

(*continued*)

Long intrinsic muscles of the vertebral column (*continued*)

Muscle	Action	Origin	Insertion	Innervation
Transversospinales				
Multifidus muscles	Extension of the trunk; contralateral rotation of the trunk (control of posture)	Intermediate sacral crest of the dorsal surface of the sacrum, mammillary and accessory processes of L1-L5, transverse processes of T1-T12, superior articular processes from C4 to C7	Spinous processes of the overlying vertebrae from one to four	Posterior rami of the spinal nerves (from C1 to L5)
Rotator muscles	Extension and contralateral rotation of the trunk (control of posture)	Superior and posterior surfaces of the transverse processes of the cervical and thoracic vertebrae and mammillary processes of the lumbar vertebrae	Base of the spinous process and inferior and lateral surfaces of the lamina of the overlying vertebra (breves) or subsequent vertebra (longi) in the cervical, thoracic and lumbar tracts of the vertebral column	Posterior rami of the spinal nerves (from C1 to L5)
Interspinales	Extension of the trunk (control of posture)	Short muscles between the spinous processes of contiguous vertebrae to the sides of the interspinous ligaments in the cervical, thoracic and lumbar tracts of the vertebral column		Posterior rami of the spinal nerves (from C1 to T3 and from T11 to L5)
Intertransversarii	Lateral inclination of the trunk (control of posture)	Short muscles between the transverse processes of contiguous vertebrae in the cervical, thoracic and lumbar tracts of the vertebral column		Anterior [C1-C8] and posterior (C1 to T1 and from T10 to L5) rami of the spinal nerves

5

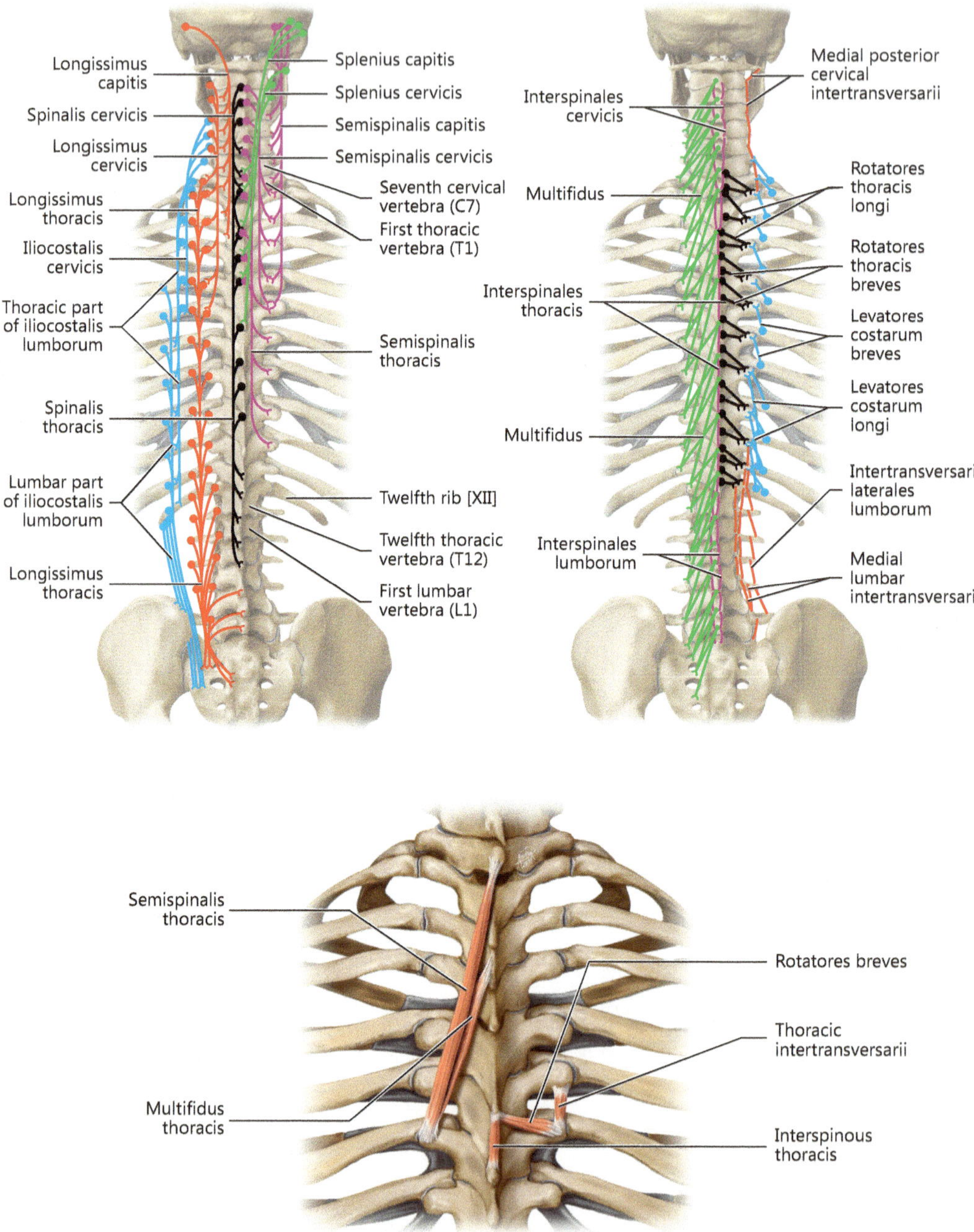

Long intrinsic muscles of the vertebral column.

Muscles of the abdomen

Muscle	Action	Origin	Insertion	Innervation
Iliopsoas	Flexion of the trunk forward (with the contralateral)	*Psoas major*: anterior surface of the transverse processes of L1-L5; lateral surface of the intervertebral bodies and the discs of T12, L1-L4 *Iliacus*: upper two-thirds of the iliac fossa, inner lip of the iliac crest; anterior sacroiliac and iliolumbar ligaments; upper part of the lateral surface of the sacrum	*Psoas major*: lesser trochanter of the femur *Iliacus*: lateral surface of the tendon of the psoas major; lesser trochanter of the femur	Branches of the lumbar plexus (principally L1, L2, with some contribution of L3) Branches of the lumbar plexus [L2, L3] and femoral nerve
Rectus abdominis	Flexion of the trunk forward (with the contralateral)	Xiphoid process (sometimes) and external surface of the fifth, sixth, and seventh costal cartilages	Superior pubic ramus	Last intercostal nerves (T6-T12 or T7-T12)
External oblique	Contralateral rotation of the trunk (by itself); flexion of the trunk forward (with the contralateral)	External surface and inferior border of the last eight ribs	Outer lip of the iliac crest, aponeurosis of the external oblique	Intercostal nerves, iliohypogastric nerve, and ilioinguinal nerve (T7-T12, and to a lesser degree L1)
Internal oblique	Ipsilateral rotation of the trunk (by itself); flexion of the trunk forward (with the contralateral)	Lateral third of the inguinal ligament, anterior superior iliac spine, intermediate line of the iliac crest, and thoracolumbar fascia	Inferior border of the last three costal cartilages, aponeurosis of the internal oblique	Intercostal nerves, iliohypogastric nerve, and ilioinguinal nerve (T7-T12, and to a much lesser degree L1)

5

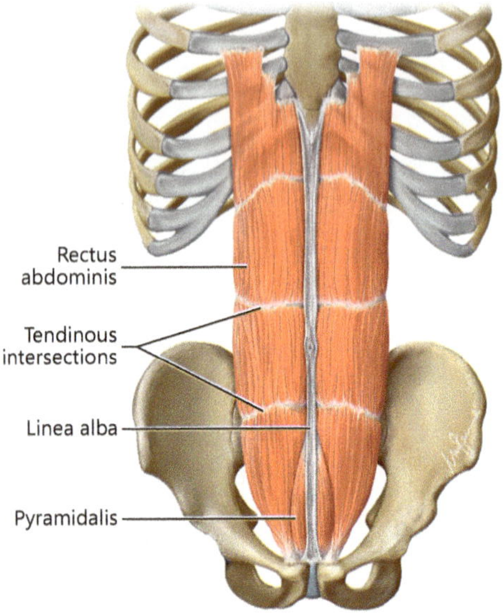

Rectus abdominis.

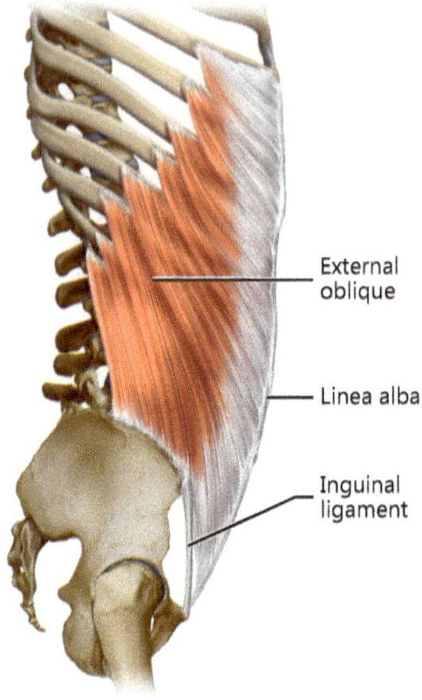

External oblique.

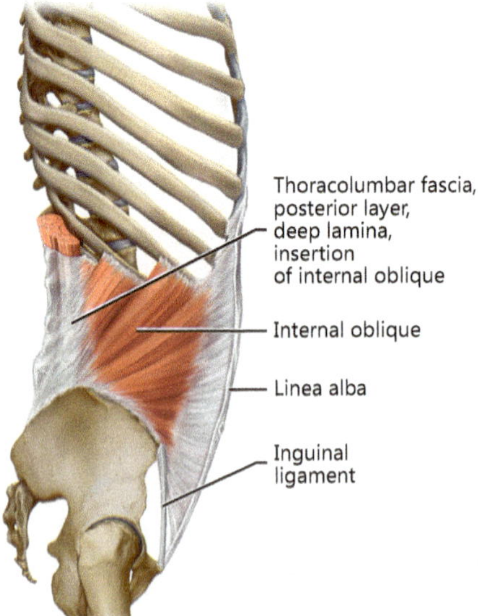

Internal oblique.

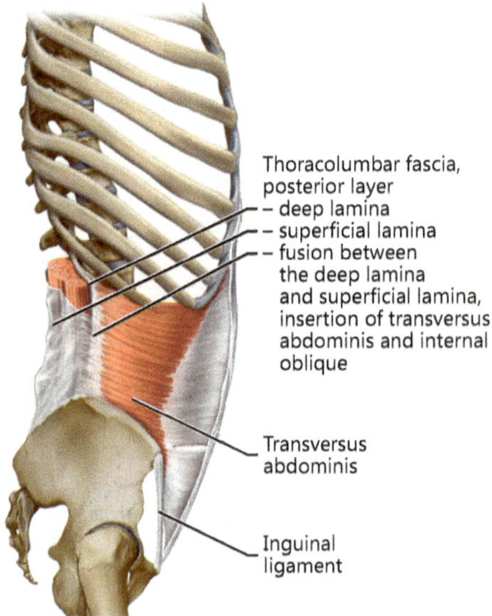

Transversus abdominis.

(For the iliopsoas, see Chapter 10 "Hip and pelvis").

Action of the muscles in the movements of the vertebral column and trunk

Extension of the vertebral column

Muscles:
- erector spinae (**7**)
  - iliocostalis lumborum (thoracic part, **1**; lumbar part, **2**)
  - longissimus (thoracis, **3**)
  - spinalis (thoracis, **4**)
- semispinalis (thoracis, **5**)
- multifidus (**6**)
- rotatores (fig. on page 182)
- intertransversarii (fig. on page 182)
- interspinales (fig. on page 186)

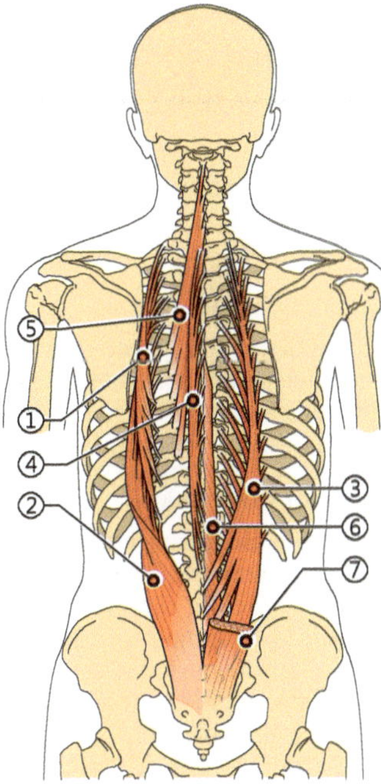

Functional aspects

- The extension of the column is the main function of the long intrinsic muscles of the vertebral column (all muscles participate when contracted bilaterally)
- The most metameric muscles (rotatores breves, interspinales and intertransversarii) extend two vertebrae (i.e., one FSU).

Extension of the trunk

- The long intrinsic muscles of the vertebral column initiate the extension of the trunk to achieve the upright position; the movement, if forced, continues successively thanks to the invention of the force of gravity and is controlled by the contraction of the abdominal muscles, which:
  - contract eccentrically throughout the movement, when the extension is against resistance (for example, when the trunk is extended to reach the light switch at the top of the bed from a prone position)
- When lifting an object from the ground from the forward flexed position:
  - there is no initial contraction of the long intrinsic muscles of the vertebral column; the thoracolumbar fascia, the elastic forces generated in the extensor muscles and the posterior intervertebral ligaments support the load and the extension movement occurs at the level of the hip joints, with the posterior rotation of the pelvis
  - successively the long intrinsic muscles of the vertebral column contract; contraction persists until the upright position is reached
  - the forces acting on the trunk during the lifting of objects from the ground, with forward flexion of the trunk, are particularly high, therefore, this type of position should be avoided, it is preferable to perform it with the back straight and having initially knees bent and the object to be lifted as close as possible to the body
- While lifting heavy loads, when strong forces are acting on the column, the abdominal muscles (primarily the transversus abdominis), the diaphragm and the intercostal muscles contract, generating an increase in intra-abdominal and intrathoracic pressure that transforms the thorax and abdomen into "semirigid cylinders":

- part of the stress due to the load is transferred, through the upper limbs, to the thorax and to the abdomen and then to the pelvis, lightening the load on the column
- there is additional strengthening of the trunk, with a moment of extensor force applied to the lumbar column through the activation of the transversus abdominis and the consequent increase in tension of the thoracolumbar fascia.

Anterior flexion of the vertebral column

Muscles:
- iliopsoas
- rectus abdominis
- external oblique
- internal oblique

Functional aspects

- In the flexion of the vertebral column, the rectus abdominis muscles act initially, and then the internal and external oblique muscles, as well as the iliopsoas
- There is a greater muscular effort in the flexion of the vertebral column from the supine position with respect to the orthostatic one.

Flexion of the trunk

- The abdominal muscles contract throughout the movement when flexion of the trunk occurs against resistance, such as that exerted by body weight:
  - they therefore represent the agonist muscles when, for example, getting up from bed from the supine position
- In the supine position, the rectus abdominis is the most active of the abdominal muscles when the head is raised, contracting in order to stabilize the thorax
- The muscles of abdomen contract isometrically and stabilize the thorax and pelvis in thrusting, traction and lifting activities
- In the upright position, the trunk flexes when lifting an object from the ground or, for example, tying shoelaces:
  - the flexion of the trunk begins with the contraction of the muscles of the abdomen and the vertebral part of the iliopsoas;
  - after the trunk has bent forward, the force of gravity intervenes to continue the flexion, which is controlled by the contraction of the long intrinsic muscles of the vertebral column until the "critical position", in which they relax and further flexion of the trunk occurs through the hip muscles
  - the posterior layer of the thoracolumbar fascia, the elastic forces generated in the extensor muscles as a result of their passive stretching and the posterior intervertebral ligaments support the trunk in a fully flexed position during the relaxation of the muscles of the vertebral column
  - if flexion is forced further, the muscles of the abdomen intervene again by contracting once the movement is completed.

Lateral inclination of the vertebral column

Muscles:
- iliocostalis lumborum (thoracic part)
- longissimus (thoracis)
- spinalis (thoracis)
- intertransversarii
- interspinales
- external oblique
- internal oblique
- quadratus lumborum
- iliopsoas

(See Chapter 10 "Hip and pelvis" for the origin, insertion and action of the quadratus lumborum and iliopsoas).

Functional aspects

- Unilateral contraction of the long intrinsic muscles of the vertebral column and the quadratus lumborum and iliopsoas with a direct action on the vertebral column
- Unilateral contraction of the external oblique and internal oblique with an indirect action on the vertebral column
- Ipsilateral contraction at the beginning of the movement and contralateral contraction when returning to the upright position
- The lateral inclination of the trunk is not frequent during everyday activity. It occurs, for example, when lifting an object laterally from a low plane or when sitting on the edge of a bed starting from lateral decubitus and vice versa.

5

Rotation of the vertebral column

Direct

Muscles:
- ipsilateral rotatores
  - iliocostalis lumborum (thoracic part)
  - longissimus (thoracis)
- contralateral rotatores
  - rotatores
  - multifidus
  - semispinalis (thoracis)

Indirect

Muscles:
- external oblique
- internal oblique
- transversus abdominis
- levatores costarum

(See Chapter 6 "Thorax and thoracic column" for the origin, insertion and action of the levatores costarum).

Functional aspects

- Ipisilateral rotation by the levatores costarum
- Contralateral rotation by the transversus abdominis
- Synergistic action of the internal oblique (ipsilateral rotation by the internal oblique and contralateral rotation by the external oblique)
- The extensor muscles of the trunk counterbalance the moment of a flexion force generated by the oblique muscles
- Contraction of the rotatores of the trunk, for example, during changes of position in decubitus and when turning to look behind.

Assessment of trunk mobility

Measurement of trunk joint mobility

Flexion of the thoracolumbar column

Measurement of the distance between the spinous processes of C7 and S2:
- first in standing position
- after the limit of the flexion of the thoracolumbar column.

The difference between the two measurements is the range of joint motion when flexing the trunk (approximately 10 cm).

Extension of the thoracolumbar column

Measurement of the distance between the spinous processes of C7 and S2:
- first in standing position
- after the limit of the extension of the thoracolumbar column.

The difference between the two measurements is the range of joint motion when extending the trunk (approximately 2.5 cm).

Alternatively, the distance between the jugular notch and the edge of the examination table can be measured after the subject, in a prone position on the examination table, with hands grasping the edges and a cushion under the abdomen, raises the trunk backward, extending the elbows to the limit of the extension movement of the thoracolumbar column.

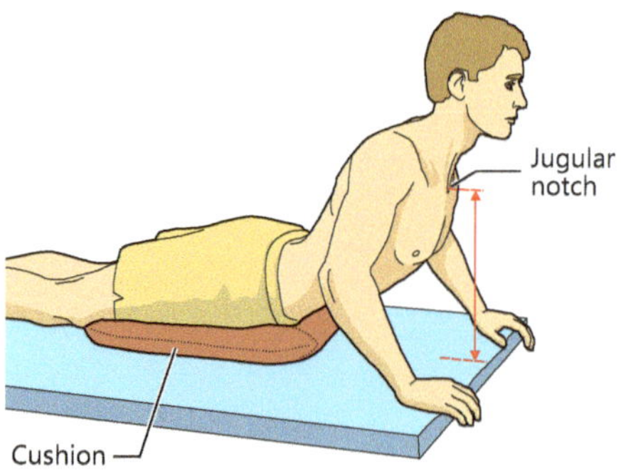

Flexion-extension of the lumbar column (modified Schober's test)

In the upright position, a point 10 cm above the spinous processes of the S2 is marked.

Measure this distance:
- after flexion of the thoracolumbar column, from the upright position, up to the limit of movement allowed
- after extension of the thoracolumbar column, from the upright position, up to the limit of movement allowed.

The difference between the two measurements is the range of joint motion when flexing the lumbar column and when extending the lumbar column, respectively.

Lateral inclination of the trunk

Measurement of the distance between the tip of the middle finger and the floor, after lateral inclination of the trunk from the upright position.

Rotation of the trunk

Visual measurement of the rotation of the trunk with the subject under examination in a sitting position with the trunk upright and arms cross over the thorax until the limit of movement allowed (45° amplitude).

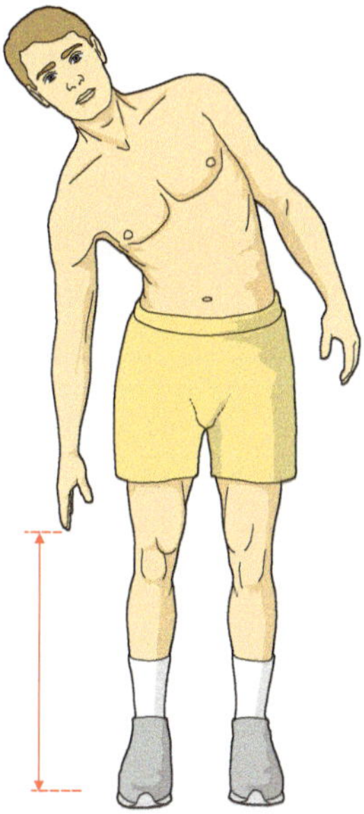

Measurement of the length of the extensor muscles of the trunk (touch the toes test)

Measurement of the distance between the tip of the middle finger of both hands and the tip of the great toe of both feet from the upright position, after flexion of the trunk and hips up to the limit of movement allowed.

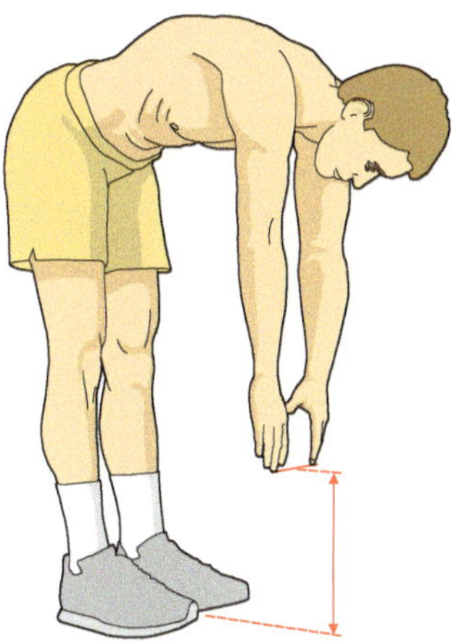

Normal joint mobility of the trunk in flexion if there is contact between the index finger and the great toe.

Measurement of the degrees of force of the flexor, extensor and rotator muscles of the trunk

Flexion of the trunk

Rectus abdominis

Starting position	Supine position on the examination table with the lower limbs flexed
Movement	Posterior inclination (retroversion) of the pelvis with flexion of the lumbar column
Degree	0 – Non-palpable contraction; no movement 1 – Weak palpable muscle contraction when the patient tries to raise the head or when coughing, without any other type of movement (palpation of the muscle next to the midline on the anterior abdominal wall, at the midpoint between the sternum and the pubis) 2 – Posterior inclination of the pelvis with flexion of the lumbar column, then flexion of the cervical column and, successively, flexion of the thoracic column; raising the head and the scapulae from the examination table with the upper limbs along the trunk 3 – As in 2 but with the arms extended in front of the trunk and the movement carried out slowly 4 – As in 2 but with the arms crossed over the chest 5 – As in 2 but with the hands behind the ears

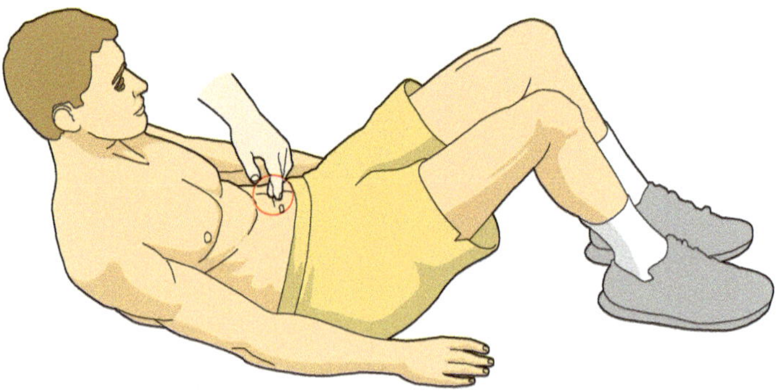

Extension of the trunk

Long intrinsic muscles of the vertebral column

Starting position	Prone position with the feet beyond the end of the examination table and a cushion under the abdomen
Movement	Extension of the trunk
Degree	0 – Non-palpable contraction; no movement 1 – Weak palpable muscle contraction when the patient tries to raise the head, without any other type of movement 2 – Raising the head and the upper part of the sternum with the upper limbs along the trunk 3 – Extension of the trunk and raising the head and the sternum, including the xiphoid process, with hands placed behind the back 4 – As in 3 but with the hands behind the lower back 5 – As in 3 but with the hands behind the head
Palpation	Adjacent to the thoracic or lumbar spinous processes (palpation of the paravertebral muscles)

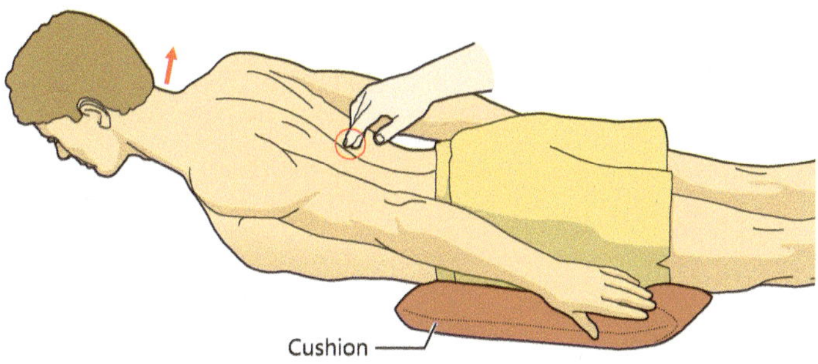

Rotation of the trunk

External oblique and internal oblique

Starting position	Supine position with the lower limbs flexed (measured against gravity)
Movement	Flexion and rotation of the trunk with the arms extended in front of the trunk; the movement is carried out slowly
Degree	4 – The arms are crossed over the trunk during the movement 5 – Elbows bent with the hands behind the ears during the movement
Palpation	External oblique: inferior border of the thoracic cage Internal oblique: medially and above the anterior superior iliac spine

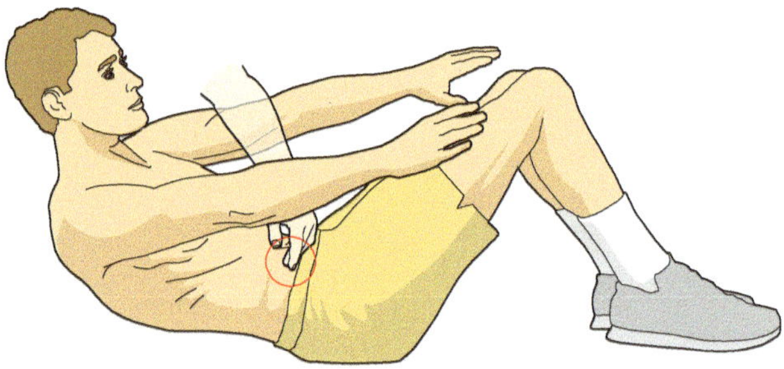

Without gravity

Starting position	Sitting position with the hands on the edge of the examination table and the feet resting on a stool (measurement without gravity)
Movement	Rotation and slight flexion of the thorax
Palpation	External oblique: inferior border of the thoracic cage Internal oblique: medially and above the anterior superior iliac spine

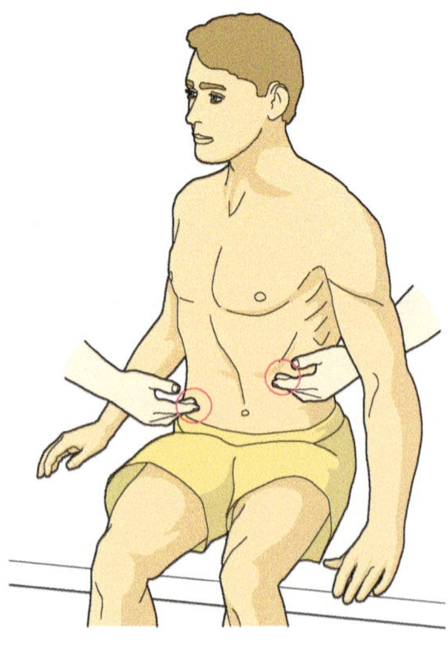

Functional mobility of the trunk

Flexion and extension of the trunk

- It contributes to increase the lumbar mobility of the vertebral column in everyday activities
- Combined with the mobility of the cervical and thoracic segments of the vertebral column, they allow the individual to reach the distal extremities of the body and objects in the surrounding space with their hands
- The last degrees of functional mobility of the lumbar column are obtained with the participation of the hips and pelvis
- The coordinated movement of the lumbar and pelvic regions ensures regular movements of the lower limbs and the trunk with wide mobility
- The coordinated group of movements between the lumbar column and the pelvis (lumbopelvic rhythm) occurs during forward flexion of the trunk to touch the toes with the hands:
  - the first part of this movement is represented by the lumbar flexion, followed by the anterior flexion of the pelvis, which concludes the movement
  - when returning to the upright position, the pelvis rotates posteriorly followed by the extension of the lumbar column
- The joint range of motion in the lumbar flexion is approximately 60° (the movement carried out when sitting down to put on socks and squatting down to pick up an object from the floor are examples of activities that require almost complete flexion of the lumbar column, corresponding to 90% and 95% of all flexion movement, respectively)
- The passage from the upright position to a sitting position and the return to the upright position requires from approximately 56-66% of the entire range of motion of lumbar flexion.

Rotation of the trunk

- It is carried out with the mobile components of the thoracic and lumbar columns and is associated with a slight lateral inclination
- The movement, freer in the upper spinal segments and increasingly reduced in the lower segments, extends the range of action of the hands beyond the opposite side of the body and allows the individual to move in different directions without moving the feet.

5

Anatomical landmarks on the surface of the trunk

1	Jugular (suprasternal) notch: rounded depression at the superior border of the sternum, between the medial ends of the clavicles
2	Xiphoid process: inferior part of the body of the sternum
3	Anterior superior iliac spine (left and right): rounded bony prominence at the anterior end of the iliac crest
4	Iliac crest: superior border of the iliac part of the hip bone; convex bony margins whose apex is located at the level of the space between the spinous processes of L4 and L5
5	Posterior superior iliac spine (left and right): rounded bony prominence at the posterior end of the iliac crest, palpable beneath the skin in the dimples located on the proximal surface of the buttocks
6	Spinous process of S2: on the central point of a line connecting the two posterior superior iliac spines
7	Inferior angle of the scapula: at the lowest point of the medial border of the scapula
8	Spine of the scapula: bony margin that obliquely crosses the upper four-fifths of the scapula
9	Spinous process of T8: on the median line between the two inferior angles of the scapula
10	Spinous process of T3: in the middle of a line between the origins of the spines of the scapula
11	Spinous process of C7: the most prominent spinous process, situated at the base of the neck

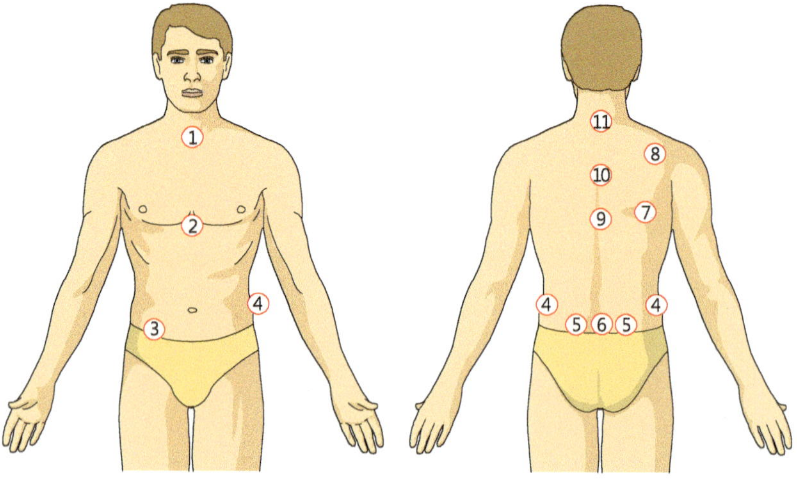

Thoracic cage

- Sternum
- Ribs
- Thoracic column.

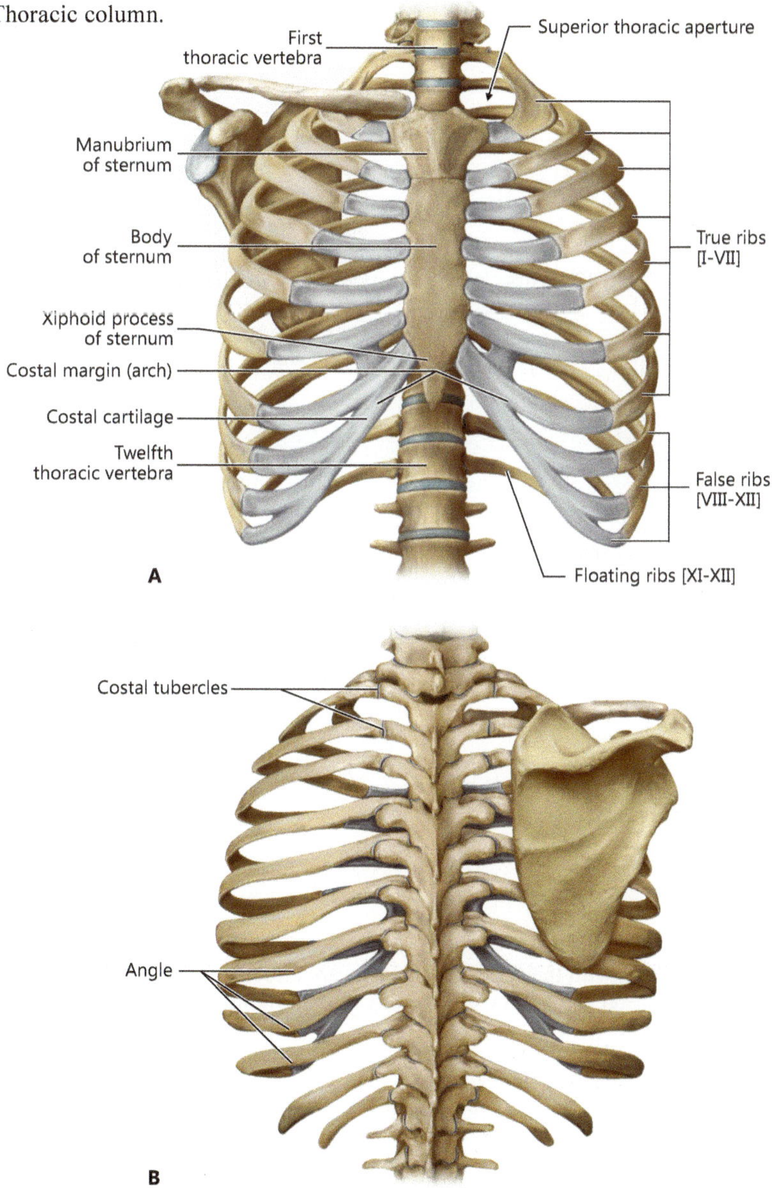

Thoracic cage, anterior view (**A**) and posterior view (**B**).

Sternum

- Manubrium
- Body
- Sternal angle or angle of Louis (dihedral angle open posteriorly between the manubrium and the body)
- Xiphoid process.

Ribs

- True ribs → first 7 pairs → Articulated directly with the sternum
- False ribs → 8th, 9th and 10th pairs → Articulated indirectly with the sternum through the 7th rib and are joined to each other and with the 7th rib through the costal cartilages
- Floating ribs → 11th and 12th pairs → Not articulated with the sternum, free in front

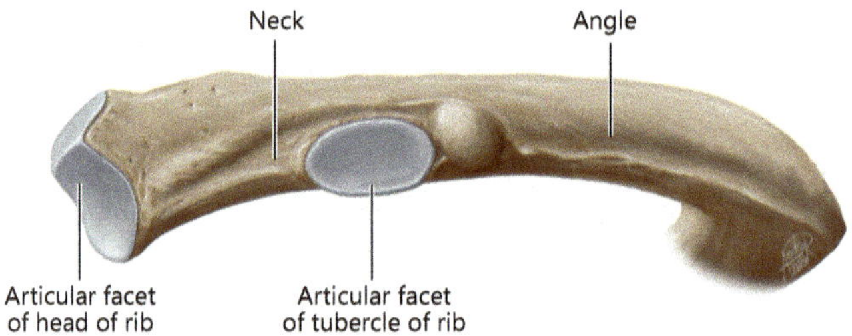

Rib, dorsal view.

Morphology

- Head (with articular facets)
- Neck
- Tubercle (with articular facet)
- Angle
- Body
- Costal cartilage.

Orientation of the ribs

- From the point of joint with the vertebrae, the ribs are directed inferiorly outward
- At the level of the costal angle, they change direction, heading superiorly inward.

During their course they describe two curves:
- external convex curve (caused by the rib's trajectory)
- torsion curve (during the rib's trajectory) by which the convex surface is directed:
  - posteriorly downward
  - anteriorly upward.

Thoracic column

Thoracic vertebrae

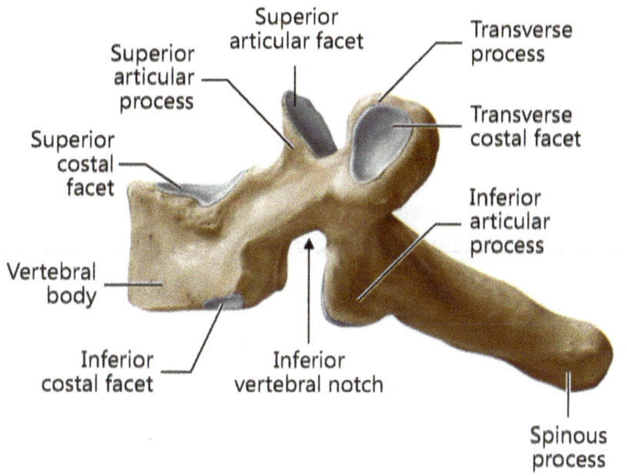

Thoracic vertebra, lateral view.

- Vertebral body – increases in height from the 1st to the 12th
- Intervertebral disc – the increase in its height is not proportional to that of the body, therefore its width is reduced compared to the height (hence the reduced mobility of the thoracic column compared to the cervical column)
- Costal demifacet:
  - superior – on the superior border of the vertebral body
  - inferior – on the inferior border of the vertebral body
  - from the 9th to the 12th thoracic vertebra, the costal facets move towards the center
  - the 10th, 11th and 12th only have one demifacet
- Spinous process – elongated and directly oblique downwards:
  - from the 2nd to the 4th thoracic vertebra, the apex of the spinous process is located two fingers lower than the transverse process
  - from the 5th to the 9th thoracic vertebra, the apex of the spinous process is located three fingers lower than the transverse process
- Transverse process – developed and directed lateroposteriorly with the costal facet of the transverse process to the anterior extremity:
  - angle variable from 35° (first thoracic vertebrae) to 55° (last thoracic vertebrae) with respect to the frontal plane
- Superior and inferior articular processes:
  - 20° angle with respect to the frontal plane
  - angle variable from 60° (first thoracic vertebrae) to 80° (T12) with respect to the horizontal plane.

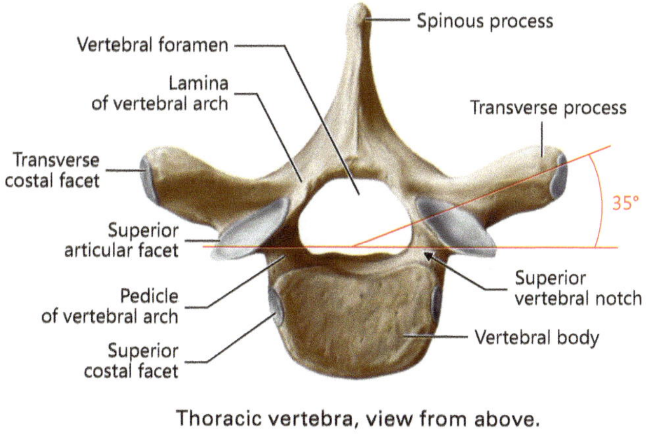

Thoracic vertebra, view from above.

Radiology

Anteroposterior projection:

- the pedicles of the vertebral arches appear as oval shadows on the sides of the column
- the vertebral canal increases in width in the craniocaudal direction.

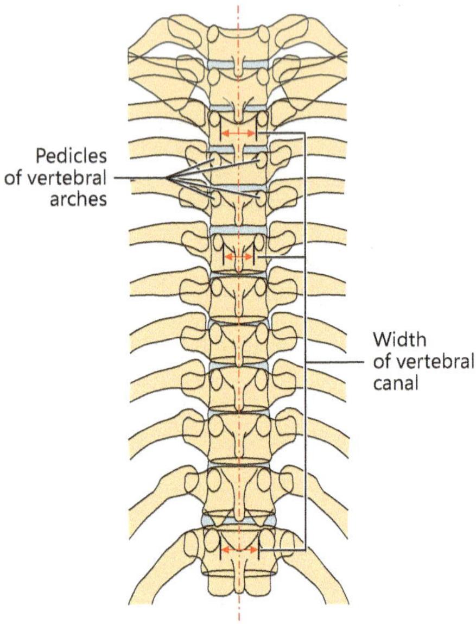

Lateral projection:

- if one traces lines perpendicular to the superior and inferior borders respectively, of the vertebral bodies of T3 and T11, the acute angle formed by the orthogonal to these perpendicular lines has a width of 25° (kyphosis angle)
- the height of the intervertebral discs increases in the craniocaudal direction.

Note: the following are considered normal: a cervical lordosis of 35°, a dorsal kyphosis of 35° and a lumbar lordosis of 40°.

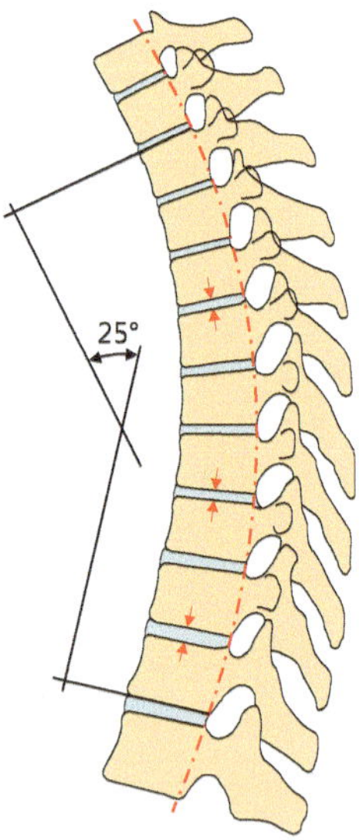

Ligaments

(See Chapter 5 "Vertebral column and movements of the trunk").

Motions

Flexion

T1-T4 moderate
T4-T8 moderate
T8-T12 good

Extension

T1-T4 moderate
T4-T8 very moderate
T8-T12 good

Lateral inclination

T1-T4 moderate
T4-T8 good
T8-T12 very good

Rotation

T1-T4 very moderate
T4-T8 good
T8-T12 very good

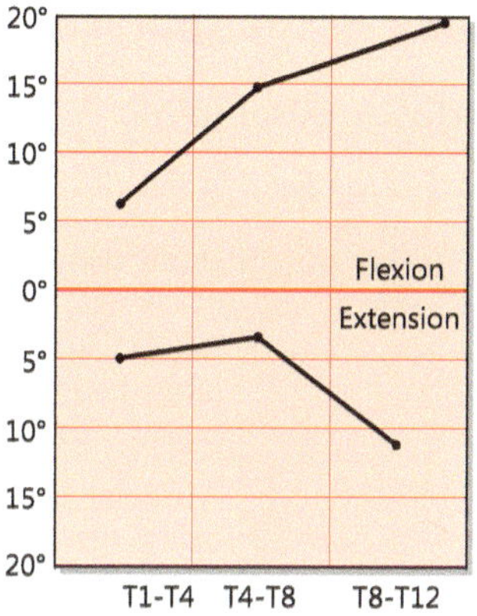

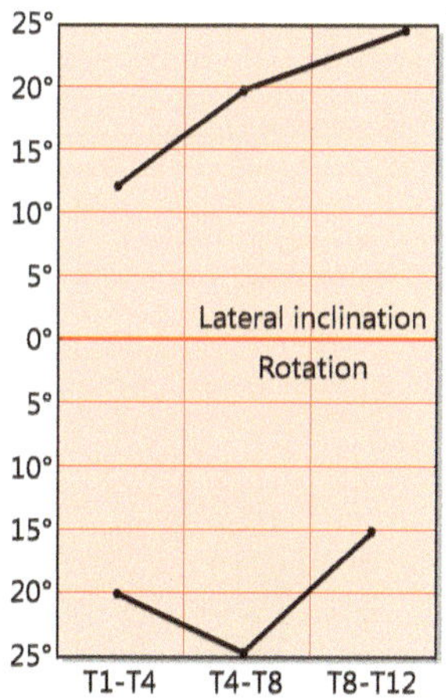

Functional considerations:

- the mobility of the thoracic column is limited by the joints with the thorax (even if the costal cartilages are sufficiently elastic)
- the T9-T12 segment has greater mobility than the superior segment, partly due to the increase in deformability associated with the greater extension of the cartilaginous components
- the flexion is limited by:
  - the posterior ligamentous structures
  - the anulus fibrosus
- the extension is limited by:
  - the superior reinforcement ligaments of the joint capsule
  - the anterior longitudinal ligament
  - the anulus fibrosus
  - the contact between the spinous processes
- the rotation causes:
  - variations in the shape of the ipsilateral and contralateral ribs (increase in the posterior curvature and flattening of the anterior curvature on the side of rotation, the opposite contralaterally)
  - the oblique position of the sternum.

From a functional perspective, the upper thoracic column is associated to the cervical column, as can be observed during the assessment of joint mobility of the cervical column, the motion of which is followed by that of the upper thoracic column. Functional alterations of the latter can radiate to the nape, shoulders and upper limbs.

6

Joints of the thoracic cage

Costovertebral joints

Joints of the head of the ribs

Articular surfaces	Demifacet located inferiorly on the posterolateral surface of the body of the overlying thoracic vertebra (inferior costal facet) Demifacet located superiorly on the posterolateral surface of the body of the overlying thoracic vertebra (inferior costal facet) Intervertebral disc located between the two demifacets Articular facet of the head of the rib divided into two parts by a ridge Exceptions: – 1st thoracic vertebra: superior facet and inferior demifacet – 10th thoracic vertebra: a single superior demifacet – 11th and 12th thoracic vertebrae: a single facet, superior and central, respectively
Type of joint	Simple plane joints (plane surfaces) 10th, 11th and 12th Double plane joints 1st-9th

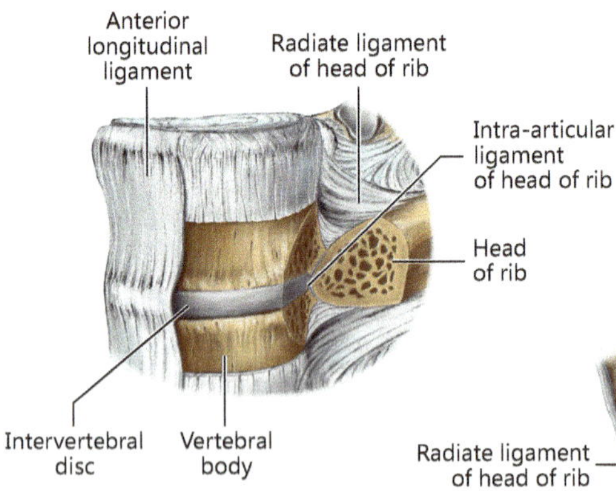

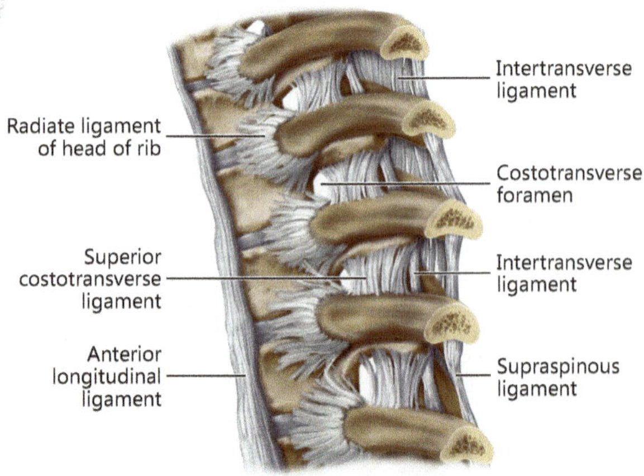

Joints of the head of the ribs.

Costotransverse joints

Articular surfaces	Articular facets of the costal tubercles (slightly convex) at the boundary between the body and neck of the ribs Articular facets of the transverse processes (costal facets) (slightly concave) located laterally Exceptions: – not present in the 11th and 12th ribs
Type of joint	Plane joints

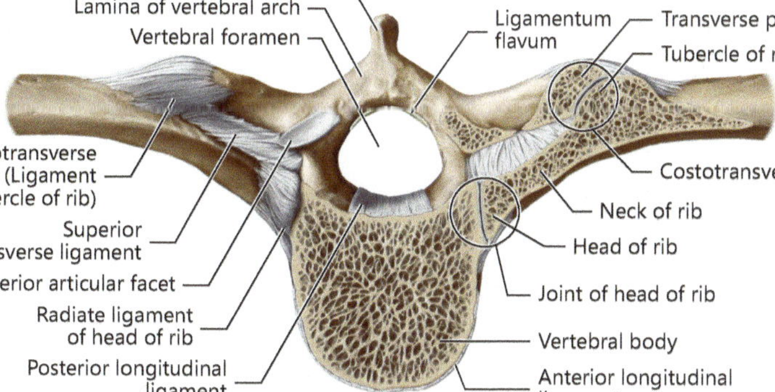

Costovertebral joints.

Ligaments

Joints of the head of the ribs:

- radiate ligament of the head of the rib (between the head of the rib and the vertebral bodies – 3 bundles: superior and inferior, directed to the bodies of the superior and inferior vertebrae; middle, directed to the intervertebral disc)
- intra-articular ligament of the head of the rib (between the crest of the head of the rib and the intervertebral disc).

Costotransverse joints:

- costotransverse ligament (between the posterior surface of the neck of the rib and the transverse process)
- lateral costotransverse ligament (between the posterior surface of the neck of the rib and the apex of the transverse process)
- superior costotransverse ligament (between the superior border of the neck of the lower rib and the inferior border of the transverse process of the superior vertebra)
- lumbocostal ligament (between the 12th rib and the transverse process of L1).

The joint of the head of the rib is closely connected, through ligaments, to the corresponding functional spinal unit (FSU), therefore treatment of rib disorders should also be extended to the corresponding FSU and vice versa.

6

Sternocostal joints

Articular surfaces	Sternal extremities of the costal cartilages of the first seven ribs Costal notches of the sternum
Type of joint	1st, 6th and 7th ribs: synchondrosis 2nd-5th ribs: plane joints

Ligaments

- Radiate sternocostal ligament (from the costal cartilages to the anterior surface of the sternum, where it widens, assuming a fan shape)
- Intra-articular sternocostal ligaments (within the sternocostal joints, from the 2nd to the 5th)
- Costoxiphoid ligaments (from the costal cartilages to the xiphoid process).

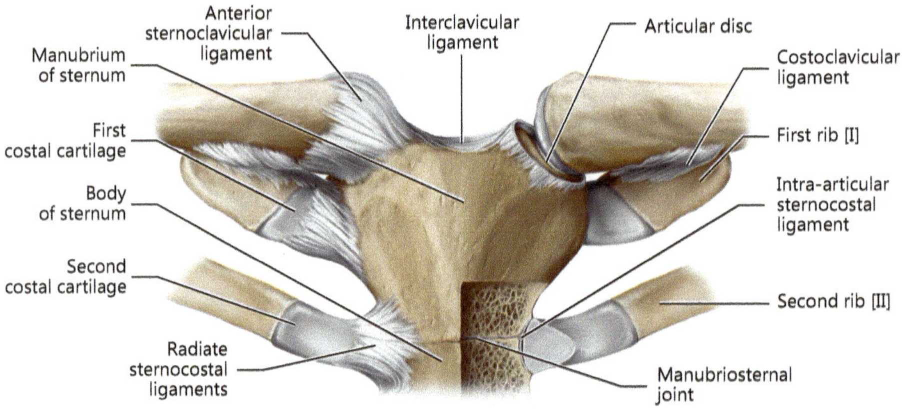

Sternocostal joints.

Interchondral joints

Articular surfaces	Costal cartilages of the 6th-7th, 7th-8th, 8th-9th, 9th-10th ribs Flat sternal facets
Type of joint	Plane joints

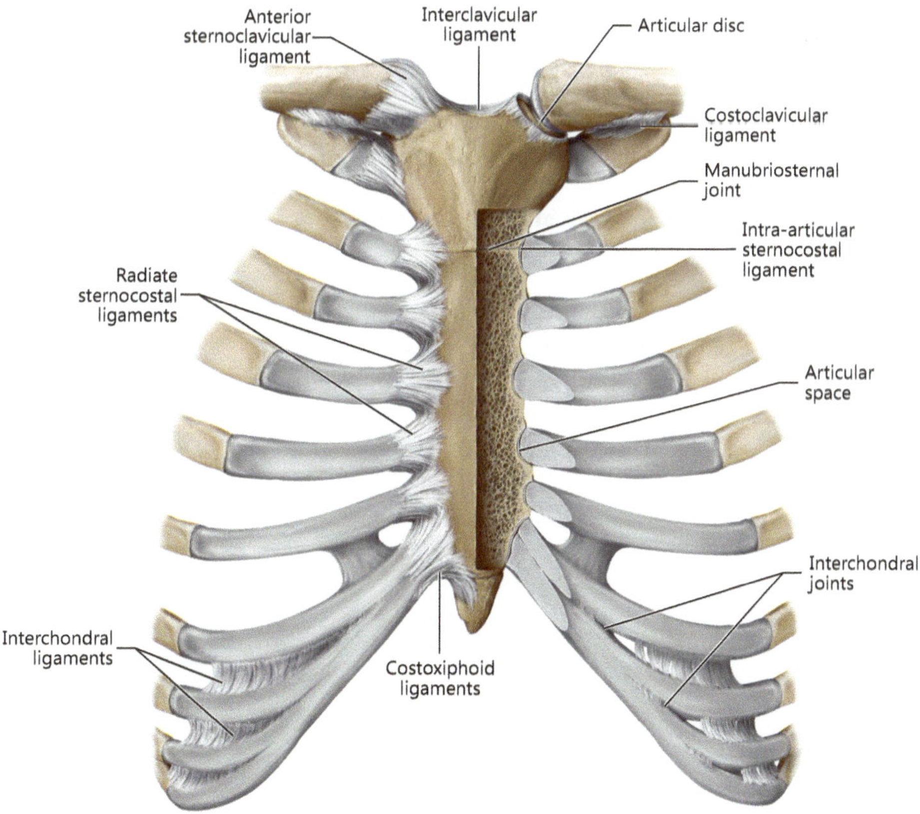

Sternocostal and interchondral joints.

Intersternal joints

- Between the manubrium and the body of sternum (amphiarthrosis)
- Between the body of sternum and the xiphoid process (synchondrosis).

Movements of the ribs

Each rib moves around three joints:
- joint of the head of the rib (posterior joint – quite rigid)
- costotransverse joint (posterior joint – quite rigid)
- sternocostal joint (anterior joint – quite deformable due to the presence of cartilaginous components).

The movement of the rib takes place around the **axis of the two posterior joints**.
It is identified by an ideal line that joins the costovertebral and costotransverse joints (on both sides) and corresponds to the longitudinal axis of the neck of the rib. Its orientation determines the direction of the rib.

Orientation of the longitudinal axis of the neck of the rib

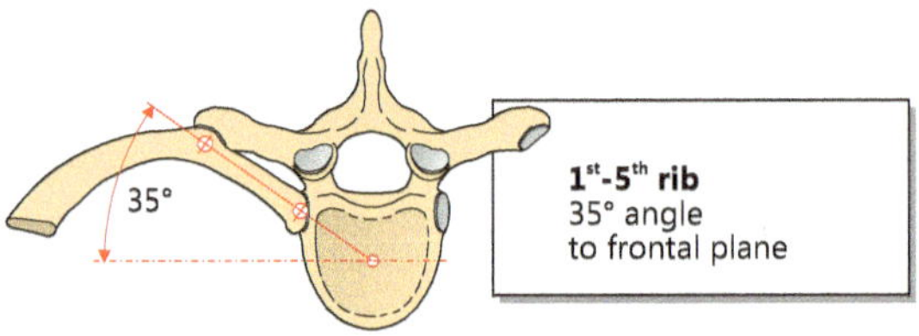

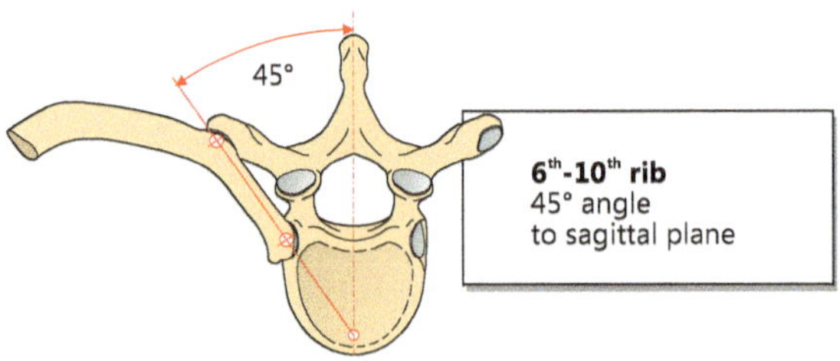

In general, the orientation of this line is:
- in an almost frontal plane in the upper ribs
- in a plane forming an angle of 45° with the frontal or sagittal plane in the intermediate ribs
- in an almost sagittal plane in the lower ribs.

During elevation of the ribs, the following occurs:

- a movement in the anterosuperior direction of the ribs, from the 1st to the 5th, which determines an increase mainly in the sagittal (anteroposterior) diameter of the thoracic cage and, to a lesser extent, in the transverse diameter
- a movement in the lateroanterior direction of the ribs, from the 5th to the 10th, which determines an increase mainly in the transverse diameter of the thoracic cage and, to a lesser extent, in the sagittal diameter.

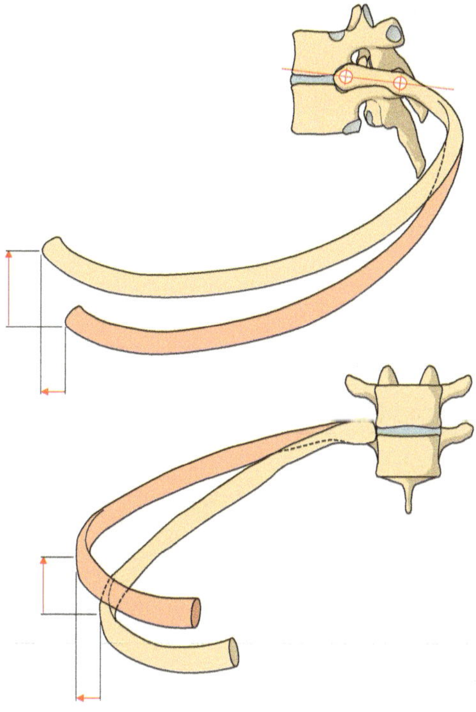

In general:

- at the level of the upper ribs, there is a greater increase in the sagittal diameter of the thoracic cage (especially between the 2nd and 3rd ribs)
- at the level of the intermediate and lower ribs, there is a greater increase in the transverse diameter with expansion of the ribs from the front to outwards at the level of the:
  - anterior axillary line, between the 4th and 6th ribs
  - midaxillary line, between the 6th and 7th ribs
  - posterior axillary line, between the 8th and 9th ribs.

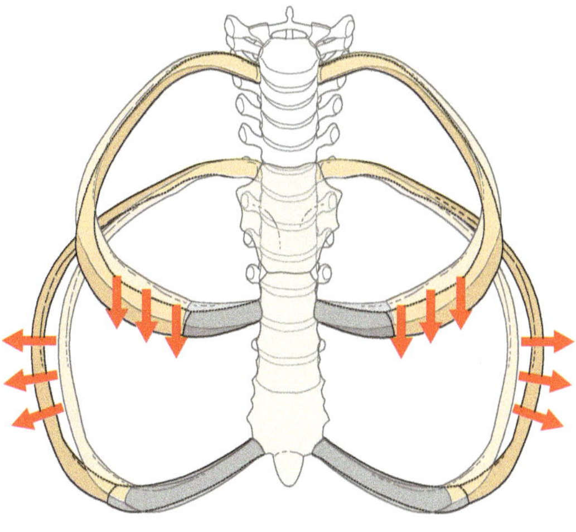

Movement of the costotransverse joints and the head of the ribs during elevation of the ribs

1st to 5th ribs	
• Costotransverse joints	Sliding downward and rotation around the intra-articular ligament of the head of the rib
• Joints of the head of the ribs	Sliding downward and rotation around the intra-articular ligament of the head of the rib
6th-10th ribs	
• Costotransverse joints	Sliding upward and backward
• Joints of the head of the ribs	Sliding downward

The lateral costotransverse ligament runs almost perpendicular to the longitudinal axis of the neck of the rib and the rotation movements of the costotransverse joints and the head of the ribs cause its traction, leading to possible alterations of the ligament insertions in the upper thoracic segments over time. On the other hand, in the lower thoracic segments, the same joints are exposed to arthritic alterations when subjected to continuous traction.

Sternocostal joints

During elevation of the ribs, there is a rotation of these joints that pushes the inferior border of the ribs upward and forward on the anterior costal part, and upward and outward on the posterior costal part.

Sternum

During elevation of the ribs, due to the effect of their movement, the sternum is displaced in the anterosuperior direction. The sternal angle (angle of Louis) also increases.

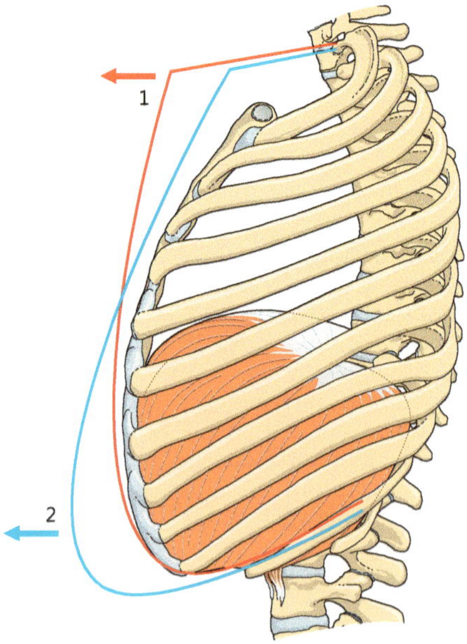

Two different interpretations of thoracic expansion (especially at the sternum level): red line (1) according to Kapandji, blue line (2) according to Forni and Cappellini.

Respiratory muscles

Inspiratory muscles

- Main muscles:
  - diaphragm
  - external intercostal muscles
  - scalene muscles

- Secondary (accessory) muscles:
  - sternocleidomastoid
  - levatores costarum
  - serratus posterior superior
  - subclavius
  - pectoralis minor and pectoralis major → see Chapter 7 "Shoulder and pectoral girdle"
  - serratus anterior → see Chapter 7 "Shoulder and pectoral girdle"
  - latissimus dorsi → see Chapter 7 "Shoulder and pectoral girdle"
  - trapezius → see Chapter 7 "Shoulder and pectoral girdle"
  - levator scapulae → see Chapter 7 "Shoulder and pectoral girdle"
  - long intrinsic muscles of the vertebral column (erectors of the trunk) → see Chapter 5 "Vertebral column and movements of the trunk".

Inspiratory muscles

Muscle	Action	Origin	Insertion	Innervation
Diaphragm	The neural stimulus coming from the respiratory centers determines the contraction of three groups of muscle fascicles, which cause the flattening of the diaphragm, which descends from the 4th to the 6th rib (2 intercostal spaces on the left, 1 or 1.5 intercostal spaces on the right) for about 5 cm. The widening of the ribs tenses the muscle fibers, favoring their contraction. The three groups of muscle fascicles (origins) act as a fixed point until the muscle encounters, by flattening, the splenic organs which oppose resistance. In this phase, the fixed point is inverted and moves towards the central tendon, which, exerting traction on the ribs, increases the three thoracic diameters.	*Sternal part*: fascicles of fibers originating from the posterior surface of the xiphoid process of the sternum *Costal part*: fascicles of fibers originating from the ribs (from the 7th to the 12th) *Lumbar part*: fascicles of fibers consisting of two crura on each side: – right medial crus: originates from the bodies of the first four lumbar vertebrae – left medial crus: originates from the bodies of the first three lumbar vertebrae – lateral crura: originates from two fibrous arches – medial lumbocostal (arch of the psoas major) and lateral lumbocostal (arch of the quadratus lumborum)	Central tendon of the diaphragm (central fibrous body)	Phrenic nerve [C3-C5] (the peripheral part of the muscle receives sensory fibers from the last six or seven intercostal nerves, T6-T12)
External intercostal muscles	The obliquity of the lever arm allows the ribs to rise. They come into action only when they are already under tension, produced by the upward traction of the ribs induced by the diaphragm	Inferior border of the superior rib. They cover externally, from the costal cartilage to the costal tubercles (before the costotransverse joint), the eleven intercostal spaces, with an oblique direction from back to front and from top to bottom and medially	Superior border of the lower rib	Intercostal nerves [T1-T12]
Levatores costarum	Each muscle elevates the underlying rib (short levator) or the successive rib (long levator). To this action is added that of ipsilateral rotation, if contracted on one side only, and that of the extension of the vertebral column, if contracted on both sides	Transverse processes from C7 to T11	Costal angles	Posterior rami of the thoracic nerves [T1-T12]

(continued)

Inspiratory muscles (*continued*)

Muscle	Action	Origin	Insertion	Innervation
Scalene muscles	They extend between the cervical column and the first ribs. With fixed point on the cervical column, they raise the first ribs acting as inspiratory muscles. They contract during normal respiration and during forced inspiration	*Anterior*: anterior tubercles of the transverse processes from C3 to C6	Tubercle of the scalene muscle on the internal border of the 1st rib and crest on the superior surface of the rib anteriorly to the groove for the subclavian artery	Anterior rami of the cervical nerves [C4-C6]
		Medius: transverse process of the axis; anterior surface of the posterior tubercles of the transverse processes from C3 to C7	Superior surface of the 1st rib between the costal tubercle and the groove for the subclavian artery	Anterior rami of the cervical nerves [C3-C8]
		Posterior: posterior tubercles of the transverse processes from C4 to C6	Lateral surface of the 2nd rib	Anterior rami of the cervical nerves [C6-C8]
Sternocleido-mastoid	It acts as an accessory inspiratory muscle, together with the suprahyoid and infrahyoid muscles, being recruited during forced inspiration, for example, during physical activity	*Sternal head*: superior surface of the manubrium of the sternum *Clavicular head*: superior surface of the medial third of the clavicle	Lateral surface of the mastoid process; lateral half of the superior nuchal line	Spinal root of the accessory nerve [XI] and branches of the cervical plexus (C2, C3 and sometimes C4)
Serratus posterior superior	It is an accessory inspiratory muscle	Transverse processes from C6 to T2	Superior border of the ribs from the 2nd to the 5th, just beyond the costal angle	Intercostal nerves [T2-T5]
Subclavius	It has a modest function as an accessory inspiratory muscle	Inferior surface of the clavicle (laterally)	Anterosuperior surface of the 1st sternocostal articulation	Nerve to the subclavius [C5, C6]

6

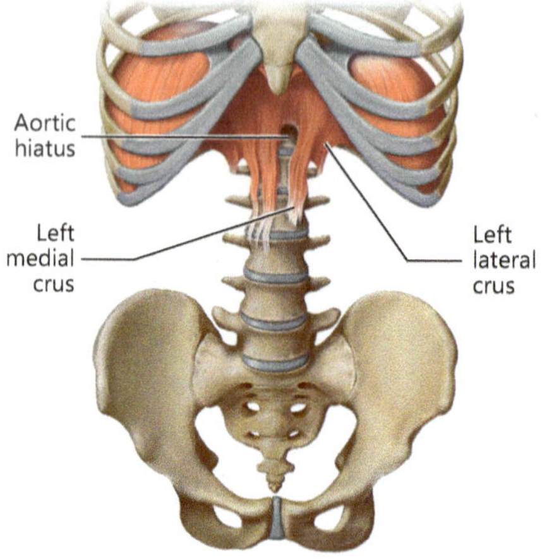

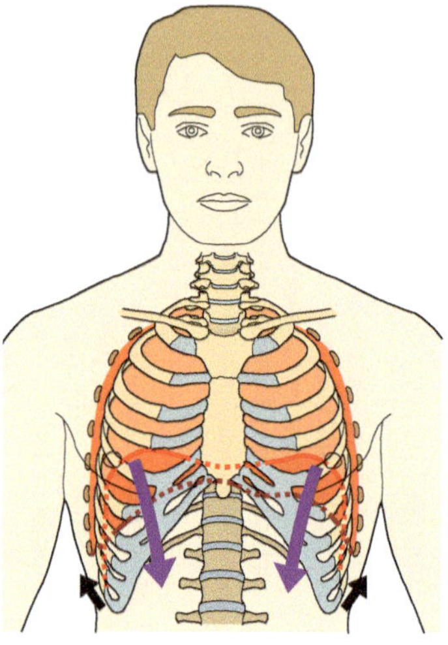

Diaphragm and its action in respiration.

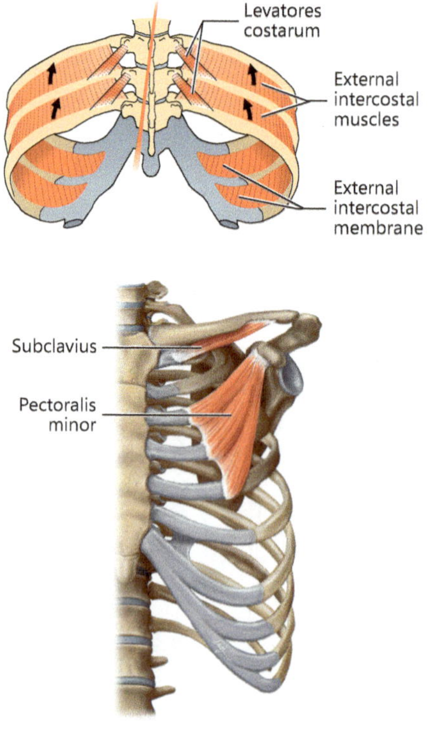

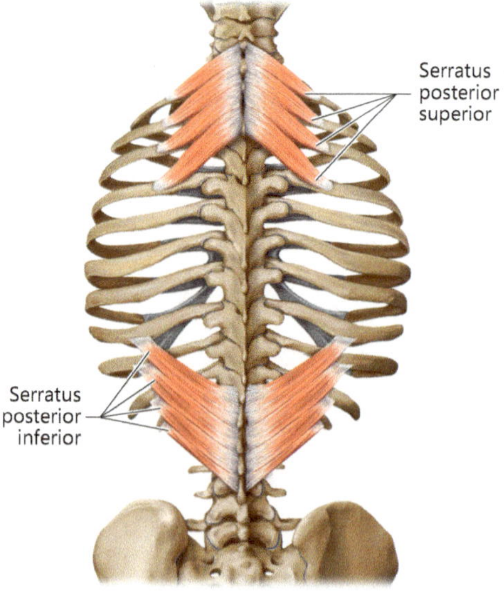

Note: The sternal part of the internal intercostal muscles (where the external intercostal muscles are missing) has an inspiratory function.

Expiratory muscles

- Main muscles:
  - internal intercostal muscles

- Secondary:
  - quadratus lumborum
  - transversus thoracis
  - subcostales
  - serratus posterior inferior
  - muscles of the abdomen → A deficiency in their muscle tone has a decisive impact on respiratory function and, from this perspective, they can be considered as major expiratory muscles. Instead, they act as secondary expiratory muscles by pushing the contents of the abdominal cavity against the diaphragm, with reduction of the thoracic cavity. (For origin, insertion, action and innervation of the muscles of the abdomen, see Chapter 5 "Vertebral column and movements of the trunk").

Expiratory muscles

Muscle	Action	Origin	Insertion	Innervation
Internal intercostal muscles	Most important expiratory muscles (with the exception of the sternal part, which has an inspiratory function). Together with the external intercostal muscles, they exert a tonic control action on the pressure gradient between the inside and outside of the thorax	Inferoposterior border of the lower rib. The fibers have an oblique direction from top to bottom and from medial to lateral	Superoposterior border of the posterior rib	Intercostal nerves [T1-T12]
Quadratus lumborum	An accessory expiratory muscle that, by acting on the lower ribs and the lumbar column, lowers the thorax and extends the vertebral column	Apex of the costal processes of the last four lumbar vertebrae; inner lip of the iliac crest and superior border of the iliolumbar ligament	Inferior border of the 12th rib and apex of the costal processes of the first four lumbar vertebrae	Subcostal nerve (last intercostal nerve) and anterior rami of the first two or three lumbar nerves (T12, L1, L2 or L1-L3)
Transversus thoracis	Downward traction of the costal cartilages, from the 2nd to the 6th	Posterior surface of the xiphoid process and the inferior part of the body of the sternum. The muscle fascicles are directed upward	Inferior border of the costal cartilages from the 2nd to the 6th	Intercostal nerves [T2-T6]
Subcostales	Accessory expiratory function	Internal surface of the ribs. The fibers have the same direction as those of the internal intercostal muscles	Costal angles within the thorax, skipping one or two ribs	Intercostal nerves [T1-T12]
Serratus posterior inferior	Downward traction of the last four ribs, but also stabilizes them; in this case, by giving the costal part of the diaphragm a fixed point, it becomes an inspiratory muscle	From the thoracolumbar fascia (from T12 to L3), inferiorly and medially. The muscle fascicles have a lateral and upward oblique direction	Last four ribs (inferoposterior border)	Intercostal nerves [T9-T12]

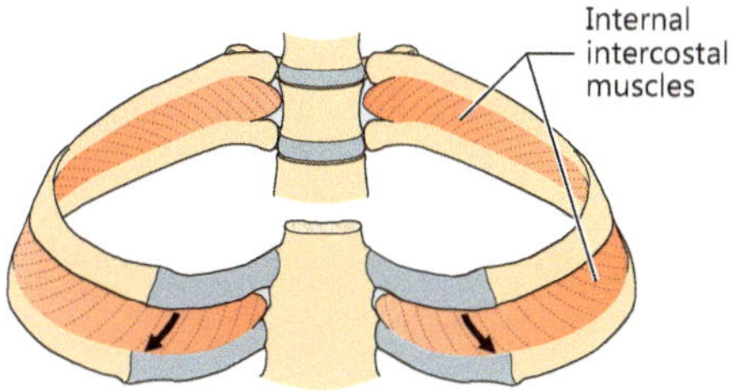
Internal
intercostal
muscles

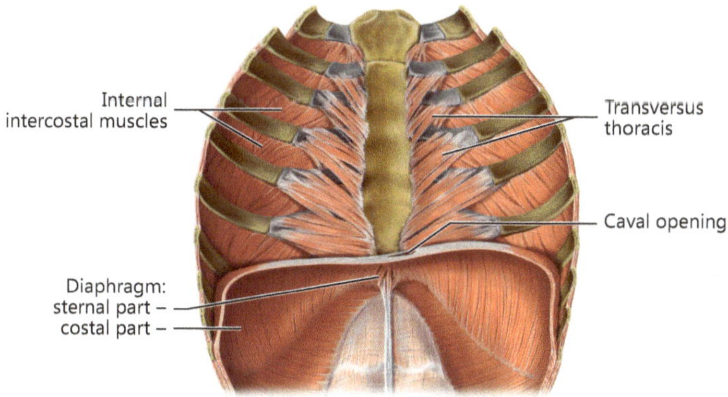
Internal
intercostal muscles
Transversus
thoracis
Caval opening
Diaphragm:
sternal part –
costal part –

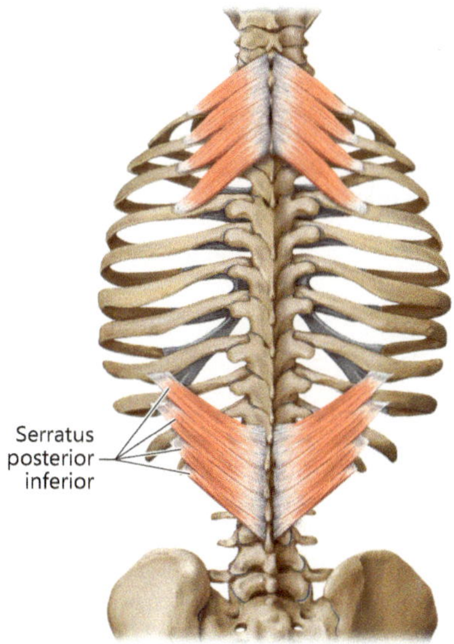
Serratus
posterior
inferior

Function of the secondary inspiratory and expiratory muscles

They only exert their action during deep breaths, for example:
- after deep effort
- in case of dyspnea.

> Coughing requires contraction of the main respiratory muscles, the secondary muscles and the muscles that stabilize respiration.

Mechanism of action of the secondary inspiratory muscles

Examples:
- when the weight of the trunk is supported by the arms, with the hands resting in front of the trunk, a distal fixed point is created for the muscles that originate from the trunk and insert on the upper limbs (for example, the pectoralis major) or head (for example, the sternocleidomastoid), corresponding to their insertion, and, therefore, the ribs and sternum are raised, with accessory inspiratory function of these muscles
- during forced inspiration, the forces transmitted to the vertebral column through the joints of the head of the ribs and costotransverse joints allow their flexion. This movement tends to reduce the expansion of the thoracic cage and is counteracted by the contraction of the long intrinsic muscles of the column, which tighten and extend the vertebral column.

Mechanism of action of the secondary expiratory muscles

Example: the muscles of the abdomen are inactive during expiration at rest. As a result of the increase in ventilation, they contract, pulling the thoracic cage downward and increasing intra-abdominal pressure. A pressing action is therefore exerted on the abdominal contents and the upward thrust of the diaphragm in the thoracic cavity, resulting in reduced lung volume and expulsion of air.

Movement of the thoracic column during respiration

When standing or sitting with the trunk upright, inspiration is accompanied by a tendency to extend the thoracic column and vice versa for expiration. It is however sufficient to rest the arms in front of the trunk to fix the shoulder girdle and prevent the extension of the thoracic column, which in this case will be characterized, always during inspiration, by a flexion movement that tends to increase the thoracic kyphosis of the column.

Respiratory mechanics

Tendency for the thoracic cage to expand (due to muscle action) as opposed to the tendency of the lungs to collapse (cartilaginous structure of the pulmonary bronchi and elastic structure of the bronchioles and pulmonary alveoli).

Inspiratory phase: stimulation of the main inspiratory muscles (diaphragm, external intercostal muscles, scalene muscles) → expansion of the thoracic cavity (elevation of the ribs, flattening of the central tendon of the diaphragm, traction of the diaphragm on the ribs, with an increase in the diameter of the thoracic cage) → decrease in the internal lung pressure (3-5 mmHg) with formation of a pressure gradient between lung pressure and atmospheric pressure → passage of air from the outside to the inside → relaxation of the pulmonary elastic fibers → increase in lung volume → collapse of the pleural cavity → increased thoracic expansion (forced inspiration, intervention of the secondary inspiratory muscles).

Expiratory phase: mainly passive (return of the elastic structures of the lungs and relaxation of the inspiratory muscles, with the exception of the external intercostal muscles, which would oppose the increase in internal pressure of the thorax, making it more gradual) but also active (action of the main expiratory muscles – internal intercostal muscles) → reduction in the diameters of the thorax → increase in the expiratory phase (forced expiration, intervention of the secondary expiratory muscles).

Palpation of the thoracic column and thorax

Spinous processes of the vertebrae

Starting from the inferior border (right or left) of the thoracic cage, the 12th rib is identified, and its course is followed medially to the joint with the 12th thoracic vertebra and thus the spinous process. Palpation continues in a cranial direction, along the series of thoracic spinous processes.

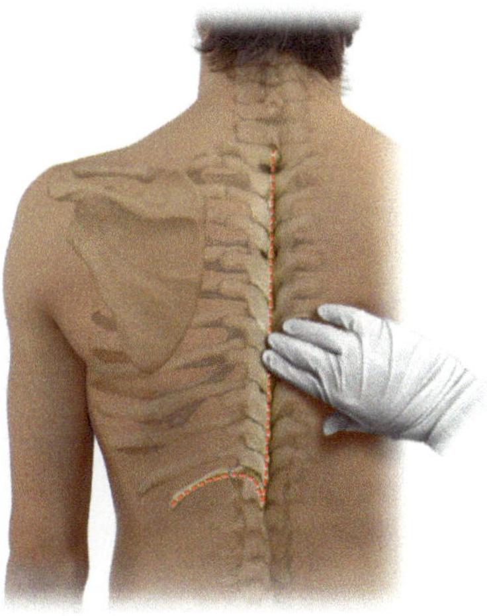

The following muscles are inserted on the spinous processes:

- trapezius
- rhomboid
- multifidus
- splenius cervicis
- rotatores
- spinal
- semispinalis thoracis.

It is not possible to distinguish the different muscle insertions, as they are very close.

Transverse processes of the vertebrae

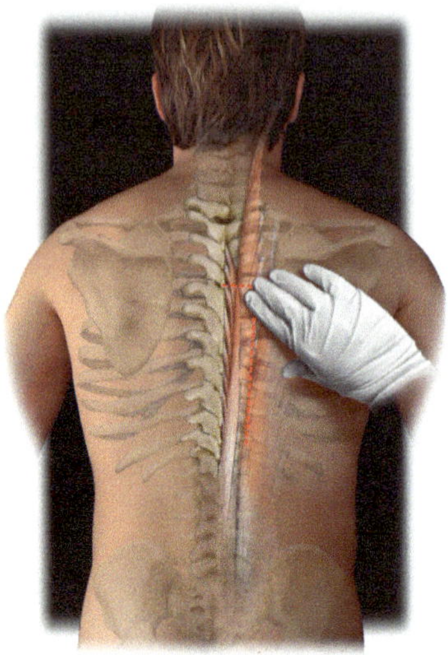

T1-T4 The lateral border of the paravertebral muscles is located at 2-3 fingers from the spinous process in the lateral direction; at this point, move 2-3 fingers upward to locate the transverse process.

T5-T9 As above, except move 3 fingers upwards, as the spinous process is more inclined downwards.

T10-T12 As for T1-T4.

The following muscles are inserted on the transverse processes:

- levatores costarum
- iliocostalis (thoracic part)
- longissimus cervicis
- longissimus thoracis.

The paravertebral muscles overlap with those located deeper, preventing their palpation.

Supraspinous ligaments

They extend between the apexes of the spinous processes and are tensed during flexion of the vertebral column, when the spinous processes move away from each other.

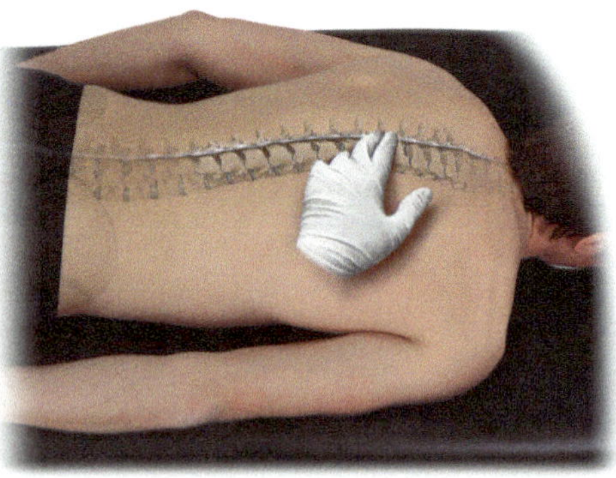

Lateral costotransverse ligament

It extends from the rib to the apex of the transverse process and can therefore be felt immediately lateral to it, after displacement of the longissimus thoracis.

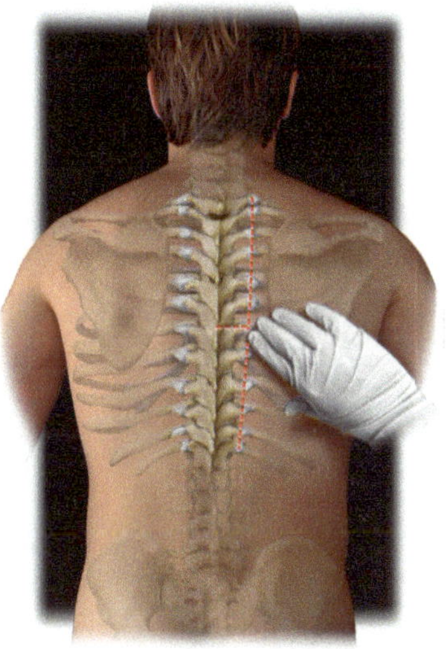

When a rib is blocked, the lateral costotransverse ligament becomes painful to palpation during deep breathing.

Costal angle

Proceed from the costovertebral joint in the lateral direction along the rib for approximately one palm of the hand, until the costal angle can be felt.

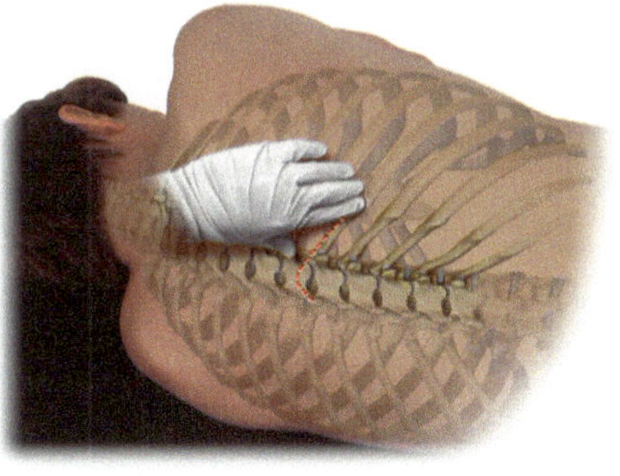

The costal angle becomes painful to palpation in case of functional alteration of the costovertebral joint.

The costal angle is used to support the palm of the hand when moving the rib in the anterolateral direction.

Sternocostal joints

They are evaluated by comparing palpation between the two sides, with the subject firstly in the supine position, and then in a seated position, since the load on these joints is greater in the latter position.

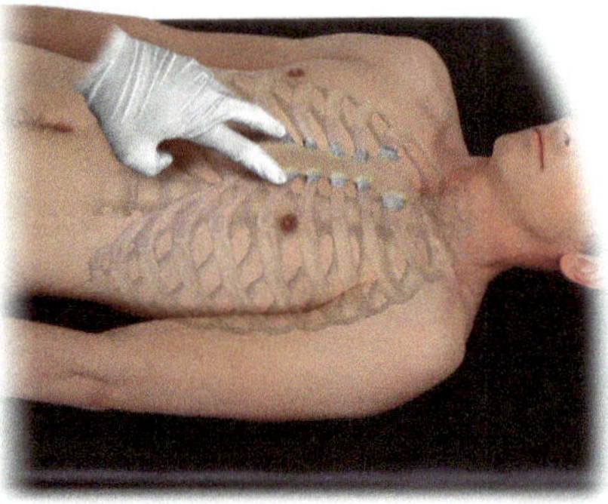

Diaphragm

Place the thumbs under the costal margin (arch), with the other fingers extended on the thorax and push in a superolateral direction. Under normal conditions, there is no particular resistance to this movement, and should be symmetrical on both sides.

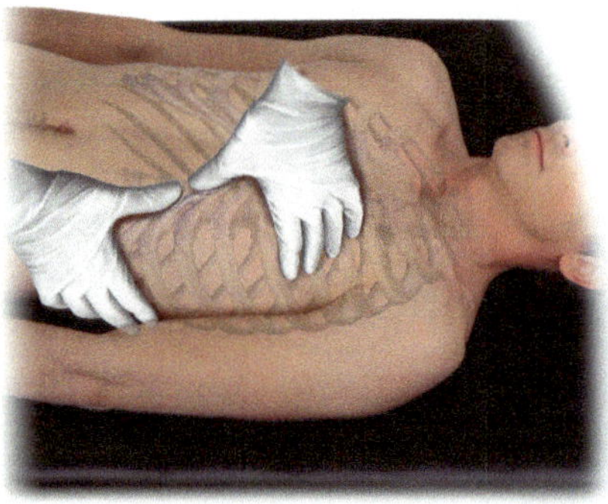

Intercostal muscles

They can be palpated with a finger that, from the anterior extremity of the ribs, proceeds in a posterior direction in the intercostal space.

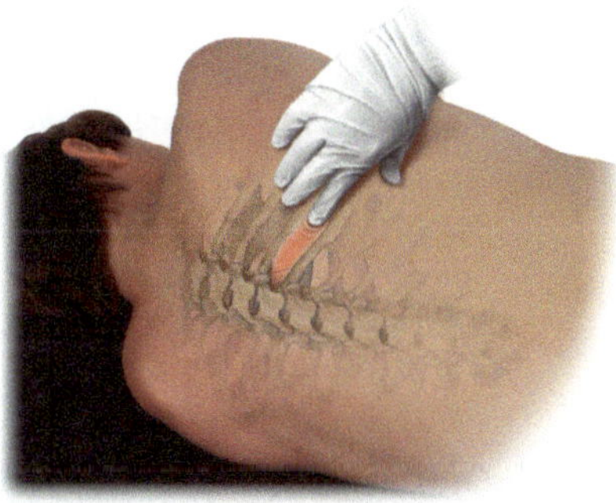

Long intrinsic muscles of the vertebral column

Elongated muscle fascicle in the paravertebral area, 2-3 fingers thick.

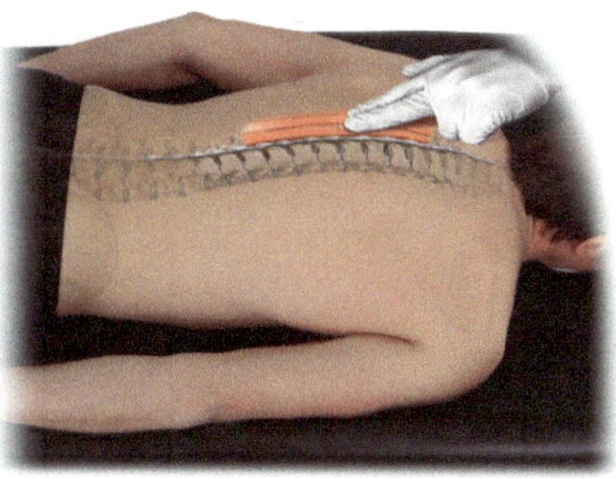

Measuring the expansion of the thorax

The circumference of the thorax is measured at the level of the joint between the body and the xiphoid process of the sternum (xiphisternal joint). Two measurements are taken:

- after complete expiration
- after complete inspiration.

The difference between the two measurements indicates the magnitude of thoracic expansion.

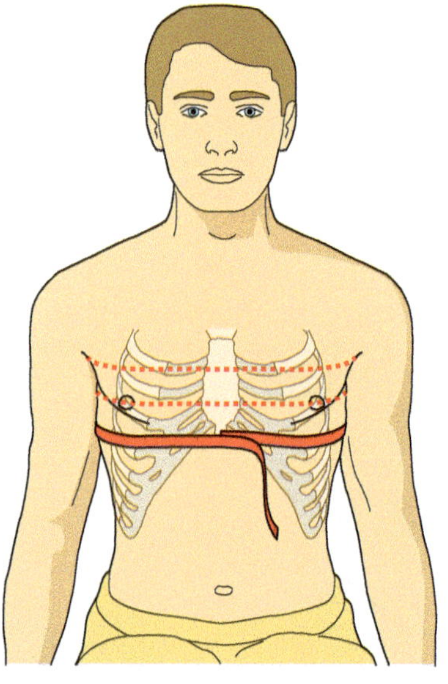

The measurement can also be performed:

- at the level of the line that joins the nipples
- in correspondence with the anterior axillary fold.

The values obtained are slightly lower than those detected at the level of the xiphisternal joint.

The normal thoracic expansion values differ greatly among individuals and, around the age of 40, begin to gradually decrease with age. Reduced thoracic expansion can be due to the involvement of the costovertebral joints that occurs in some pathological conditions or may be caused by chronic obstructive pulmonary disease.

Scapula

Superior angle
- Facing upwards and forwards
- The insertion of the levator scapulae.

Spine of the scapula
- Bony crest on the posterior surface of the scapula between the upper quarter and the lower three quarters
- It ends laterally with the acromion.

Acromion
- Accentuated relief directed outwards and forwards with which the spine of the scapula ends laterally
- The articular surface for the clavicle is on its medial margin
- It ends up with a rounded extremity (apex).

Medial border
- From the spine of the scapula down to the inferior angle of the scapula
- Insertion of the rhomboid major and rhomboid minor.

Inferior angle
- Origin of the teres major.

Lateral border
- Infraglenoid tubercle corresponding to the superior extremity, where the long head of the triceps brachii originates.

Posterior surface of the scapula
- Supraspinous fossa, where the supraspinatus originates
- Infraspinous fossa, where the infraspinatus originates.

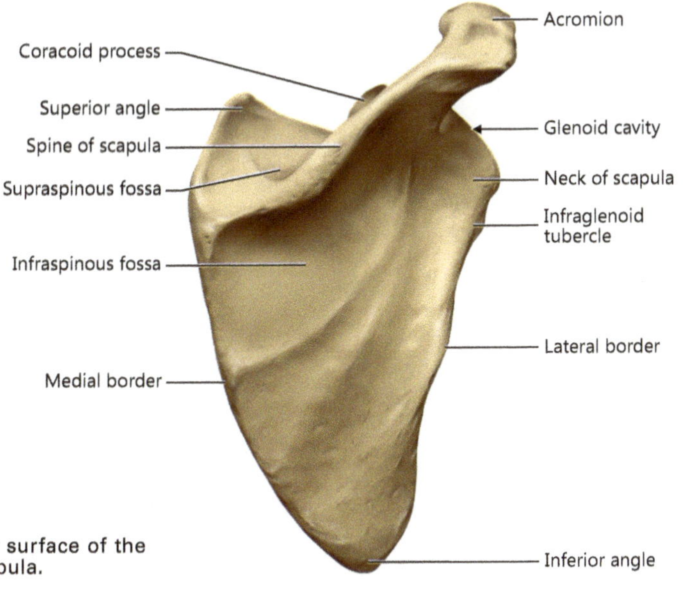

Posterior surface of the right scapula.

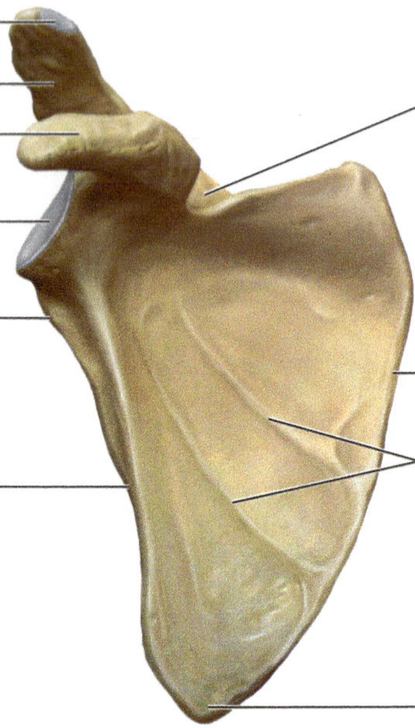

Anterior surface of the right scapula.

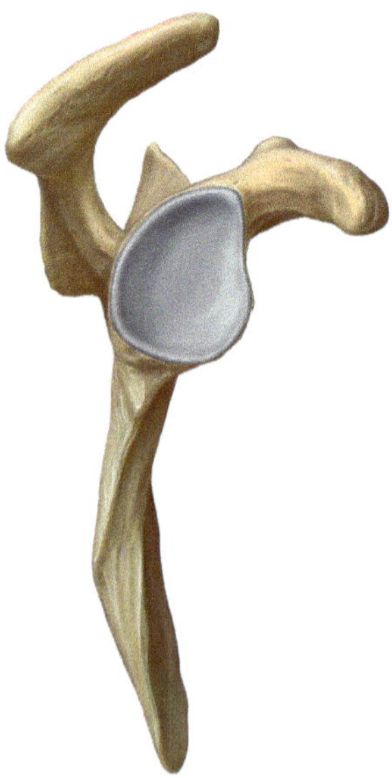

Right scapula viewed from the outside (laterally).

Superior border
- Shorter than the other borders
- Laterally presents the suprascapular notch.

Coracoid process
- Lateral to the suprascapular notch
- It raises from the superior border leading first upwards and then forwards and outwards.

The anterior (or costal) surface of the scapula
- Subscapular fossa, where the subscapularis originates.

Glenoid cavity
- It corresponds to the lateral border of the scapula
- Oval surface directed laterally, slightly concave, for the joint with the head of the humerus
- The supraglenoid tuberosity, corresponding to the upper pole, where the long head of the biceps brachii originates.

Clavicle

- Superior surface: smooth and palpable
- Sternal end (with sternal facet)
- Acromial end (with acromial facet)
- Inferior surface:
  - conoid tubercle and trapezoid line laterally (where the coracoclavicular ligament is attached)
  - subclavian groove
  - impression for costoclavicular ligament or costal tuberosity (where the costoclavicular ligament is attached).

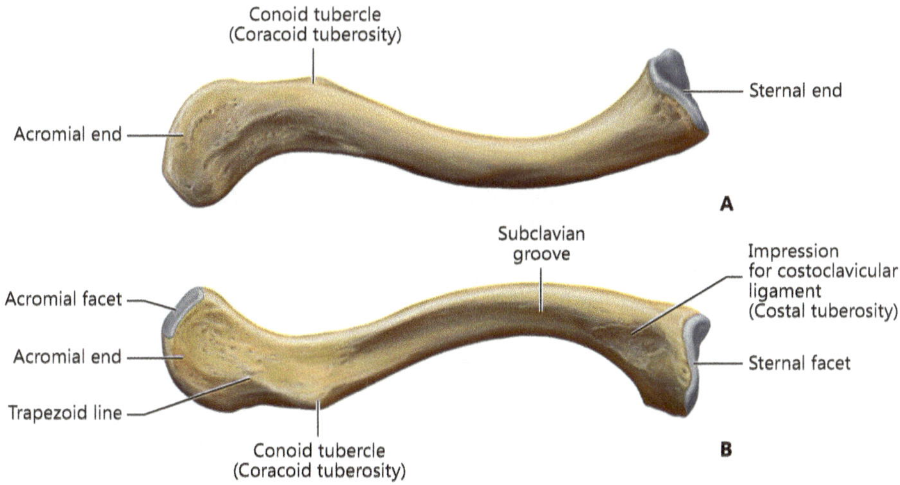

Left clavicle viewed from above (**A**) and from below (**B**).

Humerus

Proximal extremity

- Head of the humerus:
  - it is directed medially and upwards.
- Anatomical neck:
  - narrowing on the contour of the head.
- Greater tubercle:
  - below the anatomical neck laterally
  - it is directed posteriorly and laterally
  - superior facet (insertion of the supraspinatus)
  - middle facet (insertion of the infraspinatus)
  - inferior facet (insertion of the teres minor)
- Lesser tubercle:
  - below the anatomical neck medially to the greater tubercle
  - it is directed anteriorly and medially
  - insertion of the subscapularis.
- Crest of the greater tubercle:
  - from the greater tubercle downwards to the anterior border of the shaft (body) of the humerus
  - it is the lateral lip of the intertubercular sulcus of the humerus (where the tendon of the long head of the biceps brachii passes)
  - insertion of the pectoralis major.
- Crest of the lesser tubercle:
  - from the lesser tubercle downwards to the anteromedial surface of the shaft (body) of the humerus
  - it is the medial lip of the intertubercular sulcus of the humerus
  - insertion of the latissimus dorsi and teres major.

Shaft (body)

- Anteromedial surface:
  - extension of the intertubercular sulcus of the humerus in the upper part
  - insertion of the coracobrachialis on the medial part.
- Anterolateral surface:
  - deltoid tuberosity in the middle third (insertion of the deltoid).
- Posterior surface:
  - it presents the radial groove (directed from top medially down laterally), which divides it into two parts: the lateral head of the triceps brachii originates above the groove; the medial head of the triceps brachii originates below the groove.
- Anterior border
- Medial border
- Lateral margin.

Distal extremity
(See Chapter 8 “Elbow”).

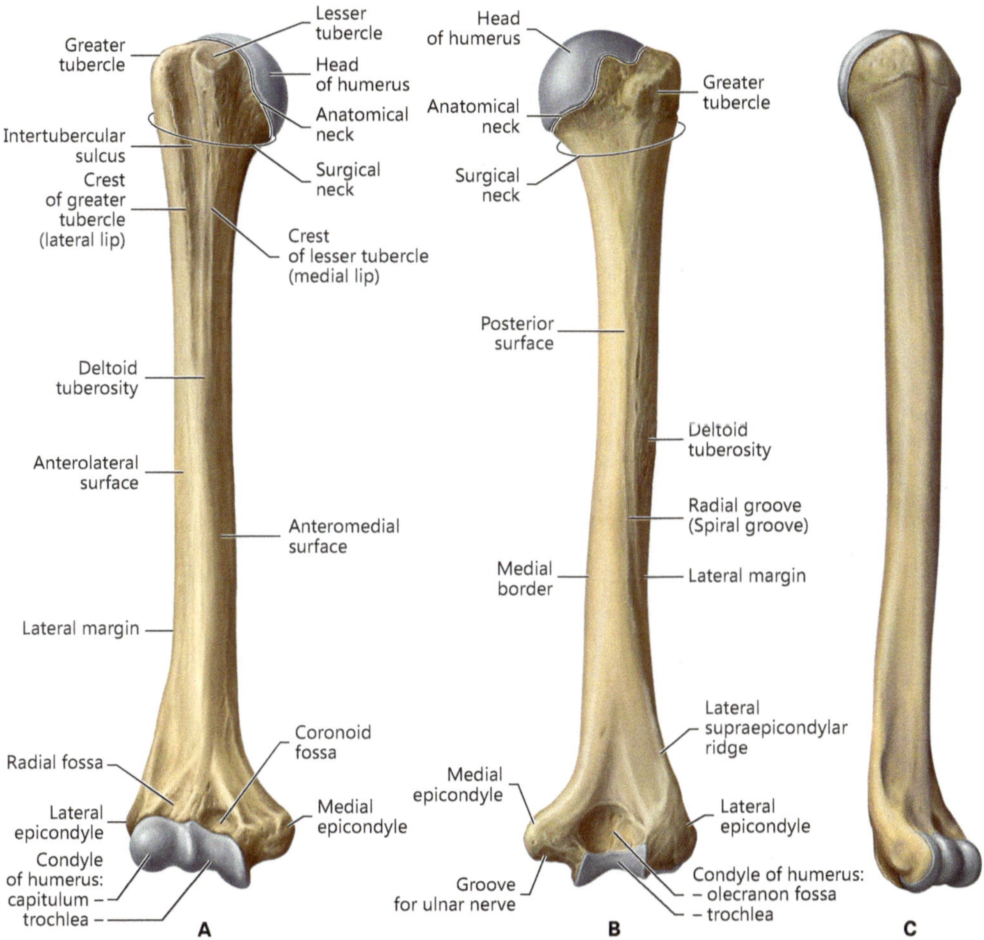

Right humerus viewed from the anterior (**A**), posterior (**B**) and lateral (**C**) surfaces.

Pectoral (shoulder) girdle

There are seven shoulder joints, five true joints and two pseudo-joints:

- acromioclavicular joint
- sternoclavicular joint
- glenohumeral (shoulder) joint
- sternocostal joint
- costovertebral joint
- scapulothoracic joint (pseudo-joint)
- coracoacromial or suprahumeral joint (pseudo-joint).

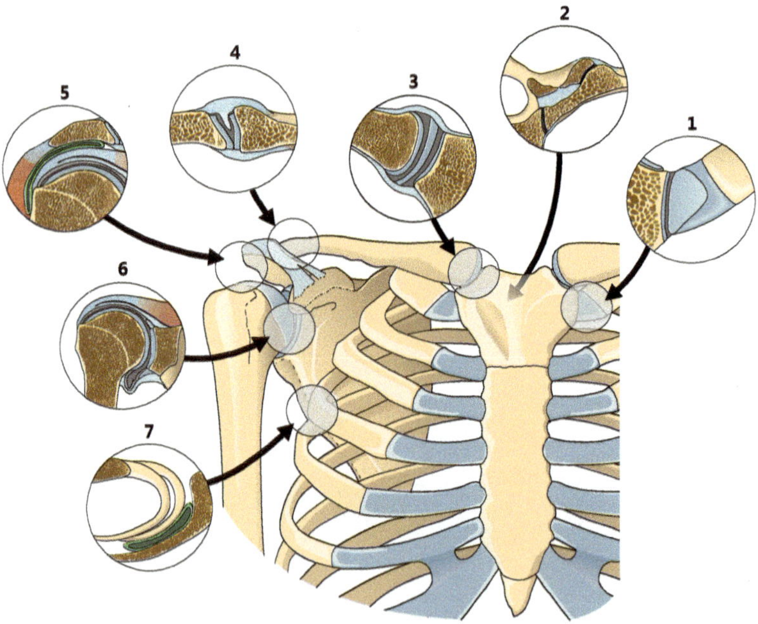

The seven joints of the pectoral girdle. **1.** Sternocostal joint; **2.** costovertebral joint; **3.** sternoclavicular joint; **4.** acromioclavicular joint; **5.** coracoacromial or suprahumeral joint (pseudo-joint); **6.** glenohumeral (shoulder) joint; **7.** scapulothoracic joint (pseudo-joint);

Acromioclavicular joint

Articular surfaces	Acromial facet on the acromial end of the clavicle (slightly concave) Articular facet for the clavicle on the medial margin of the acromion (slightly convex) The concordance is due to the presence of a disc
Capsule	It is reinforced superiorly by the acromioclavicular ligament 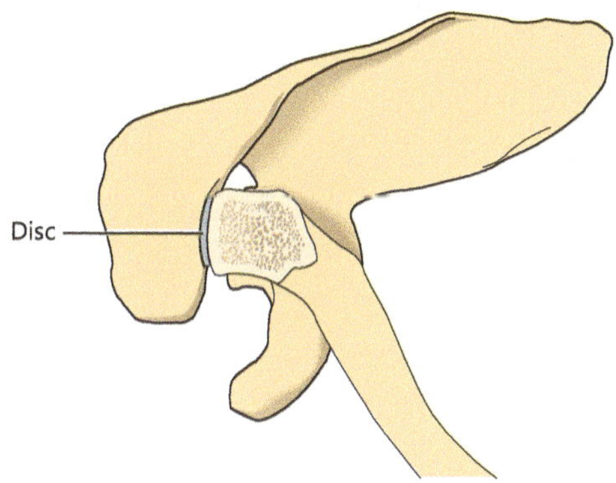 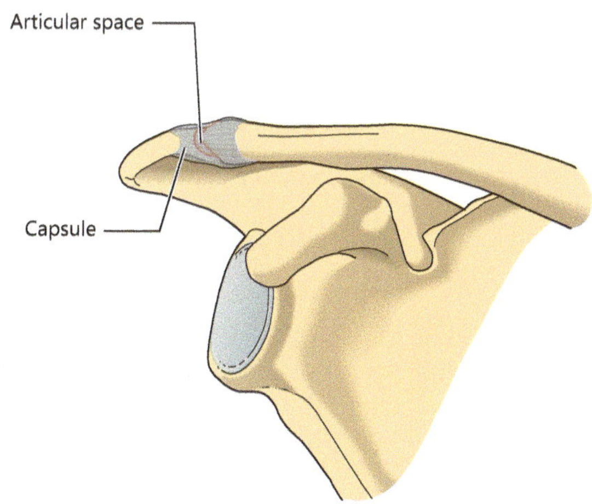
Ligaments	Acromioclavicular ligament (between the clavicle and the acromion) Coracoclavicular ligament (between the inferior surface of the clavicle and the coracoid process), divided into the trapezoid ligament (anterolateral part) and the conoid ligament (posteromedial part)

(continued)

(continued)

	These ligaments: • stabilize the clavicle and attach it tightly to the scapula (prevent sliding on the frontal and transverse planes) • limit joint movements 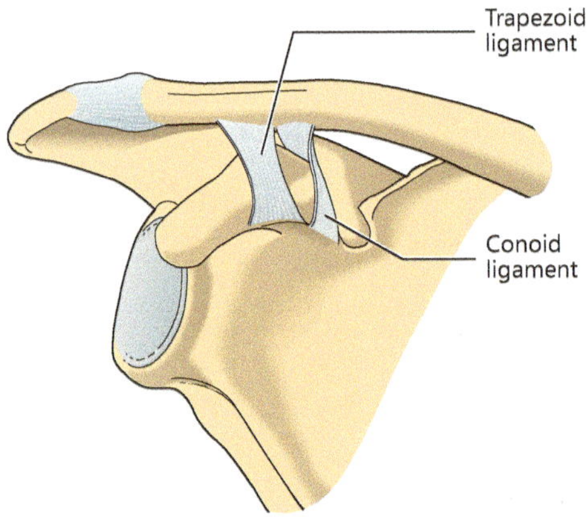
Type of joint	Plane joint
Movements	Protraction and retraction of the clavicle (anteroposterior movements on the sagittal plane) Elevation and depression of the clavicle (craniocaudal movements of low amplitude on the frontal plane) Rotation around the longitudinal axis of the clavicle Total: 3 degrees of freedom (6 types of movement) 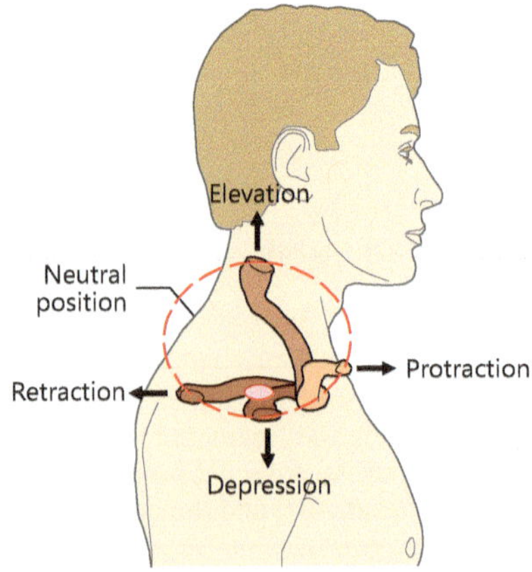

Sternoclavicular joint

Articular surfaces	Saddle-shaped sternal end of the clavicle (with the major axis directed superoinferiorly and the minor axis directed anteroposteriorly) Concordant articular surfaces of the sternum Small articular surface for the 1st rib on the inferior border of the clavicle (sternocostoclavicular joint) 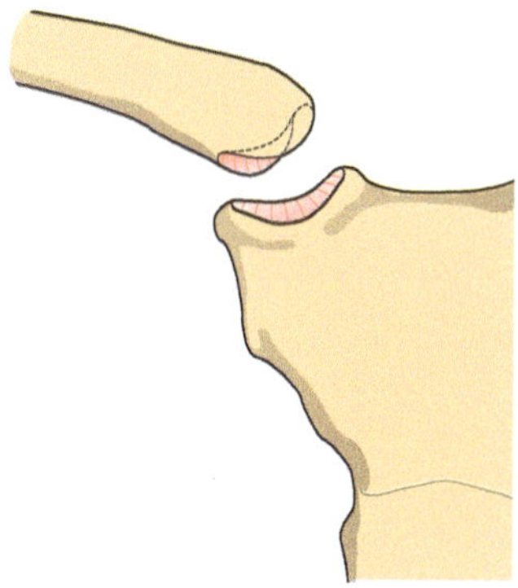
Disc	Fibrocartilaginous interposed between the articular surfaces that varies the concordance, also allowing the rotation of the clavicle
Ligaments	Interclavicular (joins the two clavicles above the sternum) Anterior and posterior sternoclavicular (between the sternum and the clavicle, anteriorly and posteriorly to the capsule) Costoclavicular (between the 1st rib and the inferior border of the clavicle, laterally to the joint; limits the elevation of the clavicle) 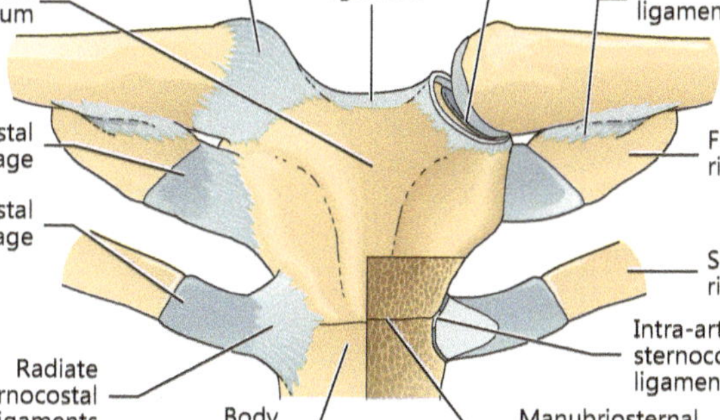

(continued)

(*continued*)

Type of joint	Double plane joint
Movements	Protraction and retraction of the clavicle (anteroposterior movements on the sagittal plane): • protraction (or antepulsion or anteposition) of approximately 3 cm • retraction (or retropulsion or retroposition) of approximately 3 cm 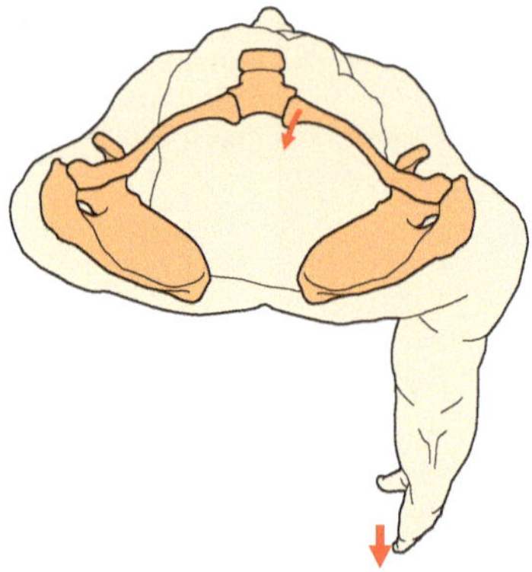 Elevation and depression of the clavicle (craniocaudal movements on the frontal plane): • elevation of approximately 10 cm: – the sternal end of the clavicle slides downwards, but the 1st rib, located just below the clavicle, limits the range of motion and therefore the elevation of the clavicle – it is always accompanied by a certain degree of rotation and a consequent minimum protraction. The rotation occurs around the axis of the clavicle and is approximately 30° • depression by approximately 3 cm: – the sternal end of the clavicle slides upwards – it is always accompanied by a certain degree of rotation and a consequent minimum retraction 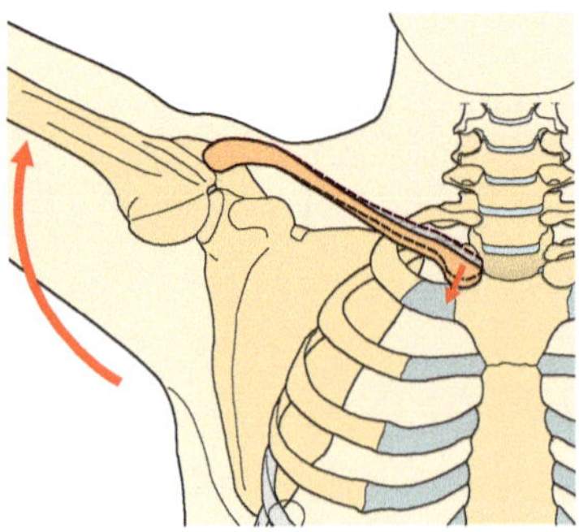 Rotation around the longitudinal axis of the clavicle of approximately 30° Total: 3 degrees of freedom (6 types of movements)

Functional aspects of the joints of the pectoral girdle

- The scapula (by means of the acromioclavicular joint) moves in synchrony with each movement of the clavicle:
  - if the various positions reached by the acromial end of the clavicle during the maximum amplitude of the clavicle's movements were joined together, the result would be an oval which is higher than it is wide, corresponding to an elevation of about 60°, a depression of 5°, and a protraction and retraction of 30° of the acromial end of the clavicle

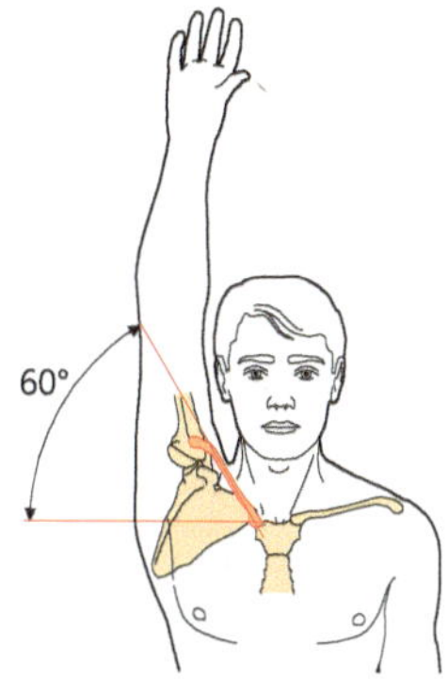

- Both joints of the clavicle aid in the movements of the scapula (the acromioclavicular joint to a lesser extent):
  - elevation of the scapula corresponds to elevation of the clavicle
  - depression of the scapula corresponds to depression of the clavicle
  - abduction of the scapula corresponds to protraction of the clavicle
  - adduction of the scapula corresponds to retraction of the clavicle

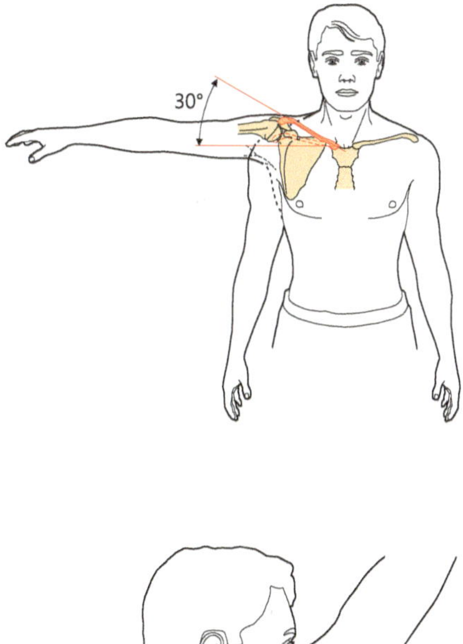

- The movements of the clavicle are combined with those of the scapula and humerus during abduction and flexion movements of the arm (see section "Movements of the glenohumeral (shoulder) joint", page 245), thereby causing the backward and lateral displacement of the glenoid cavity:
  - external rotation of the scapula (see section "Movements of the scapula", page 243)
  - simultaneous 30° elevation of the clavicle
  - rotation of the clavicle around its longitudinal axis (beings before the clavicle has reached an elevation of 30° and its amplitude is most likely less than 45°)
  - elevation of the acromial end of the clavicle from 30° to 60°.

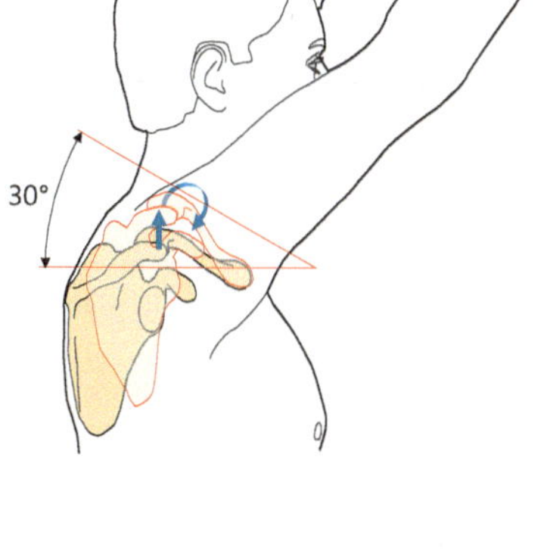

7

Glenohumeral (shoulder) joint

<table>
<tr>
<td>Articular surfaces</td>
<td>Glenoid cavity of the scapula:
• seen laterally, it presents a pear shape and its depth is not sufficient to contain the head of the humerus, since it is four times smaller than the head of the humerus
• the glenoid labrum (flat fibrocartilaginous pad), attached to the bony margin of the cavity, increases the articular surface
• the layer of cartilage covering it is thin in the center and thicker on the outside
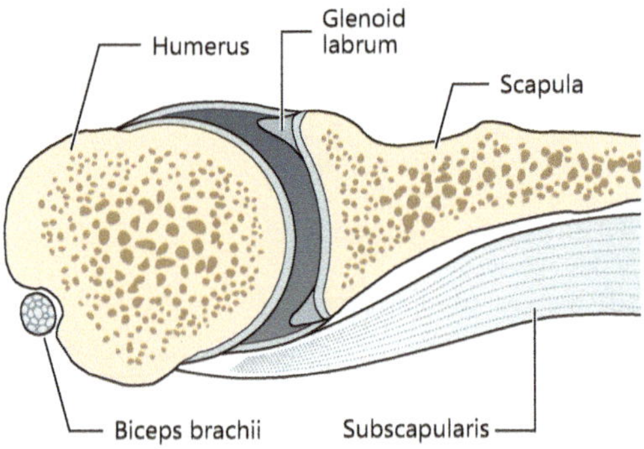

Head of the humerus:
• slightly less than one-third of a sphere
• diameter of about 3 cm
• 135° angle between the axis of the head and the axis of the diaphysis of the humerus (angle of inclination, visible on the frontal plane; the glenoid cavity's angle of inclination on the vertical axis is 15°)
• 30-40° angle between the axis of the head and the axis of the condyles of the humerus (angle of declination or retroversion, visible on transverse plane; the glenoid cavity's angle of declination is 10°)
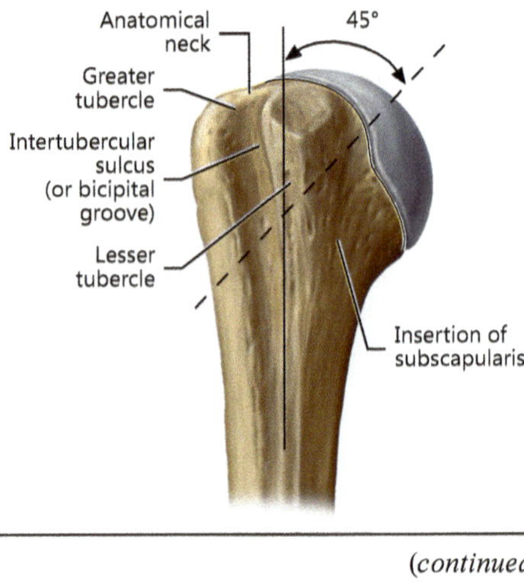
</td>
</tr>
</table>

(continued)

(*continued*)

	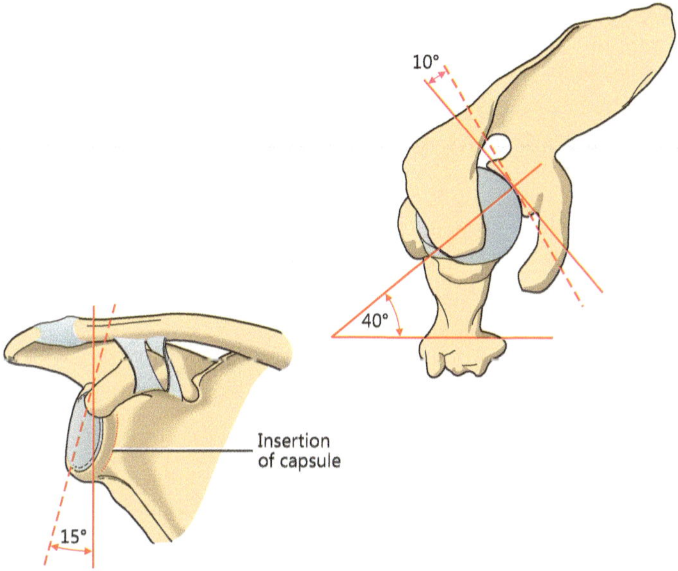
Capsule	Surrounds the articular heads, inserting proximally on the contour of the glenoid cavity and distally on the inferior border of the anatomical neck (where it joins anteriorly with the tendon of the subscapularis, superiorly with the tendon of the supraspinatus and posteriorly with the tendons of the infraspinatus and teres minor) 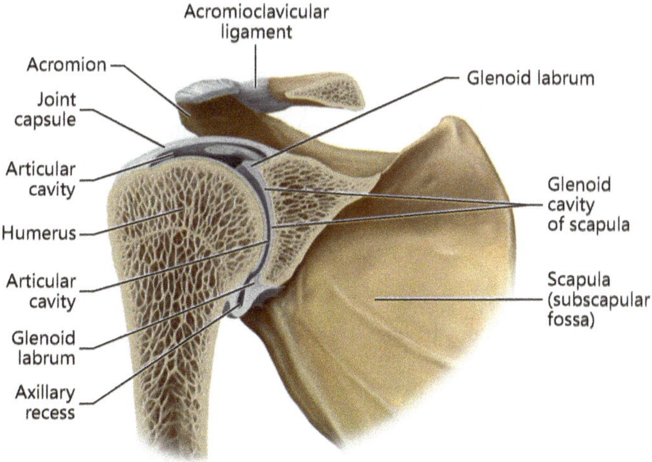

(*continued*)

(*continued*)

	Main characteristics: • laxity, which allows a considerable extension of the movements • recesses, which extend the capsule: – subscapular recess (in the anterior part, above the subscapularis, in communication with the subcoracoid bursa) – axillary recess (in the inferior part) 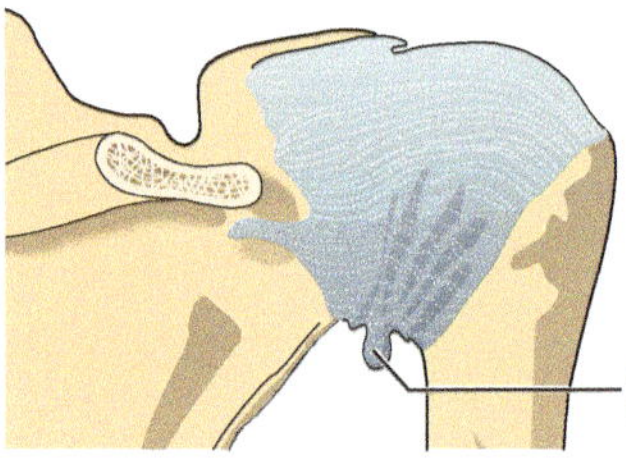 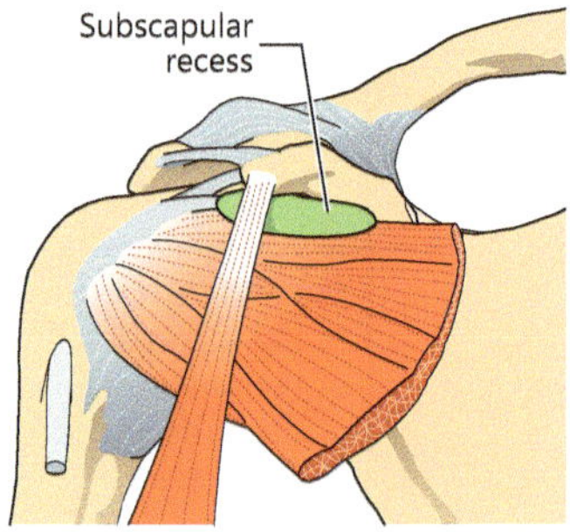
Type of joint	Ball and socket joint
Movements	In addition to the 6 types of movements occurring on the frontal, sagittal and transverse planes (3 degrees of freedom), there is a particular rotation movement that occurs around the axis of the diaphysis of the humerus

Ligaments of the glenohumeral (shoulder) joint

Ligaments	Insertion	Action
Coracoacromial	Between the lateral surface of the coracoid process and the anterior apex of the acromion	By acting synergistically with the coracohumeral ligament, it prevents downward dislocation of the shoulder; it limits the elevation of the head of the humerus, preventing upward dislocation of the shoulder

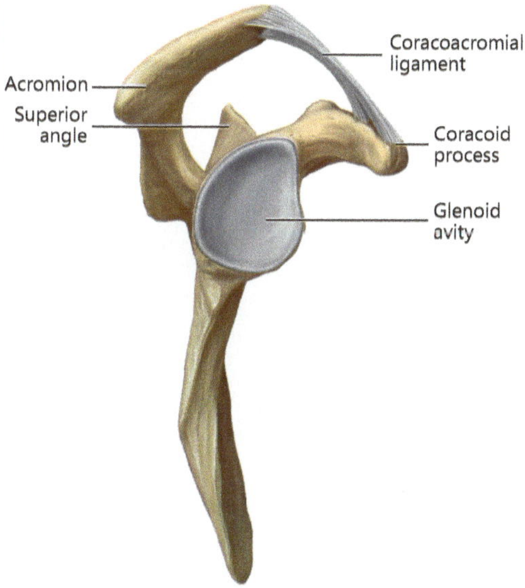

Ligaments	Insertion	Action
Coracohumeral	Anterior: between the base of the coracoid process and the lesser tubercle of the humerus Posterior: between the base of the coracoid process and the greater tubercle of the humerus	Stabilizes the joint; prevents the lowering of the head of the humerus when the arm is next to the trunk; limits the flexion, adduction and external rotation when abducted 90°

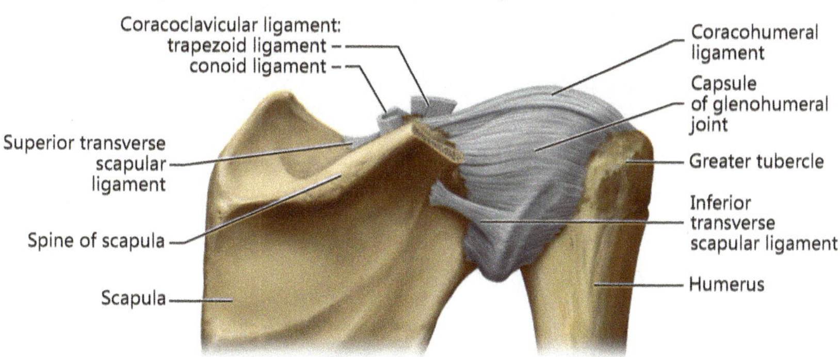

(continued)

7

(*continued*)

Ligaments	Insertion	Action
Glenohumeral (superior, middle and inferior)	Between the anterior border of the glenoid cavity and the anatomical neck of the humerus (between the superior and middle ligaments there is a weak area in the joint capsule through which the anterior dislocation of the shoulder often occurs)	Limits external rotation and prevents the lowering of the head of the humerus; the inferior part stabilizes the joint, especially during abduction and external rotation

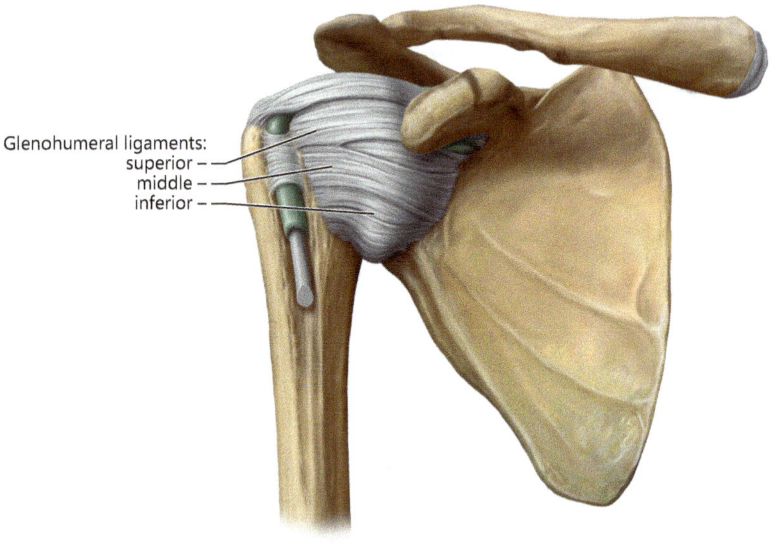

The ligaments of the glenohumeral joint have a passive restraining function on the joint. The active elements are the fixator muscles of the joint, which prevent its upward (longitudinally arranged upper limb muscles) and downward (transversely arranged upper limb muscles) dislocation.

Subacromial space

The roof of the shoulder is formed by:
- the acromion
- the coracoid process
- coracoacromial ligament.

In the subacromial space are located:
- the subacromial bursa
- the tendon of the supraspinatus
- the infraspinatus (partially)
- the tendon of the long head of the biceps brachii
- the joint capsule (superior part)
- the ligaments of the joint (superior part).

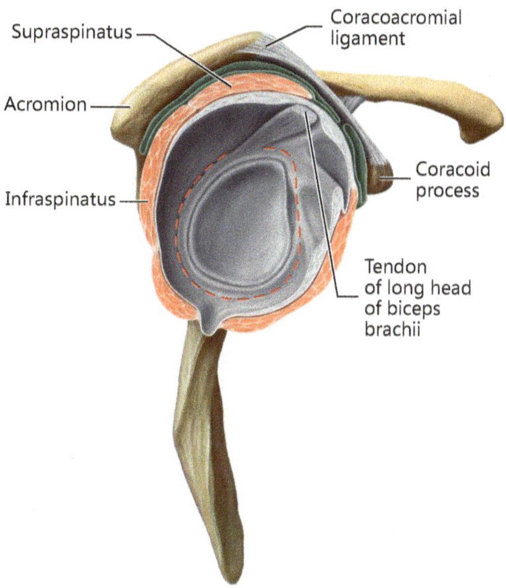

7

Subtendinous subacromial bursae

- Subacromial bursa (is located below the roof of the shoulder and reaches the acromioclavicular joint)
- Subdeltoid bursa (is located at the level of the greater tubercle of the humerus and communicates with the subacromial bursa).

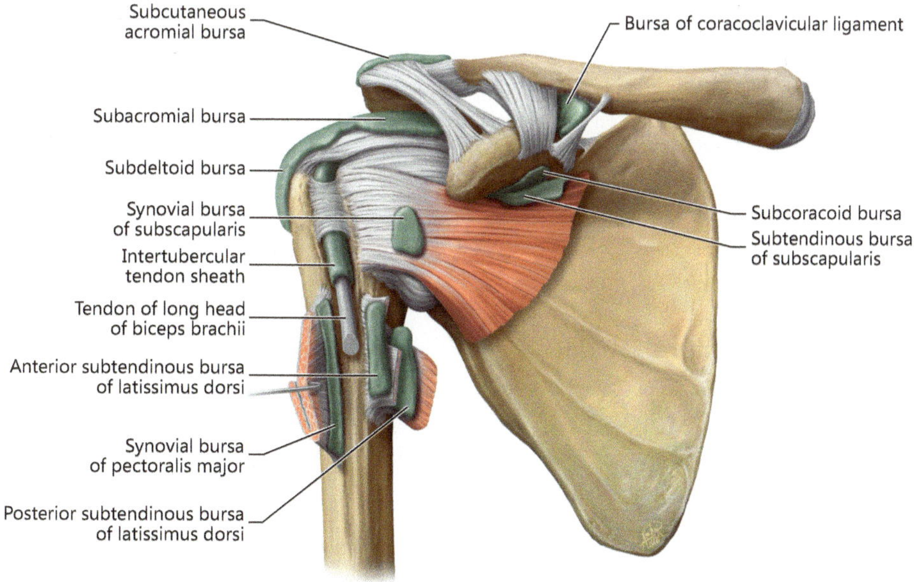

The subacromial bursa is fixed superiorly to the acromion and inferiorly to the humerus, and the rotator cuff.

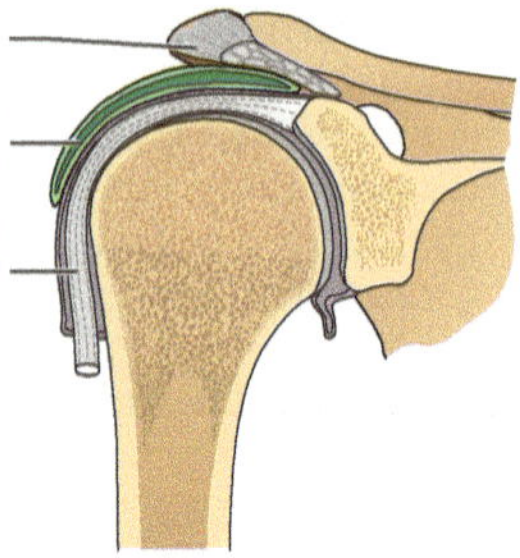

During movements of the arm, the superior insertion represents the fixed point and the inferior insertion represents the mobile point.

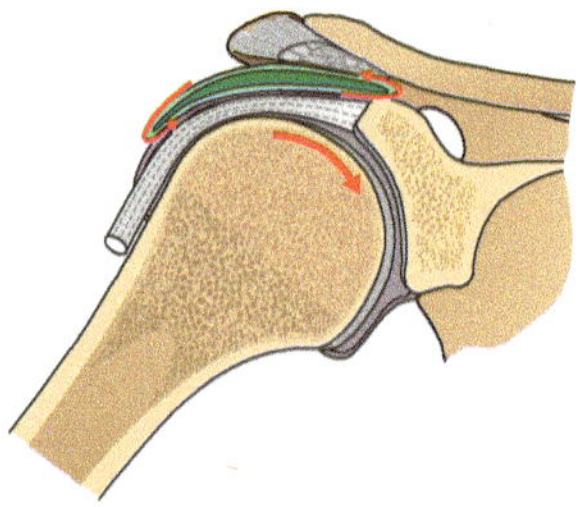

A reduction in the subacromial space can damage the subacromial bursa which, by becoming inflamed and swollen, can further reduce the subacromial space, causing a reduction in joint mobility.

In addition to these two interconnected bursae, the subcoracoid bursa (between the inferior surface of the coracoid process and the joint capsule) and the bursae of the coracobrachialis, subscapularis and biceps brachii are present (the latter two bursae are dependent of the synovium and are not represented in the figure on page 241). The bursae of the teres major, latissimus dorsi, pectoralis major, supraspinatus and infraspinatus are less constant.

Other joints of the shoulder

Coracoacromial joint — It is the coracoacromial ligament.

Scapulothoracic joint — It is the gliding of the scapula over the thorax (scapulothoracic rhythm) through the interposition of muscles, sheaths and subscapular bursa.

Sternocostal and costovertebral joints — These are indirect joints (see Chapter 6 "Thorax and thoracic column").

Movements of the clavicle

(See section "Acromioclavicular joint", page 231, and "Sternoclavicular joint", page 233).

Movements of the scapula

External rotation (extrarotation, lateral rotation)

- Lateral oscillation of the scapula
- The rotation axis, orthogonal to the plane of the scapula passing just below the spine, moves inferiorly during movement
- The amplitude of the movement is around 60°
- The inferior angle of the scapula covers a distance of approximately 10 cm in the lateral direction.

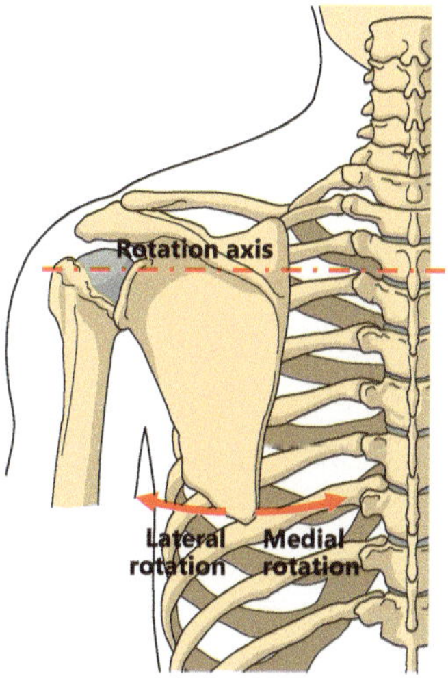

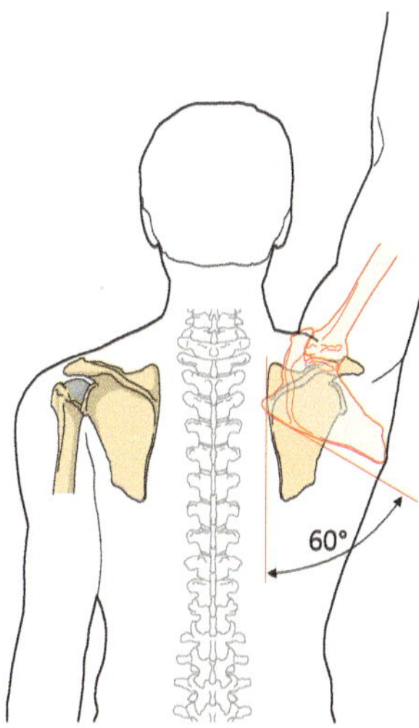

> It is the most important movement of the scapula, occurring both during abduction of the shoulder (with lateromedial elevation, in the above image) and during its flexion (with anterosuperior elevation).

Note: remember that all movements occur on the shoulder's rotation axes. Additionally, for movements it is generally customary to refer to the joint(s).

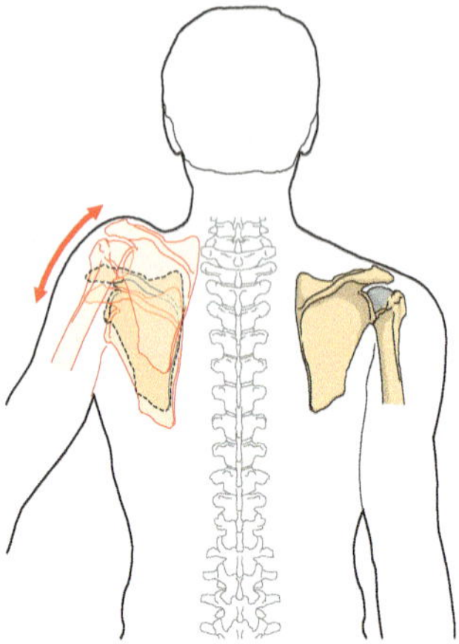

Elevation

- Upward movement of the scapula
- Elevation of approximately 10 cm.

Depression

- Downward movement of the scapula
- Depression by approximately 3 cm.

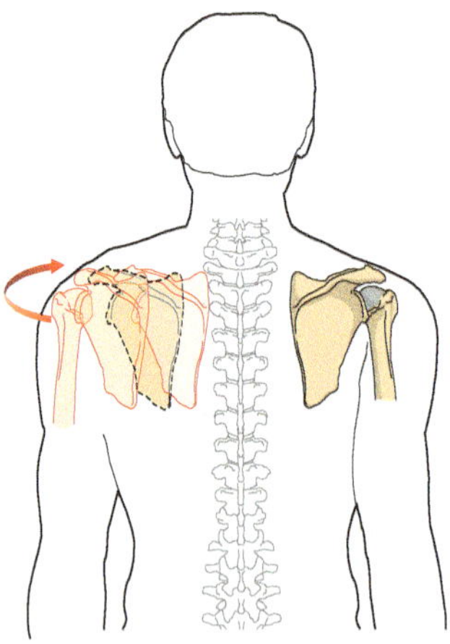

Adduction

- Approach of the medial border of the scapula to the vertebral column
- Corresponding retraction of the clavicle
- The angle between the clavicle and the scapula increases.

Abduction

- Distancing of the medial border of the scapula from the vertebral column
- Corresponding protraction of the clavicle
- The angle between the clavicle and the scapula is reduced.

Movements of the glenohumeral (shoulder) joint

The anatomical position is the starting position.

Flexion

- Occurs on the sagittal plane around the transverse (horizontal) axis
- Amplitude of approximately 180°
- Is accompanied by anterosuperior elevation.

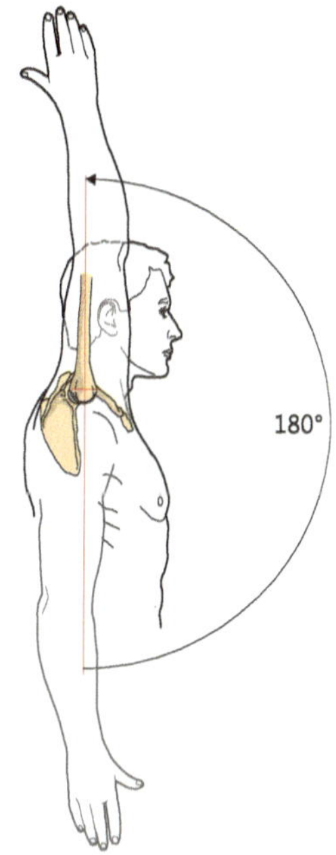

Extension

- Occurs on the sagittal plane around the transverse (horizontal) axis
- Amplitude of approximately 45-50°.

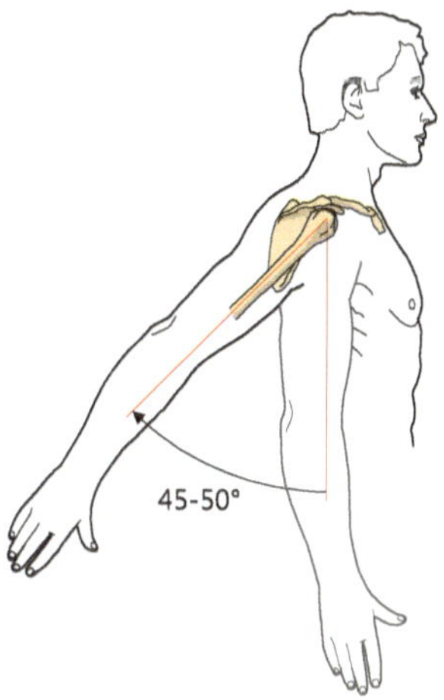

Abduction

- Occurs on the frontal plane around the sagittal axis
- Amplitude of 180°
- Is accompanied by lateromedial elevation.

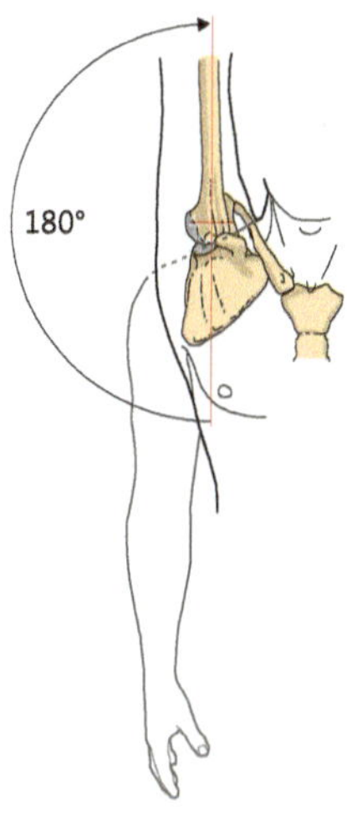

Adduction

- Occurs on the frontal plane around the sagittal axis
- Absolute:
  - when performed from the anatomical position, preceded by a slight flexion of the trunk
  - amplitude of 30-45°
- Relative:
  - when performed from any abduction position.

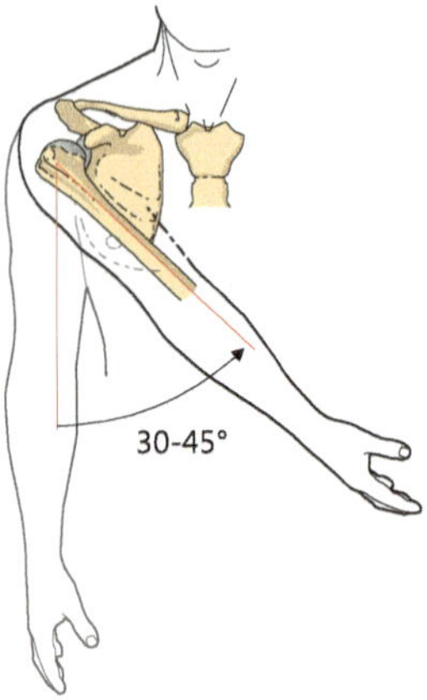

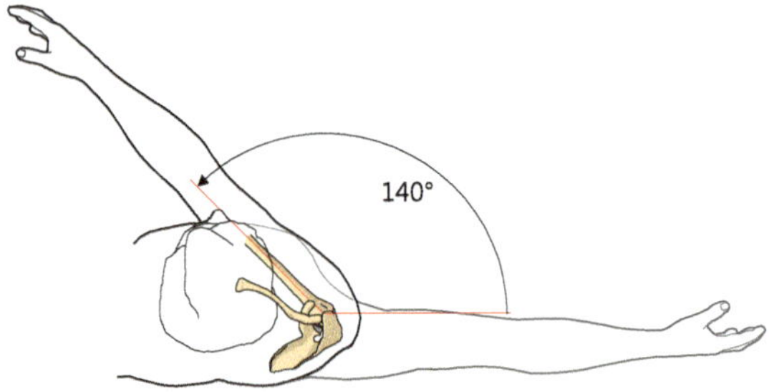

Internal rotation

- On the horizontal plane
- The starting position is 90° abduction
- Amplitude of 140°.

External rotation

- On the horizontal plane
- The starting position is 90° abduction
- Amplitude of 30°.

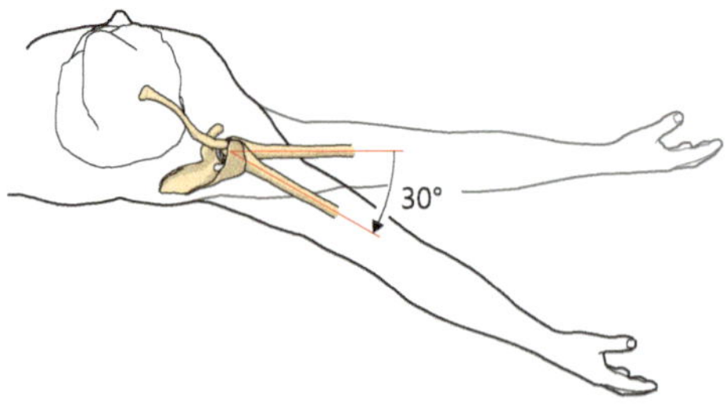

Rotation on the axis of the humeral diaphysis

- Glenohumeral joint movement around the longitudinal axis of the humeral diaphysis
- Starting position:
  - shoulder in resting position (0°)
  - elbow flexed at 90°
  - hand in any position (the pronosupination of the forearm is excluded from the movement)
- External:
  - amplitude of 80°
- Internal:
  - the arm is brought behind the trunk
  - amplitude of 95°.

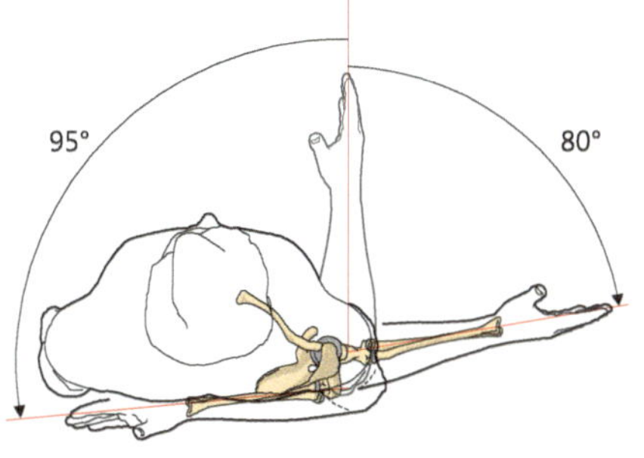

Circumduction

- Typical movement of all joints having at least two degrees of freedom (flexion-extension and abduction-adduction)
- Maximum amplitude at the level of the shoulder.

Assessment of scapular joint mobility

Movements of the scapula are assessed through the execution of movements:

- active (performed by the patient from a seated position with the arms along the trunk)
- passive (performed by the examiner on the patient in lateral decubitus).

Active movements

Evaluated movements	Execution
Elevation of the scapula 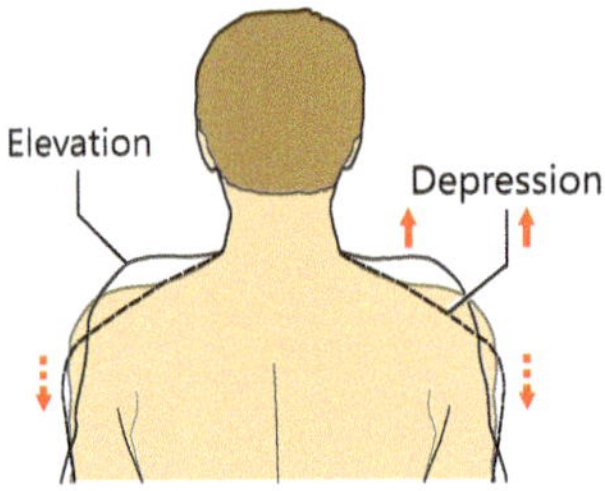	Movements of the shoulder in cranial direction, towards the ears
Depression of the scapula	Movements of the shoulders in caudal direction, towards the sides of the trunk
Abduction of the scapula 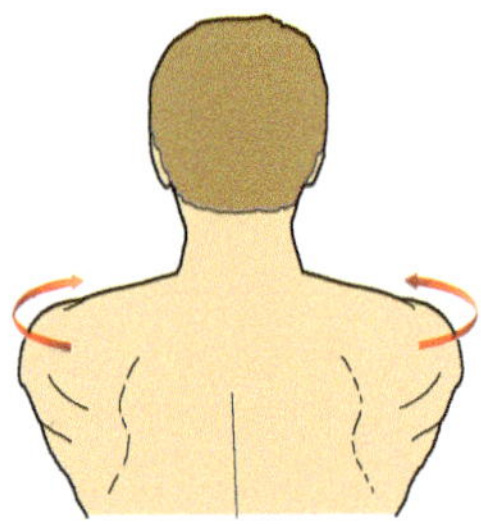	Flexion movement of the arms with anterosuperior elevation (90°): the vertebral borders of the scapulae move away from the vertebral column
Adduction of the scapula 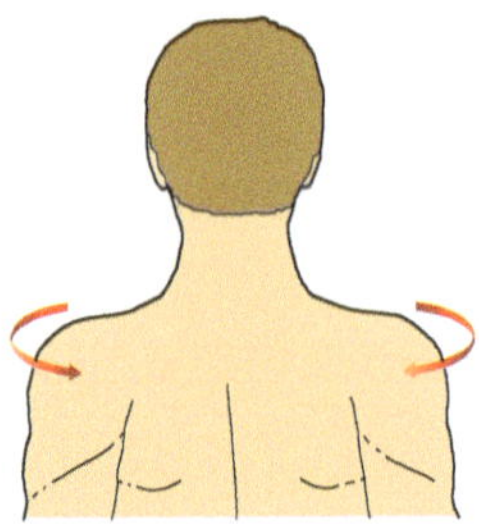	Horizontal movement of the scapulae towards the vertebral column

(continued)

Active movements (*continued*)

Evaluated movements	Execution
Internal rotation of the scapula 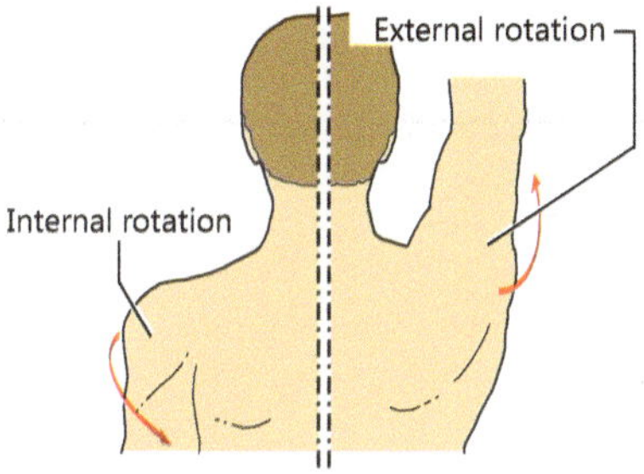	Extension and adduction movement of the arm which is carried behind the trunk: the inferior angle of the scapula is moved in a medial direction
External rotation of the scapula	Abduction movement of the arm with lateromedial elevation: the inferior angle of the scapula is moved in a lateral direction

Passive movements

Evaluated movements	Execution
Elevation of the scapula 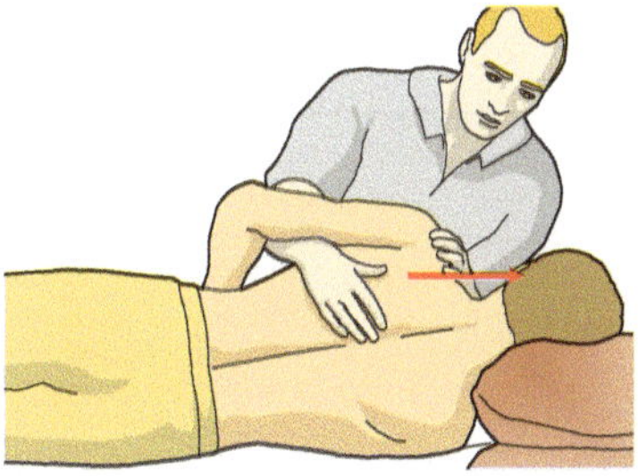	The examiner places the cupped right hand on the inferior angle of the patient's scapula, lifting it; the left hand serves as a guide for the direction of the movement
Depression of the scapula 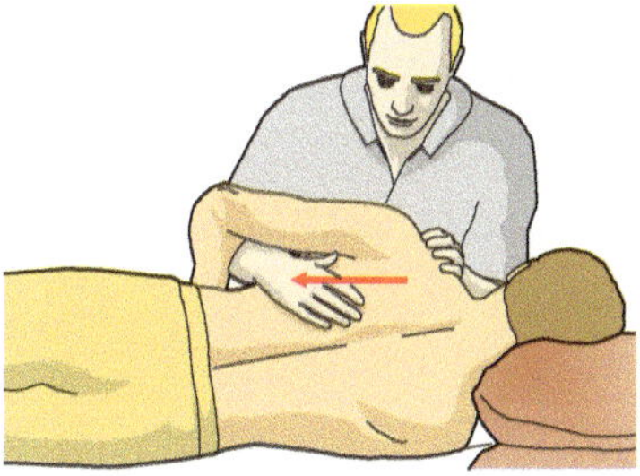	The examiner places the left hand on the apex of the shoulder and lowers the scapula; the cupped right hand, placed on the inferior angle of the scapula, controls the direction of the movement

(*continued*)

7

Passive movements (*continued*)

Evaluated movements	Execution
Abduction of the scapula 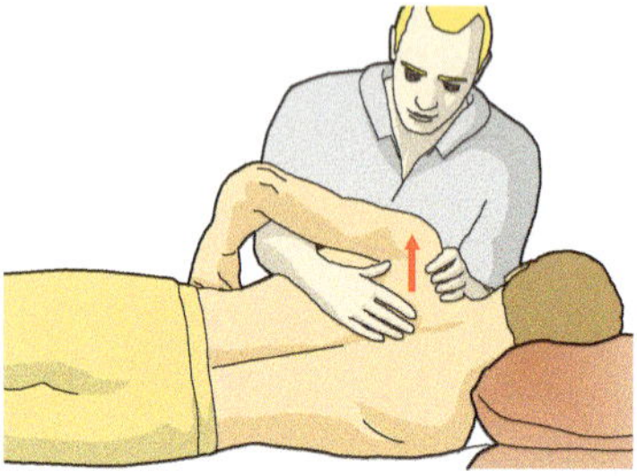	The examiner holds the vertebral border and the inferior angle of the scapula with the thumb and index finger of the right hand, abducting it; the left hand, placed on the apex of the shoulder, facilitates the abduction movement
Adduction of the scapula 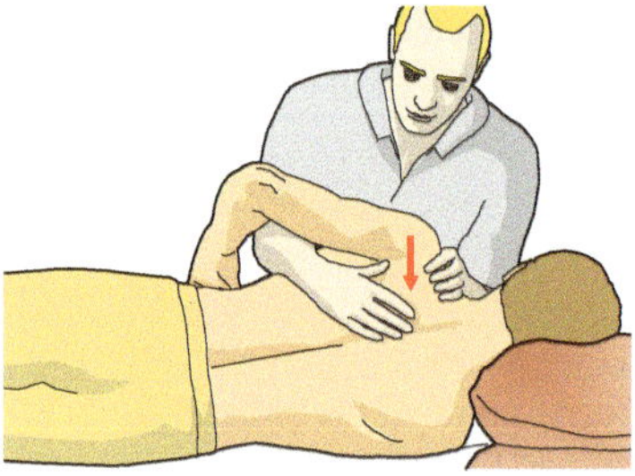	The examiner holds the axillary border and the inferior angle of the scapula with the thumb and index finger of the right hand, adducting it; the left hand, placed on the apex of the shoulder, facilitates the adduction movement

Assessment of shoulder joint mobility (glenohumeral joint)

Measuring passive mobility

Since limited mobility of the shoulder (or glenohumeral) joint can be compensated by movements of the pectoral girdle, the movements of the pectoral girdle (scapular mobility) must be distinguished from those of the glenohumeral joint when assessing and measuring the passive mobility of the shoulder. To isolate the glenohumeral joint, the scapula and clavicle should be stabilized.

Measuring passive mobility

Evaluated movements	Execution
Flexion of the shoulder with anterosuperior elevation (movement of the arm and the scapula) 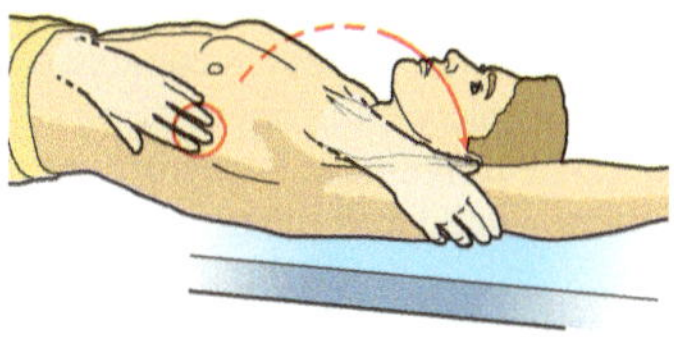	The movement is performed with the patient in the supine position, the arm along the trunk and the palm of the hand directed medially. The examiner holds the distal part of the patient's arm with one hand, bringing it forward and upward to the limit of movement allowed (180°), while the other hand stabilizes the thorax. The elbow is kept in extension to avoid movement limitations due to a passive insufficiency of the triceps brachii
Flexion of the shoulder with anterosuperior elevation (movement of the arm with the scapula held in place) 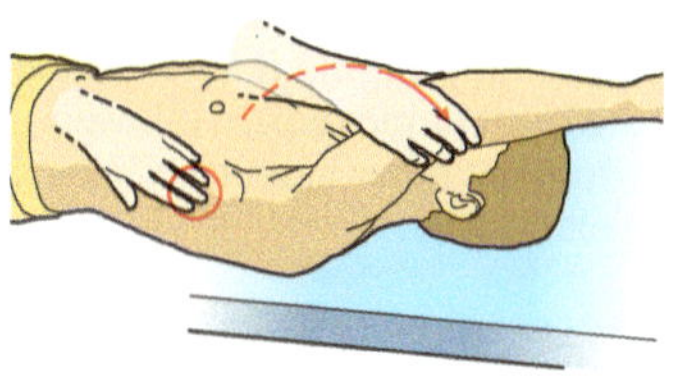	The starting position is similar to the previous one, with the examiner's hand holding the distal part of the patient's arm, bringing it forward and upward to the limit of movement allowed (120°), while the other hand is placed on the axillary border of the scapula, stabilizing it
Extension of the shoulder 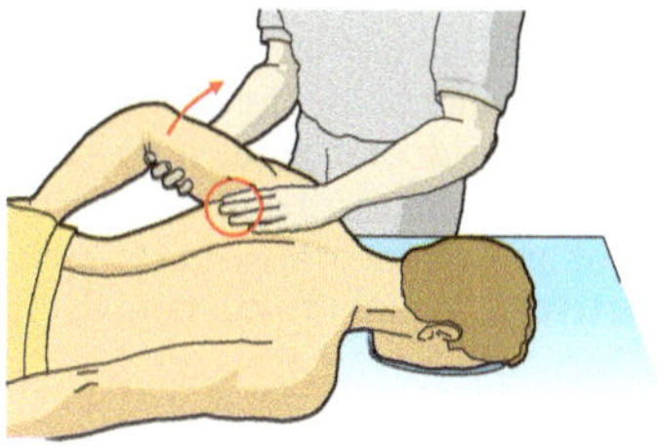	The movement is performed with the patient in the prone position, the arm along the trunk and the palm of the hand directed medially. The examiner holds the distal part of the patient's arm with one hand, bringing it backward (60°) until feels, with the other hand placed on the scapula to stabilize it, an initial displacement of the scapula. The elbow is kept in flexion to avoid movement limitations due to a passive insufficiency of the biceps brachii

(*continued*)

7

Measuring passive mobility *(continued)*

Evaluated movements	**Execution**
Abduction of the shoulder with lateromedial elevation (movement of the arm and the scapula) 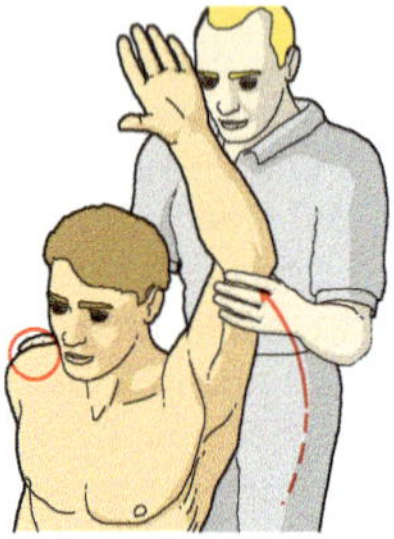	This movement is made possible by the external rotation of the arm on the horizontal plane, which prevents contact between the greater tubercle of the humerus and the acromion. It should ascertained before the evaluation whether the patient is capable of performing a complete external rotation of the shoulder. The movement is performed with the patient seated and the arm externally rotated. The examiner holds the distal part of the patient's arm with one hand, bringing it outward and upward to the limit of movement allowed (180°), while the other hand stabilizes the trunk
Abduction of the shoulder with lateromedial elevation (movement of the arm with scapular fixation) 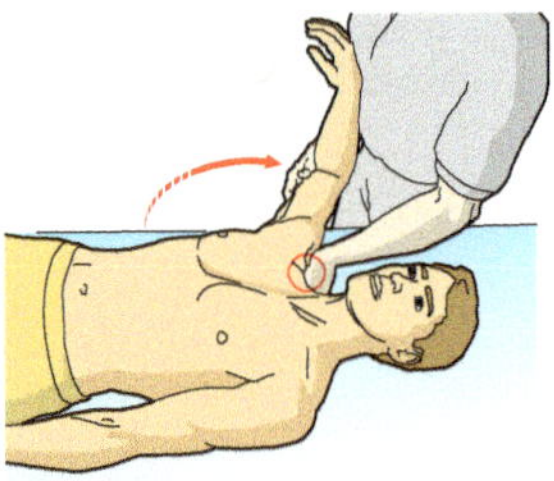	The movement is performed with the patient in the supine position, the arm along the trunk and the elbow flexed at 90°. The examiner holds the distal part of the patient's arm with one hand, bringing it outward and upward to the limit of movement allowed (90-120°), while the other hand stabilizes the scapula and clavicle
Internal and external rotation of the shoulder on the horizontal plane 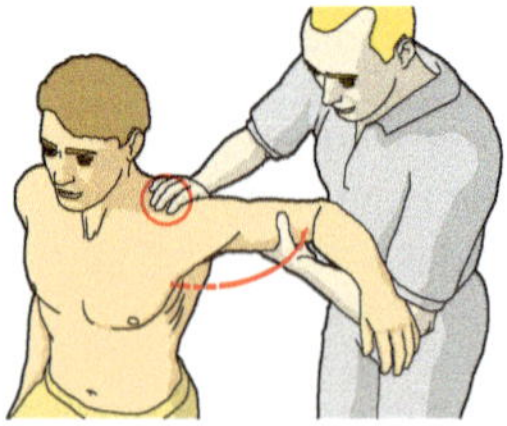 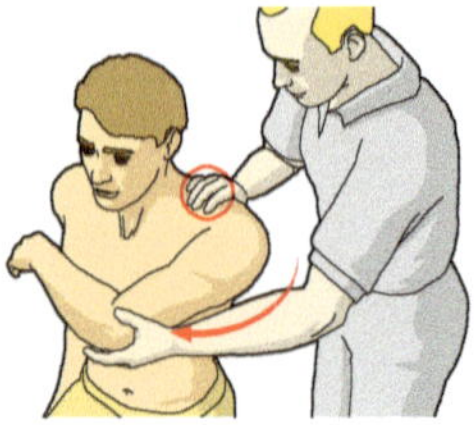	The movement is performed with the patient in a seated position, the shoulder abducted to 90° with lateromedial elevation and the elbow flexed. The examiner holds the distal part of the patient's arm with one hand, supporting it and bringing first backward and then forward to the limit of movement allowed (45° and 135°, respectively), while the other hand stabilizes the scapula

(segue)

Measuring passive mobility (*continued*)

Evaluated movements	Execution
Internal rotation of the shoulder on the axis of the humerus 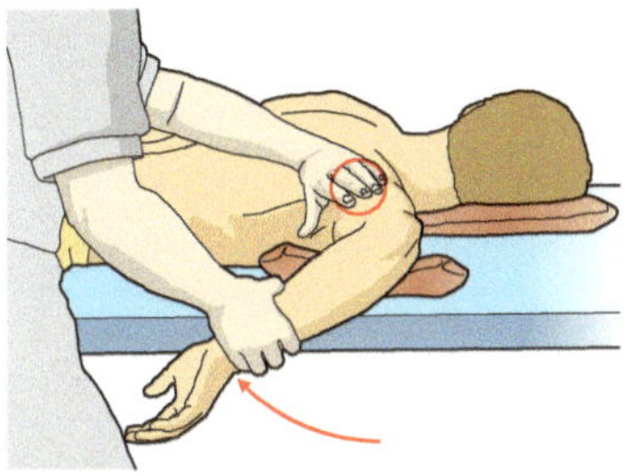	The movement is performed with the patient in the prone position, the shoulder abducted to 90° with lateromedial elevation and the elbow flexed at 90°. This starting position is contraindicated in case of previous posterior dislocation of the glenohumeral joint. The examiner holds the distal part of the forearm, bringing the palm of the patient's hand backward and upward (70°) until feels, with the other hand placed on the scapula to stabilize it, an initial displacement of the scapula
External rotation of the shoulder on the axis of the humerus 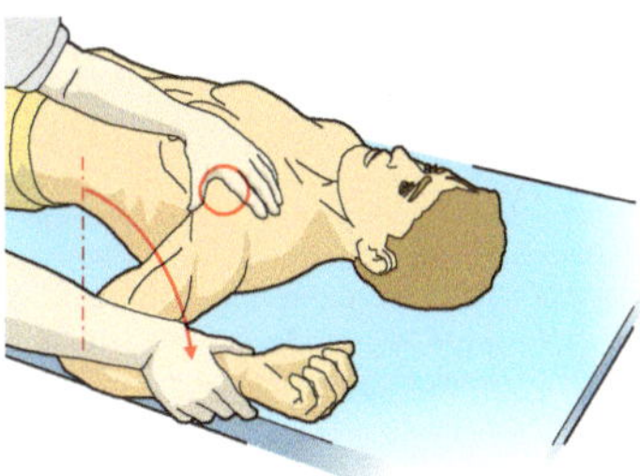	The movement is performed with the patient in the supine position, the shoulder abducted to 90° with lateromedial elevation and the elbow flexed at 90°. This starting position is contraindicated in case of previous anterior dislocation of the glenohumeral joint. The examiner holds the distal part of the forearm, bringing the dorsum of the patient's hand backward and downward (90°) until feels, with the other hand placed on the scapula to stabilize it, an initial displacement of the scapula
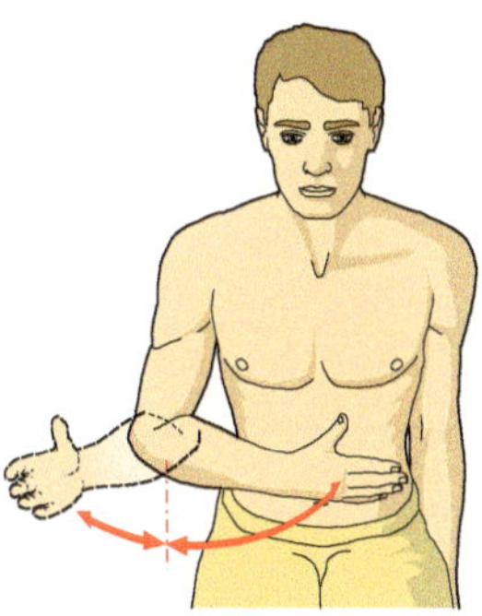	The internal and external rotation of the shoulder on the axis of the humerus can also be aided in a seated position, with 90° flexion of the elbow and 15° abduction of the shoulder during the internal rotation, 90° flexion of the elbow with arm adducted during the external rotation. The palm of the hand is brought against the abdomen in the first case and away from the abdomen in the second case

Active mobility of the joints of the upper limb

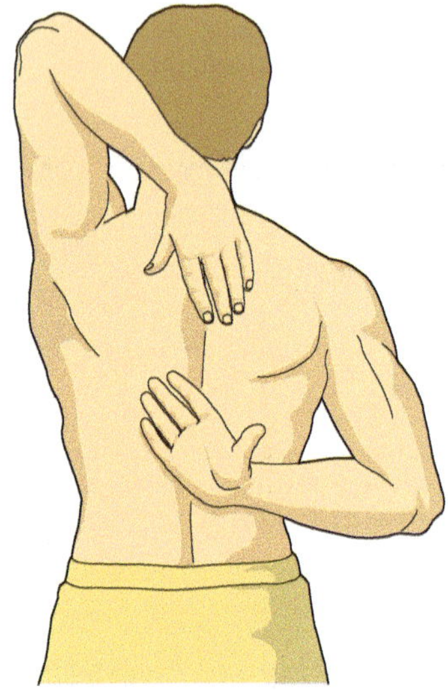

Starting position

Upright position with arms along the trunk.

Movement

The left hand is brought behind the neck and pushed downward on the vertebral column to the limit of movement allowed.

Evaluation of joint amplitude of the movements of:

- abduction and external rotation of the scapula
- flexion, abduction and external rotation of the shoulder
- flexion of the elbow
- supination of the forearm
- radial deviation of the wrist
- extension of the fingers.

Movement

The right hand is brought behind the back inferiorly and pushed upward over the vertebral column to the limit of movement allowed.

Evaluation of joint amplitude of the movements of:

- adduction and internal rotation of the scapula
- extension, adduction and internal rotation of the shoulder
- flexion of the elbow
- pronation of the forearm
- radial deviation of the wrist
- extension of the fingers.

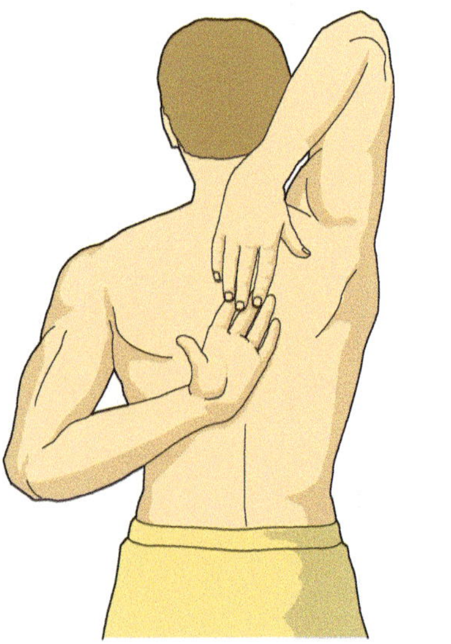

Measurement

The corresponding levels of the vertebral column reached by the tip of the middle finger of the left hand and right hand can be used as a measurement of the active mobility of the joints of the upper limb.

After returning to the starting position, the same movements are performed by inverting the hands. The difference in mobility between the two upper limbs can therefore be observed.

Functional aspects of shoulder joint mobility

Functions of the shoulder joints

To position or move the arm in space to allow use of the hand.

The shoulder joint complex is the most mobile joint complex in the body, allowing a greater range of motion than any other joint. This remarkable mobility, however, reduces the stability of the shoulder.

The glenohumeral (or shoulder) joint can be:
- abducted and adducted
- flexed and extended
- internally and externally rotated.

During functional activities, the movements of the glenohumeral joint are accompanied, at various points of the joint excursion, by movements of the scapula, clavicle and trunk. These movements increase the functionality of the shoulder and the movements of the upper limb would be limited without them.

Interdependence of shoulder and trunk movement components during the execution of functional activities

Elevation of the shoulders above the head

- This movement, which reaches an amplitude of 170-180°, can be obtained by forward flexion of the arm, on the sagittal plane, or by its abduction on the frontal plane
- The plane of the scapula anteriorly to the frontal plane forms a 30-45° angle with it
- Many daily activities are performed on the scapular plane; the latter is used as a reference plane for the diagonal elevation movements of the arm
- The plane of movement used depends on the requirements of the movement, related to a particular activity, and on the position of the hand needed to perform a certain task
- To be able to complete the elevation of the arm up to 180°, both in flexion and abduction, the movements of the glenohumeral joint must be complemented by those of the sternoclavicular and acromioclavicular joints
- The last degrees of these movements can only be achieved with the contribution of the extension and/or contralateral inclination of the trunk
- The entire shoulder joint complex functions in a coordinated manner in order to ensure regular movement and a wide range of motion of the upper limb
- The pattern of coordination of movements at the scapulothoracic and glenohumeral level is referred to as the scapulohumeral rhythm
- Individual variations are possible, depending on the contribution of all joints to the movement. These variations concern:
  - the plane of the movement of elevation
  - the amplitude of the arc of elevation
  - the extent of the load on the arm
  - individual anatomical variables

- It is estimated that the amplitude of the glenohumeral motion compared to the scapular motion during the elevation of the arm have a ratio of 2:1; i.e., two degrees of glenohumeral motion for each degree of scapular motion (for example, an abduction of 60° can be broken down into a 40° movement at the level of the glenohumeral joint and a 20° movement at the level of the pectoral girdle) (see the following section "Scapulohumeral rhythm").

Scapulohumeral rhythm

- It is involved in the elevation of the arm in flexion or abduction
- During the first 60° of flexion on the sagittal plane or the first 30° of abduction on the frontal plane, the scapulohumeral rhythm is minor:
  - the scapula tends to reach a stable condition during this phase with respect to the humerus (adjustment phase), in which it can remain stationary or rotate slightly in a medial or lateral direction
  - during this phase, the greatest contribution to the movement is always provided by the glenohumeral joint
  - the activities related to eating, which are carried out during this phase of elevation of the arm, include movements such as bringing food to the mouth or drinking from a glass:
    - these activities are performed within a joint amplitude between 5-45° of flexion and between 5-30° of abduction
- After the adjustment phase there is a predictable scapulohumeral rhythm for the entire remaining arc of motion up to 170°:
  - for each 15° of movement between 30° of abduction or 60° of flexion and 170° of abduction or flexion, 10° occurs at the level of the glenohumeral joint and 5° at the level of the scapulothoracic joint. Therefore:
    - at 90° of abduction of the shoulder, the rotation of the scapula is approximately 30° and that of the glenohumeral joint is approximately 60°
    - at 150° of abduction of the shoulder, the rotation of the scapula is approximately 50° and that of the glenohumeral joint is approximately 100°
    - at 180° of abduction of the shoulder, the rotation of the scapula is approx-

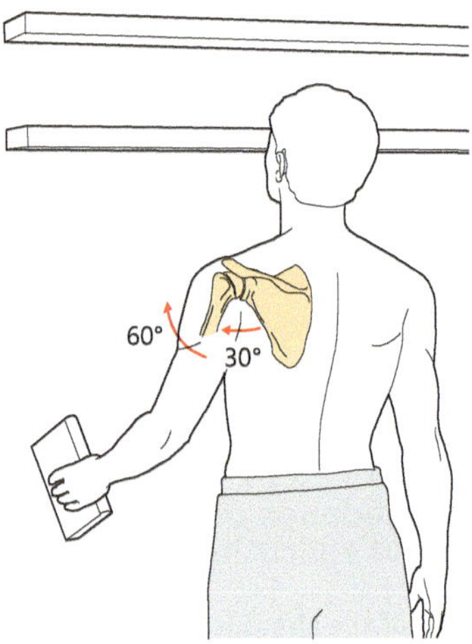

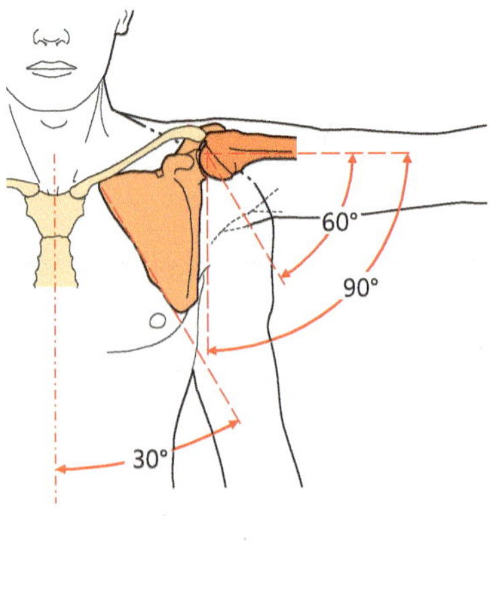

imately 60° and that of the glenohumeral joint is approximately 120°
- the movements of the scapula that characterize this phase consist of:
  - a primary movement of the lateral rotation of the scapula accompanied by secondary rotations linked to its posterior inclination (on the sagittal plane)
  - a movement of posterior rotation (on the transverse plane) with an increase of the humeral angle and elevation of the shoulder on the scapular plane
- the excursion up to 180° of the abduction of the shoulder and the ability to fully rotate the arm outward during its elevation depend on the scapulohumeral rhythm
  - in fact, when the arm reaches 90° of abduction, the full amplitude of the elevation movement cannot be achieved, as the greater tubercle of the humerus comes into contact with the superior border of the glenoid fossa and with the coracoacromial arch
  - the external rotation of the scapula brings the greater tubercle backward, allowing the humerus to move freely under the coracoacromial arch
- the complete elevation of the shoulder in flexion is also related to the scapulohumeral rhythm and to the possibility of internally rotate the humerus during joint excursion

• The last degrees of elevation of the shoulder are obtained through contralateral inclination and/or extension of the trunk.

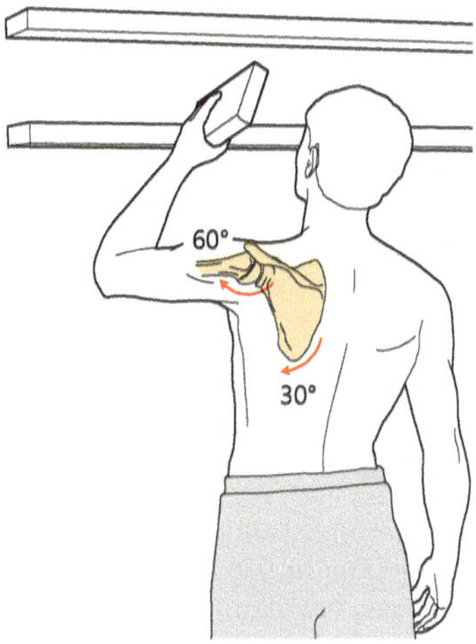

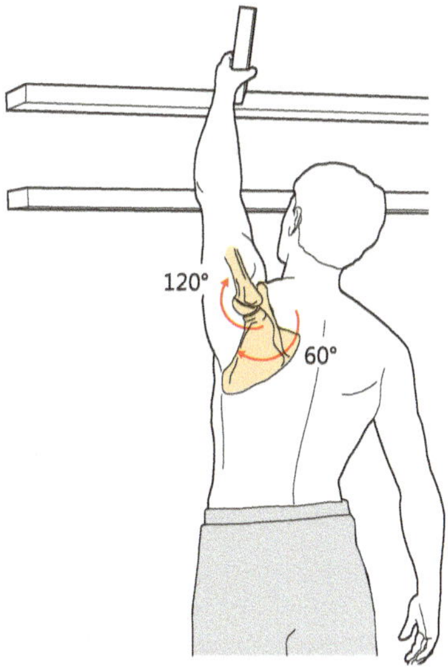

Considering the scapulohumeral rhythm, it is evident that a limitation of movement at the level of any joint of the shoulder complex implies a reduction of the functional positioning possibilities of the hand.

Extension of the shoulder

- The 60° amplitude of the extension movement of the shoulder is primarily achieved by the glenohumeral joint
- There is no significant scapulohumeral rhythm in this movement
- During the execution of functional activities, the extension of the shoulder is often accompanied by the adduction and medial rotation of the scapula
- An extension of the shoulder of a variable amplitude between 43° and 69° is required to bring a hand as high as possible to the back
- An extension of the shoulder of a variable amplitude from 28° to 48° is required to bring the hand backward and downward to the posterior perineum.

Rotation of the arm on the horizontal plane (adduction and abduction of the shoulder on the horizontal plane)

- These movements allow the arm to move around the body at the shoulder height
- By definition, rotation movements of the arm on the horizontal plane occur on the transverse plane, but many functional activities require similar movements on planes above or below the shoulder
- These can be understood as rotations of the arm on the horizontal plane when they are directed towards the frontal plane (displacement of the arm in front of the body – adduction; displacement of the arm behind the body – abduction) and are therefore related to abduction and adduction movements.

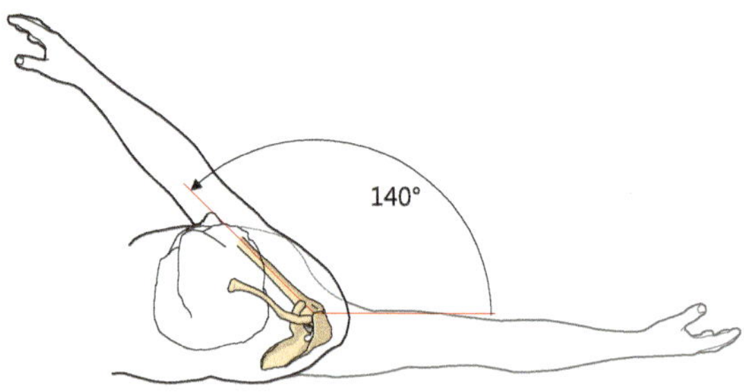

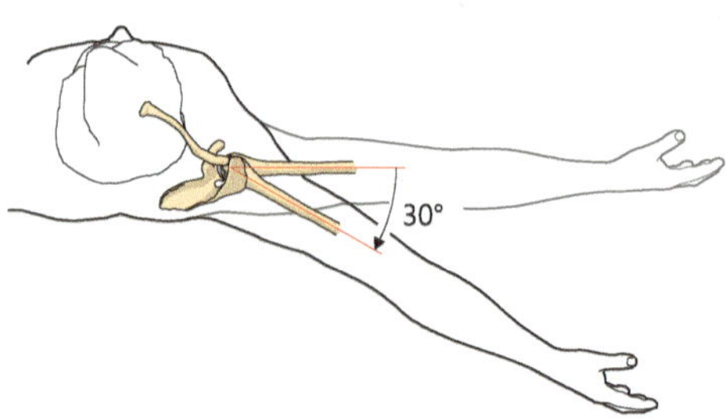

Internal and external rotation of the shoulder on the axis of the humerus

- The amplitude of movement varies with the position of the arm
- The excursion in both directions is on average 68° when the arm is placed next to the trunk
- With the shoulder abducted 90°, 70° of internal rotation and 90° of external rotation can be achieved
- The complete external rotation of the shoulder on the axis of the humerus is necessary to bring the hand behind the neck
- The internal rotation of the shoulder on the axis of the humerus is necessary:
  - to bring the hands anteriorly on the thorax to, for example, button up a shirt
  - for functional activities such as bringing food to the mouth with a fork or a spoon or drinking from a glass (5° to 25° are necessary)
- The complete internal rotation of the scapulohumeral joint, associated with movements of the scapulothoracic joint and elbow, is necessary when the hand is brought behind the back to reach the back pocket of the pants or the posterior perineum (to perform personal care) or to fasten clothing at the posterior thoracic wall.

Movements of the shoulder and elbow joints when moving the arm behind the back

- They are regulated by a coordinated pattern of movements between the glenohumeral joint and the other shoulder joints
- At the beginning of the joint excursion, the internal rotation occurs almost exclusively at the level of the glenohumeral joint, with the hand crossing the body from the front, reaching a position corresponding to that of the ipsilateral hip along the trunk
- The movement continues with the hand coming down behind the back, with the involvement of the scapulothoracic joint that increases the internal rotation of the glenohumeral joint
- At this point the elbow is flexed so that the vertebral column can be reached with the hand at the level of the thorax.

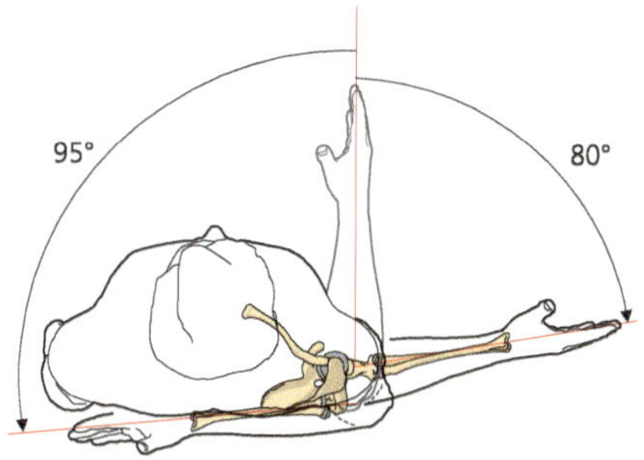

Muscles of the shoulder

Muscle	Action	Origin	Insertion	Innervation
Serratus anterior	Abduction and external rotation of the scapula	External surfaces and superior borders of the first eight, nine or ten ribs; fascia covering the corresponding intercostal muscles	Costal surface of the medial border of the scapula, including the superior and inferior angles	Long thoracic nerve [C5-C7]
Levator scapulae	Elevation and medial rotation of the scapula	Transverse processes of the first four cervical vertebrae	Medial border of the scapula, between the superior angle and the origin of the spine	Third and fourth cervical nerves [C3, C4] and dorsal scapular nerve [C5]
Trapezius				
– Descending (superior) part	Elevation of the scapula with external rotation (abduction)	Medial third of the superior nuchal line; external occipital protuberance; ligamentum nuchae	Posterior border of the lateral third of the clavicle	Spinal root of the accessory nerve [XI] and branches of the cervical plexus [C3, C4]
– Transverse (middle) part	Adduction of the scapula	Spinous processes from T1 to T5 and corresponding supraspinous ligament	Medial border of the acromion and superior border of the spine of the scapula	
– Ascending (inferior) part	Depression and adduction of the scapula (internal rotation)	Spinous processes from T6 to T12 and corresponding supraspinous ligament	Tubercle at the apex of the corresponding triangular surface of the medial end of the spine of the scapula	
Rhomboid minor	Adduction and medial rotation of the scapula	Inferior part of the ligamentum nuchae; spinous processes of C7 and T1 and corresponding supraspinous ligament	Base of the smooth triangular region at the root of the spine of the scapula	Dorsal scapular nerve [C4, C5]

(continued)

Muscles of the shoulder *(continued)*

Muscle	Action	Origin	Insertion	Innervation
Rhomboid major	Adduction and medial rotation of the scapula	Spinous processes from T2 to T5 and corresponding supraspinous ligament	Medial border of the scapula between the root of the spine and the inferior angle of the scapula	Dorsal scapular nerve [C4, C5]
Deltoid				
– Clavicular part	Flexion and internal rotation of the shoulder	Anterior border of the lateral third of the clavicle	Deltoid tuberosity on the lateral surface of the humeral diaphysis	Axillary nerve [C5, C6]
– Acromial part	Abduction of the shoulder	Lateral border and superior surface of the acromion	Deltoid tuberosity on the lateral surface of the humeral diaphysis	
– Spinal part	Extension and external rotation of the shoulder	Lower lip of the crest of the spine of the scapula	Deltoid tuberosity on the lateral surface of the humeral diaphysis	
Supraspinatus	Abduction of the shoulder	Medial two-thirds of the supraspinatus fossa	Superior facet of the greater tubercle of the humerus	Suprascapular nerve [C5, C6]
Coraco-brachialis	Flexion and adduction of the shoulder	Coracoid process of the scapula, medially to the short head of the biceps brachii	Middle third of the anteromedial surface of the humerus	Musculo-cutaneous nerve [C5-C7]
Pectoralis major	Horizontal adduction and internal rotation of the shoulder	*Clavicular head*: anterior border of the medial third of the clavicle *Sternocostal head*: medial half of the anterior surface of the sternum; cartilages of the first six/seven ribs *Abdominal head*: aponeurosis of the external oblique	*All three parts*: lateral lip of the intertubercular sulcus of the humerus	Medial and lateral pectoral nerves [C5-C8, T1]

(continued)

Muscles of the shoulder *(continued)*

Muscle	Action	Origin	Insertion	Innervation
Pectoralis minor	Forward traction and medial rotation of the scapula	External surfaces of the second to the fourth ribs, or from the third to the fifth near the costal cartilages; fascia of the corresponding external intercostal muscles	Medial border and superior surface of the coracoid process of the scapula	Medial and lateral pectoral nerves [C5-C8, T1]
Subscapularis	Internal rotation of the shoulder	Medial two-thirds of the subscapular fossa	Lesser tubercle of the humerus; anterior part of the joint capsule of the shoulder	Upper and lower subscapular nerves [C5, C6]
Infraspinatus	External rotation of the shoulder	Medial two-thirds of the infraspinous fossa	Middle facet of the greater tubercle of the humerus	Suprascapular nerve [C5, C6]
Teres minor	External rotation of the shoulder	Superior two-thirds of the lateral surface of the dorsal surface of the scapula, near to the lateral border of the scapula	Inferior facet of the greater tubercle of the humerus	Axillary nerve [C5, C6]
Teres major	Extension and internal rotation of the shoulder	Posterior surface of the inferior angle of the scapula	Medial lip of the intertubercular sulcus of the humerus	Lower subscapular nerve [C5, C6]
Latissimus dorsi	Extension, adduction and internal rotation of the shoulder	Posterior layer of the thoracolumbar fascia originating from the spinous processes of the lumbar and sacral vertebrae; corresponding supraspinous ligament; posterior surface of the iliac crest; spinous processes of the last six thoracic vertebrae anterior to the insertion of the trapezius; last three or four ribs; inferior angle of the scapula	Fundus of the intertubercular sulcus of the humerus	Thoracodorsal nerve [C6-C8]

(continued)

Muscles of the shoulder (*continued*)

Muscle	Action	Origin	Insertion	Innervation
Subclavius	Depression and protraction of the clavicle	Medial and superior surfaces of the first rib	Inferior surface of the middle third and the lateral third of the clavicle (subclavian groove)	Nerve to the subclavius [C5, C6]
Triceps	Extension and adduction of the shoulder	*Long head*: infraglenoid tubercle of the scapula *Lateral head*: posterior surface of the humerus between the radial groove and the insertion of the teres minor; lateral intermuscular septum of the arm *Medial head*: posterior surface of the humerus below the radial groove, between the trochlea of the humerus and the insertion of the teres minor; medial and lateral intermuscular septa of the arm	*All three heads*: apex, posterior surface and borders of the olecranon; some fibers continue distally, merging with the antebrachial fascia	Radial nerve [C6-C8]
Biceps brachii	Flexion, abduction, adduction and rotation of the shoulder	*Short head*: apex of the coracoid process of the scapula *Long head*: supraglenoid tubercle of the scapula	*Both heads*: radial tuberosity and antebrachial fascia (through the bicipital aponeurosis)	Musculo-cutaneous nerve [C5, C6]

Muscles attaching the pectoral girdle to the trunk

- Trapezius
- Levator scapulae
- Rhomboid major and rhomboid minor
- Serratus anterior
- Pectoralis minor
- Subclavius

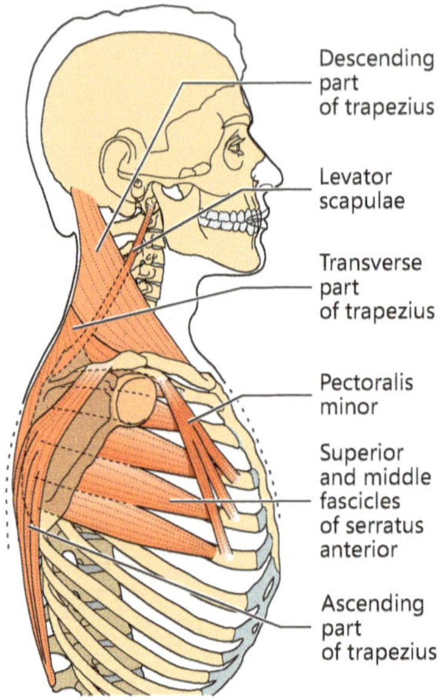

These muscle connections between the scapula and trunk are crucial for the position and coordination of the movements of the scapula, and are divided into pairs of antagonist muscles called muscle slings:

- levator scapulae-ascending part of the trapezius
- serratus anterior (superior and middle fascicles)-transverse part of the trapezius
- pectoralis minor-descending part of the trapezius
- rhomboid major and rhomboid minor-serratus anterior (inferior fascicles).

When one of the two muscles that make up the sling contracts, the other relaxes and vice versa.

These four muscle slings coordinate the following movements of the scapula, respectively:

- elevation-depression
- abduction-adduction
- forward and downward movement-backward and upward movement
- internal rotation-external rotation.

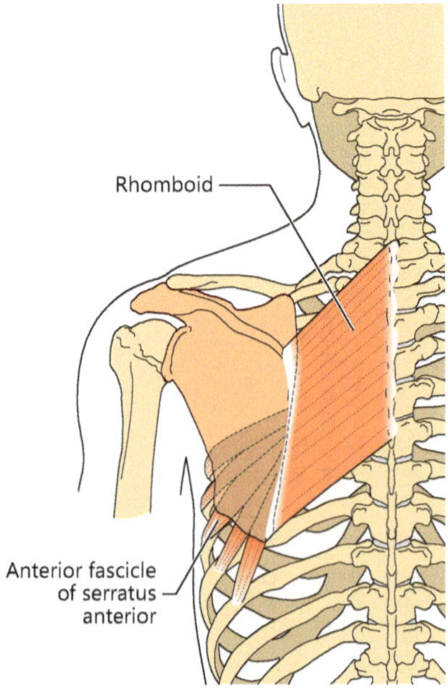

> The correct position of the scapula in relation to the thorax, which allows the coordinated execution of the movements of the arm and pectoral girdle, depends on the balance between these four muscle slings.

Actions of the muscles attaching the pectoral girdle to the trunk

Trapezius

- Descending, transverse and ascending parts → fixation of the pectoral girdle with traction on the scapula and the clavicle in a posterior and medial direction:
  - agonist synergy between the transverse part and the rhomboid major and rhomboid minor
- Descending part → external rotation of the scapula (upward and medially displacement of the acromion, with exposure of the glenoid cavity upward and externally)

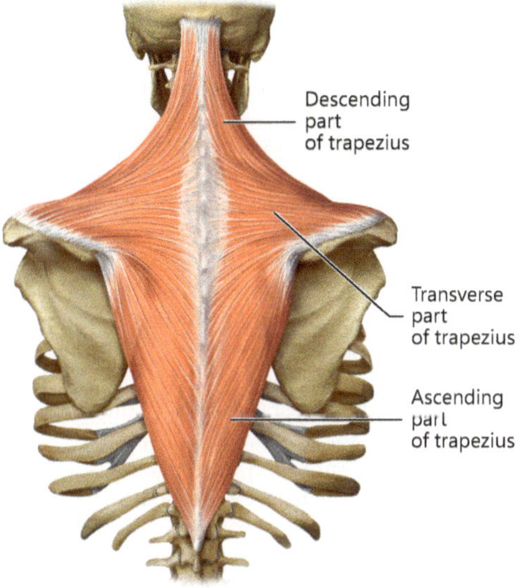

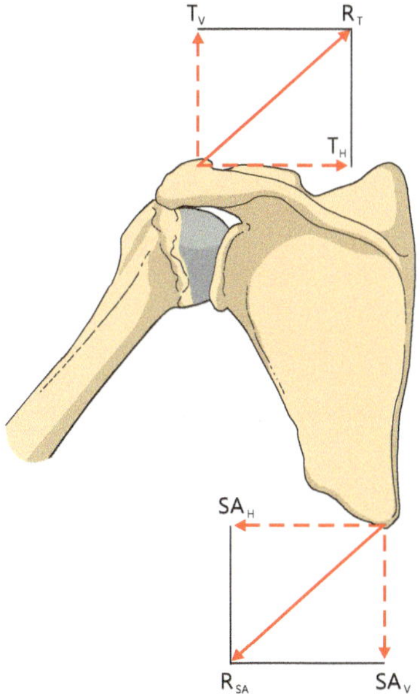

Pair of forces: descending part of the trapezius and serratus anterior. Left pectoral girdle, posterior view. The descending part of the trapezius supports the scapula with its vertical component (T_V) and brings it to its origins with its horizontal component (T_H). The serratus anterior tends to raise the scapula with its vertical component (SA_V) and to abduct it with its horizontal component (SA_H). Both resultants of the two muscles (R_T and R_{SA}) externally rotate the inferior angle of the scapula.

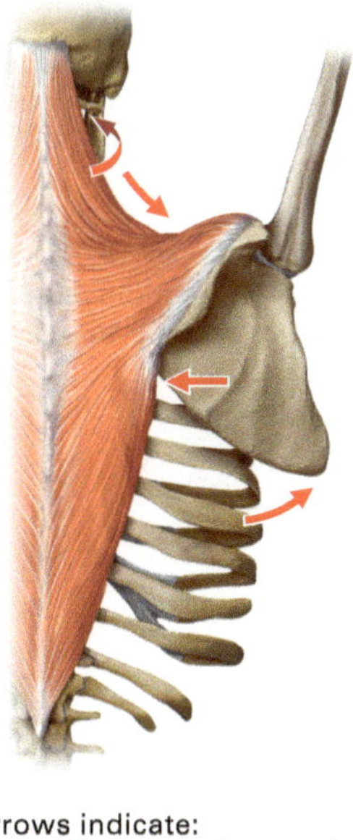

Trapezius. The arrows indicate:
- superior: ipsilateral flexion and contralateral rotation of the head;
- middle: fixation-traction action of the scapula to the column of the entire trapezius and internal rotation of the scapula due to the ascending part;
- inferior: external rotation of the scapula due to the descending part.

  - muscles
    - antagonists: rhomboid major and rhomboid minor and ascending part of the trapezius
    - synergists: serratus anterior (formation of a pair of forces, that is, two equal and parallel forces with opposite directions)
- Transverse part → displacement of the scapula towards the thorax and of its medial border towards the vertebral column
- Ascending part → displacement of the spine of the scapula downward and medially (formation of a fixed point for lateral rotation of the scapula).

Fixing of the pectoral girdle by other muscles (fixed point for the trapezius):
- unilateral action of the trapezius
  - descending part → ipsilateral inclination and contralateral rotation of the head
- bilateral action of the trapezius
  - descending, transverse and ascending parts → extension of the vertebral column
  - ascending part → elevation of the trunk when the body is suspended (agonist synergy with the latissimus dorsi).

Static function of the trapezius:
- When the upper limb is at the side of the trunk and the hand supports a weight, the trapezius unloads the sternoclavicular joint on the lateral part of the clavicle and on the medial part of the acromion.

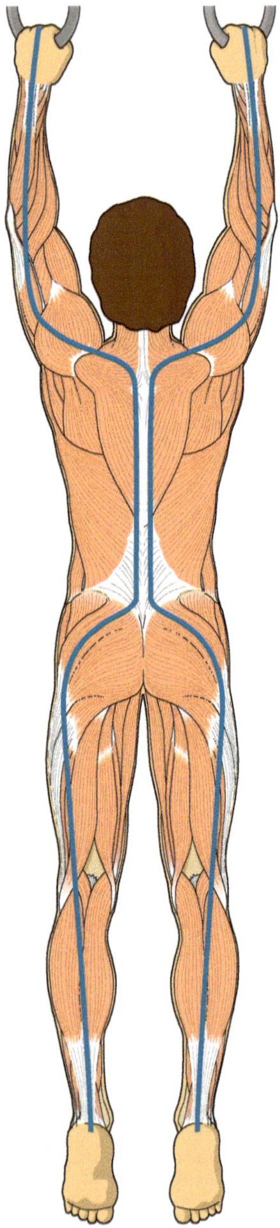

Predominant tension of the latissimus dorsi, pectoralis major (not evident) and trapezius in the body suspended from the gymnastic rings.

Levator scapulae

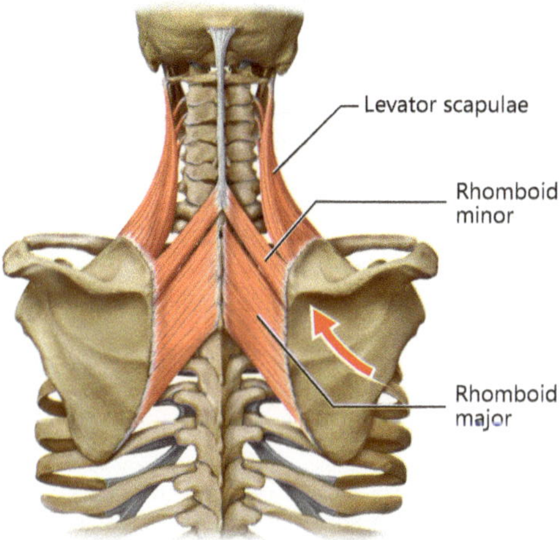

Levator scapulae and rhomboid muscles. The arrow indicates the movement of the scapula induced by the two muscles.

- Elevation and adduction (2-3 cm) of the scapula (the medial border of the scapula is directed upward) with a slight downward rotation of the glenoid cavity
  - muscles
    - synergist to the rotation: rhomboid major and rhomboid minor, ascending part of the trapezius, latissimus dorsi
    - antagonists
      - to rotation: descending part of the trapezius, serratus anterior
      - to elevation: latissimus dorsi
- Elevation of the shoulder (also with bilateral contraction)
  - synergist muscles: descending part of the trapezius, serratus anterior
- Brings the externally rotated scapula back into a neutral position (in this position of the scapula there is an eccentric relaxation of its muscle fibers)
- Mild and continuous activation as a supporting function of the scapula.

Fixation of the scapula by other muscles (fixed point for the levator scapulae):
- ipsilateral flexion and rotation of the head and neck
- slight extension of the cervical column (bilateral contraction).

Rhomboid major and rhomboid minor

- Internal and upward rotation of the inferior angle of the scapula, with elevation of the scapula and lowering of the glenoid cavity
  - antagonist muscles: descending part of the trapezius, pectoralis minor, serratus anterior
- Fixation of the scapula to the thorax (the inferior angle of the scapula is kept close to the thoracic cage).

Serratus anterior

- Superior, intermediate and inferior fascicles → rotation of the scapula outward (12-15 cm), upward and forward
  - muscles
    - agonists: descending part of the trapezius
    - antagonists: rhomboid major, rhomboid minor, levator scapulae
- Superior fascicles → internal rotation of the scapula
- Intermediate fascicles → fixation of the scapula to the thorax
- Superior fascicles → external rotation of the scapula.

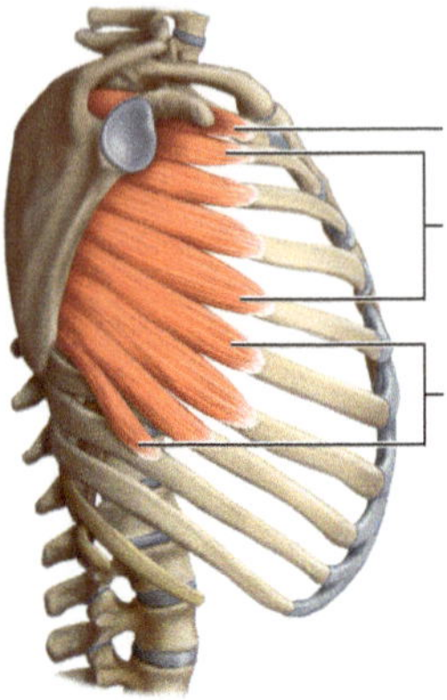

Serratus anterior.

The external rotation of the scapula occurs both during abduction of the arm with lateromedial elevation (in which there is greater activity of the trapezius compared to the serratus anterior) and during the flexion of the arm with anterosuperior elevation (in which there is greater activity of the serratus anterior compared to the trapezius).

Fixation of the scapula by the rhomboid major and rhomboid minor (fixed point for the serratus anterior):

- accessory inspiratory muscle (forced inspiration only).

Pectoralis minor

- Depression of the scapula and shoulder
- Anterior inclination (anteversion) of the scapula, the rotation of which exposes the glenoid cavity downward
- Moving away the inferior angle of the scapula from the thorax
- Fixation of the scapula during the extension of the arm.

Fixation of the scapula by other muscles (fixed point for the pectoralis minor):

- accessory inspiratory muscle (forced inspiration only).

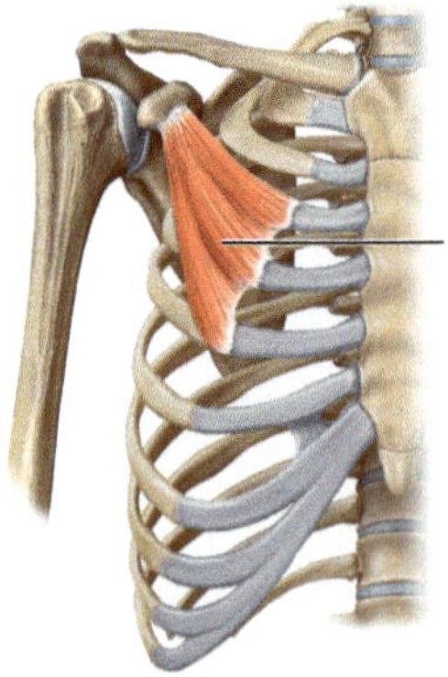

Pectoralis minor.

Subclavius

- Depression of the clavicle (with slight protraction) and shoulder, stabilizing the sternoclavicular joint

Fixation of the clavicle by other muscles (fixed point for the subclavius):

- accessory inspiratory muscle (forced inspiration only).

Muscles attaching the pectoral girdle to the humerus

- Deltoid
- Supraspinatus
- Infraspinatus
- Teres minor
- Subscapularis
- Teres major
- Coracobrachialis
- Biceps brachii
- Triceps brachii

Actions of the muscles attaching the pectoral girdle to the humerus

Deltoid

Clavicular, acromial and spinal parts

- abduction of the humerus
  - clavicular part → acts as a fixator element (by antagonism to the spinal part)
  - acromial part (the strongest part of the muscle) → responsible for the direction of force and maximal force
  - spinal part → acts as fixator element (by antagonism to the clavicular part)

Clavicular part (the most important part from a functional point of view, because it is responsible for most of the movements of the arm in front of the body)

- flexion of the humerus
- internal rotation of the humerus

Spinal part

- extension of the humerus
- external rotation of the humerus.

Also important is the static synergistic action of the acromial part of the deltoid and the descending and transverse parts of the trapezius, capable of preventing downward sliding of the humerus when the hand supports a high or medium weight for a long time.

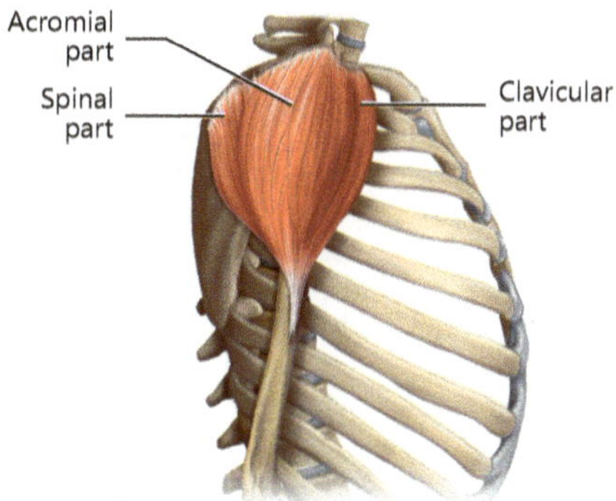

A

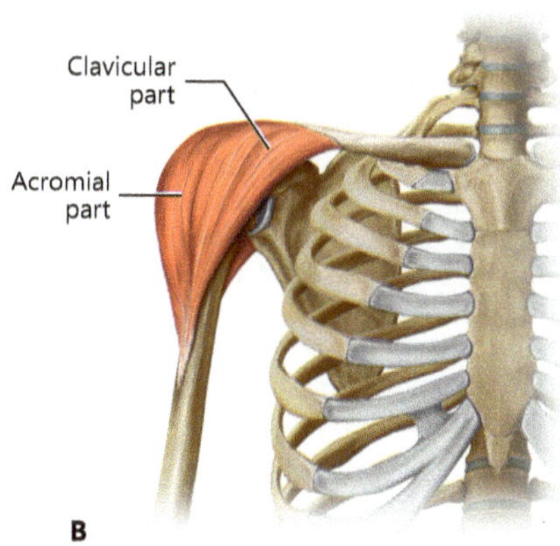

B

Deltoid. **A.** Lateral view. **B.** Frontal view.

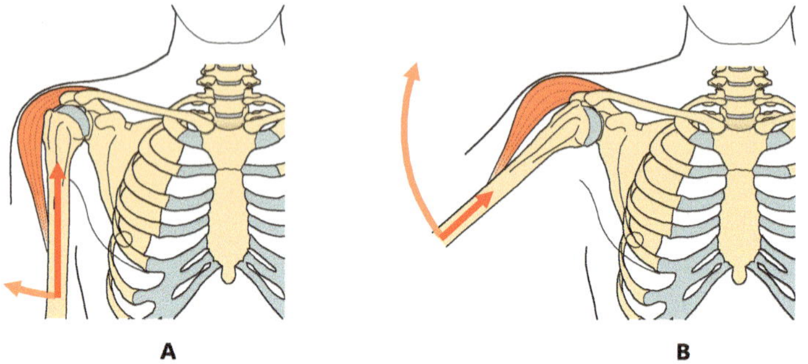

Components of the force of the deltoid. **A.** In a neutral position. **B.** In abduction.

Fixation of the humerus, for example, in the suspension on the gymnastic rings (fixed point for the deltoid):

- unilateral contraction – "flag-shaped" body arrangement
- bilateral contraction – upward translation of the trunk.

Components of the force of the acromial part of the deltoid in a neutral position:

- major vector with superior direction (the head of the humerus is brought against the roof of the glenoid cavity)
- minor vector with outward direction (abduction of the humerus)
- once the abduction of the arm has begun, the force applied to continue the abduction movement prevails over that applied to elevate the humerus.

Supraspinatus

- Abduction of the arm (progressively less during the movement)
- Depression of the head of the humerus, which is centered in the glenoid cavity.

Infraspinatus

- Extension of the humerus
- External rotation of the humerus (it is the most important external rotator muscle, developing approximately 90% of the force required for external rotation)
- External rotation of the scapula
- Depression of the head of the humerus, which is centered in the glenoid cavity.

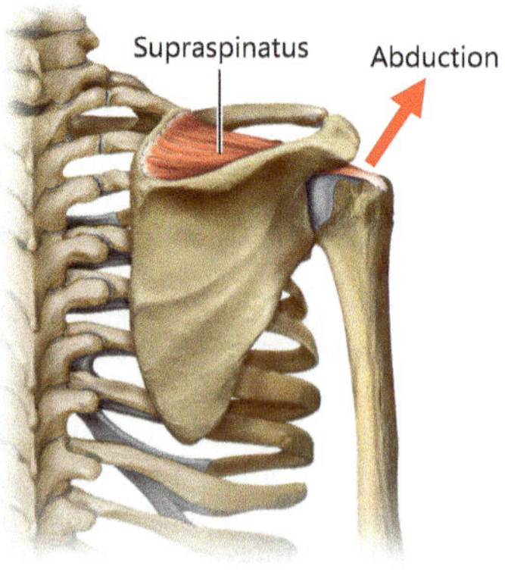

Supraspinatus.

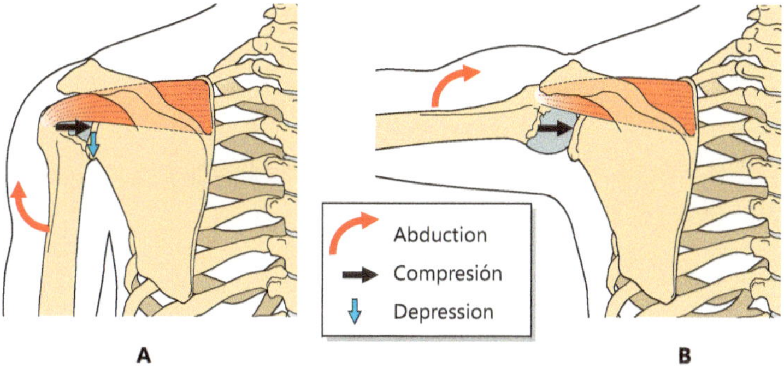

Functions of the supraspinatus. **A**. In a neutral position. **B**. In abduction.

Teres minor

- Extension of the humerus
- External rotation of the humerus
- External rotation of the scapula
- Depression of the head of the humerus, which is centered in the glenoid cavity.

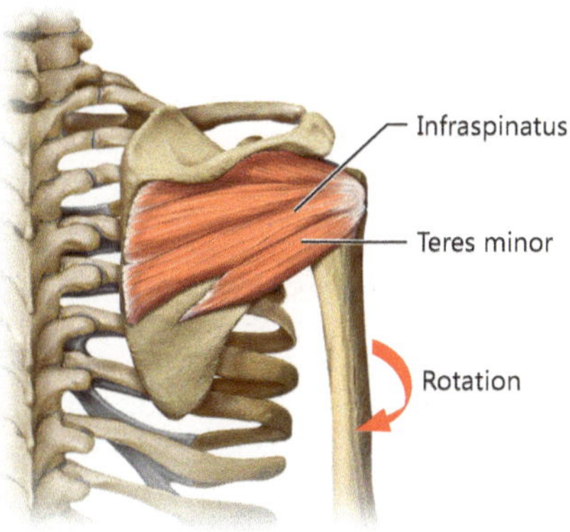

Subscapularis

- Internal rotation of the humerus (it is the most important internal rotator muscle)
- Depression of the head of the humerus, which is centered in the glenoid cavity
- Approach of the medial border of the scapula to the thoracic cage with a fixed point on the humerus.

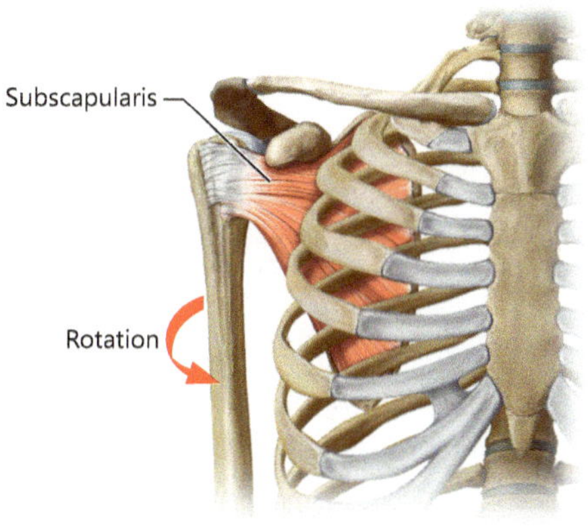

Rotator cuff

It is formed by the following muscles:

- supraspinatus (located superiorly to the glenohumeral joint)
- infraspinatus (located inferiorly to the glenohumeral joint)
- teres minor (located inferiorly to the glenohumeral joint)
- subscapularis (located anteriorly to the glenohumeral joint)

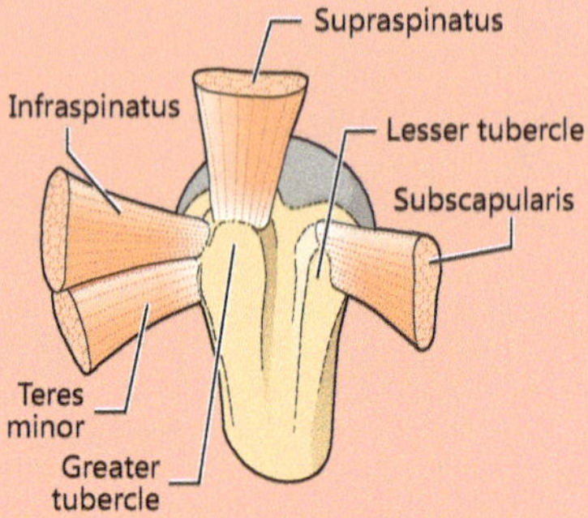

These muscles act synergistically (agonists), lowering the head of the humerus and bringing it closer to the glenoid cavity to allow its positioning. The head of the humerus is thus fixed in the glenoid cavity. In reality, there is a reciprocal movement of more or less contemporary approaching of the two joint heads that leads to the centering of the head of the humerus in the glenoid cavity.

The tendons of the rotator muscles fuse with the capsule of the glenohumeral joint, performing a significant stabilizing function in relation to this joint.

The fascicles of these muscles form a fibrous aponeurosis (subdeltoid fascia) that attaches to the spine of the scapula, the acromion and to the inferior border of the coracoid process, extending to the deltoid tuberosity.

Synergistic action of the rotator cuff and the deltoid

The acromial part of the deltoid (principal arm abductor muscle) presents, in the initial phase of the abduction movement, a force vector directed upward, which the rotator muscles oppose. Their action results in a slight lowering of the head of the humerus, which antagonizes the action of the force vector of the deltoid upward, avoiding the compression of the head of the humerus against the roof of the glenoid cavity and favoring instead its positioning.

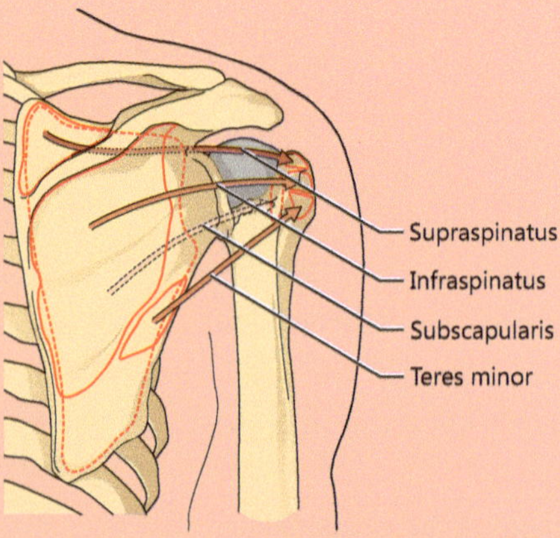

The rotator cuff (posterior view of the right humerus). Insertion, origin and muscle lines.

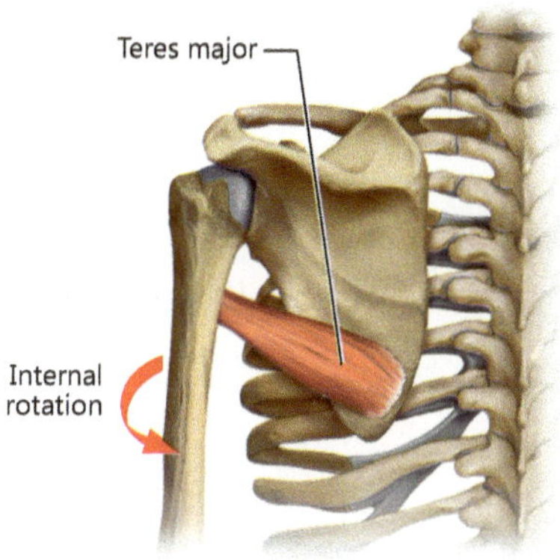

Teres major

- Extension of the arm
- Adduction of the arm
- Internal rotation of the humerus
- External rotation of the scapula with fixed point on the humerus.

Coracobrachialis

- Flexion of the arm
- Adduction of the arm
- Stabilization of the glenohumeral joint
- Depression of the scapula, with facilitation of its forward displacement (fixed point on the humerus): anteversion.

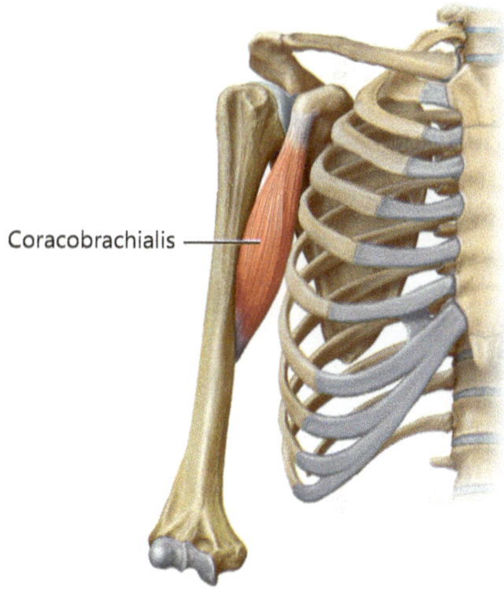

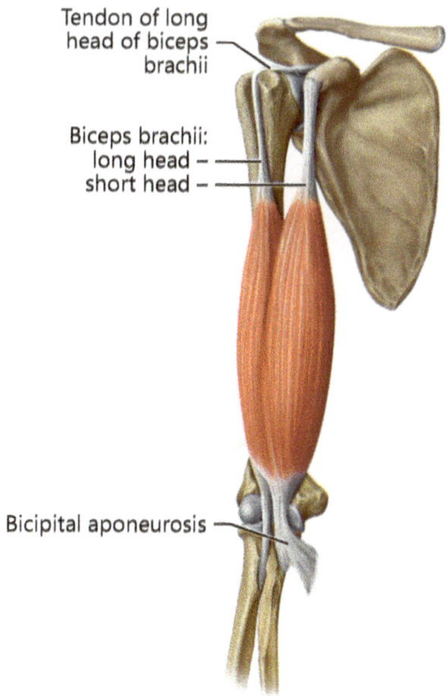

Biceps brachii.

Biceps brachii and triceps brachii

Biceps brachii:
- biarticular with action on the scapula
  - origin
    - from the supraglenoid tubercle (long head)
    - from the apex of the coracoid process (short head)
  - insertion
    - on the radial tuberosity
- short head
  - flexion of the arm
  - adduction of the arm
  - internal rotation of the humerus

- long head
  - flexion of the arm
  - abduction of the arm
  - depression of the head of the humerus in synergy with the rotator cuff.

Triceps brachii:
- biarticular with action on the scapula
  - origin from the infraglenoid tubercle (long head)
- long head
  - extension of the arm
  - adduction of the arm.

The synergistic action of the two muscles stabilizes the head of the humerus.

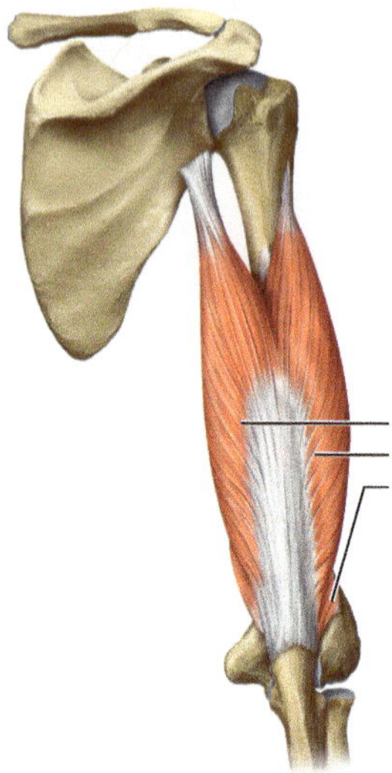

Triceps brachii.

Muscles attaching the trunk to the humerus

- Latissimus dorsi
- Pectoralis major

Actions of the muscles that join the trunk to the humerus

Latissimus dorsi

- Extension of the arm
- Adduction of the arm
- Internal rotation of the arm

(These actions lead to a lowering of the arm and are more efficient when it is abducted by 30-90°).

- With a fixed point on the humerus:
  - translation of the trunk upward when the body is in suspension
  - lateral inclination of the trunk and pelvis (ipsilateral)
  - the costal part of the muscle acts as an accessory inspiratory muscle
- Fixation of the ribs when coughing (with formation of a fixed point for the diaphragm).

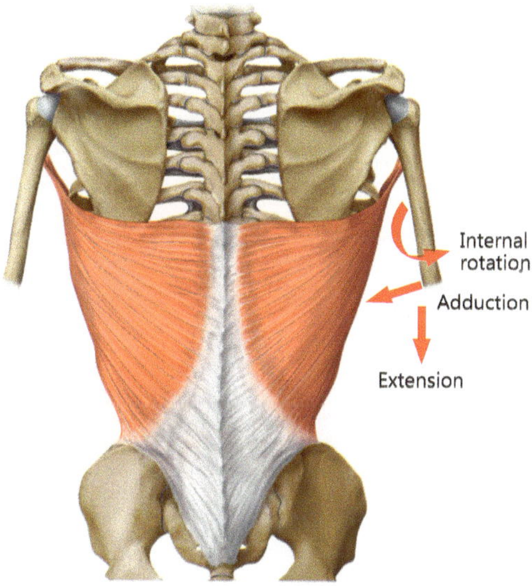

Latissimus dorsi.

Synergistic action of the latissimus dorsi and the long head of the triceps brachii during the extension of the shoulder:

- pair of forces
  - elevation of the head of the humerus towards the roof of the glenoid cavity (long head of the triceps brachii)
  - depression of the head of the humerus (latissimus dorsi).

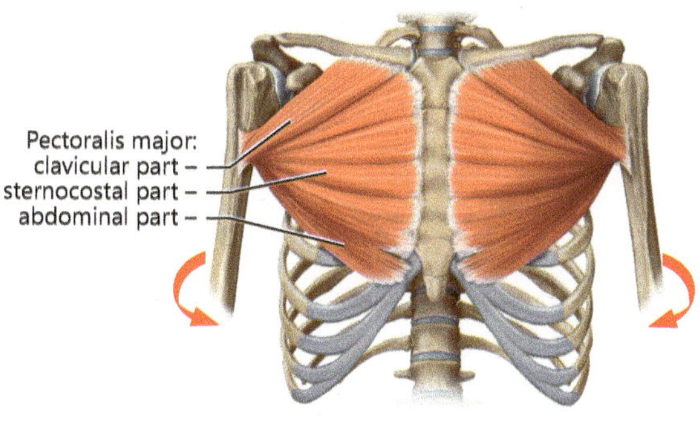

Pectoralis major. The arrows indicate the flexion, adduction and rotation actions.

Pectoralis major

- Flexion of the arm
- Adduction of the arm
- Internal rotation of the arm
- Displacement of the pectoral girdle in an inferoposterior direction with a fixed point on the humerus
- The inferior parts (sternocostal and abdominal) act as an accessory inspiratory muscle with fixed points on the humerus and scapula.

Muscles that insert on the clavicle

- Trapezius (descending part)
- Deltoid (clavicular part)
- Pectoralis major (clavicular part)
- Subclavius

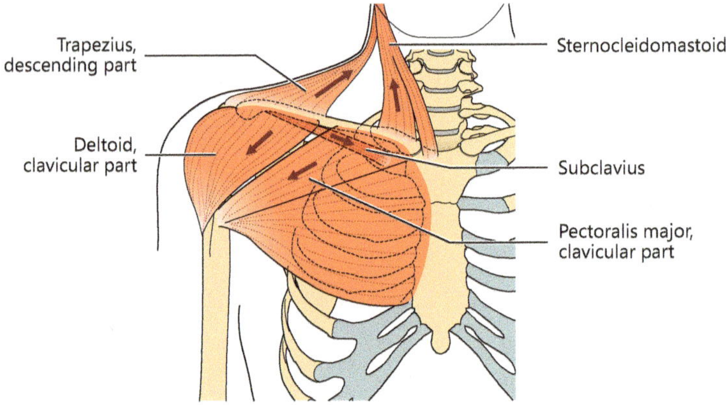

Muscles that insert on the clavicle.

The actions of these muscles can influence the position of the clavicle and, more generally, the position of the pectoral girdle (see section "Functional aspects of the joints of the pectoral girdle", page 235).

Action of the muscles in the movements of the shoulder

Abduction of the shoulder with lateromedial elevation

Abduction of the shoulder (180°) has three phases:
- Phase 1 – true abduction – from 0° to 90°
- Phase 2 – false abduction (lateromedial elevation of the arm) – from 90° to 150°
- Phase 3 – false abduction (lateromedial elevation of the arm) – from 150° to 180°.

Phase 1

Muscles originating from the scapula and inserting on the humerus come into action:
- supraspinatus (initiales abduction movement – abductor starter)
- deltoid (responsible for much of the muscular force, in this first phase of the abduction, it comes into action immediately after the supraspinatus)
- biceps brachii (long head, whose contribution is quantitatively less important than that of the other muscles).

The supraspinatus, when initiating the abduction movement of the arm, lowers the head of the humerus positioning it in the glenoid cavity, thus counteracting the action of the deltoid which, if it were able to initiate the abduction movement on its own, would cause, by pushing the head of the humerus upward, the compression of the latter against the roof of the glenoid cavity (see section "Synergistic action of the rotator cuff and the deltoid, page 272).
In fact, both muscles are temporarily synergistic in initiating abduction, controlling and correcting the direction of movement.
To this is added the fixation action of the head of the humerus in the glenoid cavity exerted by the rotator cuff and by the long head of the biceps brachii.

7

Phase 2

The following muscles come into action in the second phase of the abduction movement:
- serratus anterior
- trapezius (descending part).

These muscles constitute a pair of forces (see section "Trapezius", page 265).

Antagonist muscles:
- rhomboid major and rhomboid minor
- levator scapulae
- ascending part of the trapezius.

The movement of the scapula that occurs during abduction of the shoulder begins when it reaches an amplitude of 30-50°. The scapula is rotated counterclockwise (externally) by the serratus anterior, with upward exposure of the glenoid cavity.

The external rotation of the scapula allows the head of the humerus to move freely in the glenohumeral joint, avoiding compression against the roof of the shoulder (inferoanterior surface of the acromion) and allowing lateral elevation of the arm up to 150°. When the raised arm in abduction is adducted, the external rotation of the scapula is maintained. It is an involuntary or automatic movement defined as *Codman's paradox*.

Abduction of the shoulder associated with rotation:
- neutral of the arm → 80-90°
- external of the arm → 80-90° + 20-30°
- internal of the arm → 60°

The external rotation of the scapula moves the origin of the deltoid away from its insertions, which allows a greater force to be exerted. The maximal force of the deltoid in the abduction of the shoulder is, in fact, between 90° and 180° of abduction. Beyond this limit, the adductor resistance of the pectoralis major and the latissimus dorsi intervenes.

The external rotation of the scapula is finally accompanied by the movements of the acromioclavicular and sternoclavicular joints:
- the first 30° of rotation of the scapula corresponds to 30° of elevation of the clavicle (sternoclavicular joint)
- another 45° (rotation of the clavicle around its axis) are added to these first 30° of elevation of the clavicle

The elevation and rotation movements of the clavicle are performed by the action of the descending part of the trapezius and the sternocleidomastoid.

Antagonist muscles:
- subclavius
- deltoid
- pectoralis major

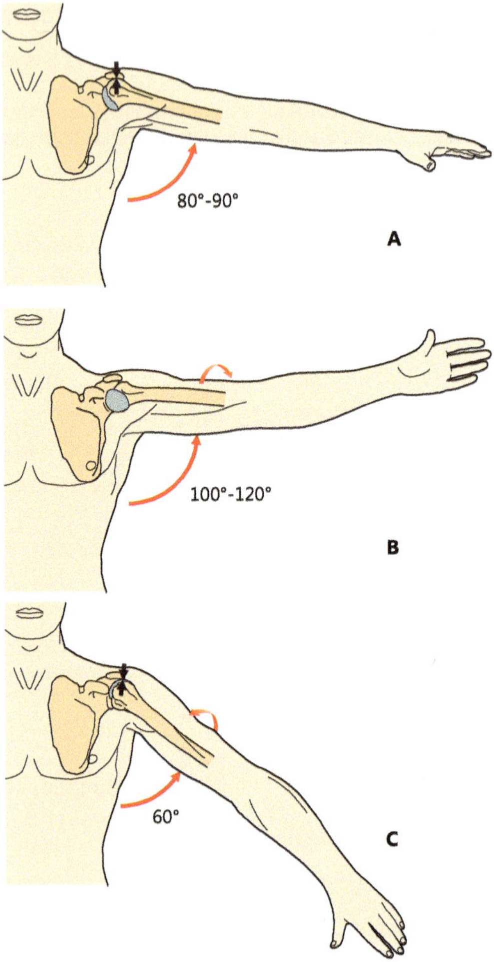

Abduction. **A.** In neutral rotation. **B.** With external rotation. **C.** With internal rotation.

The abduction of the shoulder is associated with scapulohumeral rhythm from its first degrees (see section "Scapulohumeral rhythm", page 256).

Phase 3

The muscles (motors) in action are:

- deltoid
- supraspinatus
- trapezius
- serratus anterior

The lateromedial elevation of the arm is only possible if trunk displacements, i.e., movements by the vertebral column (with simultaneous elevation of the ribs), are performed in advance:

- in unilateral abduction there is an ipsilateral rotation and a contralateral flexion of the vertebral column (due to the action of the contralateral flexor muscles of the column, which move the insertions of the motor muscles further away on the frontal plane, allowing the last 30° of abduction)
- in bilateral abduction there is an extension of the lumbar column (due to the action of the paravertebral lumbar muscles, with relaxation of the motor muscle fibers similar to that occurring in unilateral abduction).

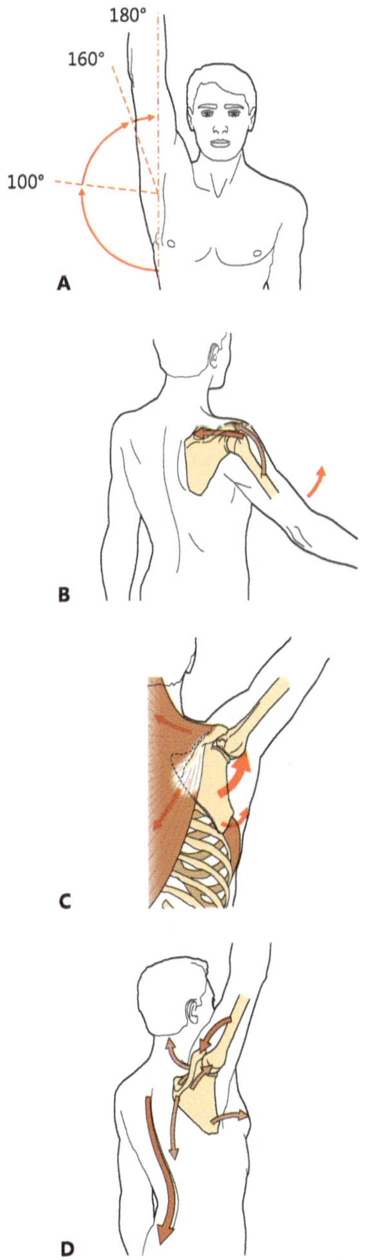

Abduction. **A**. Amplitude of movement. **B**. Phase 1 of movement. **C**. Phase 2 of movement. **D**. Phase 3 of movement.

Factors allowing maximal abduction of the shoulder with lateromedial elevation

- Elasticity of the joint capsule and the possibility of subacromial gliding
- Synergy between the rotator cuff and the deltoid
- Scapulothoracic gliding and mobility of the acromioclavicular and sternoclavicular joints
- External rotation of the scapula and humerus
- Mobility of the vertebral column

Adduction of the shoulder

Relative adduction

- It is the one originating from any position of abduction
- There is no muscle work if carried out with the trunk upright; the force of gravity is sufficient to produce the movement
- There is muscle work if the adduction is obtained:
  - by slowing down the movement (against the force of gravity; in this case there is an eccentric contraction of the abductor muscles, whereas the adductor musculature is inactive)
  - by increasing the execution speed (the adductor muscles come into action)
  - against resistance (the adductor muscles come into action).

Absolute adduction

- The starting position is the anatomical position (arms along the trunk)
- The upper limb should approach the midline, but this is not directly possible, for which there is:
  - adduction with anteposition of the arm (ventral adduction) – of greater amplitude – carried out by flexion of the arm
  - adduction with retroposition of the arm (dorsal adduction) – of lesser amplitude – carried out by the extension of the arm.

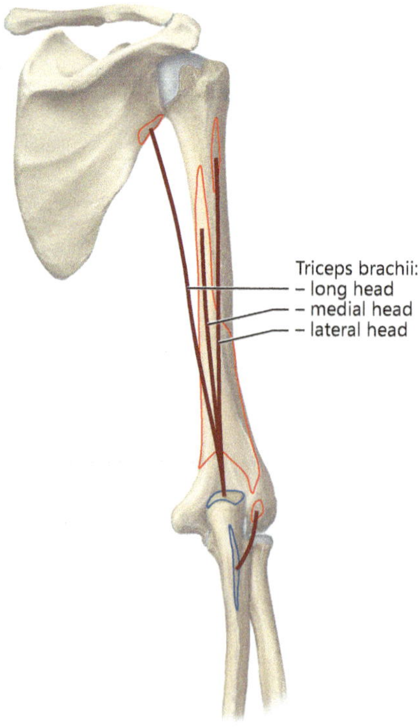

Schematic representation of the insertions of the triceps brachii. The long head has an important functional action: in the course of adduction, it keeps the head of the humerus in the glenoid cavity to counteract the dislocating action of the latissimus dorsi.

Ventral adductor muscles:
- pectoralis major
- deltoid (clavicular part)
- biceps brachii (short head)
- flexor muscles of the arm in general.

Dorsal adductor muscles:
- latissimus dorsi
- teres major
- triceps brachii (long head)
- deltoid (spinal part)
- extensor muscles of the arm in general.

During the dorsal adduction of the arm, the long head of the triceps brachii keeps the head of the humerus in the glenoid cavity, countering the displacement action produced by the latissimus dorsi on the head of the humerus itself.

Flexion of the shoulder with anterosuperior elevation

Flexion of the shoulder (180°) has three phases:
- Phase 1 – from 0° to 60°
- Phase 2 – from 60° to 120°
- Phase 3 – from 120° to 180°.

Phase 1

Involvement of the muscles that move the humerus (movements of the glenohumeral joint):
- deltoid (clavicular part)
- biceps brachii
- pectoralis major (clavicular part)
- coracobrachialis.

Antagonist muscles:
- extensors in general
- teres minor
- infraspinatus.

There is minimal rotation of the scapula in this phase.

Phase 2

Involvement of the muscles:
- serratus anterior (moves the pectoral girdle)
- trapezius (descending part) (moves the humerus).

Due to the action of the serratus anterior, external rotation of the scapula occurs (with movements of the acromioclavicular and sternoclavicular joints), which determines the exposure of the glenoid cavity forward and upward.

Once 100° amplitude is reached, movements of the thoracic column and ribs begin to be observed.

Phase 3

Involvement of the intrinsic muscles of the vertebral column:

- unilateral flexion of the arm - the movement is completed by the flexion of the vertebral column, which also determines the abduction of the arm (intrinsic flexor muscles of the vertebral column)
- bilateral flexion – the movement is completed by the extension of the lumbar column (intrinsic extensor muscles of the vertebral column).

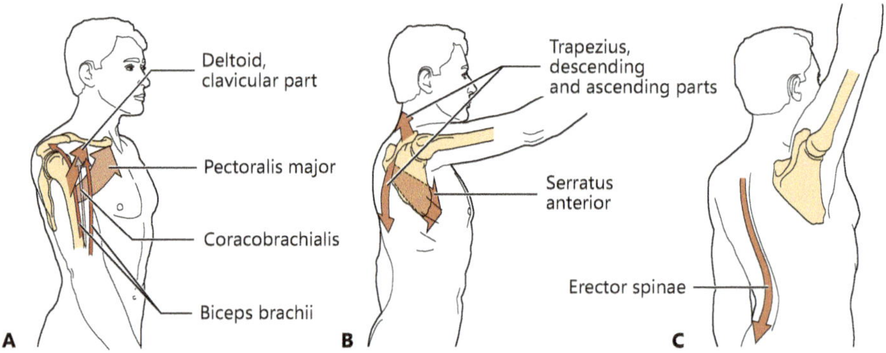

Flexion. **A.** For the movement of the glenohumeral joint. **B.** For the external rotation of the scapula. **C.** For the movement of the vertebral column.

Extension of the shoulder

Movement opposite to the flexion of the shoulder (movement of the arm backward and upward).

Extensor muscles:

- latissimus dorsi
- teres major
- teres minor
- triceps brachii (long head)
- deltoid (spinal part).

The rhomboid major and rhomboid minor and the transverse part of the trapezius are involved in the extension of the shoulder by fixing the scapula in adduction.

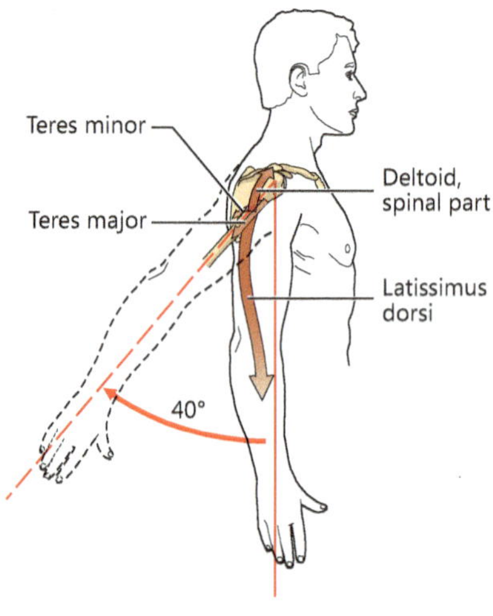

Amplitude of the movement in extension.

Rotation of the shoulder on the horizontal plane

- Starting position: arm abducted 90°
- Between the external and internal rotation, the range of motion is approximately 170° (140° internal rotation and 30° external rotation).

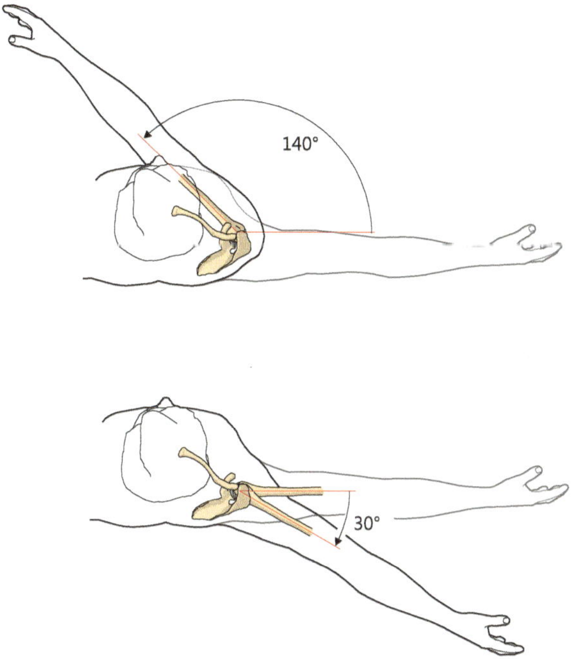

Rotation on the horizontal plane.

Internal rotator muscles:
- deltoid (clavicular part)
- subscapularis
- pectoralis major and pectoralis minor
- serratus anterior.

External rotator muscles:
- deltoid (spinal part)
- infraspinatus
- teres minor
- rhomboid major and rhomboid minor
- trapezius (transverse part).

Rotation of the shoulder on the axis of the humerus

- Starting position: arm along the trunk with the elbow flexed at 90°
- The rotation of the shoulder is measured indirectly by assessing the position of the axis of the forearm.

Internal rotation

The forearm is brought behind the back (95° rotation of the arm).

Internal rotator muscles:
- subscapularis
- pectoralis major
- biceps brachii (long head)
- deltoid (clavicular part)
- teres major
- latissimus dorsi.

External rotation

80° rotation of the arm.

External rotator muscles:
- infraspinatus
- teres minor
- deltoid (spinal part).

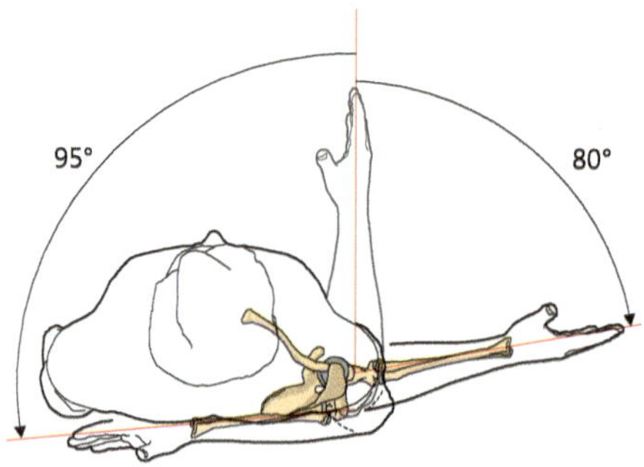

Amplitude of movement in external rotation and internal rotation.

Assessment of the length of the fibers of the pectoralis major and pectoralis minor

Pectoralis major

The shoulder is abducted on the horizontal plane up to the limit of mowement allowed, so as to obtain the complete stretch of the pectoralis major, starting from the supine position with the shoulder rotated externally and the elbow flexed at 90° with the upper limb almost adjacent to the support plane of the examination table. The left hand of the examiner blocks the trunk.

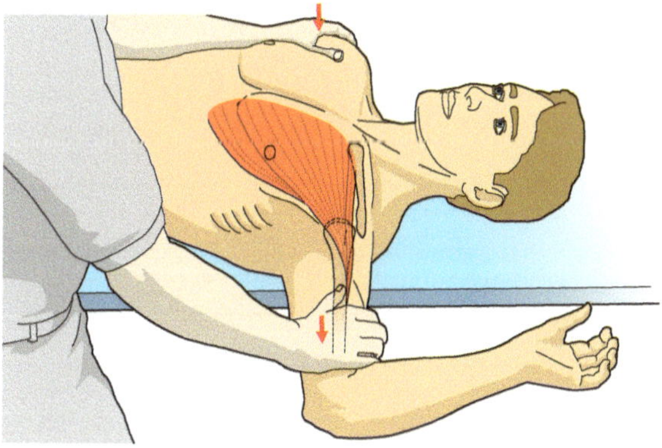

Pectoralis minor

The pectoral girdle is moved upward and backward, so as to obtain the complete stretching of the pectoralis minor, starting from the supine position with the shoulder rotated externally and flexed to 80° and the elbow flexed.

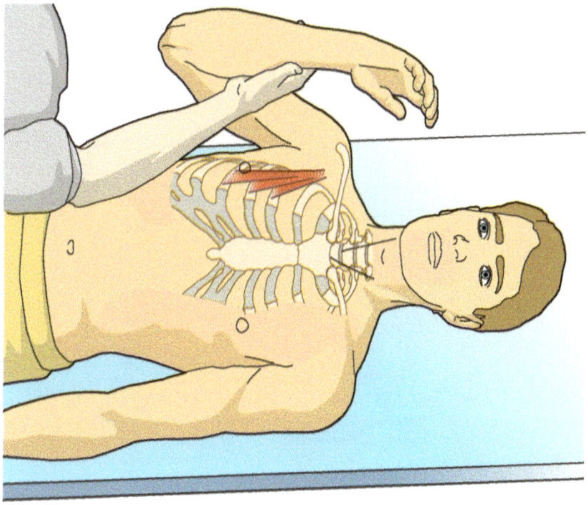

Strength assessment of the shoulder muscles

Abduction and lateral rotation of the scapula

Serratus anterior

Against gravity

The scapula is actively abducted (with protraction) from the supine position with the shoulder flexed at 90° and slightly abducted, the elbow extended and resistance applied to the distal end of the arm.

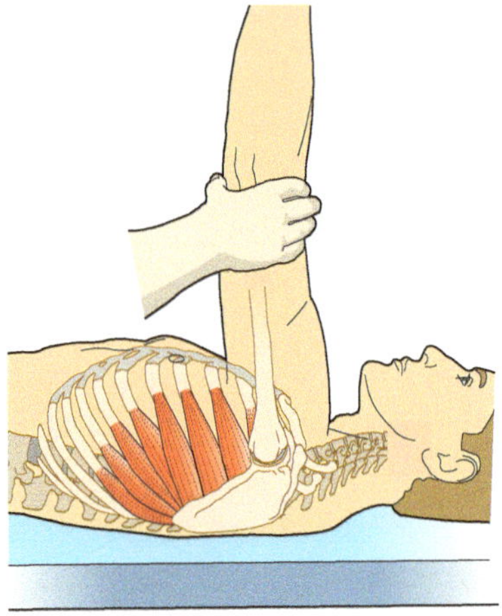

Without gravity

The scapula is actively abducted from a sitting position with the shoulders flexed at 90°, slightly abducted on the transverse plane and the elbow extended. The examiner controls the movement.

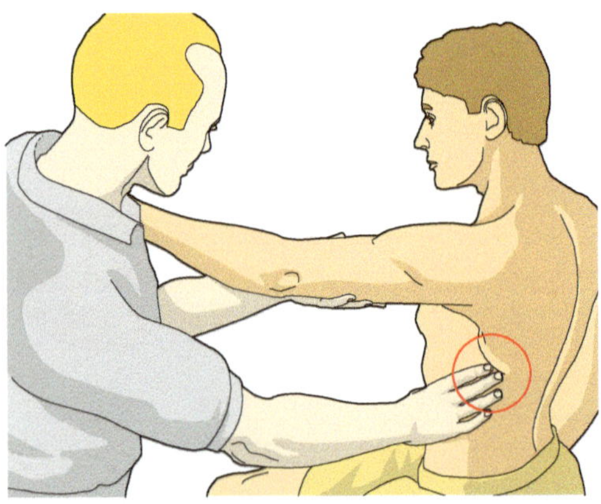

Clinical test of the serratus anterior strength

Starting position	Upright position, facing the wall and hands placed on the wall at the shoulder height
Movement	The thorax moves away from the wall with abduction of the scapulae 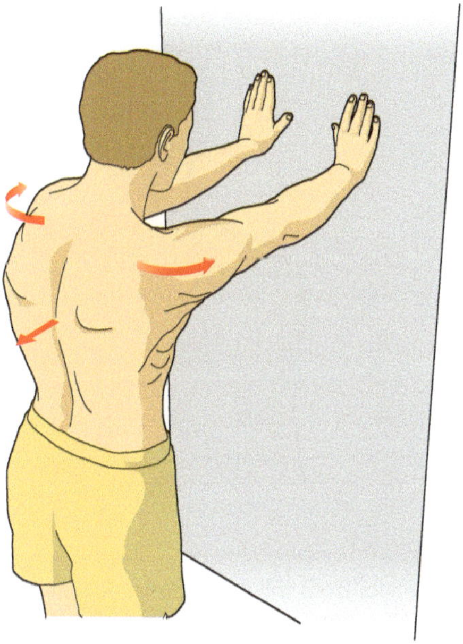
A sign of serratus anterior deficit is given by the "winged" scapula, in which the medial border and the inferior angle of the scapula appear more protruded and the scapula remains adducted and medially rotated.	

Elevation of the scapula

Levator scapulae and descending part of the trapezius

Against gravity

Elevation of one or both pectoral girdles from a sitting position with the shoulders slightly abducted and resistance applied to the apex of the shoulder.

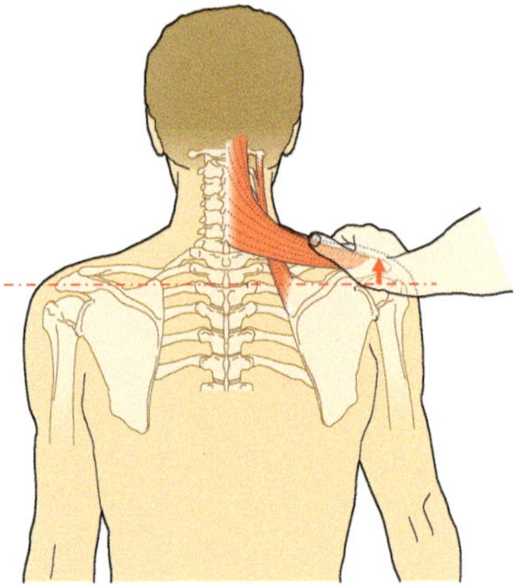

Without gravity

Elevation of the scapula from the prone position with the arms along the trunk, in neutral rotation, and the limb supported by the examiner.

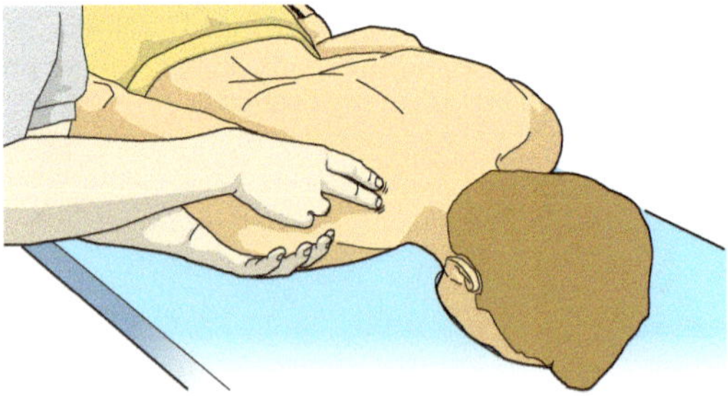

The descending part of the trapezius can be palpated at a point situated halfway along the line that joins the inion and the acromion.

Adduction of the scapula

Transverse part of the trapezius

Against gravity

Adduction of the scapula from the prone position with the shoulder flexed at 90°, in neutral rotation and resistance applied to the scapula.

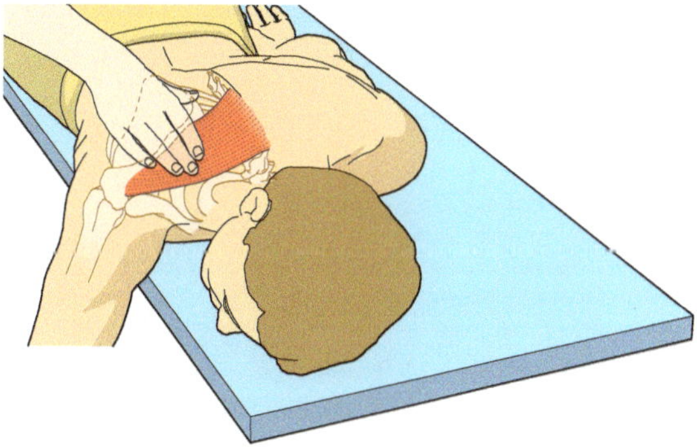

Without gravity

Adduction of the scapula from a sitting position with the shoulder flexed at 90°, slightly abducted and internally rotated, and the limb supported by the examiner.

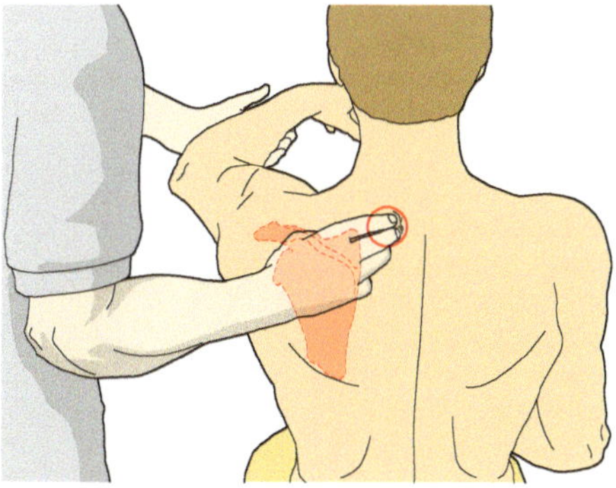

The transverse part of the trapezius can be palpated between the medial border of the scapula and the vertebrae, above the spine of the scapula.

Adduction and internal rotation of the scapula

Rhomboid major and rhomboid minor

Against gravity

Elevation of the arm from the prone position with the dorsum of the hand resting on the buttock of the non-examined side and resistance applied to the scapula.
The movement consists of raising the upper limb from the buttock and simultaneously adducting the contralateral scapula. The hand of the examiner controls the resistance to be made by the ipsilateral scapula (abducts and externally rotates).

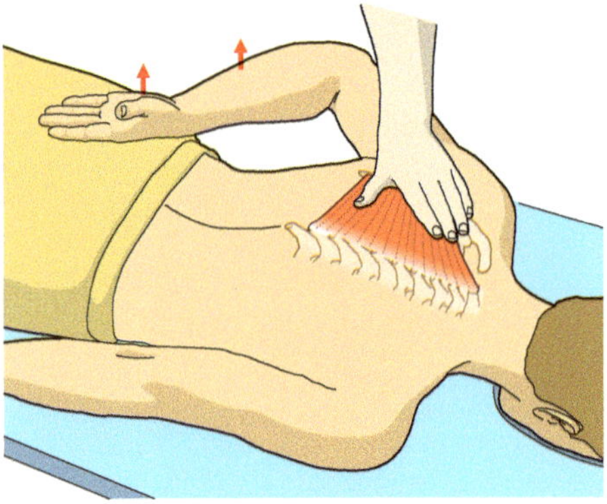

Without gravity

Moving one arm away from the back, from a sitting position with the dorsum of the hand resting on the buttock of the non-examined side.

The rhomboid major and rhomboid minor can be palpated along an oblique line between the medial border of the scapula and the vertebrae from C7 to T5. The rhomboid major can also be palpated medially to the medial border of the scapula, laterally to the ascending part of the trapezius and near the inferior angle of the scapula.

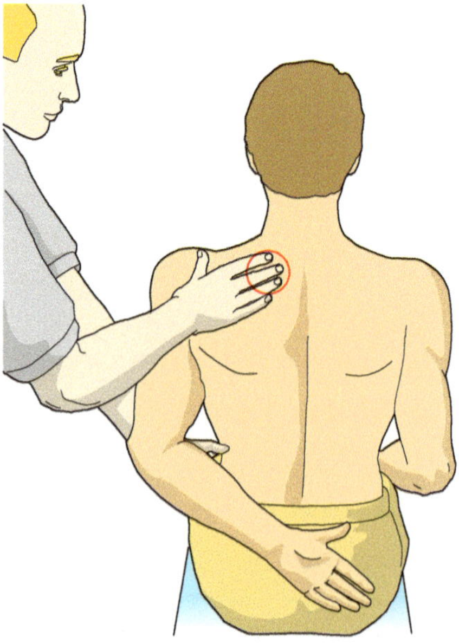

Depression and adduction of the scapula

Ascending part of the trapezius

Against gravity

Elevation of the arm from the prone position with the head rotated to the non-examined side, the shoulder abducted to approximately 130° and resistance applied to the scapula.

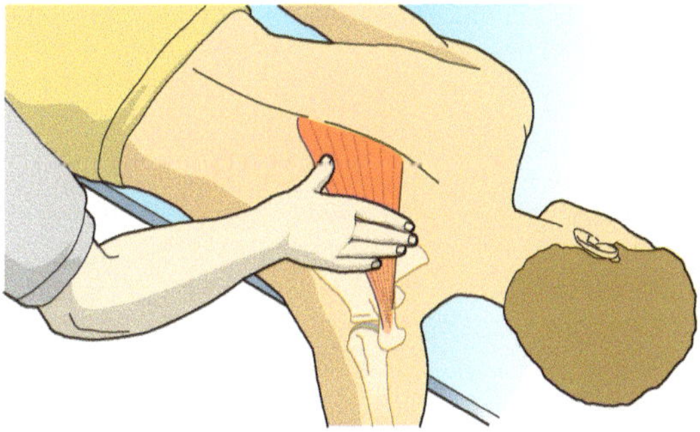

Without gravity

The scapula is lowered and abducted from the prone position with the arms along the trunk and the limb supported by the examiner.

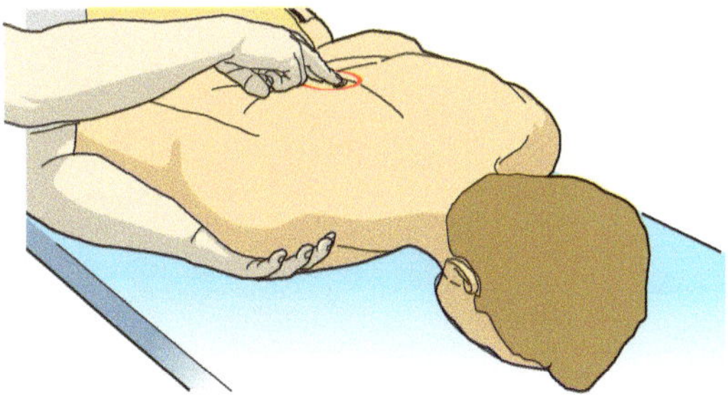

The ascending part of the trapezius can be palpated medially to the inferior angle of the scapula along a line that joins the root of the spine of the scapula with the spinous process of T12.

90° flexion of the shoulder

Clavicular part of the deltoid

Against gravity

90° flexion of the shoulder from a sitting position with the arm at the side of the trunk, slightly abducted and the palm of the hand directed medially (the resistance is applied to the anteromedial surface of the arm, just above the elbow).

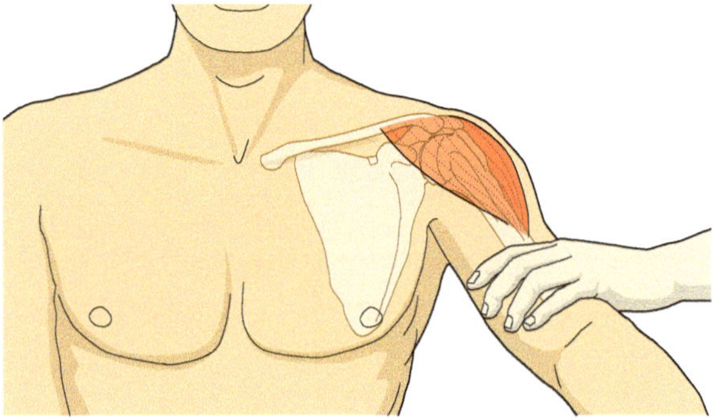

Without gravity

90° flexion of the shoulder from the lateral decubitus position on the non-examined side with the arm at the side of the trunk, slightly abducted, and the limb supported by the examiner.

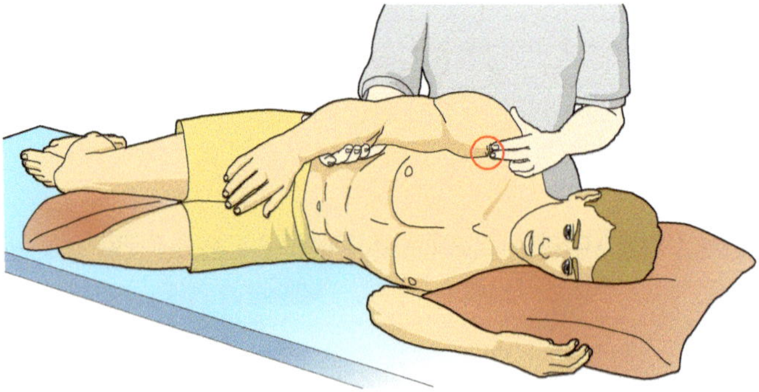

The clavicular part of the deltoid can be palpated on the anterior part of the shoulder, just distally to the lateral third of the clavicle.

Flexion and adduction of the shoulder

Coracobrachialis

Against gravity

Flexion and adduction of the shoulder from the supine position with the shoulder slightly abducted, externally rotated, the elbow flexed and resistance applied to the anteromedial surface of the distal part of the arm.

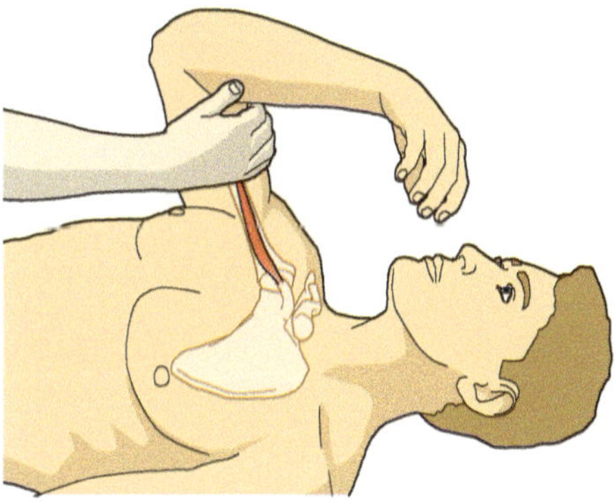

Without gravity

Flexion and adduction of the shoulder from the lateral decubitus position on the non-examined side with the shoulder slightly abducted, externally rotated, the elbow fully flexed and the limb supported by the examiner.

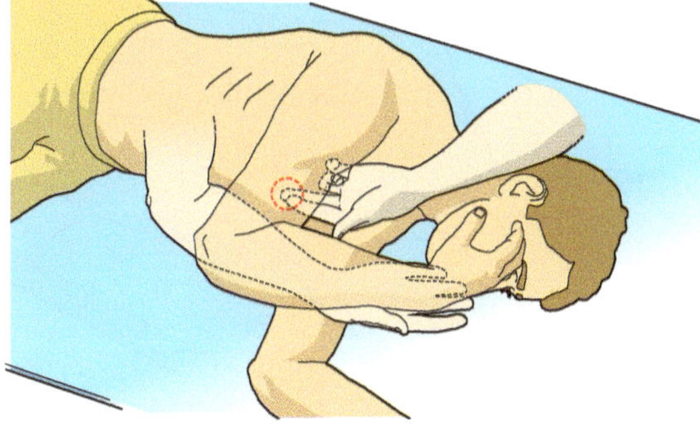

The coracobrachialis can be palpated in correspondence with the proximal third of the anteromedial surface of the arm, just anteriorly to the brachial pulse.

Extension of the shoulder

Latissimus dorsi and teres major

Against gravity

Extension of the shoulder held in adduction from the prone position with the arm at the side of the trunk, internally rotated, the palm of the hand facing upward and resistance applied to the posteromedial surface of the arm proximal to the elbow joint.

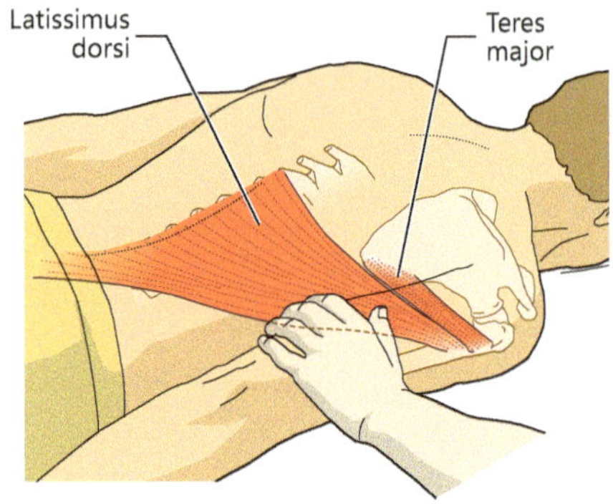

Without gravity

Extension of the arm held in adduction from the lateral decubitus position on the non-examined side, with the arm at the side of the trunk, internally rotated, the elbow extended and the limb supported by the examiner.

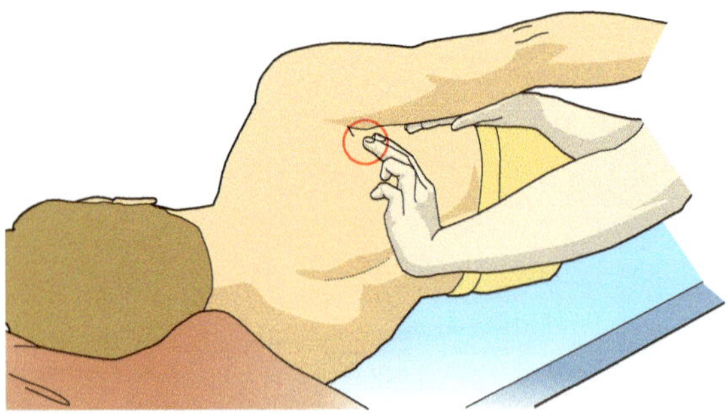

The latissimus dorsi can be palpated laterally to the inferior angle of the scapula or at the level of the posterior wall of the axilla (inferiorly and laterally to the palpation of the teres major); the teres major can be palpated on the posterior wall of the axilla laterally to the lateral border of the scapula.

90° abduction of the shoulder

Acromial part of the deltoid and the supraspinatus

Against gravity

90° abduction of the shoulder from a sitting position with the arm at the side of the trunk and resistance applied to the lateral surface of the arm proximally to the elbow.

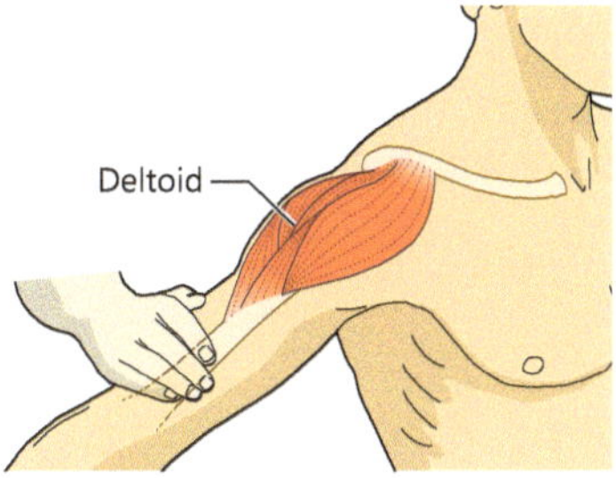

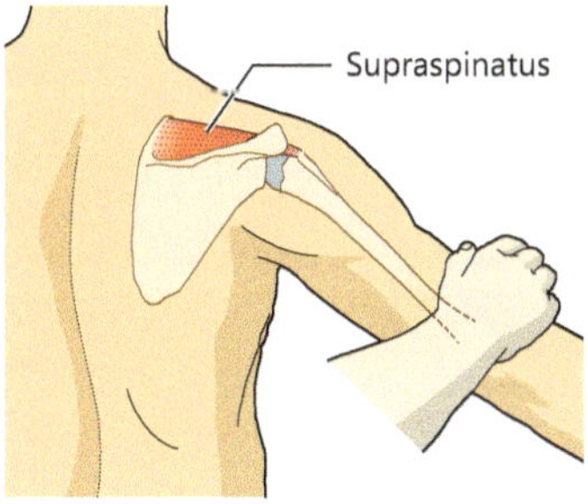

Without gravity

90° abduction of the arm from the supine position with the arm at the side of the trunk, the elbow extended and the limb supported by the examiner.

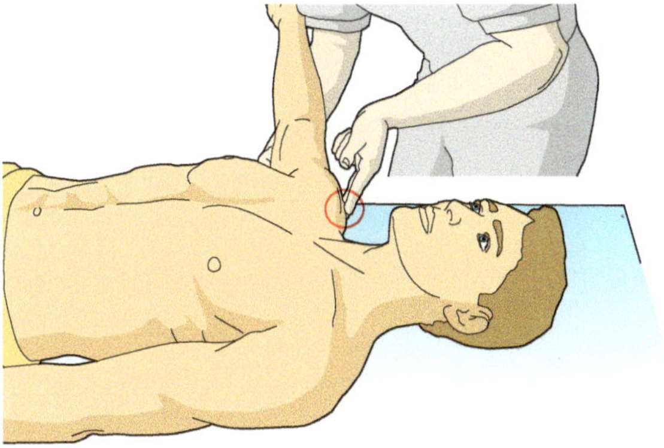

The acromial part of the deltoid can be palpated below the apex of the acromion, while the supraspinatus is situated deeper and cannot be palpated.

Internal rotation of the shoulder on the horizontal plane

Pectoralis major (sternocostal and clavicular parts)

Against gravity

Internal rotation of the shoulder on the horizontal plane from the supine position with the arm abducted at 90°, the elbow flexed and resistance applied to the anterior surface of the arm, just above the elbow joint.

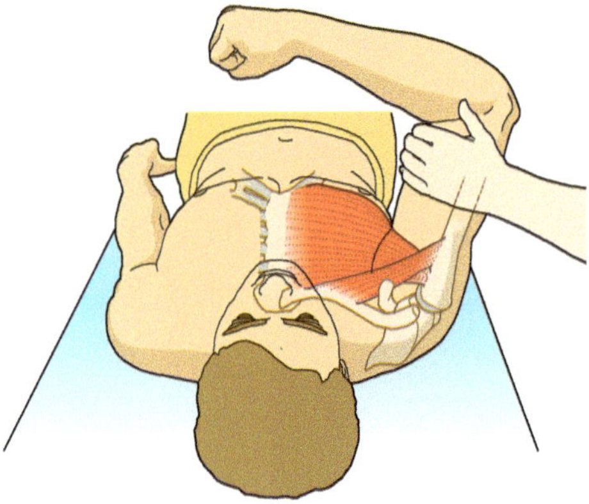

Without gravity

Internal rotation of the shoulder on the horizontal plane from a sitting position with the arm abducted at 90° and the limb supported by the examiner.

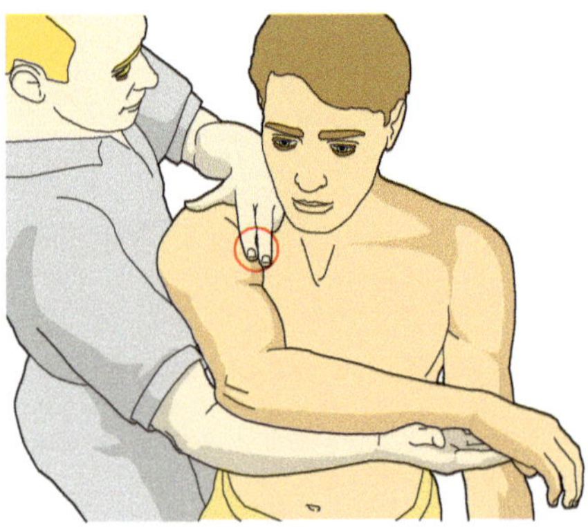

The sternocostal part can be palpated on the anterior border of the axilla, the clavicular part inferiorly to the central part of the anterior border of the clavicle.

External rotation of the shoulder on the horizontal plane

Spinal part of the deltoid

Against gravity

External rotation of the shoulder on the horizontal plane from the prone position with the arm abducted at approximately 75°, the elbow flexed and resistance applied to the postero-lateral surface of the arm, just above the elbow joint.

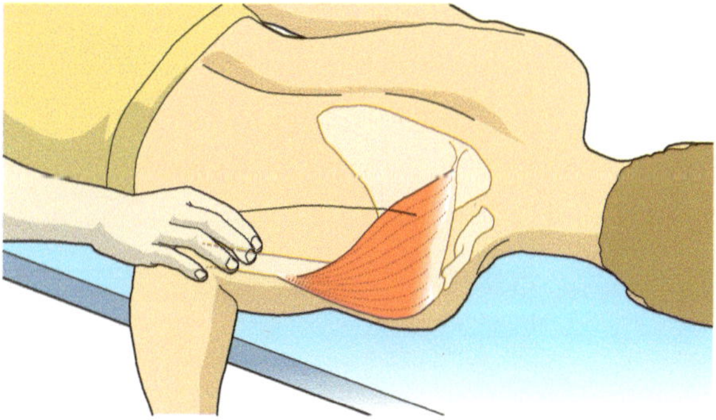

Without gravity

External rotation of the shoulder on the horizontal plane from a sitting position with the arm abducted at approximately 75°, the elbow flexed and the limb supported by the examiner.

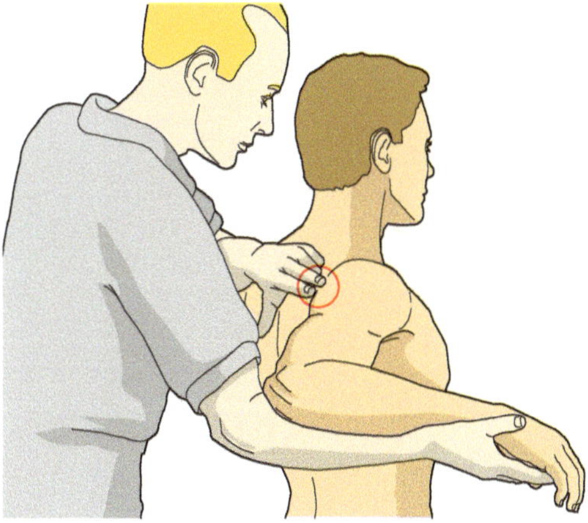

The spinal part of the deltoid can be palpated below the lateral part of the spine of the scapula.

Internal rotation of the shoulder on the axis of the humerus

Subscapularis

Against gravity

Internal rotation of the shoulder with the palm of the hand facing upward from the prone position with the shoulder abducted at 90° supported on the examination table, the elbow flexed at 90° and resistance applied just above the wrist.

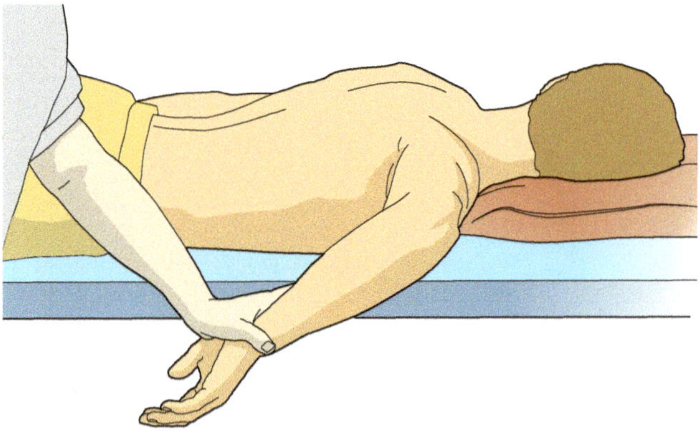

Without gravity

Internal rotation of the shoulder with the palm of the hand facing the abdomen from a sitting position with the shoulder slightly abducted, the elbow flexed at 90° and resistance applied just above the wrist. (Normally, the complete internal rotation – with the exclusive participation of the subscapularis – is carried out from the starting position with the hand resting on the lumbar column and the movement that moves it away backwards).

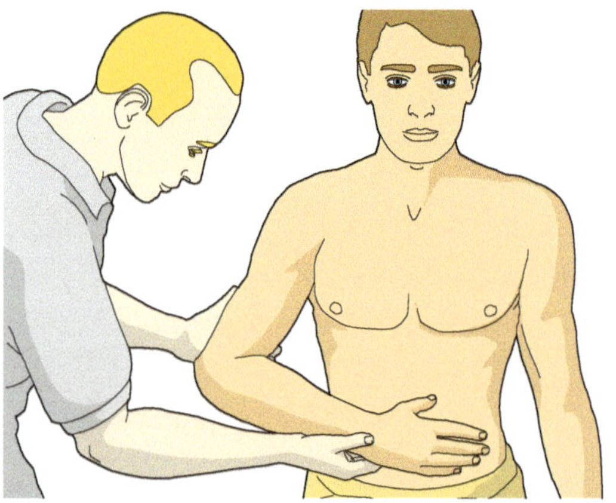

The subscapularis is situated deeper and cannot be palpated.

External rotation of the shoulder on the axis of the humerus

Infraspinatus and teres minor

Against gravity

External rotation of the shoulder with the dorsum of the hand directed upward from the prone position, the shoulder abducted at 90° and resistance applied to the posterior surface of the forearm, just above the wrist.

The infraspinatus can be palpated above the body of the scapula, just below the spine, while the teres minor cannot be palpated.

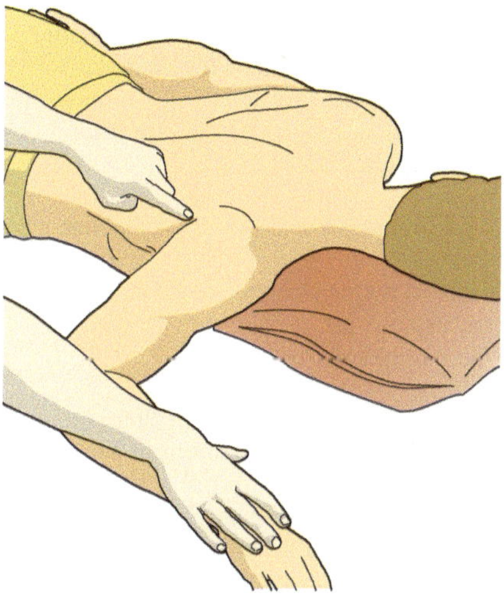

Without gravity

External rotation of the shoulder with the hand away from the trunk from a sitting position with the arm at the side of the trunk, the elbow flexed at 90° and the palm of the hand facing forward.

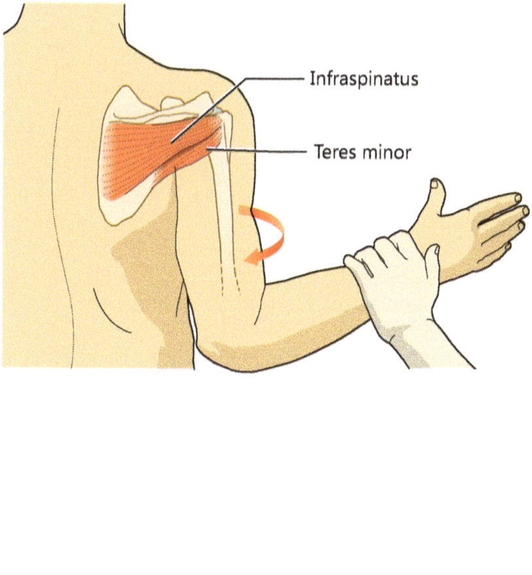

Functional aspects of the muscles of the shoulder

Elevation of the shoulder

The muscles responsible for the coordinated and regular actions leading to the elevation of the arm can be divided into four functional groups:
- stabilizers and motors of the scapula
- stabilizers of the humerus
- flexors and abductors of the humerus
- rotators of the humerus.

The first includes the following muscles:
- trapezius
- rhomboid major and rhomboid minor
- serratus anterior
- levator scapulae.

During the elevation of the arm there is:
- an initial phase of adjustment of the scapula (in which the stabilizer and motor muscles of the scapula have minimal activity)
- a subsequent phase (characterized by the scapulohumeral rhythm, with synchronous movements of the scapula and the humerus, and by a gradual increase in the activity of the first group of muscles, especially those whose main action consists of rotating the scapula externally).

The external rotation of the scapula:
- brings the glenoid cavity into a position that allows the lifting of the humerus, avoiding bone or ligament limitations
- is due to agonist action between the descending and ascending parts of the trapezius and the serratus anterior (the latter is primarily responsible for the elevation of the arm associated with flexion, the trapezius for the elevation of the arm associated with abduction).

The stabilizer muscles of the humerus fix the humeral head in the glenoid cavity and are made up of the following muscles:
- subscapularis (acts during the abduction of the arm between 0° and 150°)
- supraspinatus (acts as a fixator when the arm is declivous)
- infraspinatus (acts like the subscapularis, becoming the principal stabilizer between 150° and 180°)
- teres minor (upper part)
- biceps brachii (long head).

The flexor and abductor muscles of the humerus:
- insert proximally on the scapula and distally on the humerus.

The elevation of the humerus in abduction is due to the action of the following muscles:
- deltoid (acromial part)
- supraspinatus.

The elevation of the humerus in flexion is due to the action of the following muscles:
- deltoid (clavicular part)
- pectoralis major (clavicular part)
- coracobrachialis.

The rotator cuff fixes the head of the humerus in the glenoid cavity, creating a fulcrum around which the humerus moves during abduction or flexion.

The rotator muscles of the humerus:
- rotate the humerus externally during the elevation in abduction
- rotate the humerus internally if the elevation in flexion is associated with internal rotation (clavicular part of the deltoid).

> The elevation of the arm aims to position and move the arm in space to facilitate hand function, the activity of which leads to an increase in the activity of the muscles of the shoulder responsible for elevation of the arm, especially the stabilizer muscles of the humerus.

Adduction and extension of the shoulder

From the elevated position (in flexion or abduction), the arm returns to the side of the trunk through adduction or extension.

When these movements must occur rapidly or require greater force, for example, in activities such as closing a window, climbing a ladder or serving a tennis ball, the following muscles are the agonists:
- latissimus dorsi (also acts against resistance)
- teres major (acts only against resistance together with the rhomboid major and rhomboid minor, which rotate the scapula medially).

When the arm at the side of the trunk is brought backward on the sagittal plane, the action of the spinal part of the deltoid is added to the action of these two muscles.

Flexion and adduction of the shoulder

Many everyday activities (including personal care, such as washing, dressing, etc.) are based on the combination of these two movements, ensured by the pectoralis major (flexor and adductor of the arm).

Internal rotation of the shoulder

It occurs with the action of the following muscles:
- subscapularis (internally rotates the humerus when the arm is in front of or behind the trunk, for example, by bringing the hand to the level of the lumbar column, and its internal rotation action is not associated with other movements)
- teres major
- latissimus dorsi
- pectoralis major
- deltoid (clavicular part).

There is a functional correlation between:
- internal rotation of the arm
- pronation of the forearm.

The two actions occur simultaneously during the execution of many activities and the pronation of the forearm can be extended by internally rotating the arm.

External rotation of the shoulder

It occurs with the action of the following muscles:
- infraspinatus
- teres minor
- deltoid (spinal part).

There is a functional correlation between:
- external rotation of the arm
- action of the supinator muscles of the forearm when the elbow is extended.

The two actions occur simultaneously when, for example, the palm of the hand is rotated upward.

Palpation of the shoulder and pectoral (shoulder) girdle

Spine of the scapula

It can be easily identified by placing the hand on the superior part of the dorsum and sliding the fingers in a caudal direction until they find the superficial border. It can be palpated by sliding the fingers along its entire length both laterally, up to the acromion, and medially, up to its origin on the medial border of the scapula.

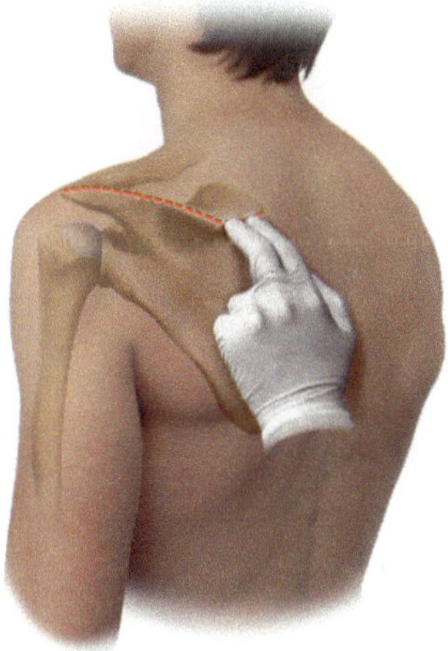

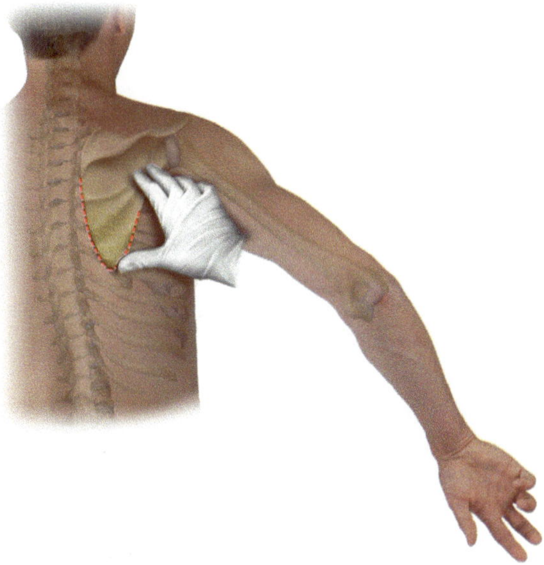

Inferior angle of the scapula

The patient is in a prone or standing position, with the arm in internal rotation so that the medial border of the scapula rises and separates from the ribs. The examiner locates the medial border of the scapula and proceeds with palpation in a caudal direction up to its extremity, where the border of the scapula forms an angle and rises superiorly and laterally: this is the inferior angle of the scapula.

Coracoid process

To facilitate palpation of the coracoid process, the patient should be placed in the supine position with the shoulder elevated with a cushion. The examiner places the thumb on the patient's clavicle and slides it first laterally, until it reaches its acromial end, then inferiorly, no more than 4 cm from the clavicle. Here the tip of the coracoid process can be palpated by compressing the surrounding tissues.

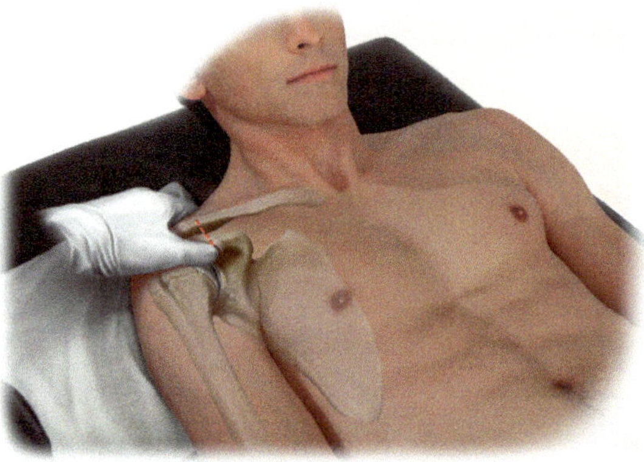

Intertubercular sulcus

The patient is seated. The examiner identifies the acromion and slides the finger downward and laterally for about 2 cm until the hard surface of the greater tubercle is encountered. The examiner brings the patient's arm into external rotation, losing contact with the protuberance of the greater tubercle, replaced by the fissure of the intertubercular groove (bicipital groove).

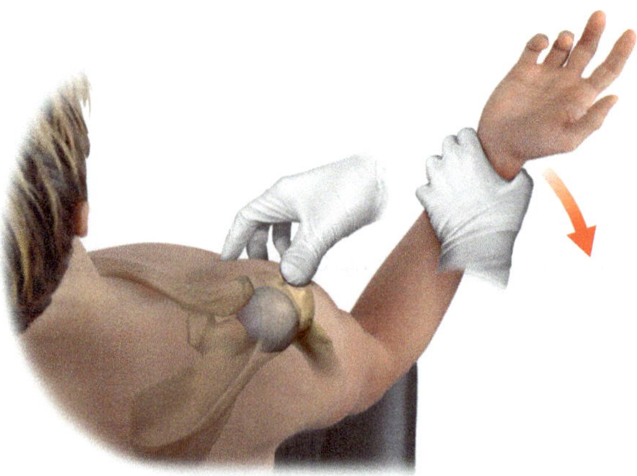

Acromion

The patient is seated with the arms in a neutral position, alongside the trunk. Extending the hand over the upper part of his back, the spine of the scapula is located. Following its border in a lateral direction, the acromion is reached, whose flat surface forms the apex of the shoulder.

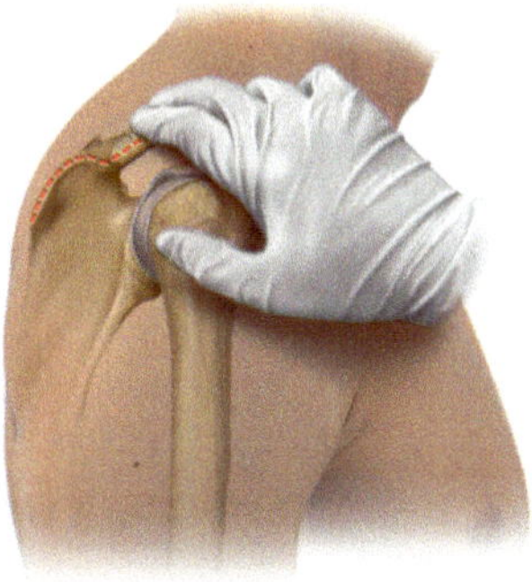

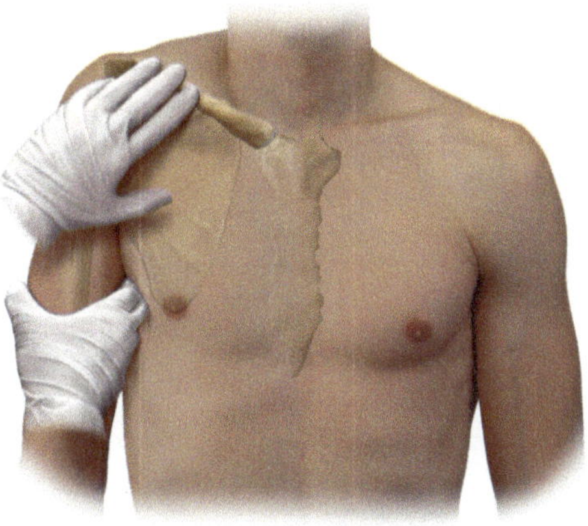

Clavicle

The patient is seated with the arms in a neutral position, alongside trunk. The acromion is identified, which represents the apex of the shoulder, and from here it continues medially and anteriorly, following the axis of the clavicle which runs superficially and is therefore easily palpable. The acromial end is slightly elevated, while the sternal end is inclined inferiorly.

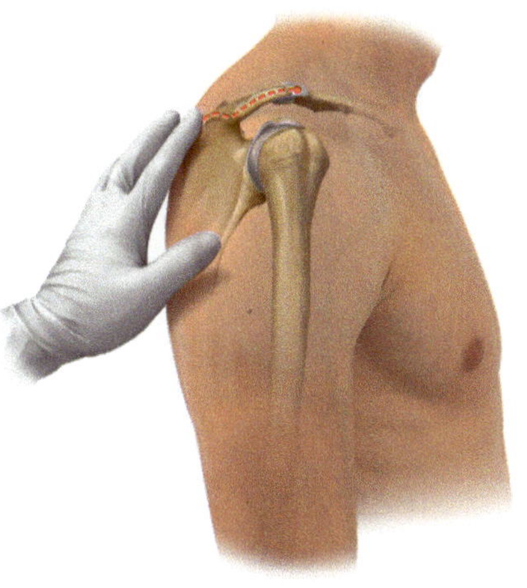

Superficial acromioclavicular ligament

The patient is seated with the arms in a neutral position, alongside the trunk. By sliding the fingers along the spine of the scapula in a lateral direction, the acromion is reached. Anterior to the acromion, the area of connection with the clavicle (superficial acromioclavicular ligament) can be explored.

Subdeltoid bursa

The patient is seated with the arms in a neutral position, next to the trunk. The examiner, standing behind the patient, palpates the anterior border of the acromion. With the other hand, the examiner lifts the patient's arm slightly, pushing the elbow backward so that the bursa comes out from under the acromion, between the deltoid and the tendons of the rotator muscles.

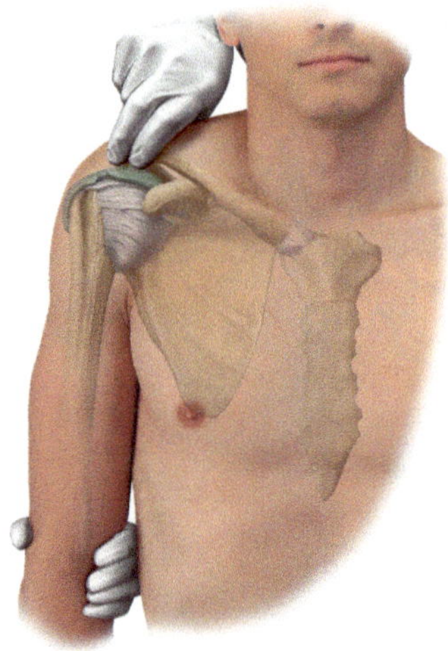

Tendon of the supraspinatus

The patient is seated, with the elbow flexed and the forearm behind the back. The examiner passively extends the patient's arm to the end of the joint course. With this movement, the tendon of the supraspinatus comes out from under the acromion, positioning itself anterior and inferior to the acromioclavicular joint.

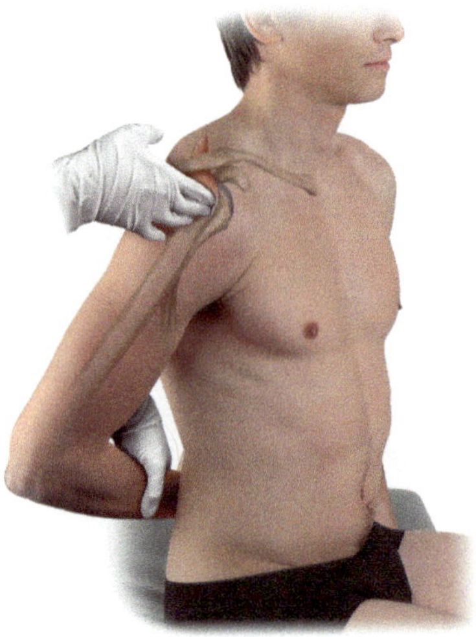

Tendon of the infraspinatus

The patient is in the prone position, with the arm hanging laterally from the examination table. The spine of the scapula and the belly of the infraspinatus below the scapula are identified. Sliding the fingers transversely to the muscle fibers, pass under the acromion and continue to feel the fine tendon insertion over the greater tubercle of the humerus.

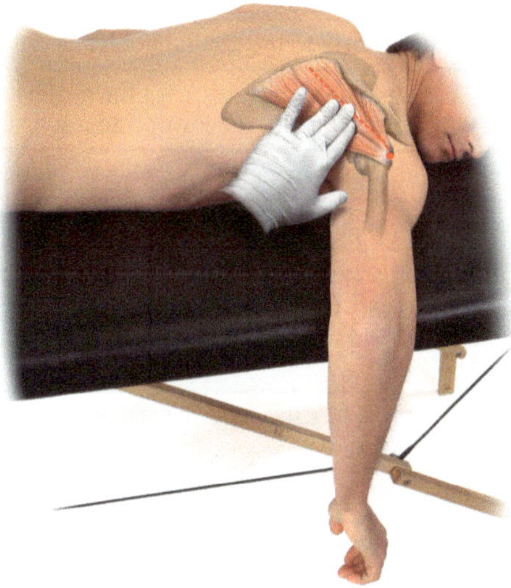

Deltoid

The patient is seated with the arm alongside the body and the elbow flexed. The examiner identifies the spine of the scapula and, from here, proceeds by palpating the deltoid, located in a superficial position, following its fibers up to the deltoid tuberosity, located in the middle third of the lateral border of the humerus. To facilitate palpation, the patient is asked to abduct the shoulder to obtain contraction of all the fibers of the deltoid.

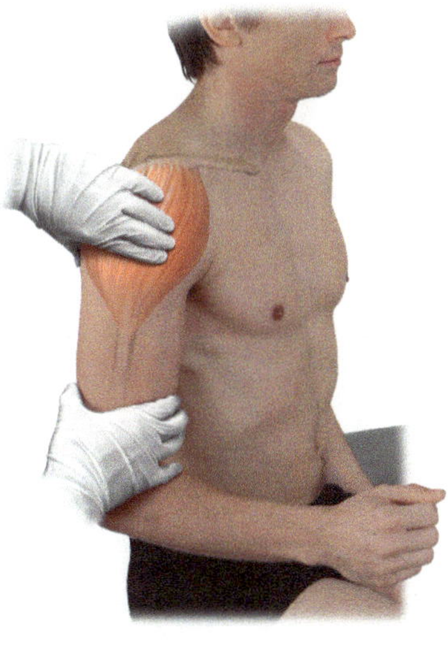

Anatomical landmarks on the surface of the shoulder and pectoral girdle

1	Inion: process marking the center of the superior nuchal line
2	Medial border of the scapula: laterally to the spinous processes of the thoracic vertebrae, 5-6 cm from them, covering the second to the seventh ribs
3	Inferior angle of the scapula: inferiorly to the medial border of the scapula
4	Spine of the scapula: bony crest passing obliquely over the posterior surface of the scapula between its upper quarter and the lower three-quarters
5	Acromion: lateral part of the spine of the scapula at the apex of the shoulder
6	Clavicle: prominent S-shaped bone in the anterosuperior part of the thorax
7	Coracoid process: prominence directed upwards and outwards distally to the passage between the middle third and lateral third of the clavicle, approximately 2.5 cm from it, in the clavipectoral triangle, deep to the anterior fibers of the deltoid
8	Brachial pulse: palpable on the medial surface of the arm at the proximal level, posterior to the coracobrachialis
9	Lateral epicondyle of the humerus
10	Olecranon
11	Spinous process of T12

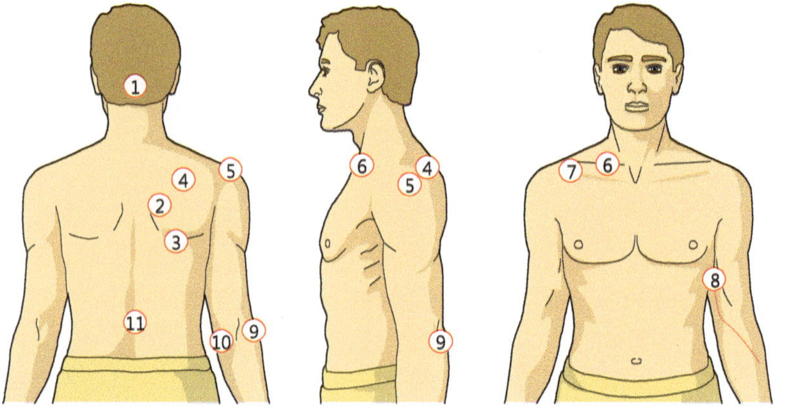

Distal extremity of the humerus

Lateral prominence – lateral epicondyle
Medial prominence – medial epicondyle.

The articular surfaces for the radius and ulna (bones of the forearm) are situated between the lateral epicondyle and the medial epicondyle:

- capitulum of the humerus (laterally) – hemispherical in shape
- trochlea of the humerus (medially) – pulley shape.

On the anterior surface of the distal extremity of the humerus are located:

- the coronoid fossa (so called because it accommodates the coronoid process of the ulna during flexion of the forearm)
- the radial fossa (located above the capitulum of the humerus, in which the head of the radius moves during flexion of the forearm).

The olecranon fossa is located on the posterior surface of the distal extremity of the humerus (so called because it accommodates the olecranon of the ulna during extension of the forearm).

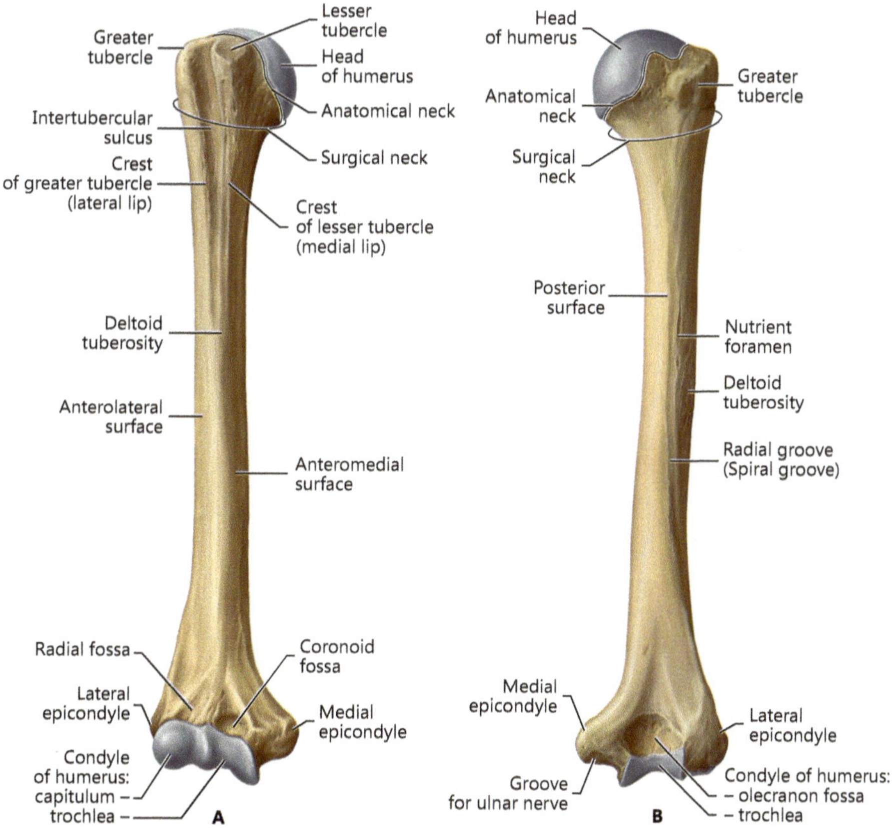

Anteromedial surface (**A**) and posterior surface (**B**) of the right humerus.

Bones of the forearm

Radius (lateral bone of the forearm)

Superior extremity (head of the radius):
- cylindrical shape (the contour of the cylinder, known as the *articular circumference of the head*, is largely covered by cartilage)
- concave articular facet (*facet of the head of the radius*) on the superior surface of the head
- neck of the radius below the head (inferolaterally to which is the radial tuberosity, where the biceps brachii inserts).

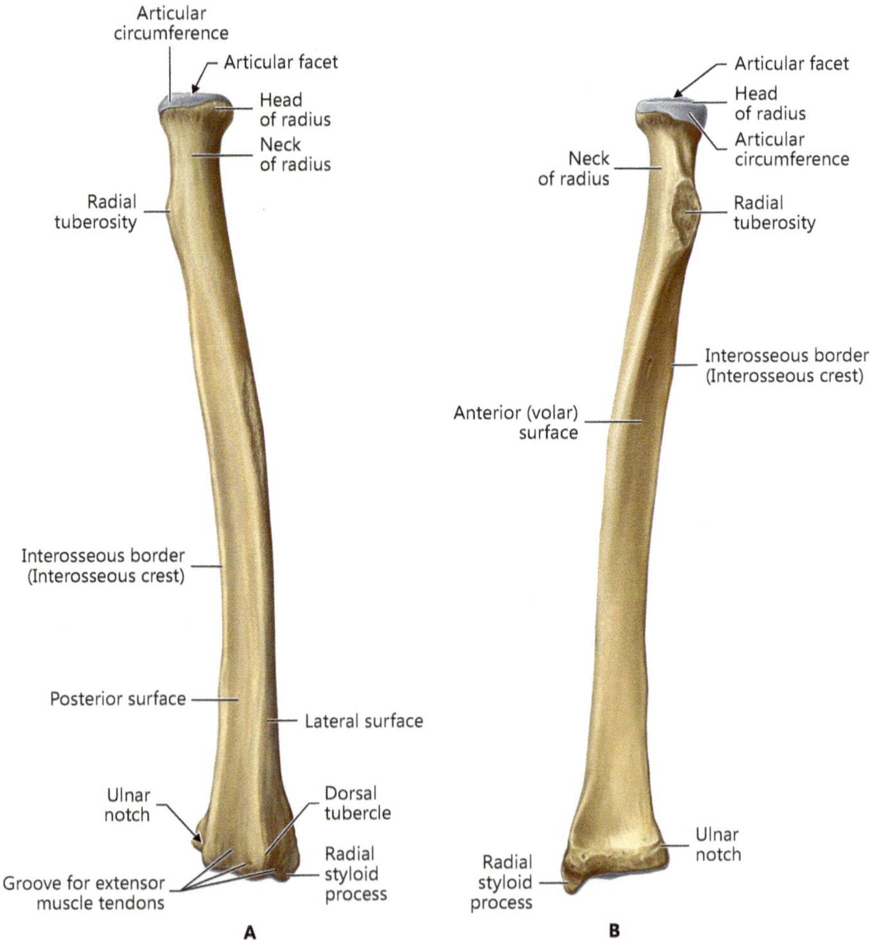

Posterior or dorsal surface (**A**) and anterior or volar surface (**B**) of the right radius.

Shaft (body):
- triangular prism shape with three surfaces:
  - anterior (volar):
    - the superior part gives insertion to the flexor pollicis longus
    - the inferior part gives insertion to the pronator quadratus
  - posterior (dorsal)
    - the middle third gives insertion to the extensor pollicis brevis and to one of the heads of the abductor pollicis longus
  - lateral
    - the superior part gives insertion to the supinator
    - the inferior part gives insertion to the pronator teres

and three borders:
  - anterior, inferiorly is located one of the three origins of the flexor digitorum superficialis
  - posterior
  - medial (interosseous border or crest), which gives insertion to the interosseous membrane.

Inferior extremity:
- medial surface
  - presents the ulnar notch (articular surface for the head of the ulna)
- posterior surface
  - the radial styloid process separates laterally
- anterior surface
- base (carpal articular surface) divided by a crest into the articular surfaces for the scaphoid and the lunate.

Ulna (medial bone of the forearm)

Superior extremity:
- superior prominence – olecranon (four surfaces and an apex)
  - anterior surface – forms the trochlear notch (together with the superior surface of the coronoid process)
  - posterior surface – insertion of the triceps brachii
  - medial and lateral surfaces – insertion of the collateral ligaments of the elbow joint and the anconeus
  - apex – olecranon beak (brought into the olecranon fossa during full extension of the forearm)
- inferior prominence – coronoid process (four surfaces and an apex)
  - superior surface – forms the trochlear notch (together with the anterior surface of the olecranon)
  - inferior surface – presents the tuberosity of the ulna, to which the brachialis inserts
  - medial surface – continues into the olecranon
  - lateral surface – presents the radial notch (which receives the articular circumference of the head of the radius and is delimited by two bony crests, the posterior of which gives insertion to the supinator)
  - apex (brought into the coronoid fossa during flexion of the forearm)
- the trochlear notch articulates with the trochlea of the humerus.

Shaft (body):
- triangular prism shape with three surfaces and three borders

- anterior (volar) surface
  - a crest gives origin to the flexor digitorum profundus
  - the inferior part gives insertion to the pronator quadratus
- posterior (dorsal) surface
  - the superior part gives insertion to the anconeus
  - the inferior part gives origin
    - medially, to the extensor carpi ulnaris
    - laterally, to the following muscles
      - abductor pollicis longus (one of the two heads)
      - extensor pollicis longus
      - extensor indicis

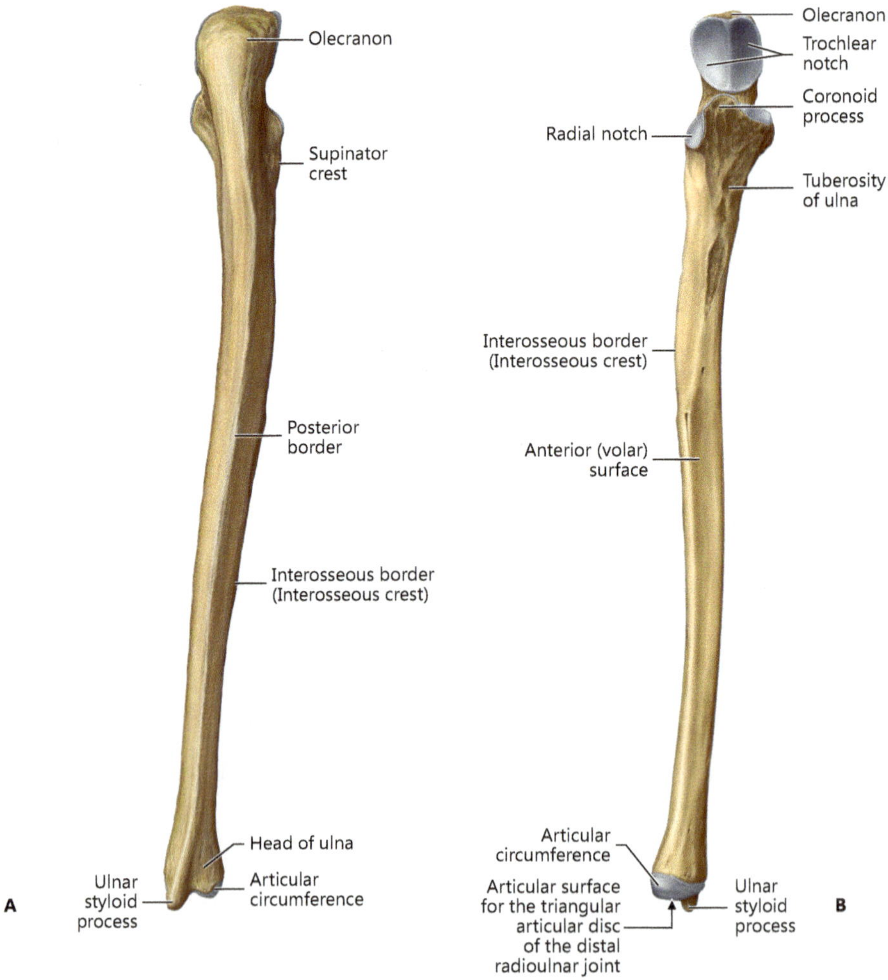

Posterior or dorsal surface (**A**) and anterior or volar surface (**B**) of the right ulna.

  - medial surface
    - the superior part gives insertion to the flexor digitorum profundus
  - anterior border
    - the superior part gives insertion to the flexor digitorum profundus
    - the inferior part gives insertion to the pronator quadratus
  - posterior border
  - interosseous border or crest – gives insertion to the interosseous membrane.

Inferior extremity (head of the ulna):
- articulates with the triquetrum of the carpus by a disc
- two articular surfaces
  - lateral (articular circumference of the head) – articulates with the radius (ulnar notch)
  - inferior (in the inferior surface of the head) – articulates with the radius
- presents the ulnar styloid process medially.

Elbow joints

- Elbow joints – complex formed by two joints:
  - humeroulnar
  - humeroradial
- proximal radioulnar joint.

The humeroulnar and humeroradial joints (the main joint of the elbow) can be considered together as the humeroradioulnar joint (compound joint whose function is performed between three bones).

The proximal radioulnar joint is the secondary joint of the elbow.

The distal radioulnar joint can also be considered, functionally, an elbow joint because it is responsible, together with the proximal radioulnar joint, for the prosupination movements of the forearm.

Humeroradioulnar joint

Articular surfaces	Capitulum of the humerus Trochlea of the humerus Articular facet of the head of the radius Trochlear notch of the olecranon
Type of joint	Hinge joint
Movements	Only flexion-extension movements are possible (one degree of freedom). The axis of the flexion-extension movement (horizontal axis) passes through the center of the epicondyles of the humerus (medial and lateral) and is oblique from medial to lateral from bottom to top and is not perpendicular to the axis of the humerus, as the trochlea of the humerus is located more distally with respect to the capitulum of the humerus and the middle third of the ulna is slightly inclined

The outward open angle, formed when the arm and forearm are extended, is called ulnar angle, whose amplitude is approximately 168°, with an interval between 158° and 180° (physiological valgus, equal to approximately 10°), and not 180° (due to the position of the two articular heads of the humerus). We are referring to cubitus valgus when the amplitude of the ulnar angle is less than 158°.

The forward open angle, formed when the arm and forearm are extended, is called the opening angle, whose amplitude is 180° in women and approximately 175° in men, where maximum extension of the arm and forearm is not possible because of the greater development of the anterior musculature (secondary sexual characteristics). In the child, the opening angle is greater than 180° (hyperextension).

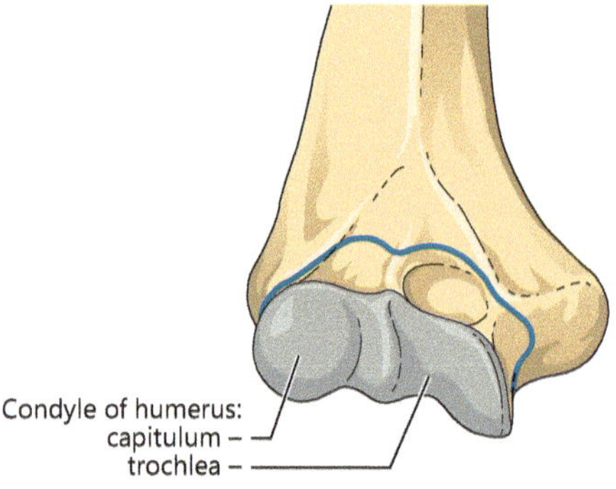

Right elbow joint. Anterior view of proximal articular surface of the humerus. The blue line indicates the boundary of insertion of the joint capsule.

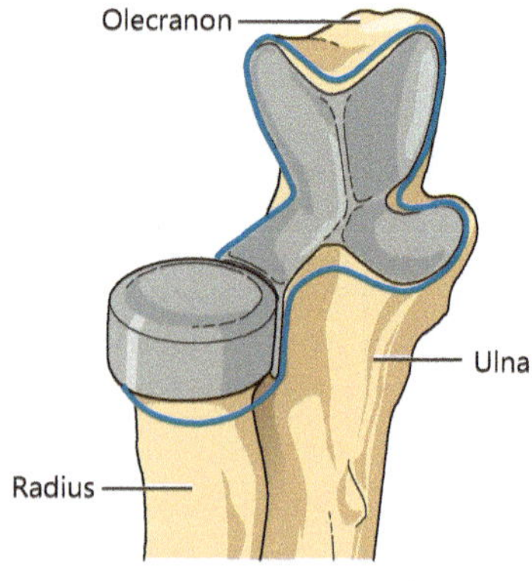

Right elbow joint. Anterior view of the distal articular surface formed by the radius and ulna. The blue line indicates the boundary of insertion of the joint capsule.

Proximal radioulnar joint

Articular surfaces	Articular circumference of the head of the radius Radial notch of the ulna (on the lateral surface of the coronoid process)
Type of joint	Pivot joint
Movements	The articular circumference of the head of the radius, covered by cartilage, rotates within an osteofibrous ring formed by the radial notch of the ulna (bony part of the ring) and by the anular ligament of the radius (fibrous part of the ring), which is fixed to the anterior and posterior borders of the notch. Only the external (supination of the forearm) and internal (pronation of the forearm) movements are possible (only one degree of freedom)

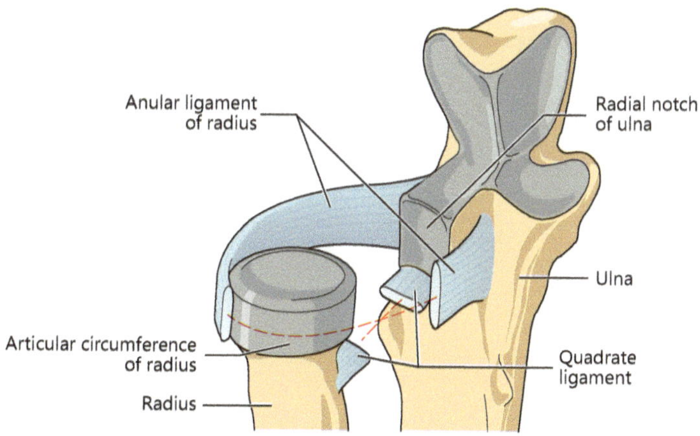

Proximal radioulnar joint.

The pronosupination of the forearm is possible at the same time by both radioulnar joints (proximal and distal). Its rotation axis (longitudinal or vertical) is directed from the center of the head of the radius (proximally) to the center of the head of the ulna (distally).
In supination position:
- the radius and the ulna are parallel to each other

In pronation position:
- the radius overlaps diagonally to the ulna

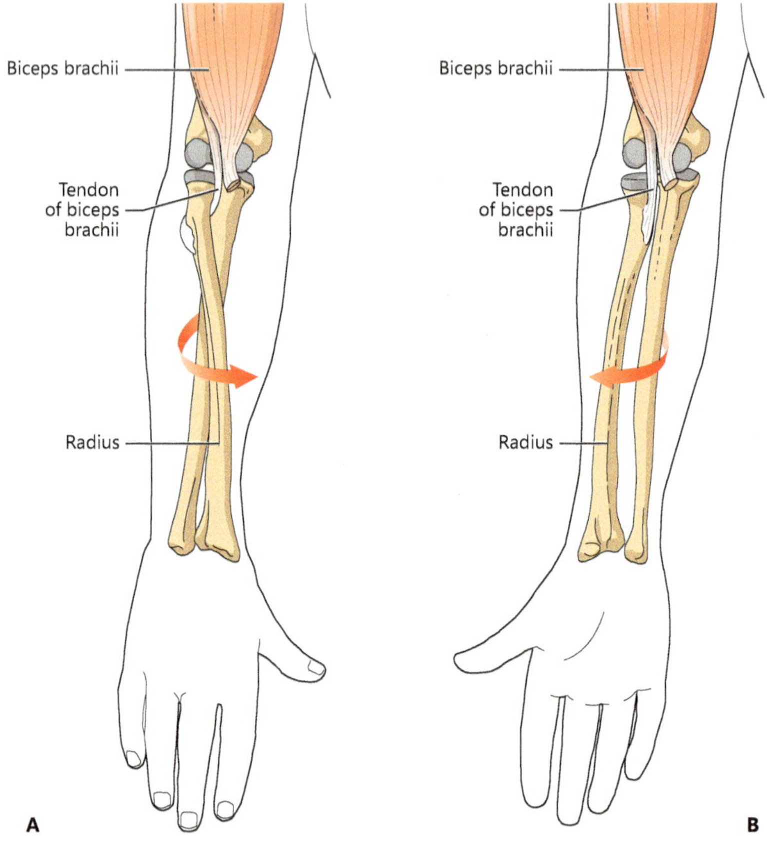

Behavior of the insertion tendon of the biceps brachii in relation to the radius in pronation (**A**) and supination (**B**).

Distal radioulnar joint

Articular surfaces	Head of the ulna (lateral articular surface on the articular circumference of the head and the inferior articular surface on the inferior surface of the head) Ulnar notch of the radius (on the medial surface of the inferior extremity of the radius)
Type of joint	Pivot joint
Movements	As in the proximal radioulnar joint, only the external (supination of the forearm) and internal (pronation of the forearm) movements are possible (only one degree of freedom)

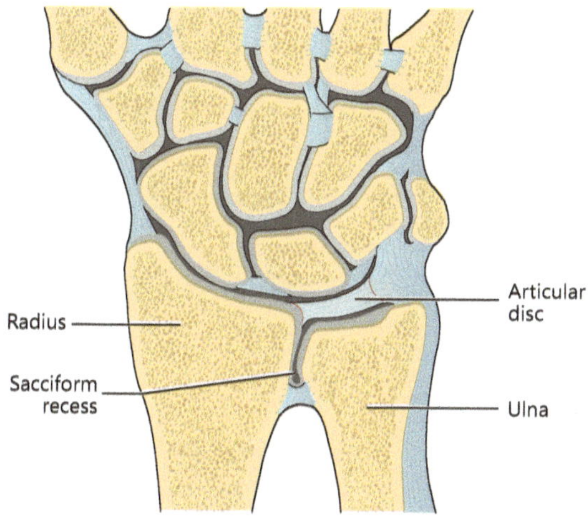

Distal radioulnar joint.

Capsule of the elbow joint

The humeroulnar, humeroradial and proximal radioulnar joints are characterized by a common joint capsule that surrounds all the articular heads.

Insertion of the capsule

On the humerus

The capitulum, trochlea and the three fossae (radial, coronoid and olecranon) of the distal extremity of the humerus are located inside the capsule, while the medial and lateral epicondyles are located outside the capsule.

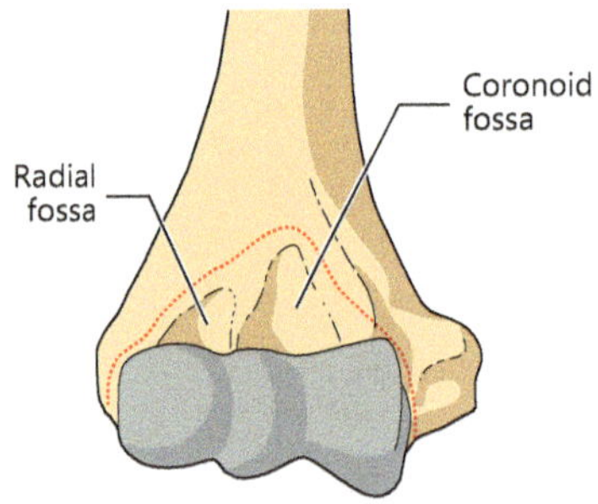

Insertion of the capsule on the anterior surface of the humerus.

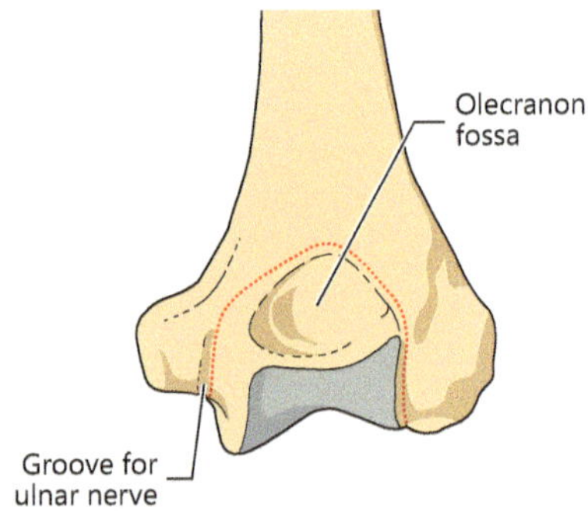

Insertion of the capsule on the dorsal surface of the humerus.

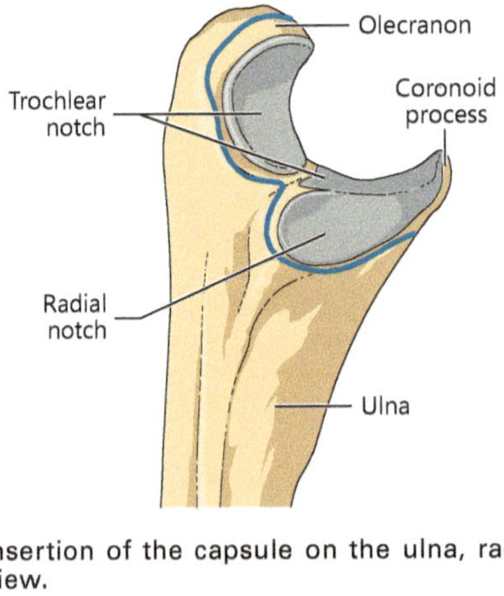

Insertion of the capsule on the ulna, radial view.

On the ulna

The olecranon and the coronoid process of the ulna (trochlear and radial notches) are located inside the capsule (the insertion of the capsule runs along the passage zone between the cartilage and the bone of the trochlear notch).

On the radius

The head of the radius (articular facet and circumference) is located inside the capsule (the insertion of the capsule passes very close to the articular circumference, just below the passage zone between the cartilage and the bone).

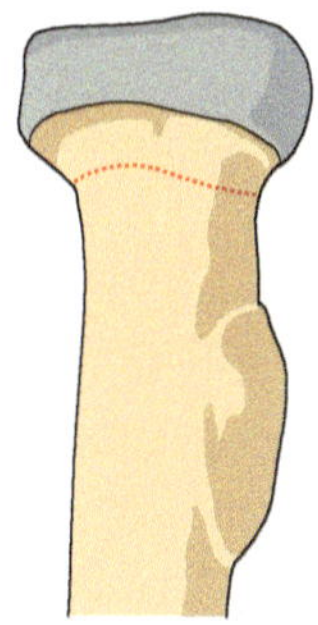

Insertion of the capsule on the radius.

Superior sacciform recess

Formed by the synovial membrane just below the anular ligament (see section "Proximal radioulnar joint", page 315), around the neck of the radius and interposed between the radius and the ulna, it facilitates the rotation of the radius over the ulna.

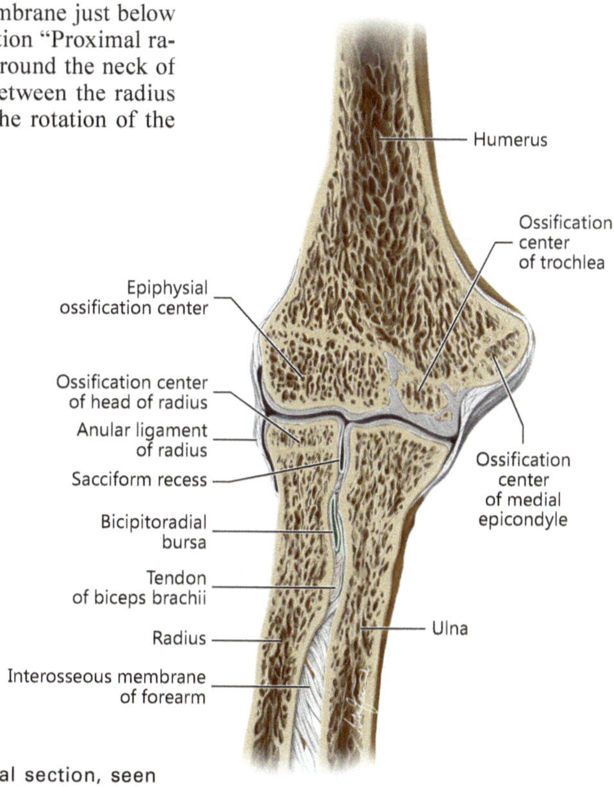

Right elbow joint. The frontal section, seen from behind, illustrates the extension of the articular cavity.

Capsule of the distal radioulnar joint

The insertion of the capsule runs along the passage zone between the cartilage and the bone.

Inferior sacciform recess

Formed by the synovial membrane and interposed between the radius and the ulna, it facilitates (together with the superior sacciform recess) the rotation of the radius over the ulna.

Ulnocarpal articular disc (or ligament)

- It has a triangular shape
- Between the inferior border of the ulnar notch of the radius (on the medial surface of the distal extremity of the radius) (base of the triangle) and the ulnar styloid process (apex of the triangle) on a horizontal plane
- Its superior and inferior surfaces, covered by cartilage, are concave (biconcave disc)
- It makes the distal extremity of the ulna concordant with the bones of the proximal carpal row.

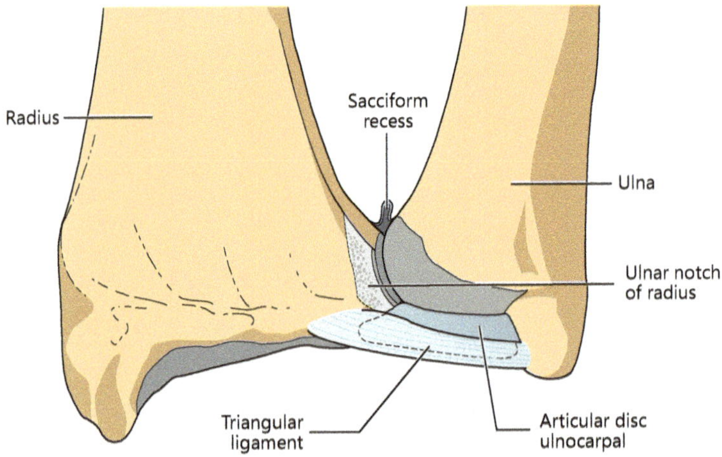

Ulnocarpal articular disc.

Ligaments of the elbow joint

- Ulnar collateral
- Radial collateral
- Anular of the radius
- Quadrate

Ulnar collateral ligament

- Anterior part (from the anterior surface of the medial epicondyle to the medial surface of the coronoid process; some fascicles reach the anular ligament of the radius)
- Posterior part (from the posterior surface of the medial epicondyle to the medial surface of the olecranon)
- Intermediate part (between the anterior part and posterior part)
- Cooper's ligament (joins the base of the anterior part with the base of the posterior part)

Function → maintains the stability of the joint on the frontal plane.

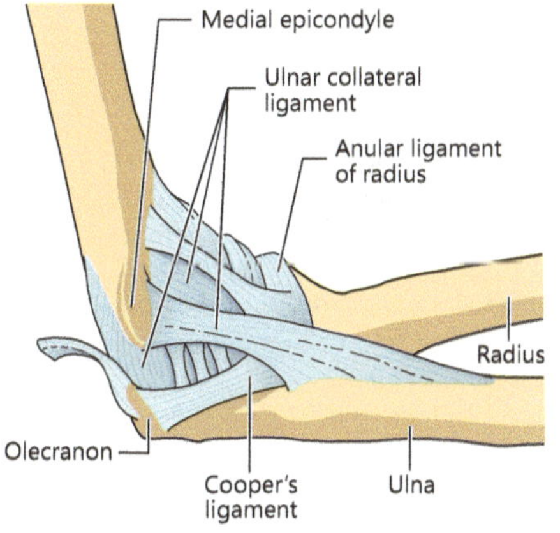

Radial collateral ligament

- Anterior part (from the anteroinferior surface of the lateral epicondyle to the anterior border of the radial notch of the ulna; some fascicles reach the anular ligament of the radius)
- Intermediate part (from the anteroinferior surface of the lateral epicondyle to the posterior border of the radial notch of the ulna)
- Posterior part (from the posterior surface of the lateral epicondyle to the lateral surface of the olecranon; some fascicles reach the anular ligament of the radius)

Function → maintains the stability of the joint on the frontal plane.

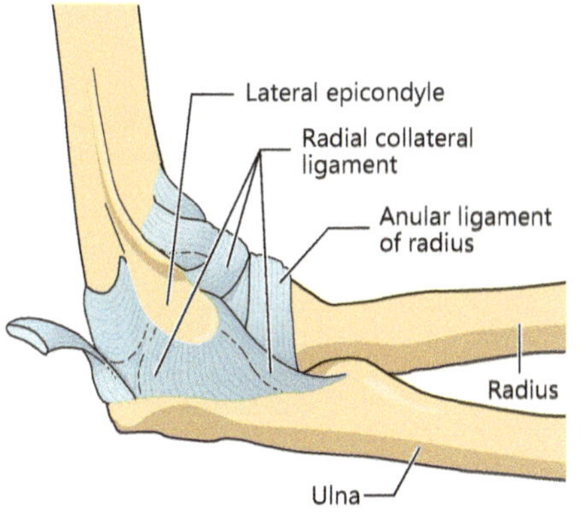

8

During elbow movements, at least one component of the collateral ligaments is under tension. Injuries to the ulnar collateral ligament occur as a result of significant strain or valgus trauma during sports activities (for example, in pitchers).

Anular ligament of the radius

- Between the anterior and posterior borders of the radial notch of the ulna
- Surrounds the articular circumference of the head of the radius in a ring shape
- It fuses with the ulnar and radial collateral ligaments (thus establishing a relationship between the humeroradial, humeroulnar and proximal radioulnar joints)

Function → maintains the articular surfaces of the proximal radioulnar joint in contact, ensuring the correct execution of the pronosupination movement.

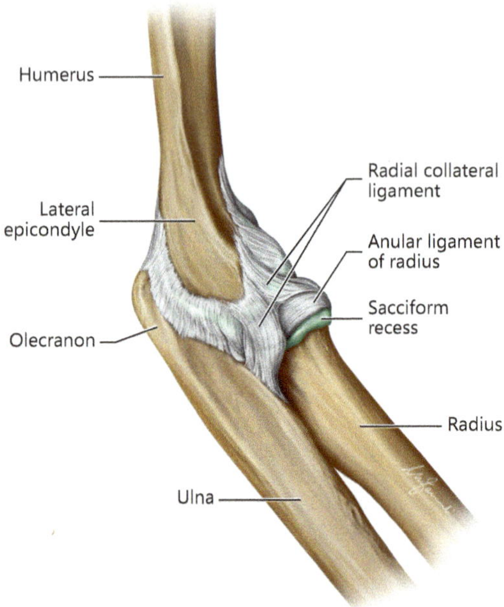

Quadrate ligament

- Between the inferior border of the radial notch of the ulna and the neck of the radius
- Anteriorly and posteriorly fixed to the inferior part of the anular ligament of the radius

Function → reinforces the joint capsule inferiorly and maintains the articular surfaces of the proximal radioulnar joint in contact by arranging its fibers differently compared to the anular ligament.

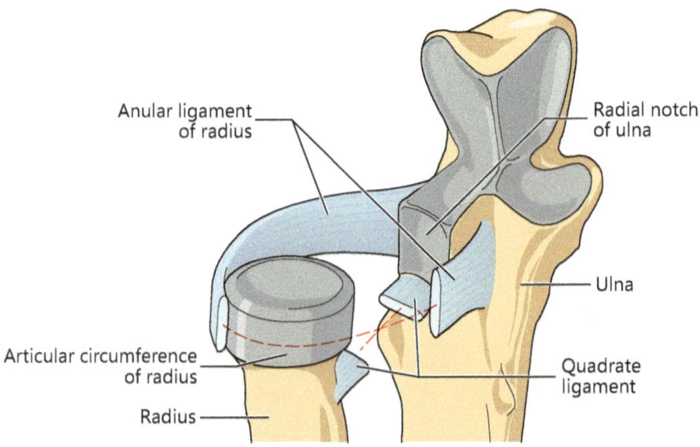

Anterior capsuloligamentous system

- Anterior ligaments (longitudinal and oblique fascicles)
- Reinforce the joint capsule and insert on the ulnar and radial collateral ligaments.

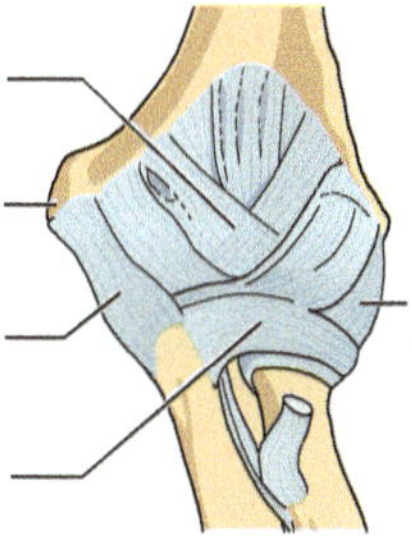

Posterior capsuloligamentous system

- Posterior ligaments (longitudinal and oblique fascicles)
- Reinforce the joint capsule and insert on the ulnar and radial collateral ligaments and anular ligament of the radius.

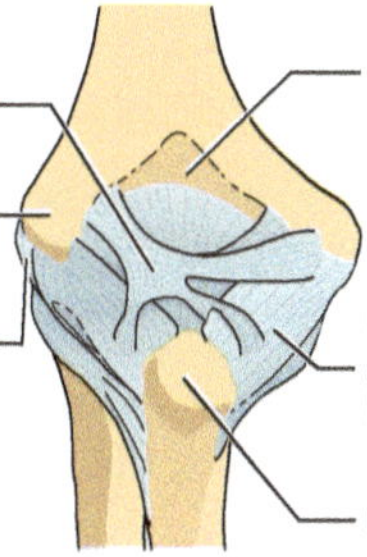

Ligaments and reinforcing structures of the proximal and distal radioulnar joints

- Interosseous membrane
- Oblique (Weitbrecht's) cord
- Inferior anterior radioulnar ligament
- Inferior posterior radioulnar ligament
- Triangular disc

Interosseous membrane

- Fibrous lamina between the radius and ulna
- Oblique direction of the fascicles, from medial to lateral and from bottom to top
  - most of the fascicles are in tension during supination
  - the structure and direction of the fascicles compensate the tensile stresses exerted by the different directions
- Origin of the flexor and extensor digitorum profundus muscles.

Function → prevents the downward displacement of the radius with respect to the ulna.

Oblique cord

- Nastriform structure between the ulna and the radius in proximal position (inserts below the radial notch of the ulna and the radial tuberosity)
- Oblique direction of the fibers, opposite to that of the fascicles of the interosseous membrane.

Inferior anterior radioulnar ligament

- Between the ulna and the radius in distal position
- Oblique direction of the fibers, from lateral to medial and from bottom to top.

Inferior posterior radioulnar ligament

- Between the ulna and the radius in distal position
- Oblique direction of the fascicles, from lateral to medial and from bottom to top.

Triangular disc

- See section "Ulnocarpal articular disc (or ligament)", page 320.

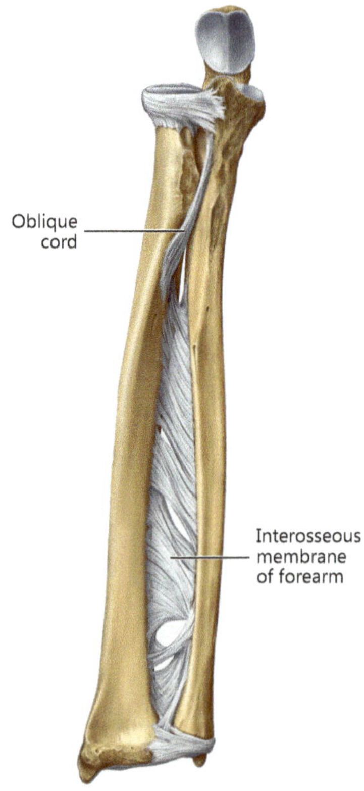

Movements of the elbow joint

Flexion-extension of the humeroulnar and humeroradial joints

Flexion of the elbow

The reference position is given by the upper limb along the side, with the palm of the hand facing forward, and the movement brings the anterior surface of the forearm closer to that of the arm.

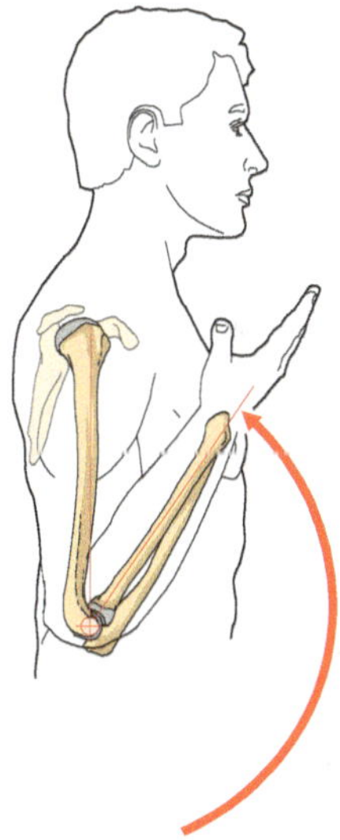

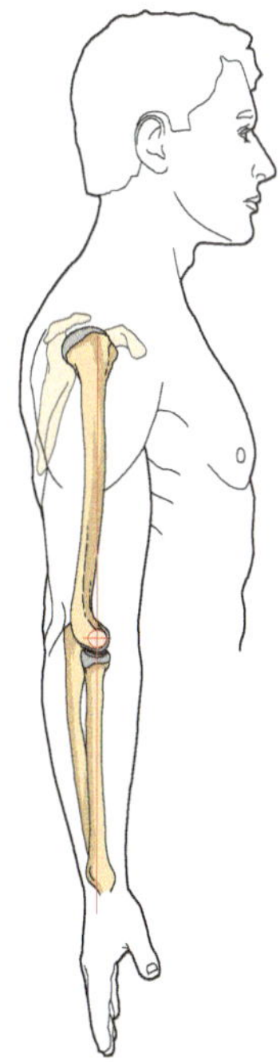

Extension of the elbow

- Relative – return of the elbow to the starting position from any position of flexion
- Absolute (hyperextension) (starting from the reference position).

Amplitude of the flexion-extension movement

The amplitude of the flexion movement is:

- 145° (active movement)
- 160° (passive movement)

The amplitude of the extension movement:

- corresponds to the amplitude of the reference position (achieved as a result of the distancing of the anterior surface of the forearm from that of the arm with the return to the starting position), equal to 175-180°
- absolute is approximately 10° (with an interval of 5-15°), which must be added to the 180° of the reference position.

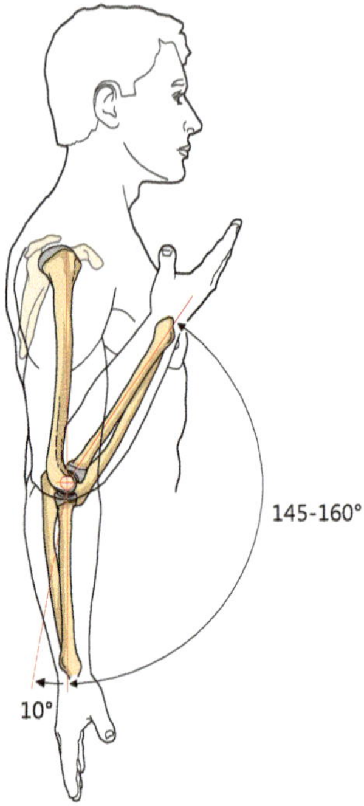

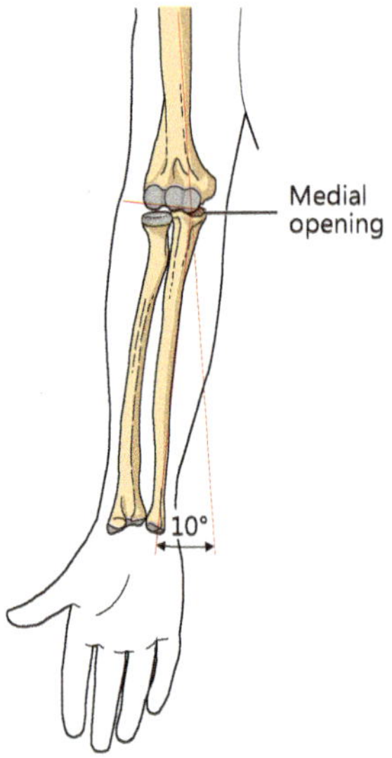

Axis

The flexion-extension movement occurs:

- on the sagittal plane
- around an oblique axis (which, below the lateral and medial epicondyles, crosses the condyle and the trochlea of the humerus).

Factors limiting flexion-extension movement

Active flexion is limited by:

- contact between the soft tissues of the anterior regions of the arm and forearm
- muscle contraction
- tension of the fibers of the anconeus and triceps brachii.

Passive flexion is limited by:

- contact between the head of the radius and the coronoid process of the ulna, respectively, with the radial and coronoid fossae of the humerus
- tension of the fibers of the flexor muscles of the forearm:
  - biceps brachii
  - brachialis

– brachioradialis
- tension of the posterior capsuloligamentous system.

Extension is limited by:
- ulnar and radial collateral ligaments
- tension of the anterior capsuloligamentous system
- contact between the olecranon beak and the olecranon fossa of the humerus.

Pronosupination of the proximal and distal radioulnar joints

During the movement of pronosupination:
- the articular circumference of the head of the radius rotates on the osteofibrous ring formed by the radial notch of the ulna and the anular ligament
- the condyle of the humerus rotates on the articular facet of the head of the radius
- the articular circumference of the head of the ulna rotates on the ulnar notch of the radius
- there is movement of the articular disc of the distal radioulnar joint.

Pronation

- The radius rotates around the ulna
- The distal third of the ulna moves laterally
- At the end of the movement, the radius is positioned obliquely in relation to the ulna.

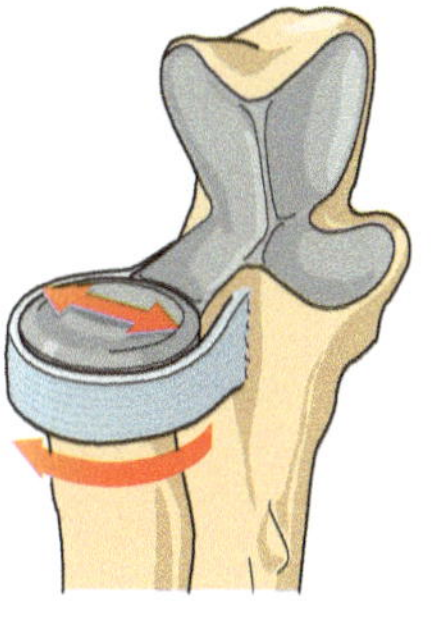

Supination

- The distal third of the ulna moves slightly in a medial direction
- At the end of the movement, the radius and ulna are parallel.

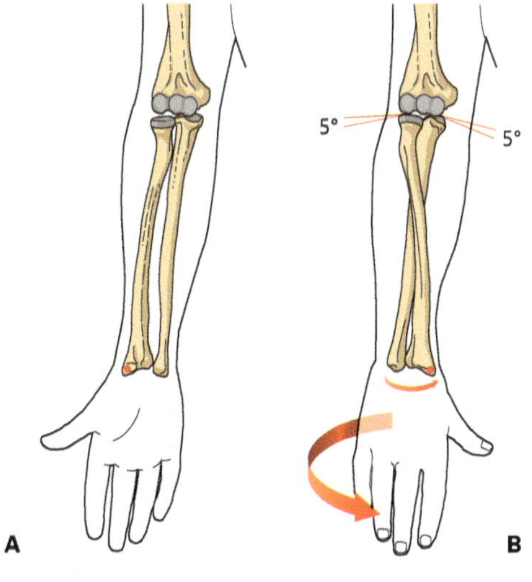

Left hand in the supine position (**A**) and prone (**B**) position.

Reference position

The reference (starting or indifferent) position is given by:

- the limb aligned with the trunk
- the elbow flexed at 90°
- the palm of the hand directed medially.

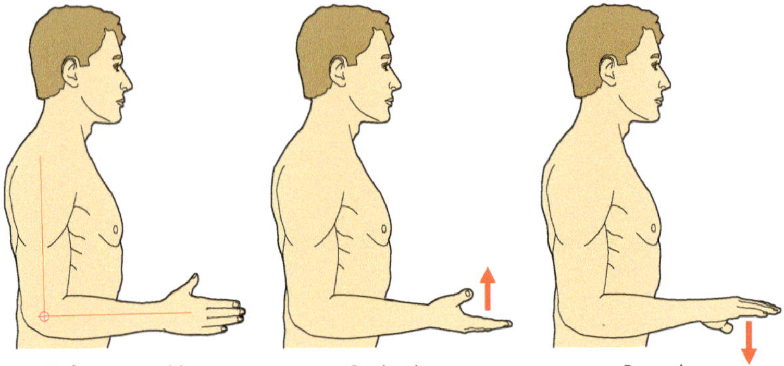

The intermediate position between pronation and supination (reference position), which is common during everyday activities, is characterized by the greatest possible contact between the surfaces of the proximal and distal radioulnar joints.

Amplitude of the prosupination movement

The amplitude of the pronation movement is 85° (the movement is stopped due to the contact produced when the radius and ulna overlap).

The amplitude of the supination motion is 90°.

Thanks to the involvement of the shoulder joint, the global movement of pronosupination can reach an amplitude of:

- 360° when performed with the forearm extended and the arm aligned with the trunk or abducted at 90°
- 270° when performed with the forearm extended and the arm flexed at 90°
- 180° when performed with the forearm extended and the arm at the maximum lateromedial elevation.

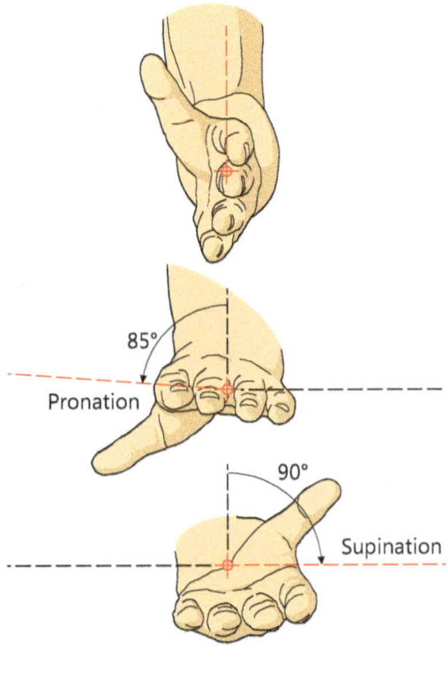

Axis

Pronosupination movement occurs around a vertical axis (which passes proximally through the condyle of the humerus and the center of the head of the radius and distally through the ulnar styloid process).

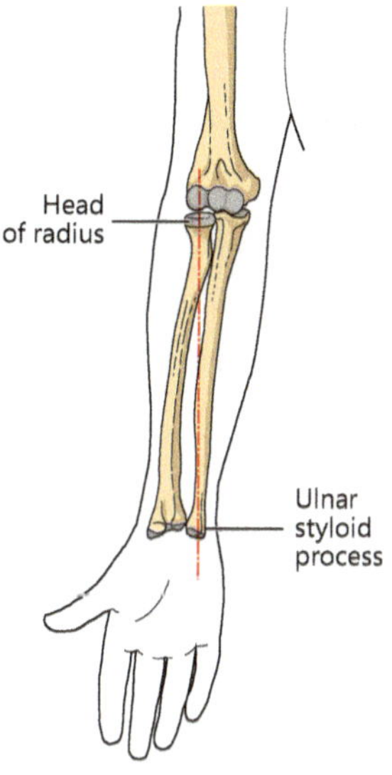

Factors limiting pronosupination movement

Pronation is limited by:

- contact between the radius and the ulna
- the inferior posterior radioulnar ligament
- tension of the posterior capsuloligamentous system
- supinator muscles
- the flexor digitorum profundus and the flexor pollicis longus.

Supination is limited by:

- the interosseous membrane
- the oblique (Weitbrecht's) cord
- the inferior anterior radioulnar ligament
- the quadrate ligament
- tension of the anterior capsuloligamentous system
- pronator muscles.

Assessment of elbow joint mobility

Flexion-extension of the elbow

Starting position	Supine position with the arm aligned with the trunk and the elbow extended: • a towel placed under the distal extremity of the humerus favors joint mobility • due to the tension of the biceps brachii fibers, the position equivalent to 0° (corresponding to the elbow extended at 180°) may not be obtained in males with hypertrophic musculature • in females (due to reduced muscle development compared to males) or in children (due to smaller olecranon size) a hyperextension of the elbow of 15° may be observed
Movement	The examiner moves the forearm upward and backward (bringing the hand closer to the shoulder) to the limit of the elbow flexion movement, and then upward and forward (moving the hand away from the shoulder) to the limit of the elbow extension (or hyperextension) movement 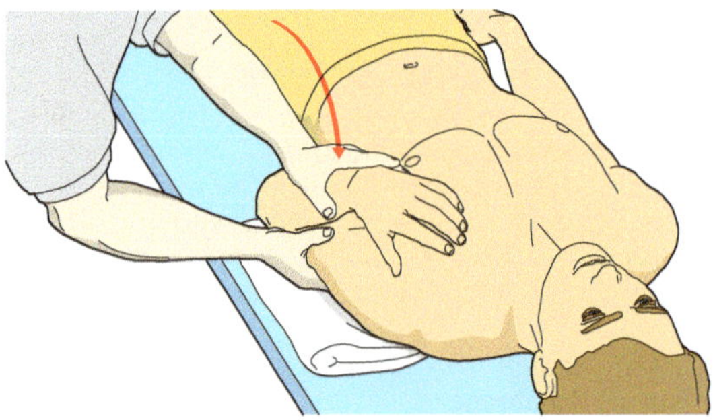 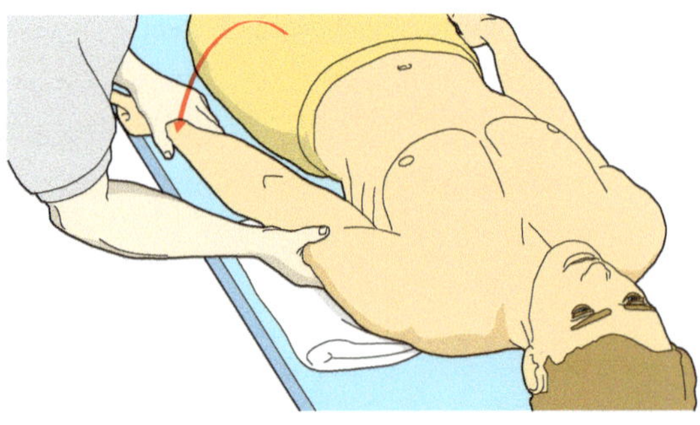

Pronosupination of the elbow

Starting position	Supine position with the arm aligned with the trunk, the elbow flexed at 90° and in an intermediate position between pronation and supination (the palm of the hand directed medially)
Movement	From the intermediate position, the forearm is rotated first externally, orienting the palm of the hand upward, up to the limit of the movement of supination, and then internally, orienting the palm of the hand downward, up to the limit of the movement of pronation of the elbow 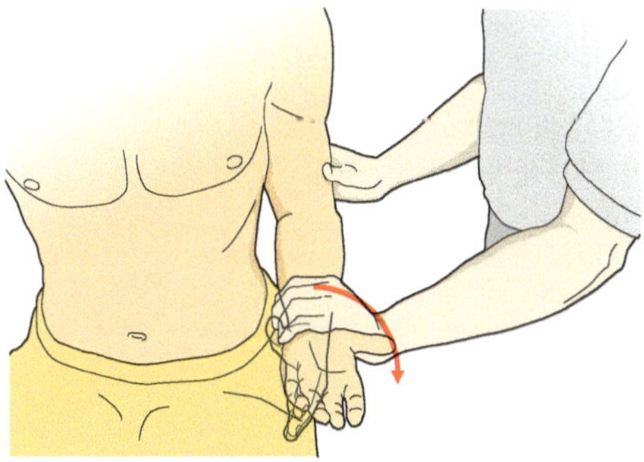 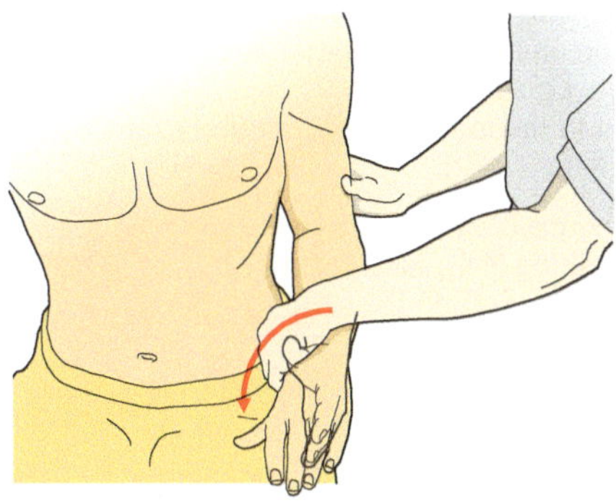

Functional aspects of the elbow joint

Functions of the elbow:
- assists the hand
  - moving it away from the body (extension of the elbow)
  - moving it towards the body (flexion of the elbow)
  - improving its spatial orientation and mobility (through supination and pronation of the forearm)
  - by contributing, together with the forearm, to many of its movements, both specialized or based on strength, in daily activities
- to ensure the strength necessary for lifting objects and for activities requiring the elevation or lowering of the body.

Normal amplitude of elbow movements:
- from 0° extension (equivalent to 180° extension of the forearm in the reference position) to 150° flexion
- from 80° to 85° pronation of the forearm
- from 90° to 95° supination of the forearm.

The majority of everyday activities require excursions inferior to those indicated, for example, many activities of personal care can be carried out by:
- **flexion** of between 30° and 130°
- pronosupination between 50° of **pronation** and 50° of **supination**.

The joint amplitude necessary depends on:
- the characteristics of the objects for manual use and their position
- the subject's posture (activities such as writing, pouring liquid from a bottle, reading a newspaper, performing personal hygiene activities are some examples).

Combined movements of elbow **flexion** between 45° and 136° and of pronosupination between 59° of **supination** and 47° of **pronation** are required for activities related to nutrition like:
- drinking from a glass
- bringing food to the mouth using a knife or fork
- cutting food with a knife.

Complete excursions of elbow movements may be required for everyday activities such as:
- combing or washing of the hair (combined movements of **flexion, pronation** and **supination**)
- reaching a fastener behind the neck with the hands (combined movements of **flexion** and **pronation**)
- using the telephone (**flexion** of 135-140°)
- tying shoelaces (**flexion** of 16°)
- throwing a ball (**extension**)
- walking with the help of crutches (**extension**)
- lifting the body with the arms while seated on a chair (**flexion** of 15°)
- playing tennis (**extension**).

When flexion-extension of the elbow is limited, compensatory movements may occur at the level of:
- vertebral column (thoracic and lumbar segments)
- shoulder
- wrist

These compensatory movements ensure functional elbow mobility between 75° and 120° of **flexion**.

Muscles of the elbow

Muscle	Action	Origin	Insertion	Innervation
Biceps brachii	Flexion and supination of the elbow	*Short head*: apex of the coracoid process of the scapula *Long head*: supraglenoid tubercle of the scapula	Radial tuberosity Antebrachial fascia (through the bicipital aponeurosis)	Musculocutaneous nerve [C5, C6]
Brachialis	Flexion of the elbow	Distal half of the anteromedial and anterolateral surfaces of the humerus	Tuberosity of the ulna	Musculocutaneous nerve [C5, C6]
Brachioradialis	Flexion of the elbow	Proximal two-thirds of the lateral margin of the humerus; lateral intermuscular septum of the arm	Radial styloid process	Radial nerve [C5, C6]
Triceps brachii	Extension of the elbow	Long head: infraglenoid tubercle of the scapula *Lateral head*: posterior surface of the humerus between the radial groove and the insertion of the teres minor; lateral intermuscular septum of the arm *Medial head*: posterior surface of the humerus beneath the sulcus of the radial nerve, between the trochlea of the humerus and the insertion of the teres minor; lateral and medial intermuscular septa of the arm	*All three heads*: apex, posterior surface and borders of the olecranon; some fibers proceed distally, merging with the antebrachial fascia	Radial nerve [C6-C8]
Supinator	Supination of the elbow	Lateral epicondyle of the humerus; radial collateral ligament of the elbow joint; anular ligament of the radius; supinator crest on the shaft (body) of the ulna	Proximal third of the anterior and lateral surfaces of the radius	Posterior interosseous nerve, branch of the radial nerve [C6, C7]

(continued)

8

Muscles of the elbow *(continued)*

Muscle	Action	Origin	Insertion	Innervation
Pronator teres	Pronation of the elbow	*Humeral head*: anterior surface of the medial epicondyle of the humerus; medial border of the humerus; brachial fascia *Ulnar head*: medial surface of the coronoid process of the ulna	*Both heads*: middle part of the lateral surface of the radius	Median nerve [C6, C7]
Pronator quadratus	Pronation of the elbow	Distal quarter of the anterior surface and of the anterior border of the ulna	Distal quarter of the anterior surface and of the anterior border of the radius	Anterior interosseous nerve, branch of the median nerve [C7, C8]
Anconeus	Extension of the elbow	Posterior part of the lateral epicondyle of the humerus and the radial collateral ligament of the elbow joint	Posterior and lateral surfaces of the olecranon	Radial nerve [C6-C8]

As for the muscles of the forearm involved in elbow movements, the origins, insertion and innervation are described in Chapter 9 “Wrist and hand”, where they perform their main actions.

Anterior muscles of the arm and forearm

The flexor muscles of the forearm, also called epitrochlear, with the exception of the biceps brachii and brachialis, because of their origin from the epitrochlea (or medial epicondyle) of the humerus, are arranged in two layers:

- superficial (from lateral to medial)
  - biceps brachii (superficial)
  - pronator teres
  - flexor carpi radialis
  - palmaris longus
  - flexor digitorum superficialis
  - flexor carpi ulnaris
- deep
  - brachialis (situated deep below the biceps brachii)
  - flexor pollicis longus (situated laterally)
  - flexor digitorum profundus (situated medially)
  - pronator quadratus (situated more deeply compared to the previous one).

(The coracobrachialis, which acts on the shoulder, is also included among the muscles situated anteriorly on the arm).

Posterior muscles of the arm and forearm

They are arranged in two layers:

- superficial (from lateral to medial)
  - extensor digitorum
  - extensor digiti minimi
  - extensor carpi ulnaris
  - triceps brachii
  - anconeus

(These muscles, with the exception of the triceps brachii, are also called epicondyle muscles, because of their origin from the lateral epicondyle of the humerus)

- deep (from lateral to medial)
  - supinator
  - abductor pollicis longus
  - extensor pollicis brevis
  - extensor pollicis longus
  - extensor indicis.

Lateral muscles of the forearm

Also known as radial muscles, are represented by:

- extensor carpi radialis brevis
- extensor carpi radialis longus
- brachioradialis.

Action of the muscles in the movements of the elbow

Flexion of the elbow

Flexor muscles of the elbow (from greatest to least muscular work):
- biceps brachii
- brachialis
- brachioradialis
- extensor carpi radialis longus
- pronator teres.

Auxiliary flexor muscles of the elbow:
- extensor carpi radialis brevis
- flexor carpi radialis
- palmaris longus.

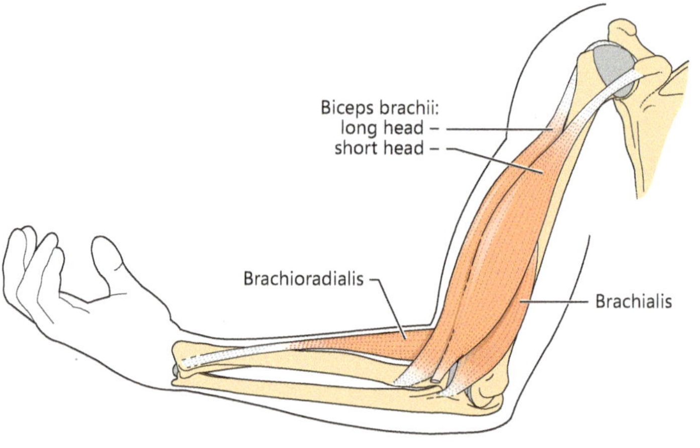

Mode of insertion and lever arms of the three main elbow flexor muscles.

The strength of these muscles varies according to the position in which the flexion of the elbow is carried out, with the exception of the brachialis which, being only a flexor of the forearm, keeps its strength constant. In pronation of the forearm, the tendon of insertion on the radial tuberosity of the biceps brachii wraps around the neck of the radius, resulting in a reduction in the efficiency of the muscle during flexion (see figure on page 316); in this position there is, instead, a greater strength of the other flexor muscles of the forearm, as their insertions are tighter.
The position of the arm influences the strength of the flexor muscles of the elbow, which is greater when the arm is raised.
The force developed by the flexor muscles of the forearm can also be twice compared to that exerted by the extensor muscles of the forearm (see section "Extension of the elbow", page 341).

Action of the flexor muscles of the elbow

Biceps brachii

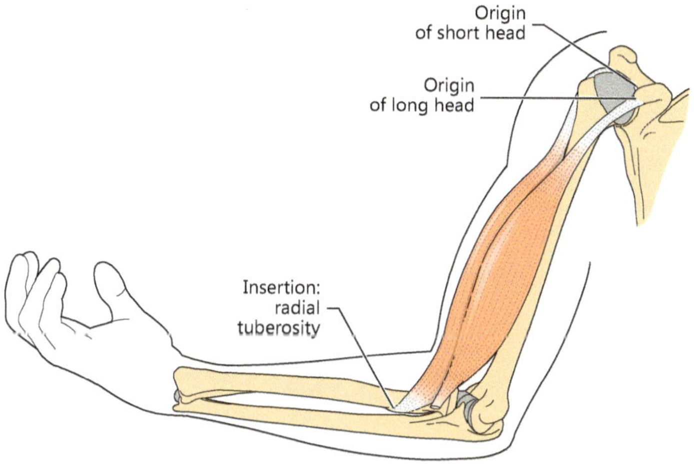

- First flexor of the elbow (based on muscular force)
- Optimal action of the muscle with the forearm flexed at 90° in the supine position
- Second supinator of the forearm (based on muscular force, equal to 2-4 times that of the other supinator muscles), especially against resistance and with the elbow flexed at 90° (representing the most powerful supinator muscle in this case)
- With fixed point on the radius, it brings the scapula forward and down
- Abductor of the shoulder above 90° (long head)
- Adductor of the shoulder (short head).

8

Brachialis

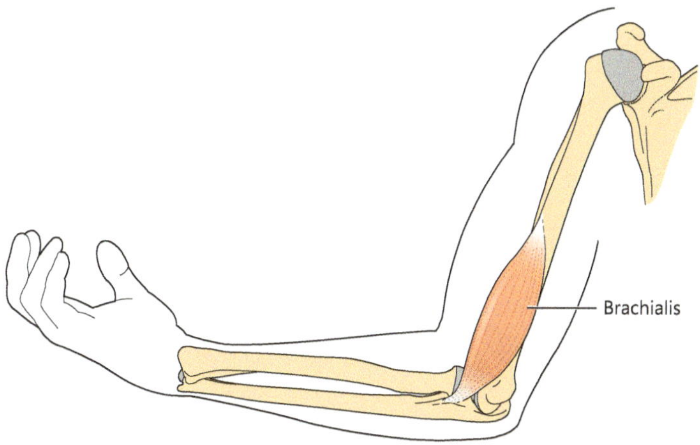

- Pure flexor of the elbow
- Maximum force in slow movements or against resistance of flexion of the elbow.

Brachioradialis

- Third flexor of the elbow (based on muscular force)
- Optimal action with the forearm in an intermediate position between pronation and supination
- Supinator against resistance (from a position of maximum pronation to an intermediate position)
- Pronator against resistance (from a position of maximum supination to an intermediate position)
- Supination action is less when flexion of the elbow increases.

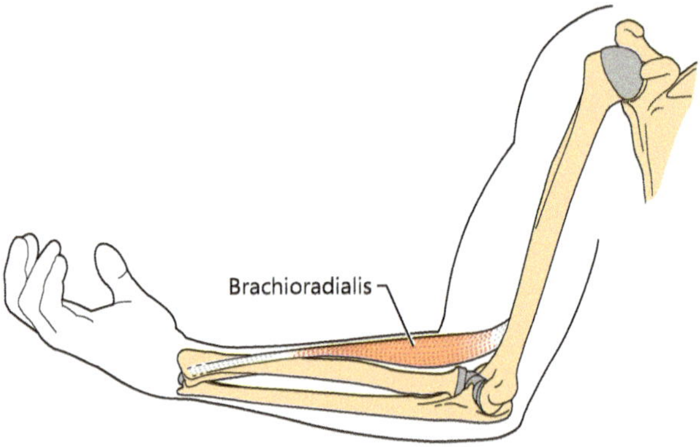

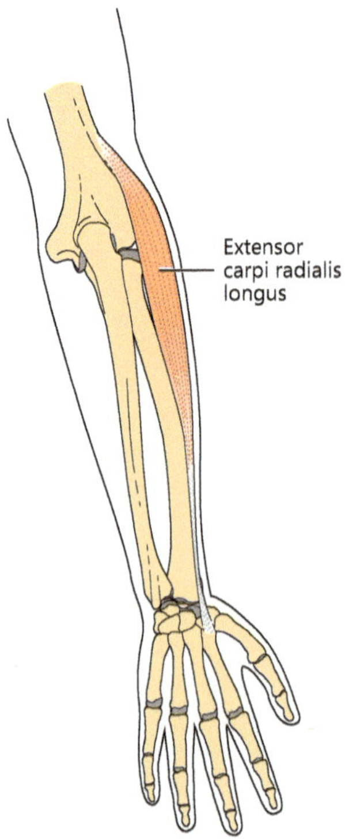

Extensor carpi radialis longus

- Weak flexor of the elbow (fourth based on force developed)
- Weak supinator of the elbow (with the forearm extended)
- Weak pronator of the elbow (with the forearm flexed)
- Second extensor (or dorsal flexor) of the hand
- First radial abductor of the hand.

Pronator teres

- Weak flexor of the elbow against resistance (fifth based on force developed)
- Pronator (second to the pronator quadratus), especially against resistance and when fast action is required
- Antagonizes the supinator action of the biceps brachii.

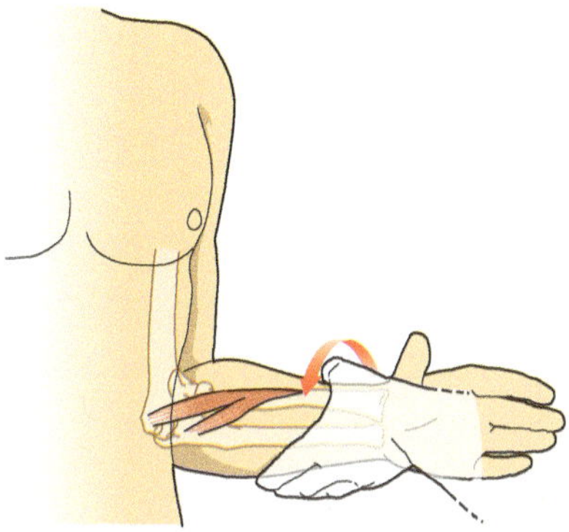

Extensor carpi radialis brevis

- Weak flexor of the elbow
- Extensor (dorsal flexor) of the hand (principal action, second to the extensor carpi radialis longus and third based on force developed)
- Radial abductor (brings the wrist from ulnar abduction to the intermediate position between ulnar abduction and radial abduction).

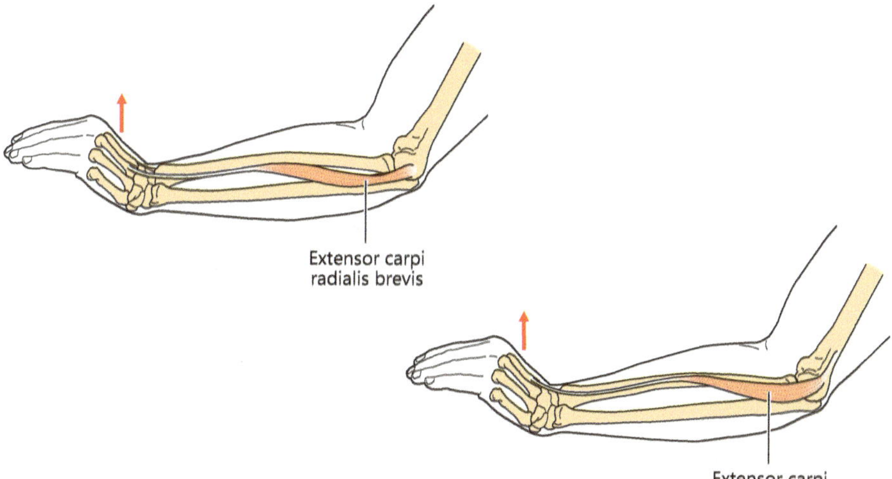

Inflammation of the extensor carpi radialis brevis in corrispondence with its origin in the lateral epicondyle is known as lateral epicondylitis (or "tennis elbow"), which can be localized by palpation of the muscle and the execution of maneuvers that provoke elongation or contraction. Medial epicondylitis (or "golfer's elbow") is a tendinopathy that affects the entire area of the origin of the flexor muscles represented by the medial epicondyle; its assessment is possible during contraction of the flexor muscles of the elbow, possibly against resistance.

Flexor carpi radialis

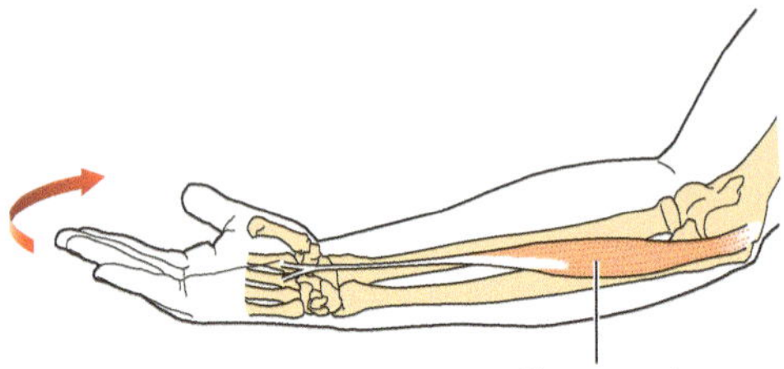

- Weak flexor of the elbow
- Weak pronator of the elbow
- Radial abductor of the hand (principal action, with the hand in palmar flexion) (fourth based on force developed)
- Palmar flexor of the hand (fifth based on force developed).

Palmaris longus

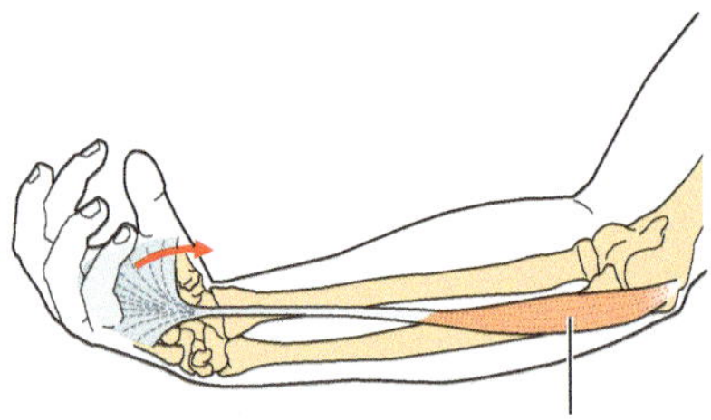

- Weak flexor of the elbow
- Very weak pronator of the elbow
- Palmar flexor of the hand (principal action)
- Extends the palmar aponeurosis.

(For the origin and insertion of the extensor carpi radialis longus, extensor carpi radialis brevis, flexor carpi radialis brevis and palmaris longus, see Chapter 9 "Wrist and hand").

Extension of the elbow

Extensor muscles of the elbow:
- triceps brachii
- anconeus

Action of the extensor muscles of the elbow

Triceps brachii

- Extensor of the elbow (principal action, the greatest force is developed from the medial head)
- Fixator of the head of the humerus (together with the biceps brachii), adductor and extensor of the elbow (actions of the long head).

Anconeus

- Mild extensor of the elbow (synergistic action with that of the triceps brachii).

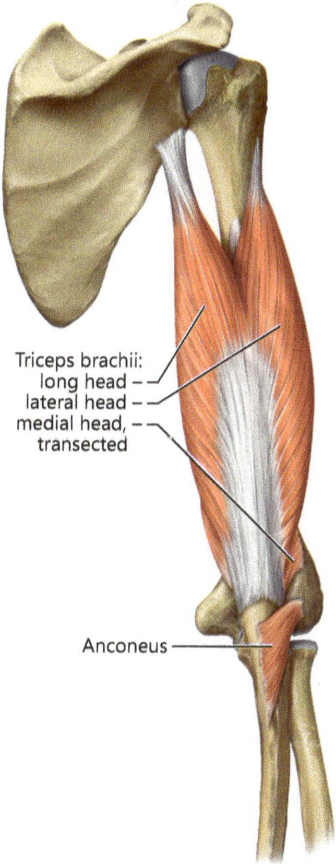

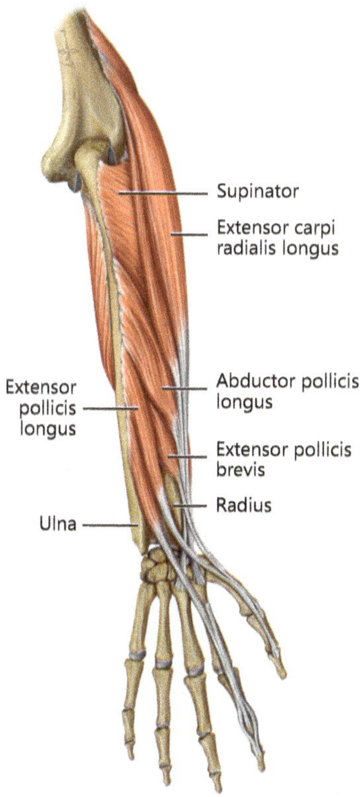

Supination of the elbow

Supinator muscles of the elbow (from greatest to least muscular work):
- supinator
- biceps brachii
- abductor pollicis longus
- extensor pollicis longus
- brachioradialis
- extensor carpi radialis longus.

If the biceps brachii is excluded, the supinator muscles of the elbow have a common origin in the lateral epicondyle of the humerus and is located posteriorly to the interosseous membrane. The last two muscles (brachioradialis and extensor carpi radialis longus) are in a lateral position.

Action of the supinator muscles of the elbow

Supinator

- Pure supinator of the elbow (independently of the position of the forearm, flexed or extended)
- If the elbow is extended, it initiates the movement of supination (supported in a second moment by the biceps brachii)
- Stabilizes the elbow joint (by being connected to the anular ligament of the radius, to the joint capsule and to the radial collateral ligament).

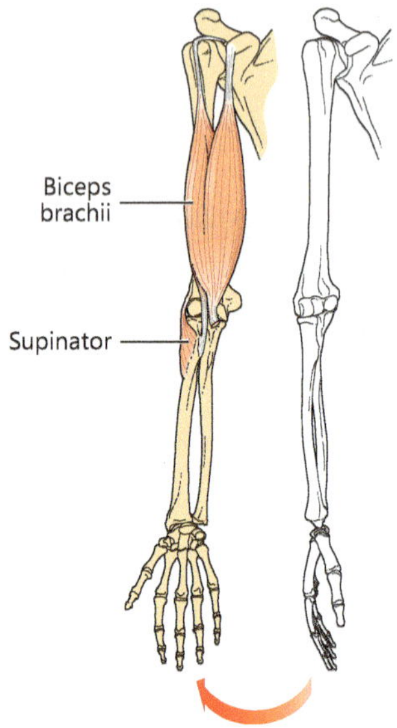

Biceps brachii – see section "Flexion of the elbow", page 337.

Abductor pollicis longus

- Weak supinator of the elbow
- Abductor of the first metacarpal (principal action)
- Palmar flexor of the hand
- Radial abductor of the hand.

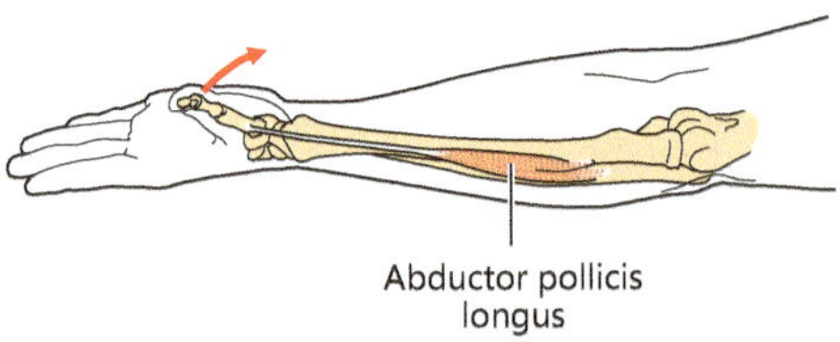

Extensor pollicis longus

- Weak supinator
- Extensor (dorsal flexor) of the hand
- Extensor of the thumb (principal action).

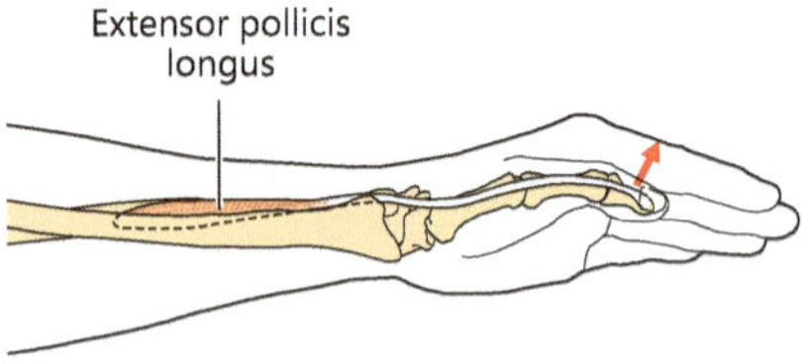

Brachioradialis – see section "Flexion of the elbow", page 338.

Extensor carpi radialis longus – see section "Flexion of the elbow", page 338.

(For the origin and insertion of the abductor pollicis longus, extensor pollicis longus and extensor carpi radialis longus, see Chapter 9 "Wrist and hand").

Pronation of the elbow

Pronator muscles of the elbow (from greatest to least muscular work):
- pronator quadratus
- pronator teres
- flexor carpi radialis
- extensor carpi radialis longus
- brachioradialis
- palmaris longus

The pronator muscles of the elbow have a common origin in the medial epicondyle of the humerus and are located anteriorly to the interosseous membrane, with the exception of the pronator quadratus which is located distally on the forearm.

Action of the pronator muscles of the forearm

Pronator quadratus
- First pronator of the elbow.

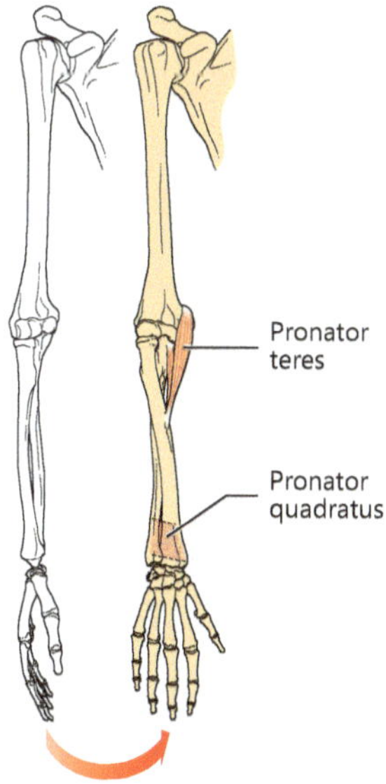

Pronator teres – see section "Flexion of the elbow", page 339.

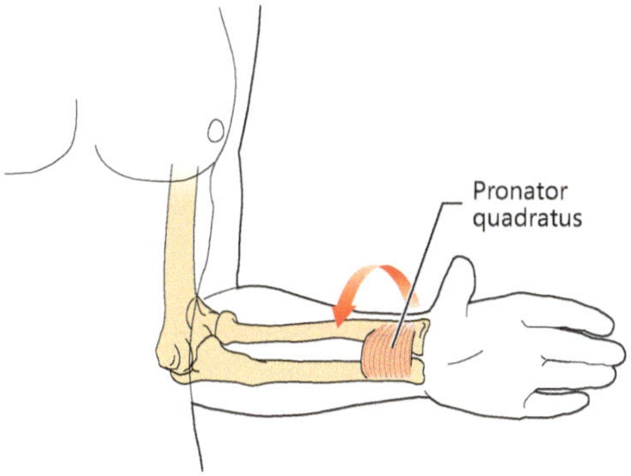

Flexor carpi radialis – see section "Flexion of the elbow", page 340.
Extensor carpi radialis longus – see section "Flexion of the elbow", page 338.
Brachioradialis – see section "Flexion of the elbow", page 338.
Palmaris longus – see section "Flexion of the elbow", page 340.

Assessment of the length and stretch of the fibers of the biceps brachii and triceps brachii

Biceps brachii

Starting position	Supine position with the shoulder extended and the elbow flexed in pronation
Movement	The forearm is brought to maximum extension, thus obtaining the complete stretching of the fibers of the biceps brachii 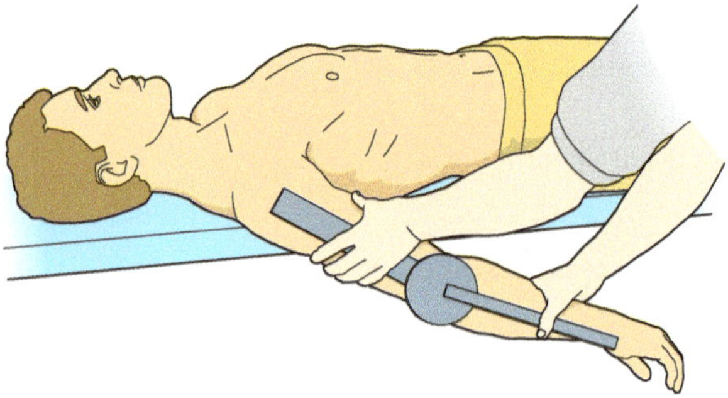

Triceps brachii

Starting position	Seated position with the shoulder flexed at 180° (anteroposterior elevation) and rotated externally with the elbow extended
Alternative starting position	Supine position with the shoulder flexed at 90° and the elbow (this position is used in case of reduction of the joint amplitude of the flexion movement of the arm)
Movement	The forearm is brought to maximum flexion, thus obtaining the complete stretching of the fibers of the triceps brachii 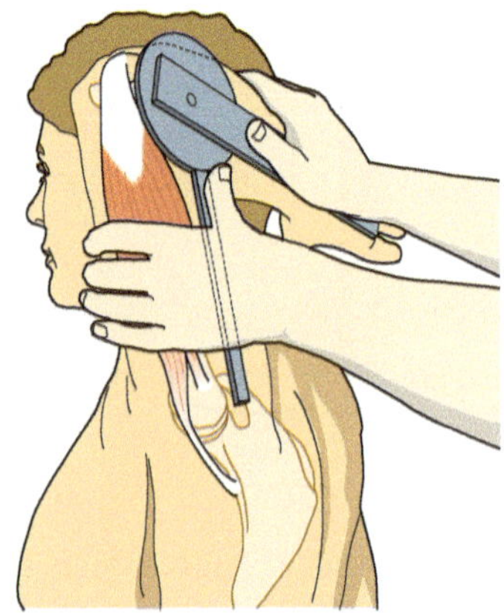

Assessment of muscle strength

Flexion of the elbow

Biceps brachii

Against gravity

Active flexion of the elbow from the supine position with the arm at the side of the trunk, the elbow extended in supination and the resistance applied to the anterior surface of the forearm, just above the wrist joint.

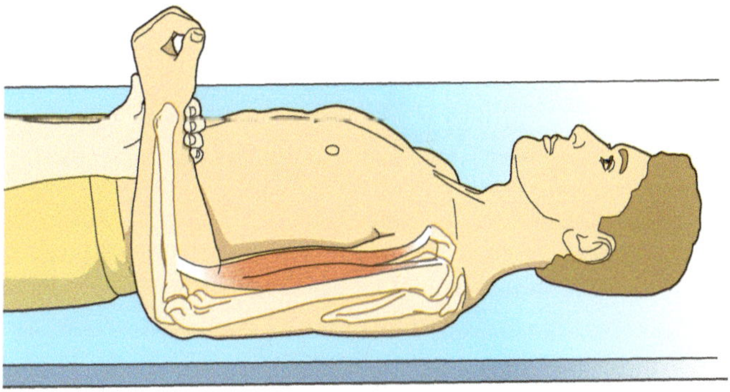

Without gravity

Active flexion of the elbow from a seated position with the shoulder abducted at 90° and the elbow extended in supination and resting on a surface (or, alternatively, from the lateral decubitus position with the upper limb supported by the examiner).

The biceps brachii can be palpated in the anterior part of the cubital fossa.

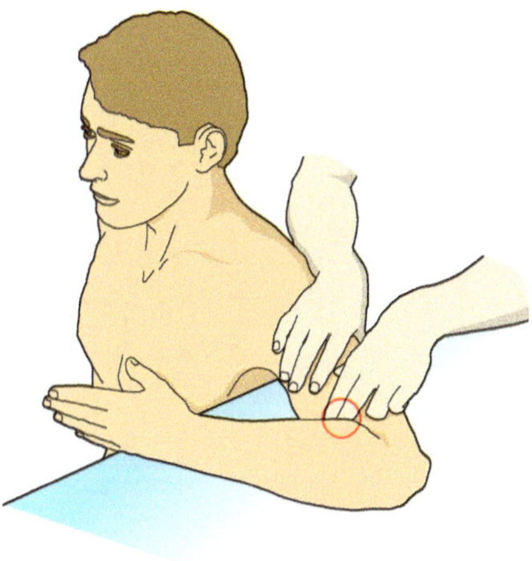

Brachialis and brachioradialis

Against gravity

Active flexion of the elbow from the supine position with the arm at the side of the trunk, the elbow extended in pronation and the resistance applied to the posterior surface of the forearm, just above the wrist joint.

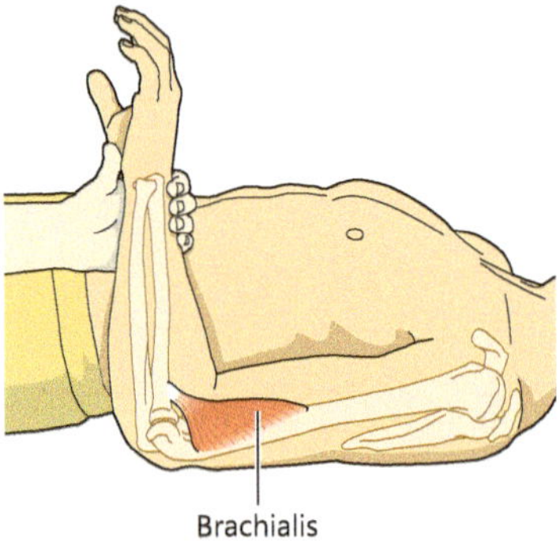

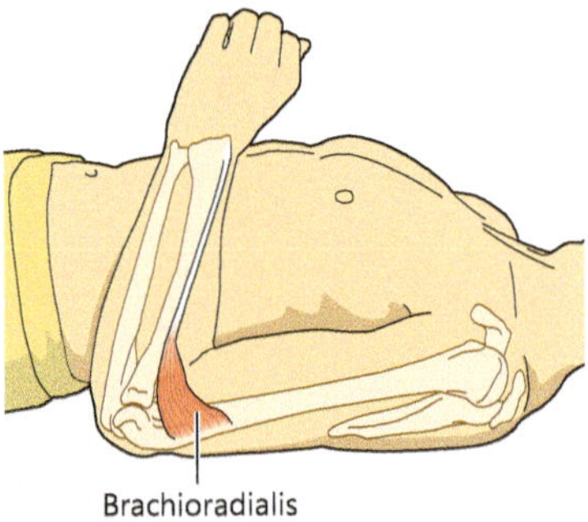

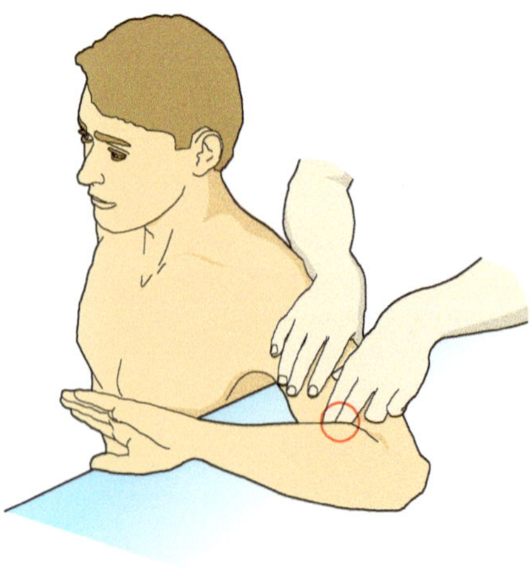

Without gravity

Active flexion of the elbow from a seated position with the shoulder abducted at 90° and the elbow extended in pronation and resting on a surface (or, alternatively, from the lateral decubitus position with the upper limb supported by the examiner).

The brachialis can be palpated medially to the tendon of the biceps brachii, the brachioradialis can be palpated on the anterolateral surface of the forearm, just below the elbow crease.

Extension of the elbow

Triceps brachii

Against gravity

Active extension of the elbow from the supine position with the arm flexed at 90° and rotated internally, the elbow flexed in supination and the resistance applied to the posterior surface of the forearm, just above the wrist joint.

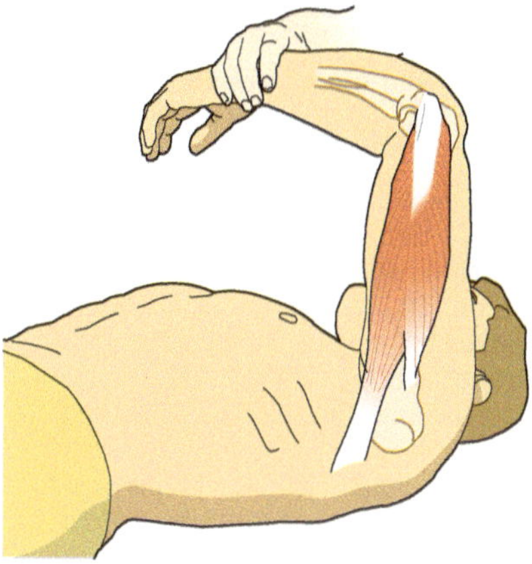

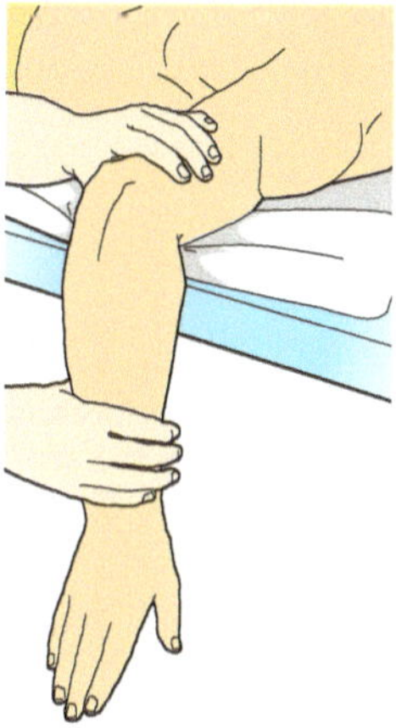

In the presence of weakness in the muscles of the shoulder, the active extension of the elbow can be assessed starting from the prone position with the shoulder abducted, the elbow flexed and the hand hanging vertically from the edge of the examination table and the resistance applied to the posterior surface of the forearm above the wrist joint.

Without gravity

Active extension of the elbow from a seated position with the shoulder abducted at 90° and the elbow flexed in supination and resting on a surface (or, alternatively, from the lateral decubitus position with the upper limb supported by the examiner).

The triceps brachii can be palpated just above the olecranon of the ulna.

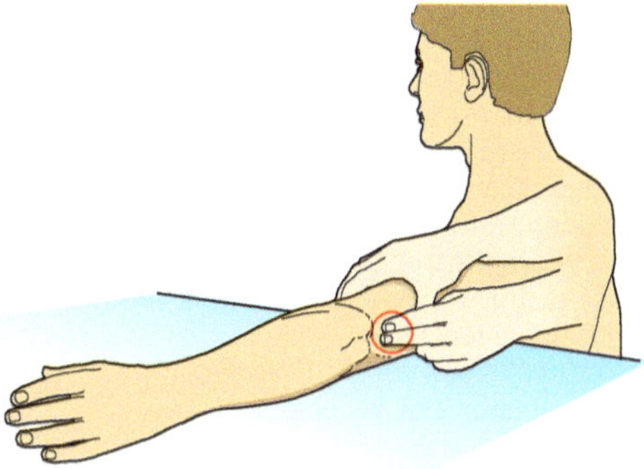

Supination of the elbow

Supinator and biceps brachii

Against gravity

Active supination of the forearm from a seated position with the arm at the side of the trunk, the elbow flexed at 90° in pronation, and the resistance applied to the posterior surface of the distal extremity of the radius with counterpressure on the anterior surface of the ulna.

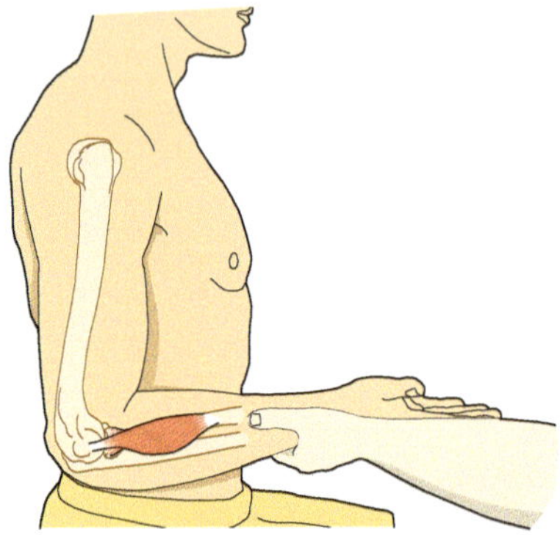

The biceps brachii can be palpated on the anterior surface of the cubital fossa, the supinator can be palpated on the posterior surface of the forearm, distally to the head of the radius.

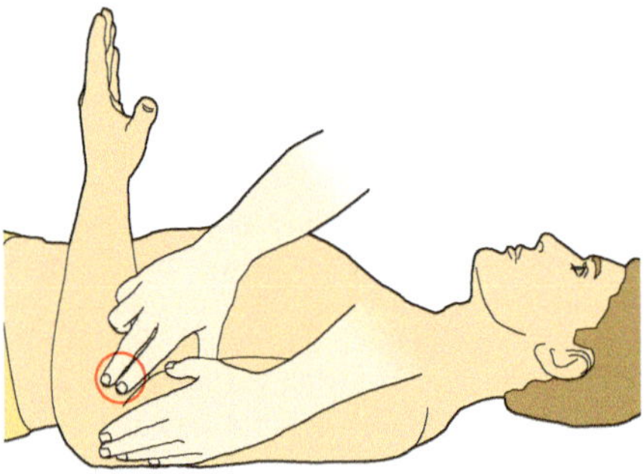

Without gravity

Active supination of the forearm from the supine position with the arm at the side of the trunk and the elbow flexed at 90° in pronation (or, alternatively, from a seated position with the shoulder flexed at 90° and the elbow flexed at 90° in pronation).

Isolation of the supinator

Active supination of the forearm, performed slowly, starting from a seated position with the arm at the side of the trunk and the elbow extended in pronation (when the elbow is extended, the biceps brachii is not able to perform supination) or, alternatively, from the supine position with the arm flexed at 90° and the elbow completely flexed in pronation (in this case, there is a maximum shortening of the fibers of the biceps brachii which is not able to develop effective tension).

The supinator can be palpated during movement.

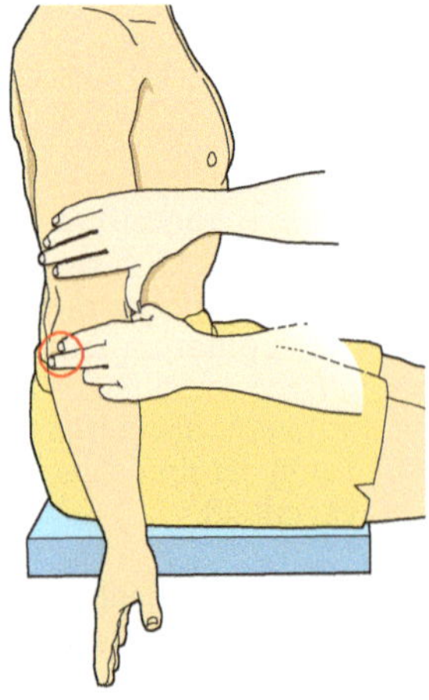

Pronation of the elbow

Pronator teres and pronator quadratus

Against gravity

Active pronation of the forearm from a seated position with the arm at the side of the trunk, the elbow flexed at 90° in supination, and the resistance applied to the anterior surface of the distal extremity of the radius, with counterpressure on the posterior surface of the ulna.

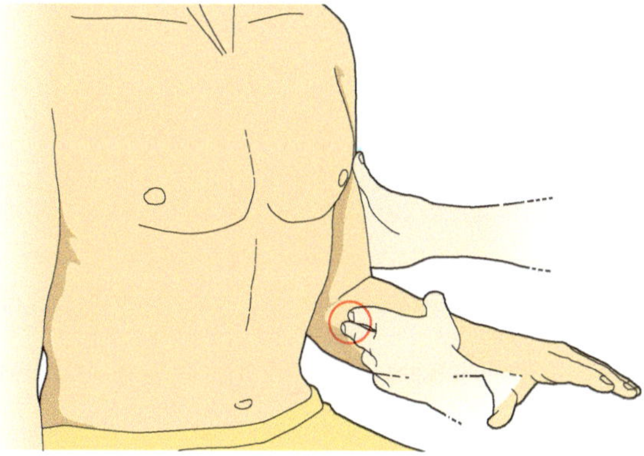

The pronator teres can be palpated on the proximal third of the anterior surface of the forearm, along a diagonal that joins the lateral epicondyle of the humerus with the intermediate point of the lateral border of the radius, whereas the pronator quadratus is situated deeper and cannot be palpated.

Without gravity

Active pronation of the forearm from the supine position with the arm at the side of the trunk and the elbow flexed at 90° in supination (or, alternatively, from a seated position with the arm flexed at 90° and the elbow flexed at 90° in supination).

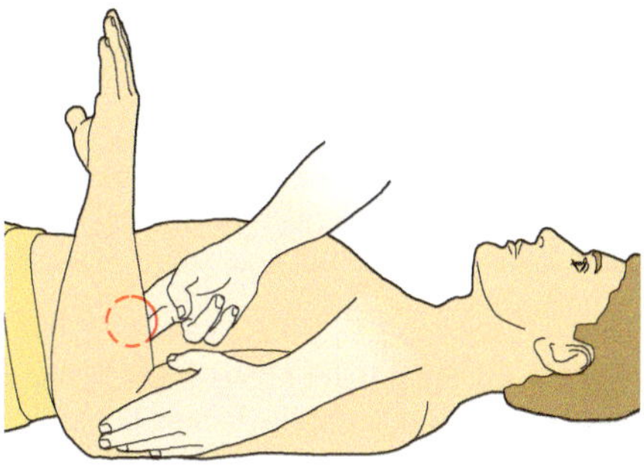

Functional aspects of the muscles of the elbow

Flexion of the elbow

It is performed mainly by the action of the following muscles:
- biceps brachii
- brachialis
- brachioradialis.

Their role in the functional activities is determined by:
- position
  - of the elbow
  - of the forearm
- intensity of the load applied
- speed of the movement.

The force arm of these muscles – that is, the distance between the point of application of the force and the center of rotation – (from greatest to least): brachioradialis → biceps brachii → brachialis.

The flexion of the elbow is privileged compared to other movements of the elbow by:
- number of participating muscles
- overall diameter of the muscle mass of the flexor region, with greater resultanting muscular force.

Function of the biceps brachii

- Works more efficently with the forearm flexed at 90° (45° angle of insertion)
- As it is also a supinator of the forearm, in addition to a flexor, its action is exemplified by activities that involved the execution of both types of movement, such as:
  - using a corkscrew or a screwdriver:
    - in these movements there is agonism with the triceps brachii (i.e., contraction of both muscles), which acts as a fixator of the forearm flexed at 90° through its action as an extensor
- The maximum flexion force is reached when the forearm is in an intermediate position between pronation and supination
- It does not supinate the forearm when it is extended, unless the supination encounters strong resistance
- It does not flex the forearm when it is prone.

The biarticularity of the biceps allows for its elongation, with the glenohumeral (shoulder) joint extended (retroposition) while the elbow is flexed.

The pre-elongation of the biceps brachii from this position attributes greater efficiency to movements of partial static condition such as traction (in sports, this technique is used in tug-of-war), and to dynamic movements such as the loading of a punch, in throwing, etc.

If the biceps brachii and the triceps brachii are antagonists to one another in the above described movements (the triceps brachii pushes, the biceps brachii pulls), they collaborate in other movements, such as when tightening a screw (co-contraction).

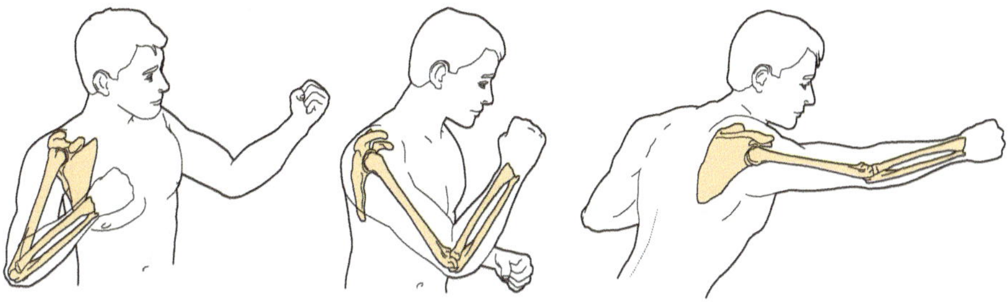

Loading of a punch by the shoulder and its terminal phase.

In this case, the biceps brachii needs to maintain an angle of around 90° in order to supinate with greater efficacy. This position is reached, predominantly, by the extensor action of the triceps brachii, which acts as a fixator in this case.

Function of the brachialis

- It is active in every position of the forearm, with or without resistance
- Inserting at the proximal extremity of the ulna and at the distal extremity of the humerus, it is not influenced by changes of position of the forearm caused by the rotation of the radius, nor by the position of the arm
- Being exclusively a flexor muscle, it can act alone when movements of supination and pronation of the forearm are not required (however, there are activities in which all flexor muscles are recruited, for example, when using a hammer).

Function of the brachioradialis

- Contributes to the flexion movement when speed and force of execution are required with the forearm in a partial or fully pronated position
- Its action is exemplified by activities such as drinking from a glass, typing or playing the piano.

8

Extension of the elbow

Function of the triceps brachii

- Adductor and extensor of the shoulder (long head)
- Extensor of the elbow
  - its efficacy as an extensor of the elbow is influenced by the position of the arm, as the long head is biarticular due to its origin on the scapula
  - when the shoulder and the elbow are flexed and there is an attempt to extend the elbow, there is an elongation of its fibers (that is, a separation of its muscular insertions) which makes the contraction more effective, as occurs in the thrust movements that take place:
    - during forward displacement of heavy objects
    - in the terminal phase of a throw or a punch
    - during activities such as sawing wood
    - when lifting up from the ground by holding with the upper limbs (in particular if the shoulders are flexed and adducted). In this latter case, the extensor thrust of the triceps brachii is associated with the adductor traction of the pectoralis major, which is longer or smaller extent in relation to the abduction or adduction of the shoulders, as

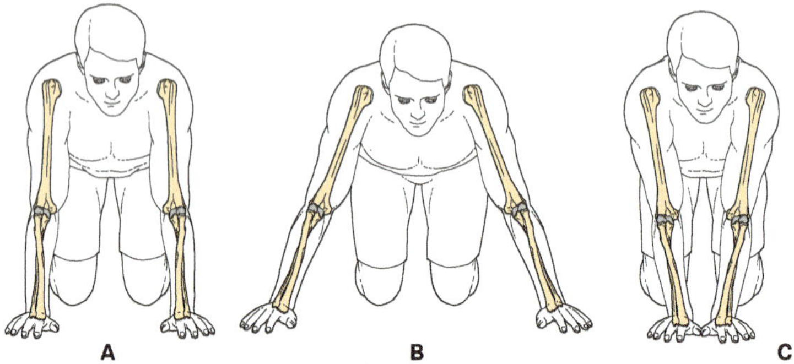

A, Balanced work of the pectoralis major and triceps brachii; **B**, predominant work of the pectoralis major; **C**, predominant work of the triceps brachii.

abduction separates, whereas adduction brings the insertions of the pectoralis major closer

- when the elbow is extended, the force of contraction is minimal (in this case, the axial component of decomposition of the muscular strength, which is more effective when the forearm is flexed at 20-30°, tends to displace the forearm backward, with luxation of the elbow; its action is, however, balanced by the rotatory component, which is in fact three times greater compared to the angular component; for greater degrees of flexion of the forearm, the angular component tends to diminish)
- the medial head of the triceps brachii muscle is always active during the extension of the elbow
- the lateral head and the long head are brought into play when a greater muscular force is required which, although notable (in relation to the small diameter of the fibers), becomes less important compared to the action speed of the muscle (obtained by the minimum power arm derived from the insertion of the ulna to the olecranon).

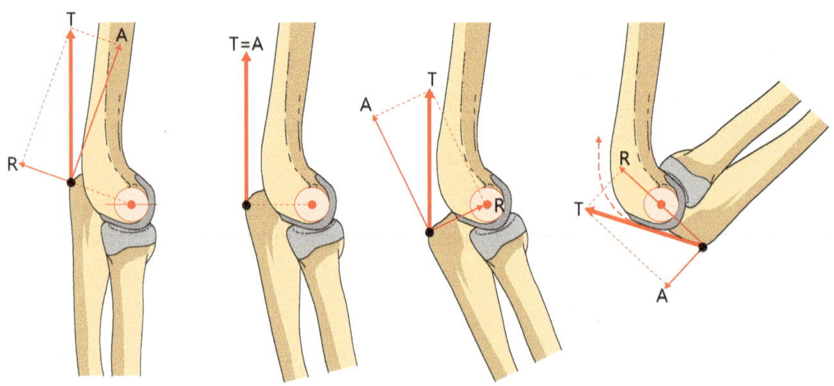

The triceps brachii (T) could cause a posterior dislocation of the elbow when this is at its maximum extension, better when flexed at 20°-30°. This is because the axial component (A) exerts traction on the ulna, favored by a possible thrust produced axially on the forearm. R = Rotation component.

Supination of the elbow

- Occurs by the action of the following muscles:
  - supinator
  - biceps brachii
- The supinator, acting alone, is capable of performing supination of the elbow from any position
- The biceps brachii participates in the supination of the elbow if force and speed are required
- In the majority of everyday activities, varying intensities of force and different combinations of flexion and supination of the forearm are required:
  - these associations are necessary for keeping or moving the hand close to the body and rotating it so that the palm is facing upwards
- There is a functional correlation between the supinator muscles of the forearm and the external rotators of the arm when the elbow is extended; starting from this position, the supination of the elbow and the external rotation of the arm occur simultaneously in the course of various activities
- Supination may also be carried out by the brachioradialis if the forearm is in a pronated position
- Other muscles may participate in supination or reinforce it. These are the abductor pollicis longus and the extensor pollicis longus as well as the extensor carpi radialis longus. All of the supinator muscles, with the exception of the biceps brachii, originate from the lateral epicondyle of the humerus and adjacent regions.

Pronation of the elbow

- Occurs by the action of the following muscles:
  - pronator teres
  - pronator quadratus
- The main action is performed by the pronator quadratus
- The pronator teres participates in the pronation of the elbow if force and speed are required, for example, in movements such as throwing a ball or using a racket
- The action of the pronator muscles accompanies many everyday activities such as writing, washing, dressing, etc.
- There is a functional correlation between the pronator muscles of the forearm and the internal rotators of the arm, as the pronation of the forearm and the internal rotation of the arm occur simultaneously in the course of various activities
- Pronation may also be carried out by the brachioradialis if the forearm is in a supinated position
- Other muscles may participate in supination or reinforce it. These are the flexor carpi radialis, extensor carpi radialis longus, brachioradialis and palmaris longus. All the pronator muscles originate from the medial epicondyle of the humerus and adjacent regions.

Palpation of the elbow

Head of the radius

The patient has the arm in slight flexion. The lateral epicondyle is identified and from here proceed distally, through the small depression between the humerus and the radius. The head of the radius is easily identified because it is the only bony structure present in the area. During pronosupination movements of the forearm, the head of the radius can be felt acting as a point of rotation.

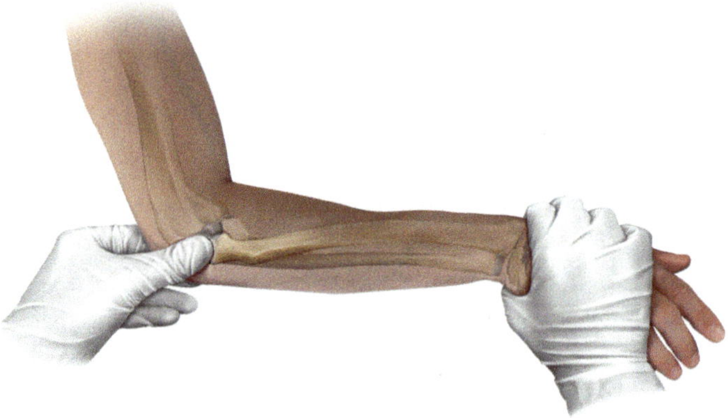

Shaft (body) of the ulna

The examiner holds the patient's upper limb flexed at the elbow with one hand, while the other hand palpates the posterior elbow area to identify the olecranon. From here proceed by sliding the fingers over the border of the ulna, along the entire length of the forearm.

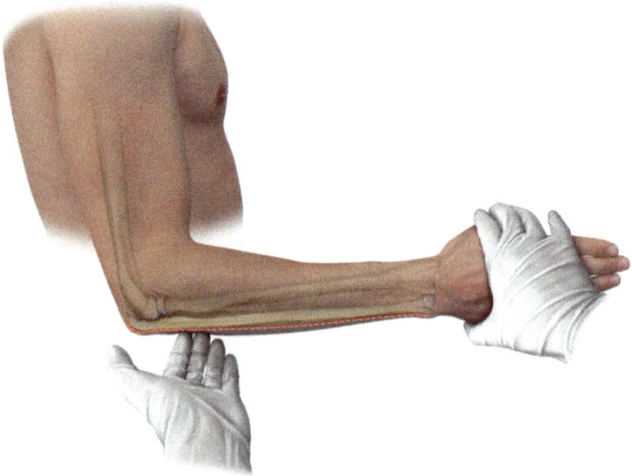

Olecranon

The patient is seated, with the elbow flexed. The examiner takes the patient's hand and proceeds to palpate the large tuberosity located superficially at the elbow joint. By passively extending and reflexing the elbow, it is possible to access the olecranon fossa on the humerus.

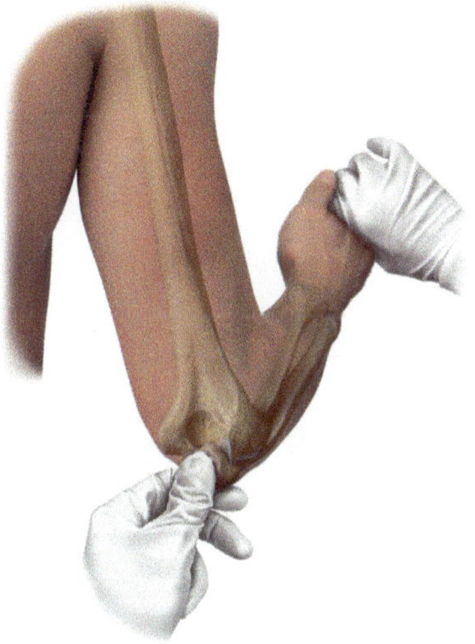

Lateral supraepicondylar (supracondylar) ridge

Taking the patient's hand, the olecranon is identified with the elbow flexed. From here move laterally over the lateral epicondyle to explore the lateral supraepicondylar (supracondylar) ridge proceeding in a proximal direction until it disappears under the muscles of the forearm.

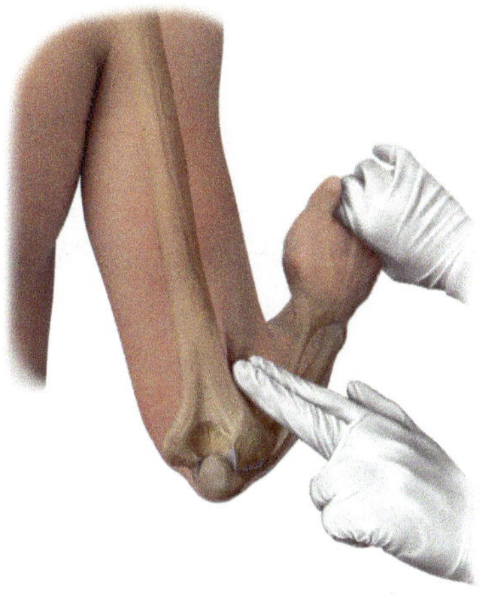

Lateral epicondyle of the humerus

The examiner holds the patient's upper limb flexed at the elbow with one hand while palpating the posterior elbow area with the other to identify the olecranon. From here slide laterally until the bony protrusion of the lateral epicondyle is found.

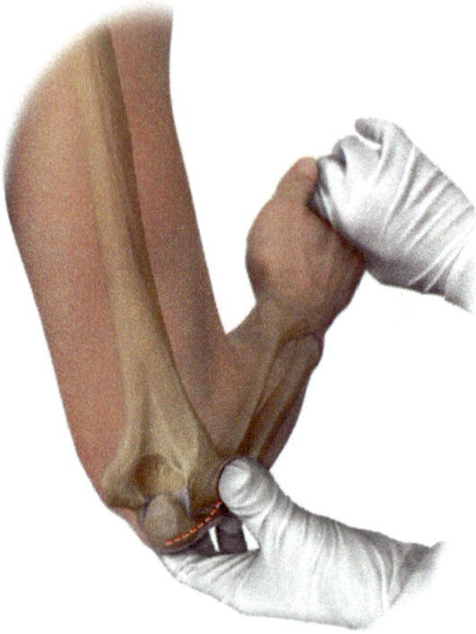

Medial epicondyle of the humerus

Taking the patient's hand, the olecranon is identified with the elbow flexed. From here slide the fingers medially and, after reaching a small depression, move up towards the medial epicondyle.

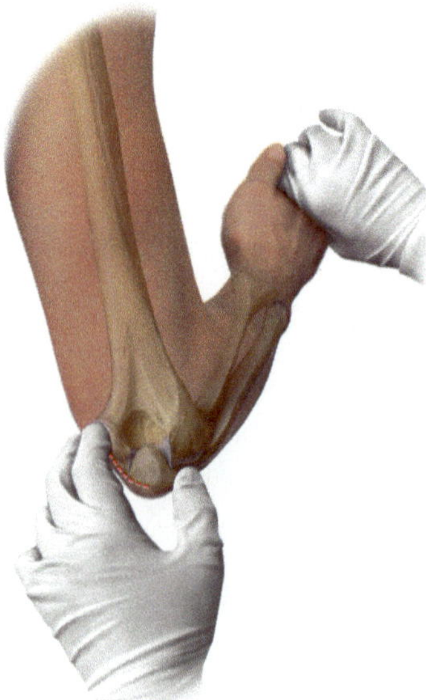

Common tendon of the flexor muscles

Extending the hand over the anterior surface of the forearm, between the brachioradialis and the ulna, the patient is asked to perform a series of isometric wrist flexions, interspersed with a rest. During flexion it is possible to palpate the contracted muscle bellies and identify their tendinous insertion.

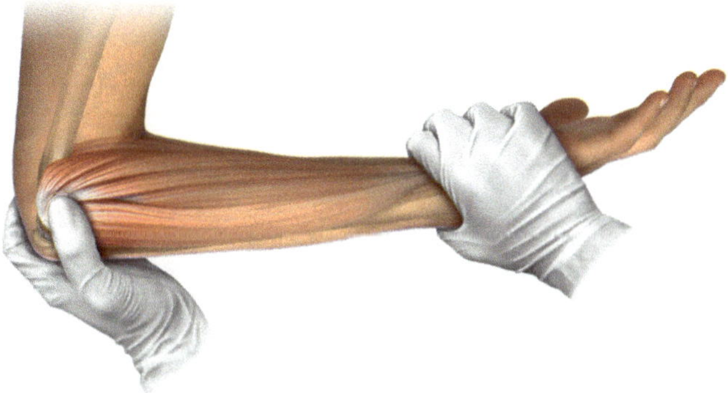

Extensor carpi radialis longus and extensor carpi radialis brevis

Taking the patient's hand, the examiner asks the patient to perform an isometric adduction of the wrist. During abduction, the fibers of the extensor carpi radialis longus and extensor carpi radialis brevis contract: their course is followed in a cranial direction, until reaching the tendinous origin at the lateral supraepicondylar (supracondylar) ridge of the humerus.

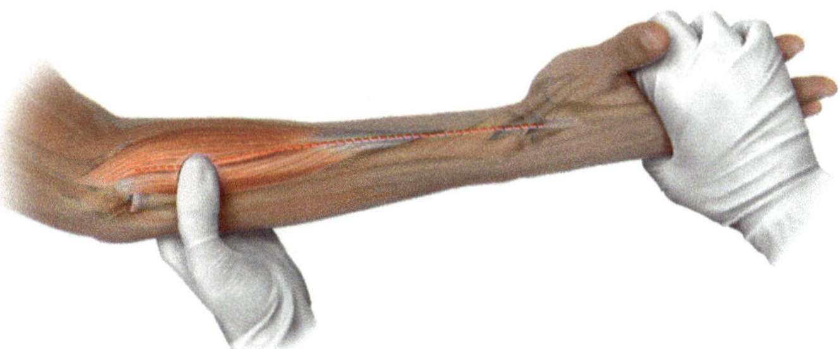

Anatomical landmarks on the surface of the elbow and forearm

1	Acromion: process by which the spine of the scapula extends laterally to the apex of the shoulder
2	Medial epicondyle: medial prominence of the distal extremity of the humerus
3	Lateral epicondyle: lateral prominence of the distal extremity of the humerus
4	Olecranon: rough prominence on the proximal extremity of the ulna
5	Head of the radius: superior extremity of the radius distal to the epicondyle of the humerus
6	Radial styloid process: downward extension on the lateral part of the posterior surface of the inferior extremity of the radius
7	Head of the third metacarpal: distal extremity of the third metacarpal
8	Head of the ulna: inferior extremity of the ulna

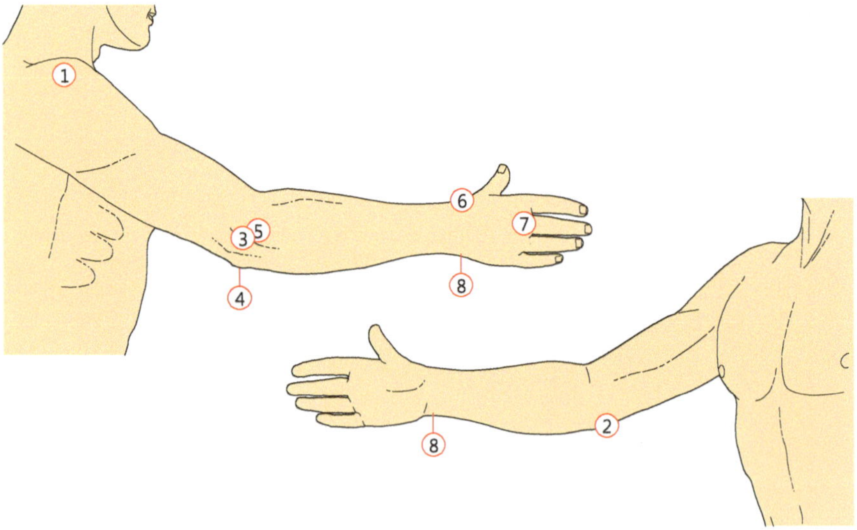

Distal extremities of the radius and ulna

(See Chapter 8 "Elbow").

Bones of the hand

Carpal bones

Eight short bones located in two rows:
- proximal (from external to internal):
  - scaphoid (or navicular)
  - lunate
  - triquetrum
  - pisiform
- distal (from the outside to the inside):
  - trapezium
  - trapezoid
  - capitate
  - hamate.

Metacarpals

Five long bones numbered from the outside to the inside [I-V], each formed by:
- a proximal extremity (base)
- a shaft (body)
- a distal extremity (head).

Skeleton of the digits

- 1st digit (thumb): proximal and distal phalanges
- 2nd, 3rd, 4th and 5th digits (index, middle, ring and little fingers): proximal, middle and distal phalanges.

Each phalange is formed by:
- a proximal extremity (base)
- a shaft (body)
- a distal extremity (head).

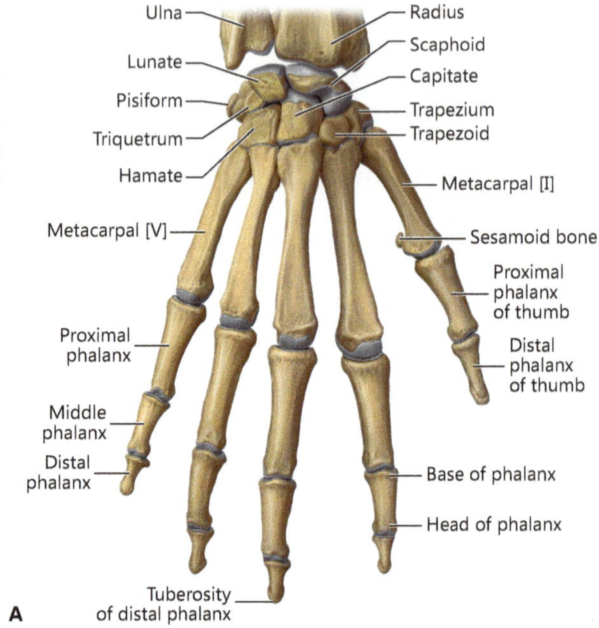

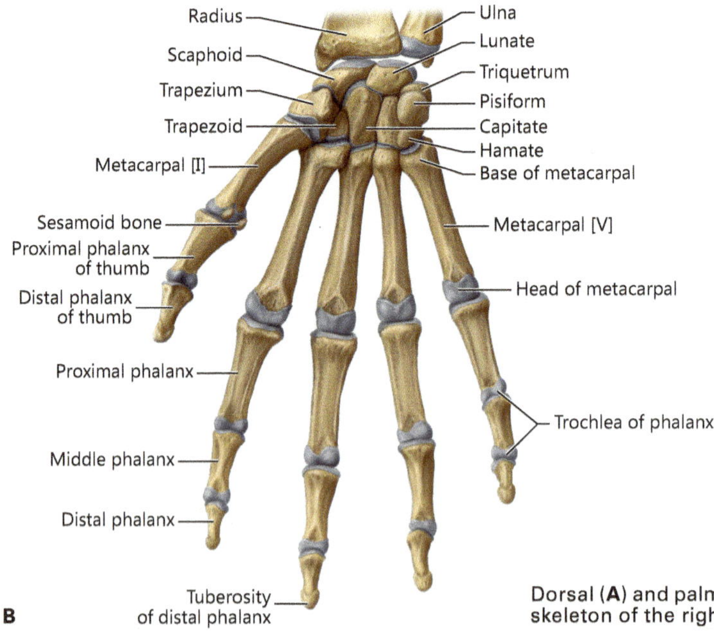

Dorsal (**A**) and palmar (**B**) views of the skeleton of the right hand.

Joints of the wrist and hand

Wrist

- Radiocarpal – fundamental joint of the wrist
- Distal radioulnar – functionally attributable to the forearm (see Chapter 8 "Elbow") and anatomically to the wrist
- Midcarpal – functionally attributable to the wrist and anatomically to the hand.

Hand

- Intercarpal (carpal joint)
- Carpometacarpal
- Intermetacarpal
- Metacarpophalangeal
- Interphalangeal.

Radiocarpal joint

Type of joint	Condyloid
Articular surfaces	Carpal articular surface of the inferior extremity of the radius → constitutes the external two-thirds of the proximal articular surface Proximal articular surface: inferior surface of the articular disc (biconcave disc extending between the internal inferior border of the radius and the lateral border of the base of the ulnar styloid process) → constitutes the internal third of the proximal articular surface The proximal articular surface has a concave ellipsoidal shape (oval cavity or glenoid cavity elongated in the transverse direction) The distal articular surface (articular surface of the carpus) is formed by the proximal surfaces of the scaphoid, lunate and triquetrum, joined together by the interosseous ligaments (the scaphoid and part of the lunate correspond to the radius, part of the lunate and the triquetrum to the articular disc) The distal articular surface has a convex ellipsoidal shape (condyle) 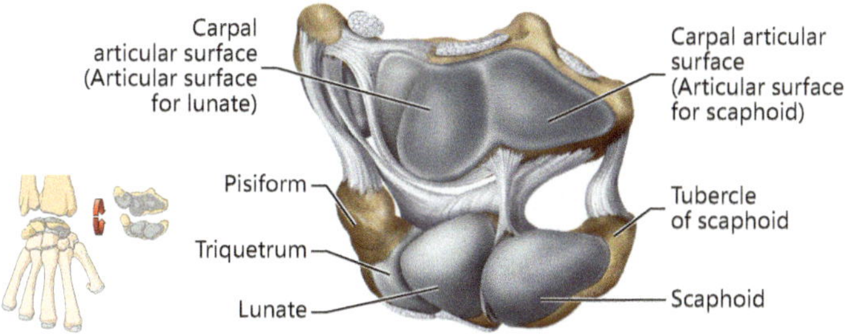

9

Flexion-extension and abduction-adduction movements (two degrees of freedom, four possible movements) of the hand are possible. The former reach greater amplitude thanks to the curvature of the condyle, which is more accentuated (the convex surface of the carpus is 1.5 times larger than the concave articular surface of the radius and the triangular disc along the radioulnar axis and 2 times larger along the dorsopalmar axis).

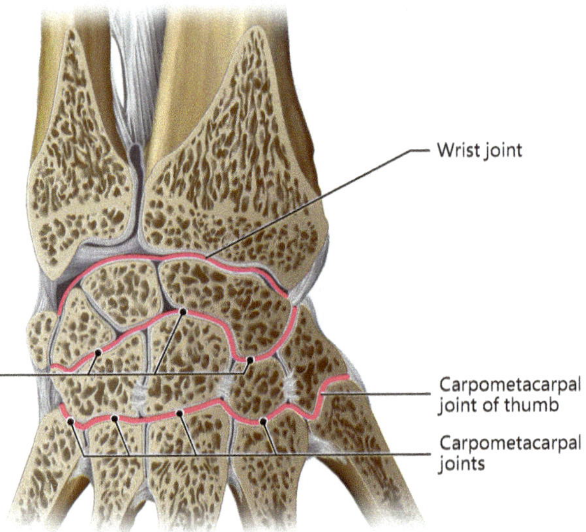

The wrist.

The abduction of the hand (radial abduction or true abduction) consists of the lateral movement of the hand away from the axis of symmetry of the wrist; the adduction of the hand (incorrectly called ulnar abduction) consists of the medial movement of the hand away from the axis of symmetry of the wrist.

Midcarpal joint

Type of joint	Between the proximal and distal rows of carpal bones, it is formed by two juxtaposed condylar joints (lateral and medial)
Articular surfaces	Lateral condylar joint: • condyle – distal surface of the scaphoid divided by a sagittal crest into two articular surfaces that correspond to the trapezius and trapezoid • glenoid cavity – constituted by the proximal surfaces of the trapezium and trapezoid (because of their flat surfaces they can also be called plane joints) Medial condylar joint (inverse to the above): • condyle – head of the capitate (proximal surface) and apex of the hamate (proximal surface) • glenoid cavity – concave surface constituted by the medial surface of the scaphoid and the distal surfaces of the lunate and triquetrum The joint interline has an "S" shape arranged horizontally along the shortest axis of the hand

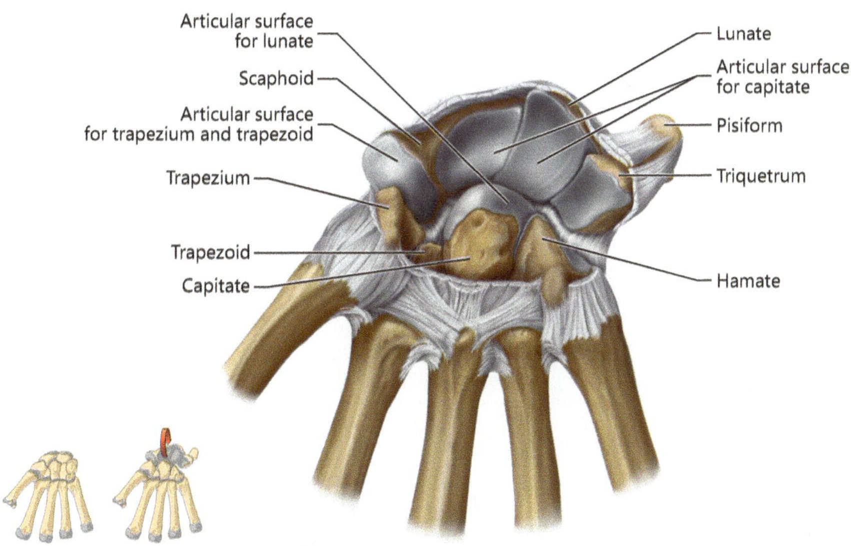

Right midcarpal joint. The articular surface is formed by the bones of the proximal carpal row and the distal carpal row.

Only generic and limited sliding movements are possible between the articular surfaces, which are carried out in different directions and facilitate flexion-extension and abduction-adduction (lateralization) movements of the hand.

Intercarpal joints

- Reciprocal joints between the bones of the proximal carpal row
- Reciprocal joints between the bones of the distal carpal row
- Reciprocal joints between the bones of the proximal carpal row and the bones of the distal carpal row (see section "Midcarpal joint", page 363).

Reciprocal joints between the bones of the proximal carpal row

- Between scaphoid and lunate – flat, vertical, sagittally oriented articular surfaces (plane joint)
- Between lunate and triquetrum – flat, vertical, sagittally oriented articular surfaces (plane joint)
- Between triquetrum (anterior surface) and pisiform – flat articular surfaces (plane joint)

Only small sliding movements of the articular surfaces are possible.

Reciprocal joints between the bones of the distal carpal row

- Between trapezium and trapezoid – flat, vertical, sagittally oriented articular surfaces (plane joint)
- Between trapezoid and capitate – flat, vertical, sagittally oriented articular surfaces (plane joint)
- Between capitate and hamate – flat, vertical, sagittally oriented articular surfaces (plane joint)

Only small sliding movements of the articular surfaces are possible.

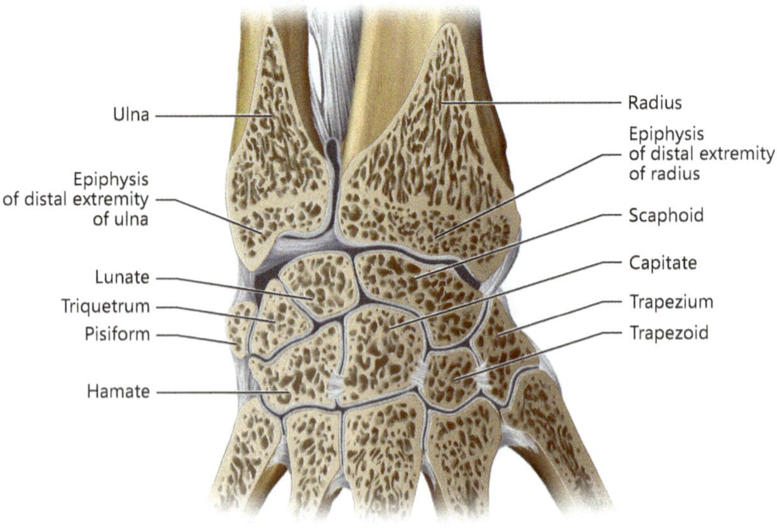

Right joints of hand. The frontal section plane passes through the distal part of the forearm and the proximal part of the hand. The complex system of articular cavities delimited by the radiocarpal, intercarpal and carpometacarpal joints is shown. The section plane is seen from the dorsal side.

Carpometacarpal joints

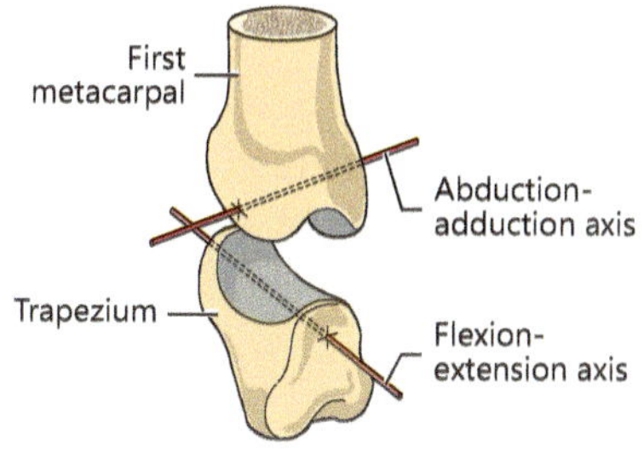

Saddle joints of the thumb.

Joints between bones of the distal carpal row and the bases of the five metacarpals:

- carpometacarpal joint of the 1st digit (thumb)
- carpometacarpal joints of the 2nd, 3rd, 4th and 5th digits (index, middle, ring and little fingers).

Carpometacarpal joint of the thumb

- Between the distal surface of the trapezium and the base of the first metacarpal
- The articular surface:
  - of the trapezium is concave in the transverse direction
  - of the first metacarpal is convex in the transverse direction (the trapezium also has a minor convexity orthogonal to its predominant concavity and the first metacarpal has a minor and marginal concavity orthogonal to its predominant convexity)
- Type of joint: saddle
- Allowed movements: flexion-extension and abduction-adduction of the thumb in addition to circumduction.

Carpometacarpal joints of the 2nd, 3rd, 4th and 5th digits

- Between the distal articular surfaces of the trapezoid, capitate and hamate and the bases of the metacarpal bones from the 2nd to the 5th digit
- Flat articular surfaces
- Type of joint: plane
- Allowed movements: modest sliding of the articular surfaces which, when occurring on different planes, are similar to the movements of modified saddle joints (this is especially true for the carpometacarpal joints of the 4th and 5th digits and is evident in movements such as making a fist and the opposition between the thumb to the little finger).

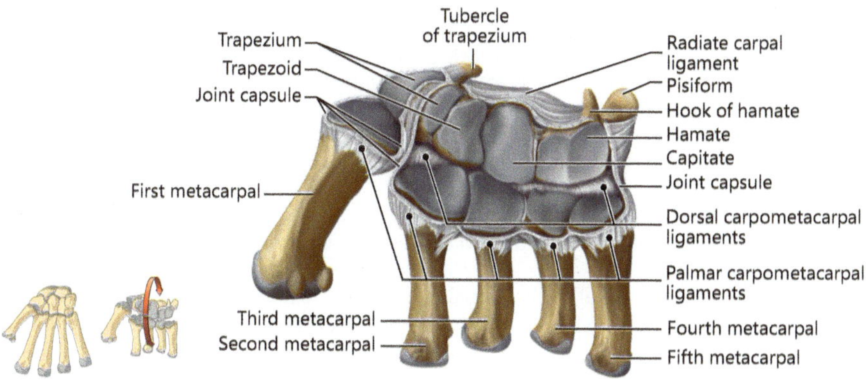

Right carpometacarpal joint. Here we can see the inverted articular surface, formed by the bones of the distal carpal row and the proximal extremities of the metacarpals.

Intermetacarpal joints

- Between the bases of the metacarpals from the 2nd to the 5th digits
- Flat articular surfaces
- Type of joint: plane
- Allowed movements: modest sliding of the articular surfaces.

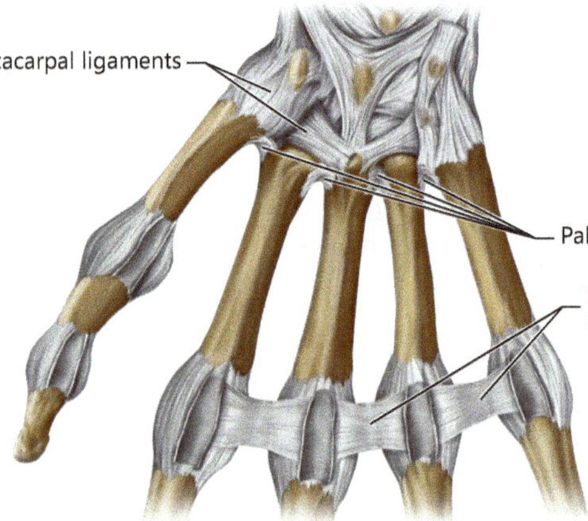

Intermetacarpal joints (palmar or volar view).

Metacarpophalangeal joints

Joints between the heads of the metacarpals and the bases of the proximal phalanges:
- metacarpophalangeal joints of the 2nd, 3rd, 4th and 5th digits
- metacarpophalangeal joint of the thumb.

Metacarpophalangeal joints of the 2nd, 3rd, 4th and 5th digits

- Convex surfaces of the heads of the metacarpals (wider on the palmar side)
- Concave surfaces of the bases of the proximal phalanges (extended anteriorly by the accessory fibrocartilaginous ligaments)
- Type of joint: condylar
- Allowed movements: flexion-extension and abduction-adduction.

Metacarpophalangeal joint of the thumb

- Surface of the head of the first metacarpal less convex compared to the heads of the other metacarpals
- Concave surface of the base of the proximal phalanx of the thumb (extended anteriorly by the accessory fibrocartilaginous ligament, which includes two sesamoid bones located laterally)
- Type of joint: condylar
- Allowed movements: flexion-extension and abduction-adduction, but to a lesser extent compared to other metacarpophalangeal joints.

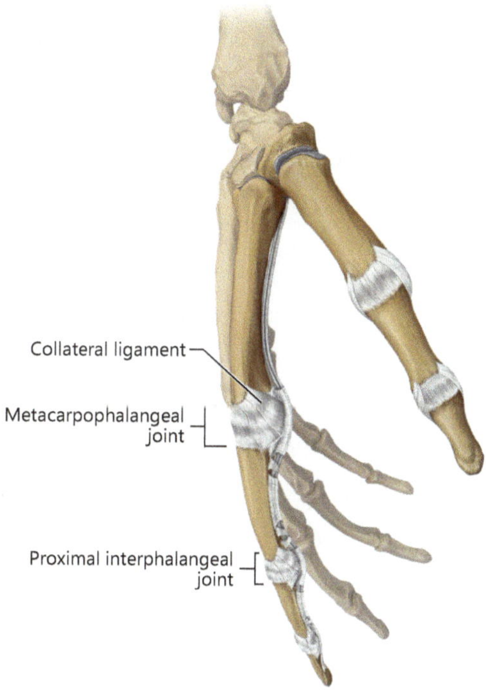

Metacarpophalangeal and interphalangeal joints on the right side, viewed from the radial side.

Interphalangeal joints

- Between the proximal phalanx and the middle phalanx and between the middle phalanx and the distal phalanx of the 2nd, 3rd, 4th and 5th digits
- Between the proximal phalanx and the distal phalanx of the thumb
- Articular surfaces represented by the:
  - heads of the proximal phalanges
  - bases of the middle phalanges (extended by the fibrocartilage)
  - heads of the middle phalanges
  - bases of the distal phalanges (extended by the fibrocartilage)
- The heads have a trochlear shape, more extended on the palmar side, with a medial groove and two lateral protuberances (convex surfaces)
- The bases have a median crest and two lateral depressions (concave surfaces)
- Type of joint: hinge joint
- Allowed movements: flexion-extension of the middle and distal phalanges (one degree of freedom, two allowed movements).

Capsules and ligaments of the joints of the wrist and hand

Joint capsules of the wrist and hand (distal radioulnar, wrist, midcarpal, intercarpal, carpometacarpal and intermetacarpal joints).

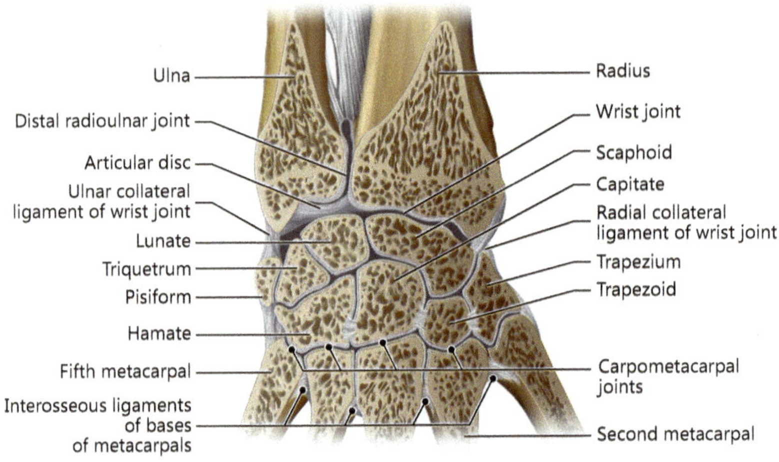

Joint capsules of the hand.

Joint capsules of the digits (metacarpophalangeal and interphalangeal joints).

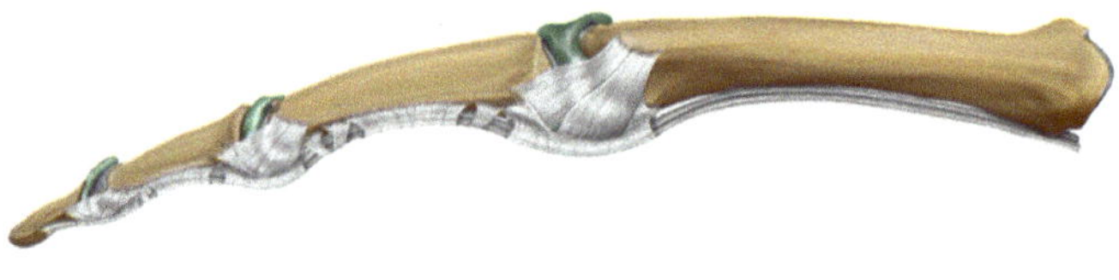

A

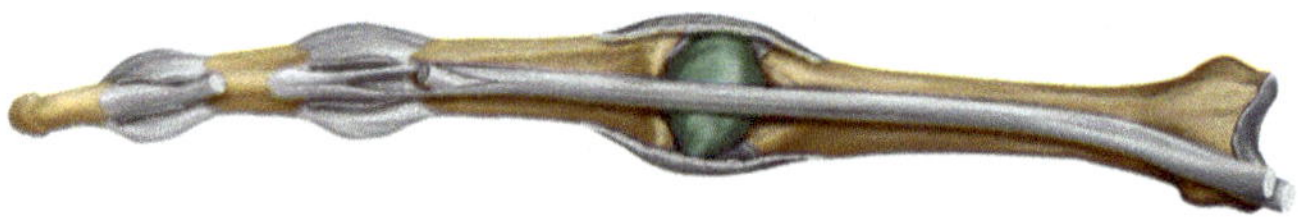

B

Metacarpophalangeal and interphalangeal joints. **A**, Lateral view; **B**, palmar or volar view after removal of the capsule.

Ligaments of the wrist and hand

They control the movements of the hand and can be subdivided into:

- collateral
- dorsal
- palmar (volar)
- interosseous.

The first limit the **abduction-adduction** movements of the hand, the second limit the **flexion** movements (palmar flexion) of the hand, the third limit the **extension** movements (dorsal flexion) of the hand; the interosseous ligaments have a stabilizing function.

Collateral ligaments

- Radial collateral ligament of the wrist joint – between the radial styloid process and the scaphoid and trapezium – restrains the ulnar abduction of the hand
- Ulnar collateral ligament of the wrist joint – between the ulnar styloid process and the triquetrum and pisiform – restrains the radial abduction of the hand.

Dorsal ligaments

- Dorsal radiocarpal – between the radius and the lunate and triquetrum – restrains the palmar flexion of the hand
- Dorsal ligament of the midcarpal joint (arcuate ligament of the wrist):
  - proximal fascicles with transverse course between the triquetrum and scaphoid – stabilize the midcarpal joint
  - distal fascicles with transverse course between the triquetrum, trapezium and trapezoid – stabilize the bones of the distal carpal row
- Dorsal intercarpal – between the bones of the proximal carpal row and the bones of the distal carpal row – stabilize the bones of the distal carpal row
- Dorsal carpometacarpal
- Dorsal of the base of the metacarpals
- Dorsal carpal ligament (extensor retinaculum) – located on the dorsal part of the wrist joint – from the deep surface originate the septa that delimit six osteofibrous canals in which pass, from the outside to the inside, the tendons of the abductor pollicis longus and extensor pollicis brevis, extensor carpi radialis longus and extensor carpi radialis brevis, extensor pollicis longus, extensor digitorum, and extensor indicis, extensor digiti minimi, extensor carpi ulnaris.

9

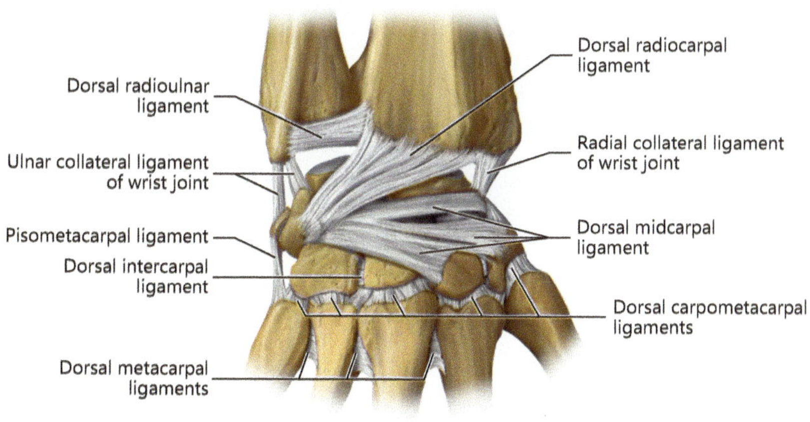

Dorsal ligaments.

The midcarpal joint is characterized by various ligaments, to a lesser degree at the level of the bones of the proximal row and to a greater extent at the level of the bones of the distal row. The latter are firmly connected to each other and to the metacarpals. The bones of the proximal row are therefore relatively mobile, while those of the distal row are rigid and block-bound to the metacarpals.

Palmar (volar) ligaments

- Palmar radiocarpal – between the radial styloid process and the lunate and capitate – restrains the extension (dorsal flexion) of the hand
- Palmar ulnocarpal – between the ulnar styloid process and the capitate – restrains the extension of the hand
- Radiate carpal – between the capitate and hamate, the scaphoid, triquetrum and trapezium
- Palmar intercarpal – between the bones of the proximal carpal row and the bones of the distal carpal row – stabilize the bones of the distal carpal row
- Pisohamate – between the pisiform and hamate
- Palmar carpometacarpal
- Palmar ligaments of the bases of the metacarpals (palmar metacarpal ligaments)
- Palmar carpal – located above the wrist joint.

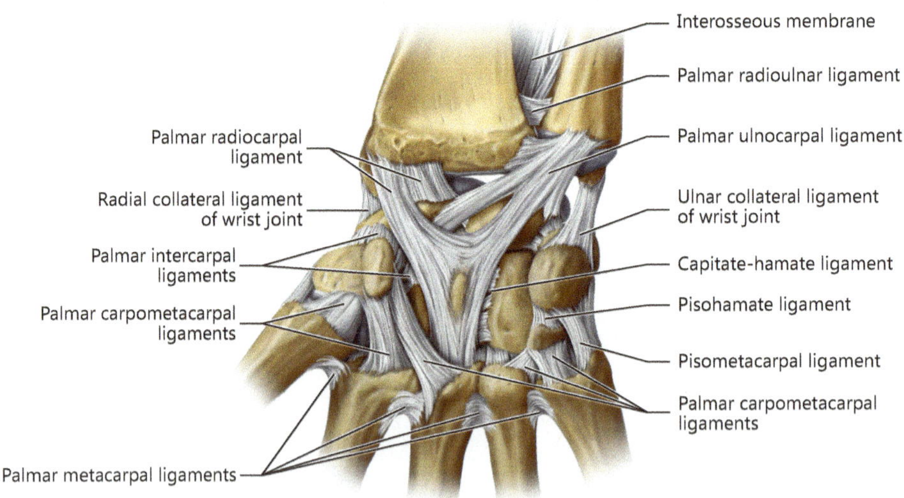

Ligaments of the right carpus, palmar (volar) view.

Flexor retinaculum

Also called transverse carpal ligament, it is made up of two parts:

- proximal – between the scaphoid and pisiform
- distal – between the trapezium and hamate.

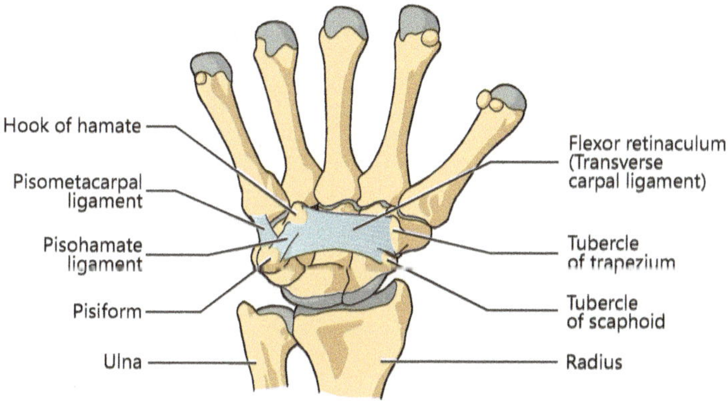

Flexor retinaculum (transverse carpal ligament).

The deep surface, covering the carpal groove, delimits the carpal tunnel and gives rise to a fibrous septum that divides the tunnel into a lateral part, where the tendon of the flexor carpi radialis runs, and a medial part, where the tendons of the flexor digitorum superficialis and flexor digitorum profundus (each with four tendons, and flexor pollicis longus) pass, together with the median nerve.

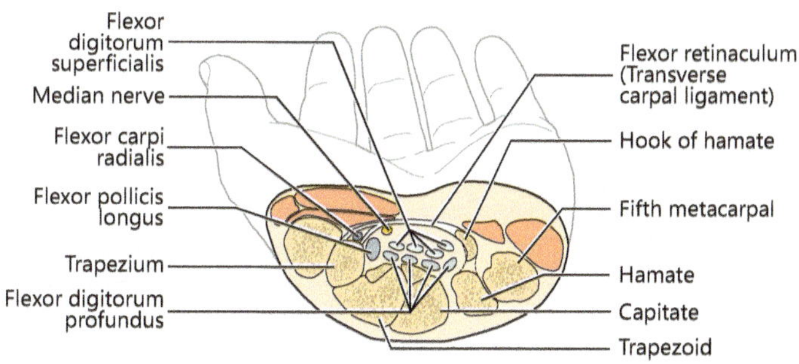

Carpal tunnel (transverse section through the bones of the distal carpal row).

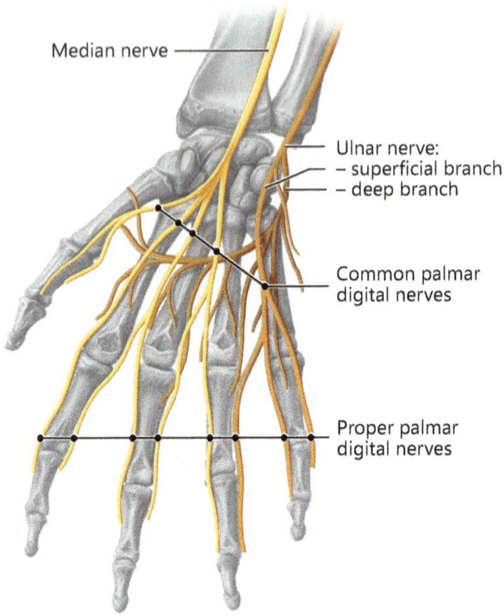

Course of the median nerve.

Carpal tunnel syndrome is characterized by hypoesthesia, or paresthesia, of the region innervated by the median nerve, stiffness of the digits of the hand and weakness of hand grip due to the impossibility of a correct opposition between the thumb and the other digits. This symptomatology is caused by compression of the median nerve due to edema associated with inflammation of the tendons (tenosynovitis) of the flexor muscles, caused by functional overload.

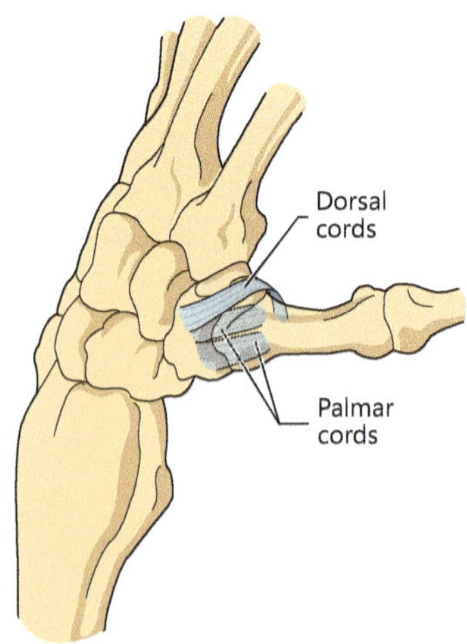

Ligaments of the carpometacarpal joint of the thumb (dorsal view).

Interosseous ligaments

- Carpal
- Metacarpal

Ligaments of the carpometacarpal joint of the thumb

They are in direct contact with the capsule, which is lax and therefore allows the execution of wide movements, and are arranged in such a way that in each position of the thumb at least one of the ligaments are in tension.

Ligaments of the metacarpophalangeal and interphalangeal joints

Metacarpophalangeal joints

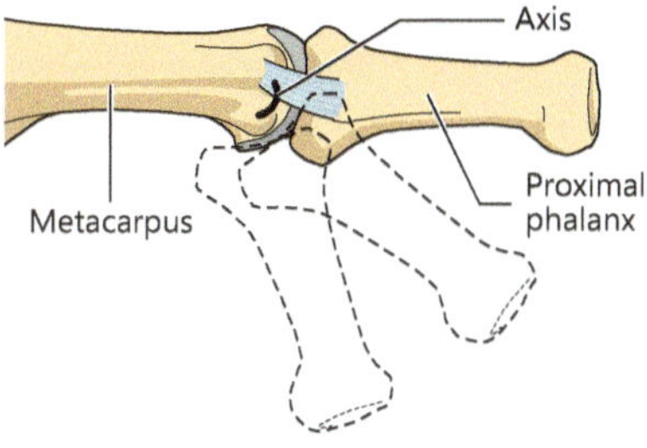

Collateral ligament of the metacarpophalangeal joint (the dashed lines represent the palmar flexion movements).

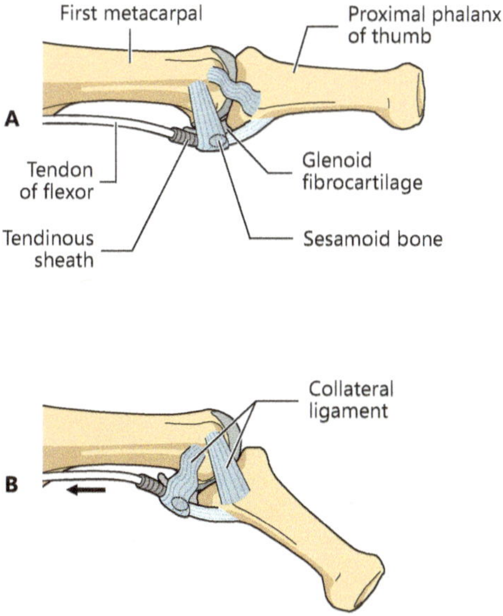

Collateral ligament of the metacarpophalangeal joint of the thumb. **A**, In neutral position; **B**, in flexion.

- Accessory volar ligament (or glenoid fibrocartilage) – anteriorly increases the concave surface of the base of the proximal phalanges
- Palmar ligaments of the metacarpophalangeal joints – reinforce the capsule of the metacarpophalangeal joints
- Collateral ligaments of the metacarpophalangeal joints – originate in the posterior region of the heads of the metacarpals and run laterally, inserting in the base of the proximal phalanges at the palmar level – they are stretched during flexion of the proximal phalanges, limiting their flexion and preventing their abduction
- Transverse ligaments of the metacarpophalangeal joints – they are located in the palmar region between the heads of the metacarpals from the 2nd to the 5th – they stabilize the heads of the metacarpals
- Metacarpoglenoid ligaments of the metacarpophalangeal joint of the thumb – they are fixed to the sesamoid bones incorporated in the accessory volar ligament that anteriorly extends the concave surface of the base of the proximal phalanx of the thumb
- Dorsal ligament of the metacarpophalangeal joint of the thumb – limits the flexion of the proximal phalanx
- Collateral ligaments of the metacarpophalangeal joint of the thumb – the insertion, in addition to the base of the proximal phalanx at the palmar level (radial ligament), is at the level of the accessory volar ligament and the sesamoid bones it contains, following a mainly palmar course (ulnar ligament) – they laterally stabilize the

joint, remaining in tension both during flexion and maximum extension of the proximal phalanx of the thumb and, vice versa, they are relaxed when flexion is slight, thereby allowing lateral and circumduction movements (flexion + abduction) of the proximal phalanx of the thumb.

Interphalangeal joints

- Fibrocartilaginous ligament that anteriorly extends the articular surface of the bases of the middle and distal phalanges – increases the flexion of the middle and distal phalanges (also favored by the larger anterior area of the articular surface of the heads of the proximal and middle phalanges and by the laxity of the capsules of the interphalangeal joints)
- Phalangoglenoid (or anterior) ligament – anterior to the capsule of the interphalangeal joints – limits the extension of the middle and distal phalanges
- Collateral ligaments – they are tensed both during flexion and maximum extension of the middle and distal phalanges, which limit lateral movements (the ulnar collateral ligament of the interphalangeal joint of the thumb is tensed before the radial ligament, as the head of the proximal phalanx of the thumb is wider at the ulnar level, causing an increase in the rotation position of the thumb, whose palmar surface is mostly oriented towards the palm of the hand, improving the grip).

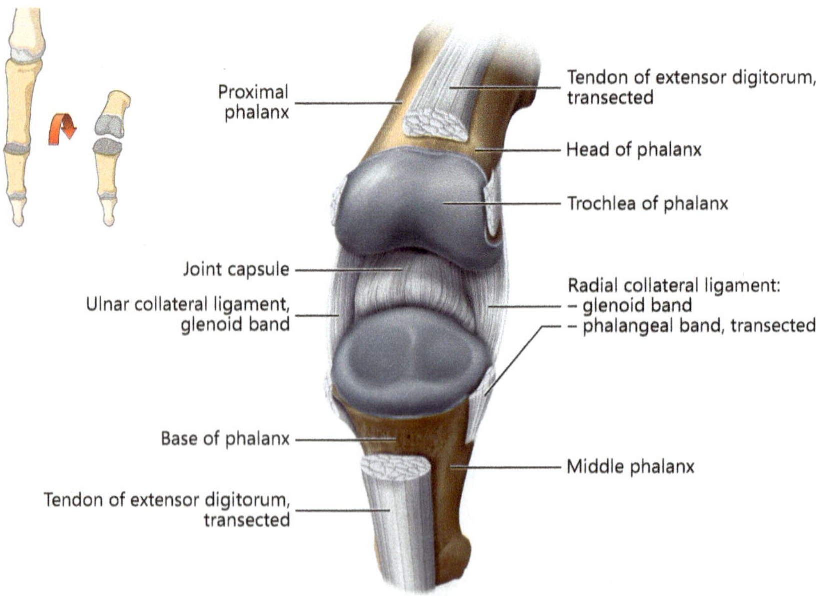

Proximal interphalangeal joint. The trochlea of the proximal phalanx has been turned over to show the base of the middle phalanx.

Subdivision of the joints of the wrist and hand into columns

From a functional perspective, the joints of the wrist and hand can be subdivided into three longitudinal columns:

- lunate column (central)
- scaphoid column (radial)
- triquetrum column (ulnar).

Lunate column

Radius → lunate → capitate → 3rd metacarpal → 3rd digit.

The palmar ligaments between the radius and lunate and between the radius and capitate are tensed during dorsal flexion of the hand, while the dorsal ligaments between the radius and lunate push the lunate towards the radius during palmar flexion.

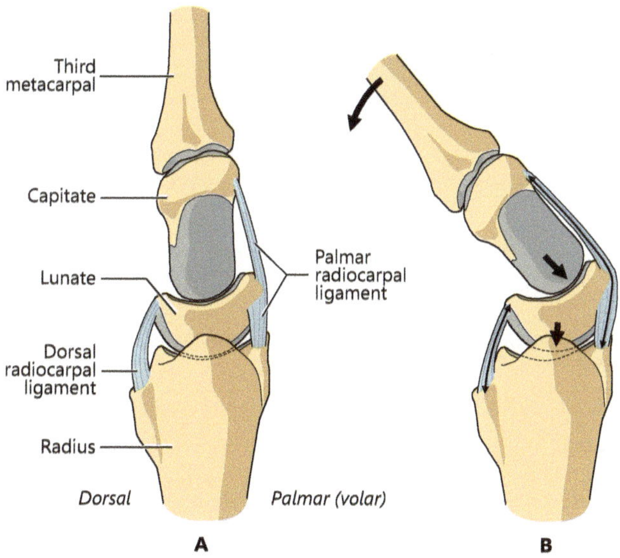

A, Lunate column (left hand, radial view). **B**, Behavior of the ligaments of the lunate column during extension (dorsal extension).

9

Scaphoid column

Radius → scaphoid → trapezium → 1st and 2nd metacarpals → 1st and 2nd digits.

The palmar ligaments between the radius and scaphoid and between the scaphoid and trapezium are tensed during the dorsal flexion of the hand, preventing any movement of the scaphoid, fixed between the trapezium and radius, while the dorsal ligaments between the scaphoid and radius are relaxed.

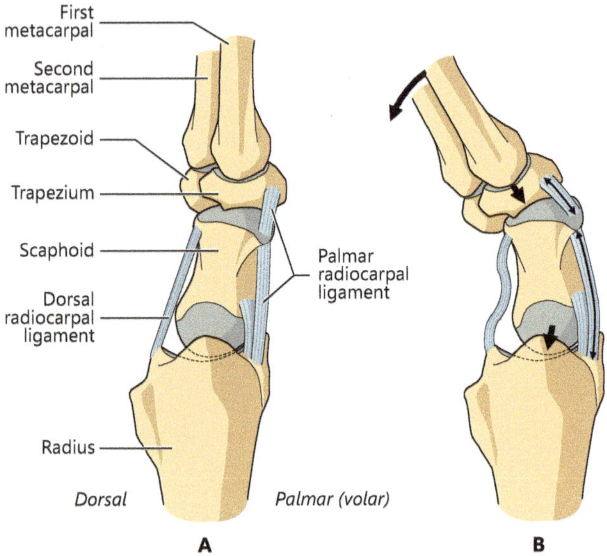

A, Scaphoid column (left hand, radial view). **B**, Behavior of the ligaments of the scaphoid column during extension (dorsal extension).

Triquetrum column

Ulna → triangular disc → triquetrum → hamate → 4th and 5th metacarpals → 4th and 5th digits.

The palmar ligaments between the radius and triquetrum and between pisiform and hamate are tensed during dorsal flexion of the hand, as well as the dorsal ligaments between the hamate and triquetrum, while the dorsal ligaments between the radius and triquetrum and the ulna and triquetrum are relaxed.

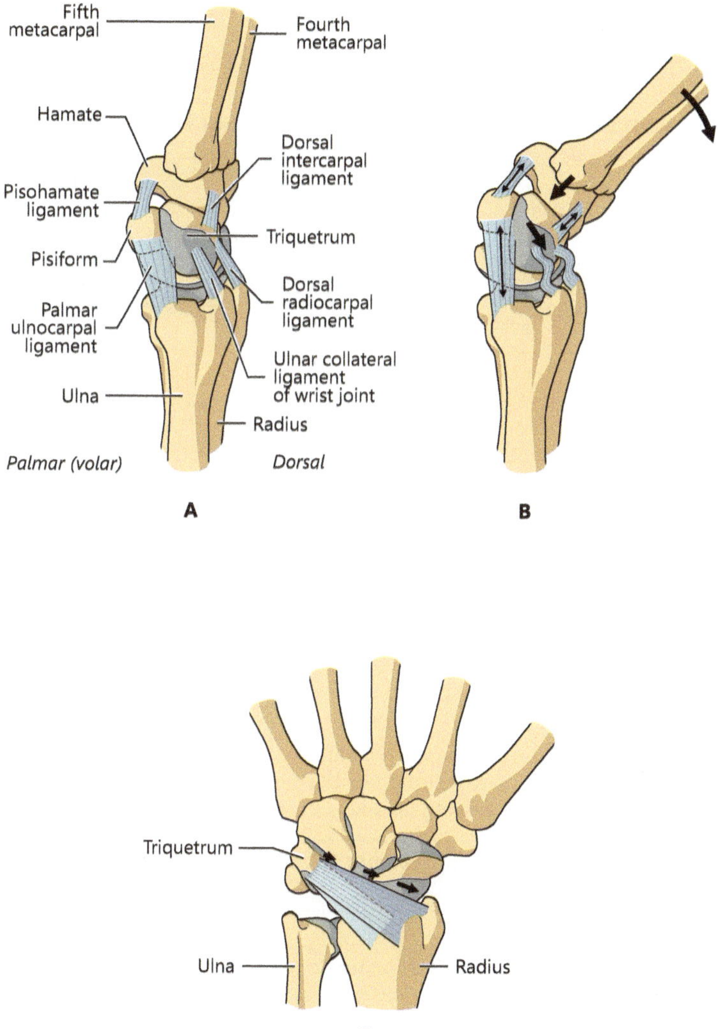

A, Triquetrum column (left hand, ulnar view). **B**, Behavior of the ligaments of the triquetrum column during extension (dorsal extension). **C**, Traction exerted on the triquetrum (dorsal view).

Movements of the wrist

The wrist and midcarpal joints, although anatomically different, form a functional unit.

Flexion (palmar flexion) and extension (dorsal flexion) of the wrist

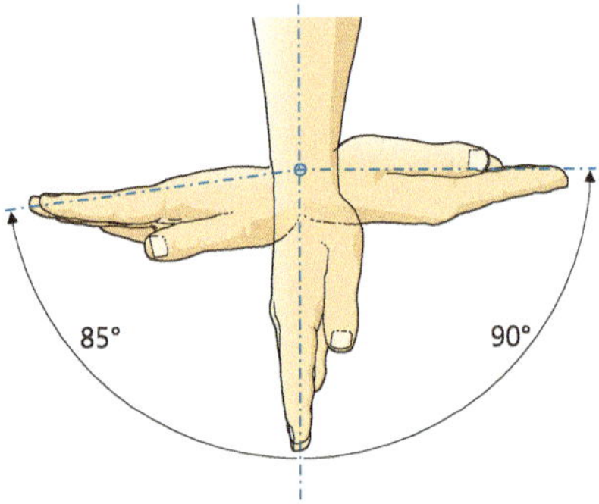

Dorsal flexion and palmar flexion of the wrist.

Amplitude:
- 85-90° → palmar flexion (50° – wrist joint; 35-40° – midcarpal joint)
- 85° → dorsal flexion (35° – wrist joint; 50° – midcarpal joint).

Maximum amplitude of the flexion movement:
- palmar, can be obtained by extending the digits of the hand
- dorsal, can be obtained by flexing the digits of the hand.

> Activities of daily living in general require 40° of amplitude in dorsal flexion and 30° in palmar flexion.

Rotation axis around which the flexion-extension movements occur:
- line joining the radial and ulnar styloid processes.

Radial abduction (true abduction) and ulnar abduction (adduction) of the wrist

Amplitude:

- 15° → radial abduction
- 45° → ulnar abduction

In total: 60° of abduction (37° – wrist joint; 23° – midcarpal joint; the latter is the sum of 15° of ulnar abduction and 8° of radial abduction).

The lower amplitude of radial abduction is due to blockade of the scaphoid under the radial styloid process, which has a greater distal protrusion with respect to the ulnar styloid process. The lower distal protrusion of the ulna and the characteristics of the shape and position of the pisiform and triquetrum, which are more distant from the ulnar styloid process, make the ulnar abduction wider.

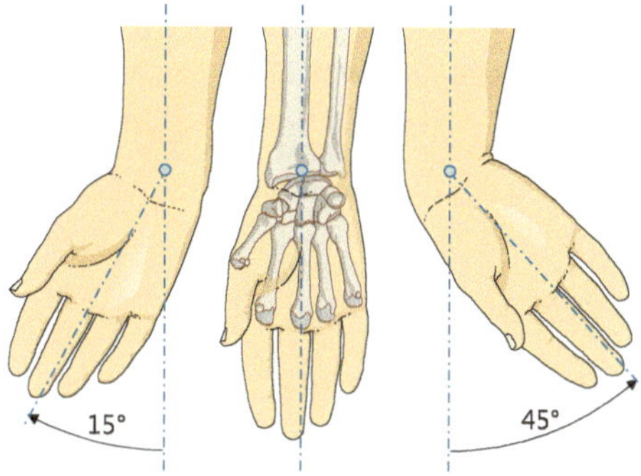

Radial abduction and ulnar abduction of the wrist.

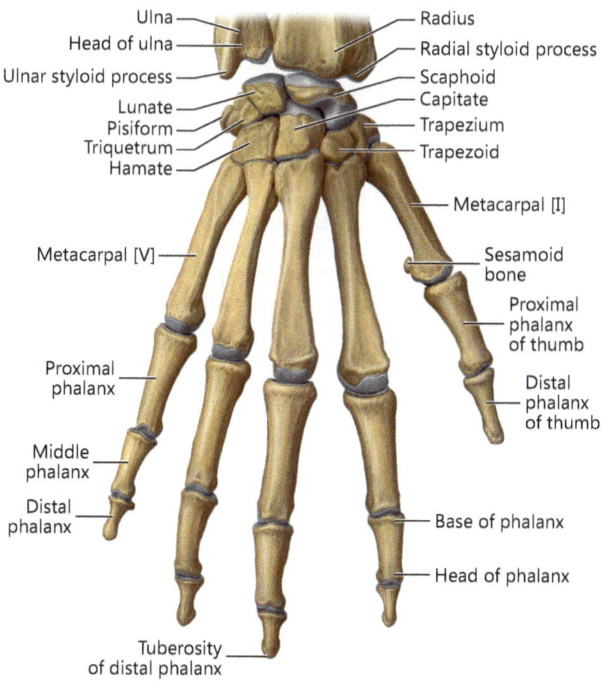

Dorsal surface of the skeleton of the right hand. A sesamoid bone is observed in the metacarpophalangeal joint of the thumb.

> Activities of daily living in general require 10° of amplitude in radial abduction and 20-40° in ulnar abduction.

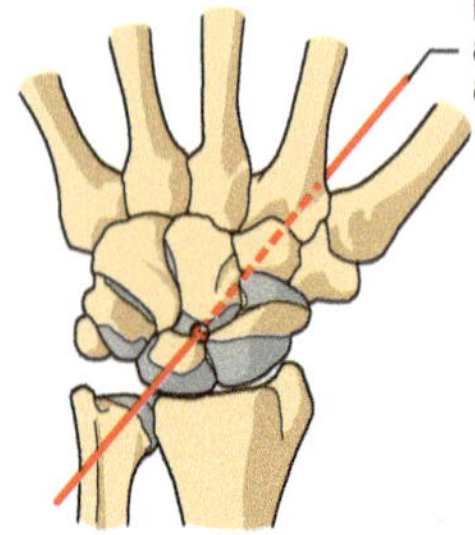

Rotation axis around which the abduction movements occur:
- sagittal line which passes from the most distal point of the axis of the forearm through the capitate and lunate.

Movements of the digits

Movements of the thumb

The following joints primarily contribute to the movements of the thumb:
- carpometacarpal (or trapeziometacarpal) of the thumb
- metacarpophalangeal of the thumb
- interphalangeal of the thumb.

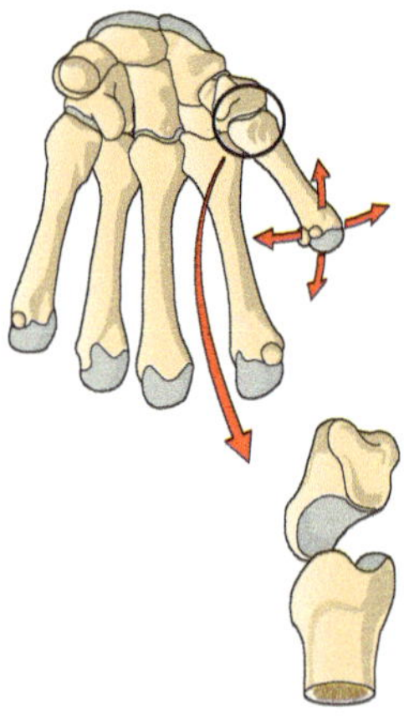

Saddle joints of the thumb.

Movements of the carpometacarpal joint of the thumb

Axes of rotation

The axes of rotation are oblique and the flexion-extension and abduction-adduction movements do not occur exactly in the sagittal and frontal planes. The flexion-extension movements occur on a frontal oblique plane around an oblique sagittal rotation axis. The abduction-adduction movements occur on a sagittal oblique plane around a frontal oblique rotation axis. The center of the flexion-extension axis passes through the trapezium, while the center of the abduction-adduction axis passes through the base of the first metacarpal. From a kinematic perspective, flexion-extension movements resemble abduction-adduction movements and, vice versa, abduction-adduction movements resemble flexion-extension movements.

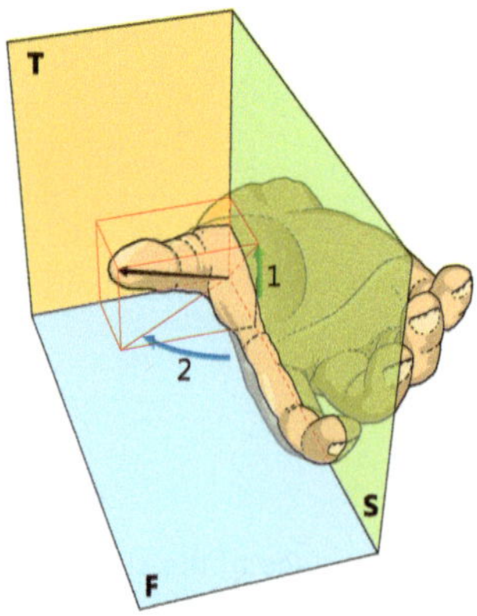

Assessment

The first metacarpal moves around a rectangular reference triad made up of the transverse (**T**), frontal (**F**) and sagittal (**S**) planes. From a reference position in which the first metacarpal is in contact with the second metacarpal (approximately in the **F** plane), the flexion is the forward movement of the first metacarpal (arrow 1) and the extension is the reverse movement, while the abduction moves away the first metacarpal from the second metacarpal (arrow 2) and the adduction is the reverse movement.

Carpometacarpal flexion-extension of the thumb

Flexion

• Reference position	Anatomical position with the thumb in contact with the 2nd metacarpal and the proximal phalanx of the 2nd digit
• Rotation axis	Oblique sagittal, with an angle of 15° in relation to the non-oblique sagittal axis, and orthogonal in relation to the abduction-adduction axis
• Movement	Forward, upward and inward (with rotation of the metacarpus around its own axis)
• Amplitude	15°

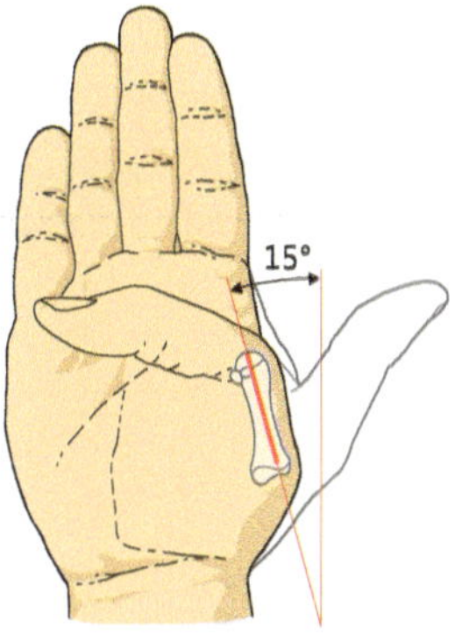

Carpometacarpal flexion of the thumb (palmar view of the hand).

Extension

• Movement	Backward, upward and outward
• Amplitude	40°

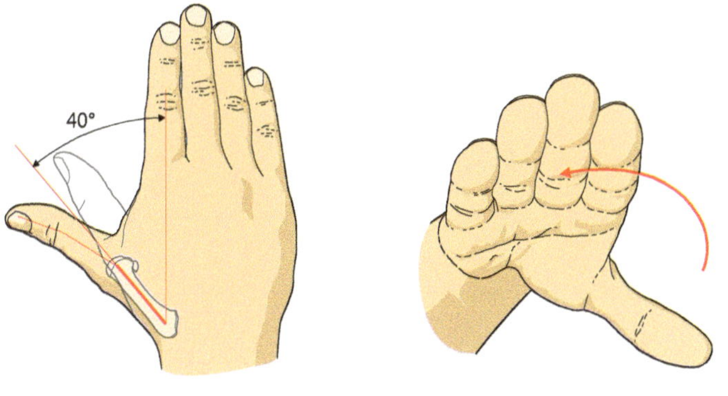

On the left, carpometacarpal extension of the thumb (dorsal view of the hand). On the right, carpometacarpal extension of the thumb (frontal view of the hand). The arrow indicates the direction of flexion.

Carpometacarpal abduction-adduction of the thumb

Abduction

- Reference position — The same as with flexion-extension movements
- Rotation axis — Oblique frontal, with an angle of around 30° in relation to the non-oblique frontal axis, and orthogonal in relation to the flexion-extension axis
- Movement — Forward, upward and inward
- Amplitude — 40-50° (70° passively)

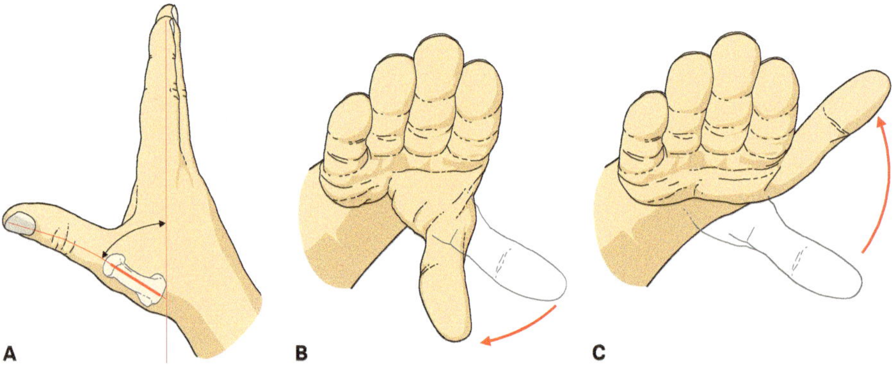

A, Carpometacarpal abduction of the thumb (right hand seen from the side of the thumb). **B**, The downward arrow indicates the carpometacarpal abduction of the thumb (frontal view of the hand). **C**, The upward arrow indicates the carpometacarpal adduction, or rather, hyperadduction of the thumb (frontal view of the hand).

Adduction

- Movement — Return to the reference position from abduction

Hyperadduction

- Movement — Adduction from the reference position
- Amplitude — 20°-30°

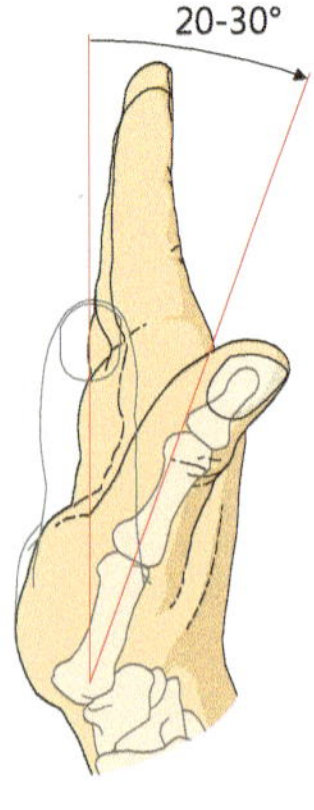

Hyperadduction of the carpometacarpal joint of the thumb (left hand seen from the side of the thumb).

The carpometacarpal circumduction movement of the thumb, derived from a combination of abduction-extension and adduction-flexion movements, allows for the opposition and retroposition movements of the thumb to the other finger (contact between the thumb and the other digits of the hand), as is characteristic of the human hand.

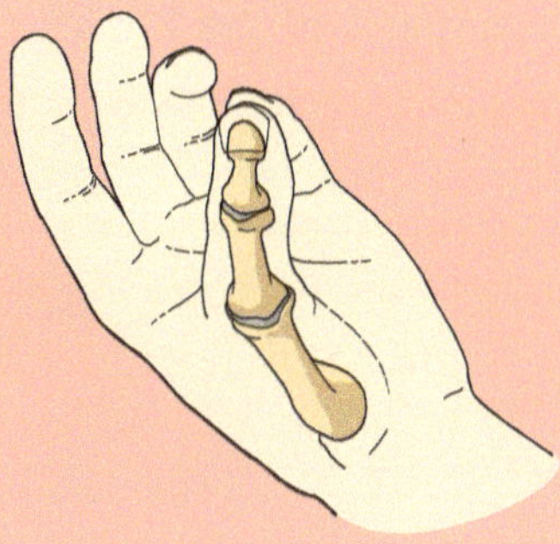

Movements of the metacarpophalangeal joint of the thumb

Metacarpophalangeal flexion-extension of the thumb

Flexion

- Amplitude 45°-60°

Extension

- Amplitude 0°

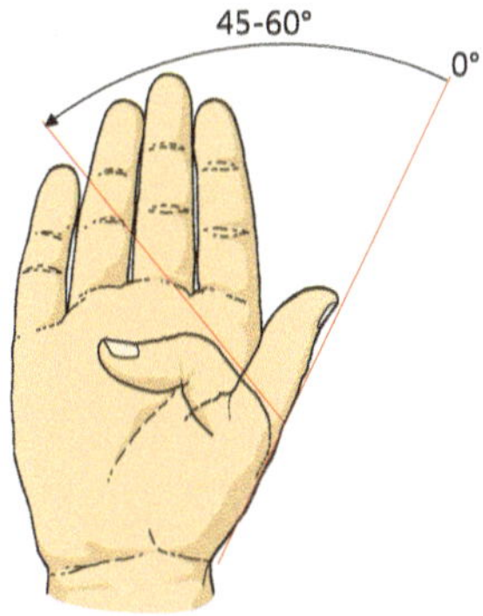

Flexion and extension of the proximal metacarpophalangeal joint.

Metacarpophalangeal abduction-adduction of the thumb

- Amplitude Almost nothing

The opposition movements of the thumb to the other digits (allowed by the carpometacarpal joint of the thumb) are based, at the level of the metacarpophalangeal joint of the thumb, on the internal and external rotation (active or passive) of the proximal phalanx with respect to the first metacarpal (axial rotation), which occurs by opposing the pulp of the thumb to the distal phalanx of the ring finger and leveraging on this.

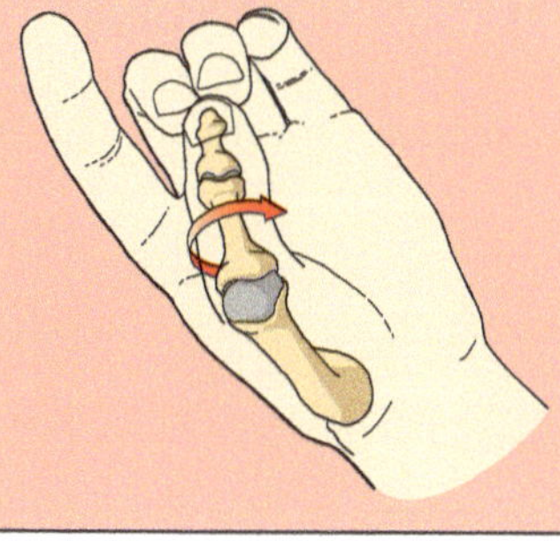

Movements of the 2nd, 3rd, 4th and 5th digits

Metacarpophalangeal flexion-extension of the 2nd, 3rd, 4th and 5th digits

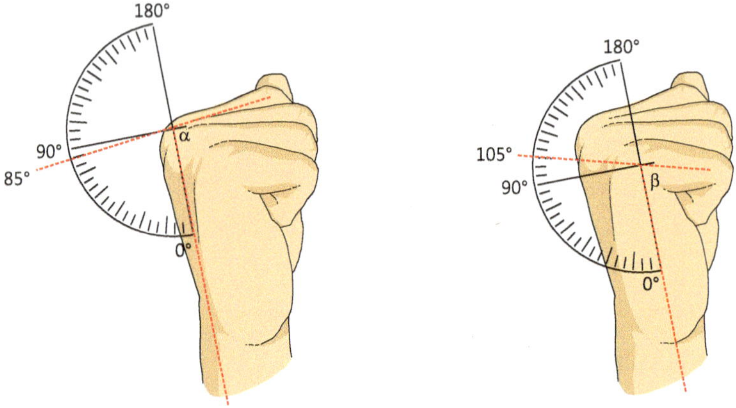

Closing the hand to make a fist, a significant difference can be observed between the angular amplitude of the metacarpophalangeal joint of the index finger (0-85°) and that of the little finger (0-105°).

Flexion

- Movement — Nearing of the proximal phalanx to the palm of the hand
- Amplitude — 90° (increases from the 2nd to the 5th digit)

Extension

- Movement — Return to the starting position

Hyperextension

- Active – about 20-30°
- Passive – up to 90° (in some subjects)

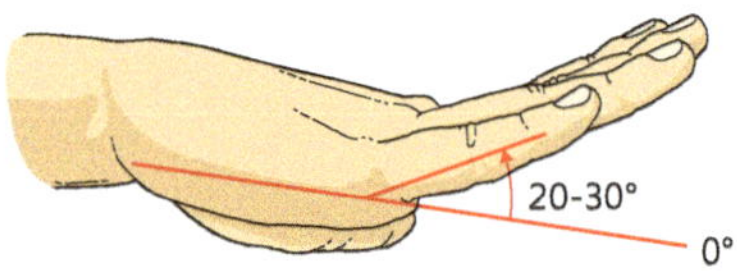

Active hyperextension of the proximal metacarpophalangeal joint.

Metacarpophalangeal abduction-adduction of the 2nd, 3rd, 4th and 5th digits

Abduction

- Movement — Separation of the 2nd, 4th and 5th digits from the 3rd digit (the 3rd digit refers to radial or ulnar abduction)
- Amplitude — 20-30° (maximum for the 3rd digit)

Adduction

- Movement — Return to starting position

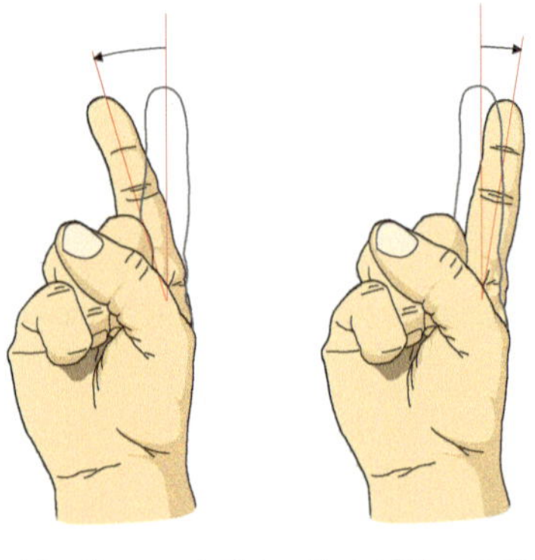

Adduction and abduction of the metacarpophalangeal joint of the 2nd digit.

The abduction and adduction movements are limited or non-existent if the proximal phalanges of the 2nd, 3rd, 4th and 5th digits are flexed.

Metacarpophalangeal axial rotation of the 2nd, 3rd, 4th and 5th digits

- Passive (up to 50-60°)

The passive external axial rotation of the 2nd digit is almost non-existent, unlike the internal rotation which is, on the contrary, quite wide (45°).

Movements of the interphalangeal joints of the 1st, 2nd, 3rd, 4th and 5th digits

Flexion-extension of the interphalangeal joints of the 1st, 2nd, 3rd, 4th and 5th digits

Flexion

- Amplitude > 90° (middle phalanx)
  60-70° (distal phalanx)
  Increases from the 2nd to the 5th digit
  Thumb → about 90° (active flexion)

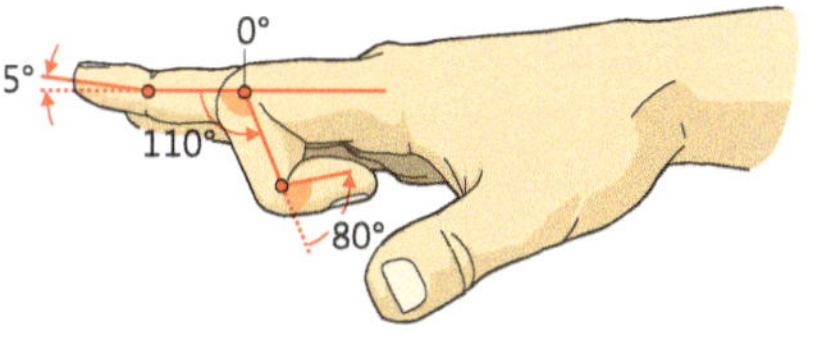

Axis of the interphalangeal joints.

Extension

- Amplitude Almost nothing, since the movement is represented by the return to the starting position and hyperextension is prevented by the accessory volar ligament

  Distal phalanx → passive extension and modest active hyperextension
  Thumb → passive hyperextension of 30° and active hyperextension of about 5-10°.

When the digits are flexed, the axis joining the bases of the middle or distal phalanges (from the 2nd to the 5th digit) have a downward, oblique and medial orientation. The axis joining the bases of the proximal phalanges (from the 3rd to the 5th digits) has the same orientation as well. However, if you look at the tips of the 5th, 4th and 3rd digits (when in a position of flexion), you can see how they are oriented laterally downward, in the direction of the scaphoid. This arrangement of the digits of the hand is of vital importance for the opposing movement of the thumb to the other fingers.

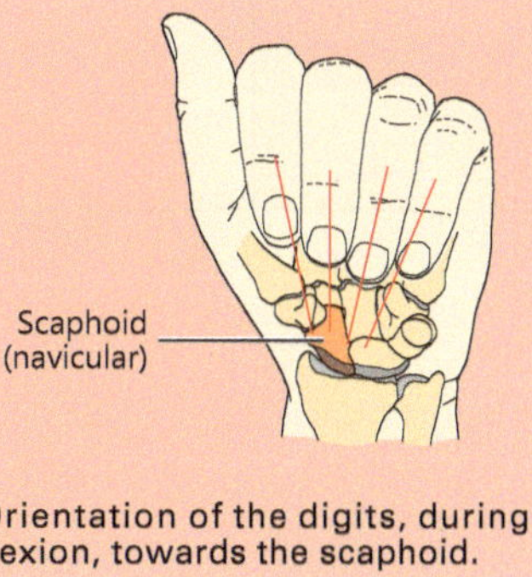

Orientation of the digits, during flexion, towards the scaphoid.

Assessment of the wrist and hand joint mobility

Flexion-extension of the wrist

Starting position	Seated position with the forearm prone and resting on the examination table and the hand off the edge of the examination table
Movement	The examiner flexes and then extends the hand up to the limit of movement allowed. The movements are approximately 80-85° for dorsal flexion and 85-90° for palmar flexion

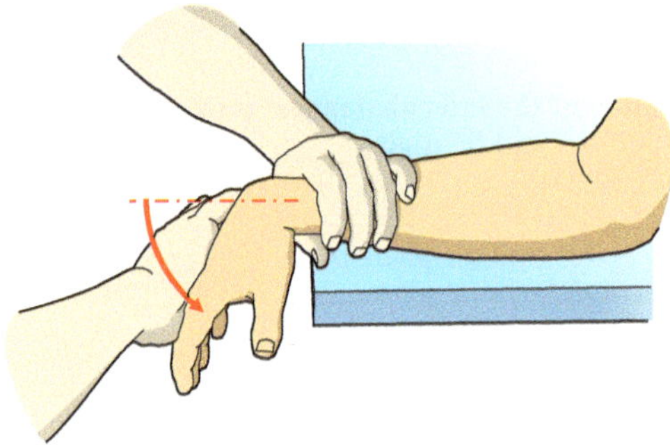

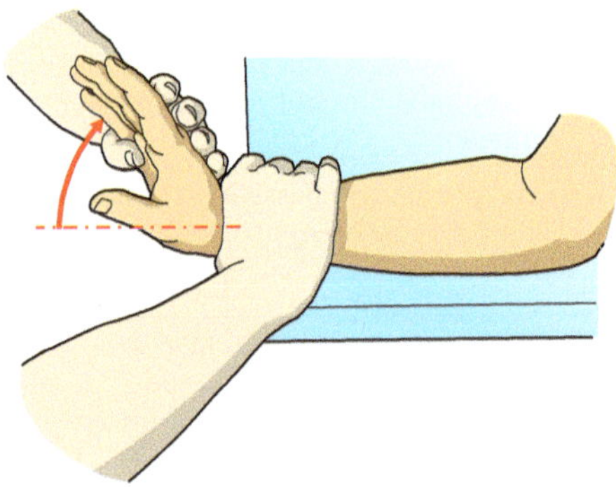

Radial abduction and ulnar abduction of the wrist

Starting position	Seated position with the forearm prone and resting on the examination table and the hand off the edge of the examination table
Movement	After holding the metacarpus by the radial part, the examiner moves the hand in the ulnar direction up to the limit of movement allowed (45-50°); after holding the metacarpus by the ulnar part, the examiner moves the hand in the radial direction up to the limit of movement allowed (15-20°) 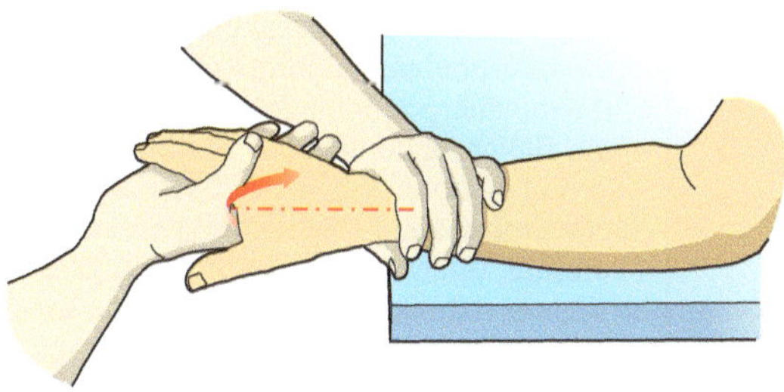 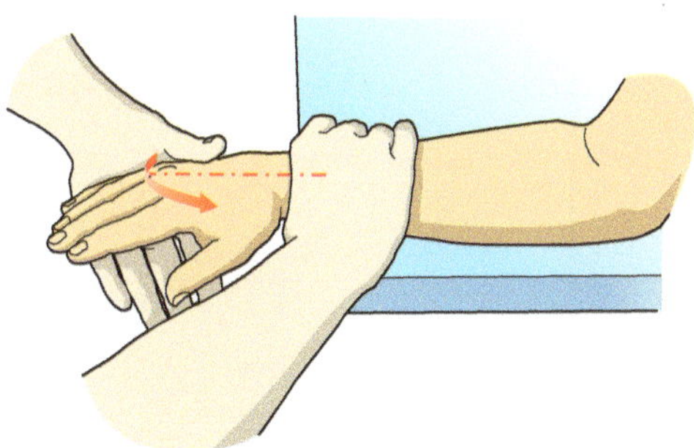

Metacarpophalangeal flexion-extension of the 2nd, 3rd, 4th and 5th digits

Starting position	Seated position with the forearm resting on the examination table in an intermediate position between pronation and supination
Movement	The examiner holds the proximal phalanx of each of the last four digits by flexing and then extending to the limit of movement allowed, which is 90° and 45°, respectively. Each digit is flexed towards the palm of the hand, with a progressively increasing range of motion from the 2nd to the 4th digit (allowing the extension of the interphalangeal joints so that the flexion movement of the metacarpophalangeal joints is not limited by the tension of the extensor tendons of the 3rd digit), then extended in the dorsal direction (allowing the flexion of the interphalangeal joints so that the extension movement of the metacarpophalangeal joints is not limited by the tension of the flexor tendons of the 3rd digit). It should be noted that the active flexion of the proximal phalanx (metacarpophalangeal flexion) exceeds 90° in many subjects. Therefore, under normal conditions, passive flexion should always be greater than 90° in the 2nd digit and greater than 100° in the 4th and 5th digits. However, extension is often less than 45°, especially if the interphalangeal joints are not previously stabilized in flexion. 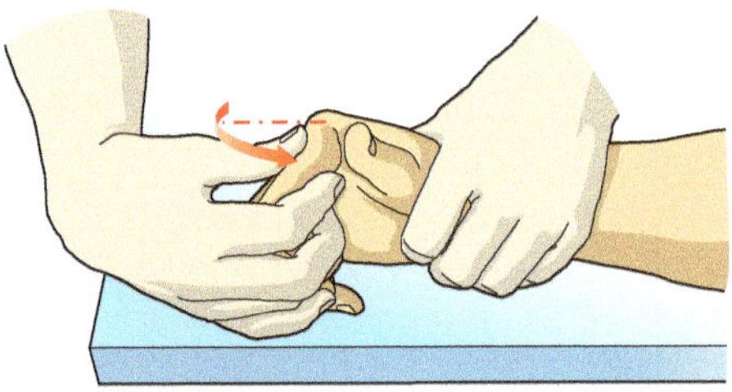 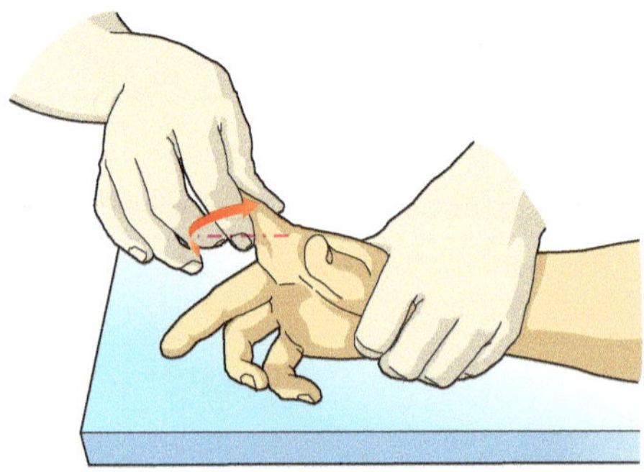

Metacarpophalangeal abduction-adduction of the 2nd, 3rd, 4th and 5th digits

Starting position	Seated position with the forearm prone and resting on the examination table with the fingers in anatomical position
Movement	After holding both sides of the proximal phalanx of each digit, the examiner moves it laterally, moving the digit away from the midline of the hand, up to the limit of abduction, and then medially, moving the digit closer to the midline of the hand, up to the limit of adduction 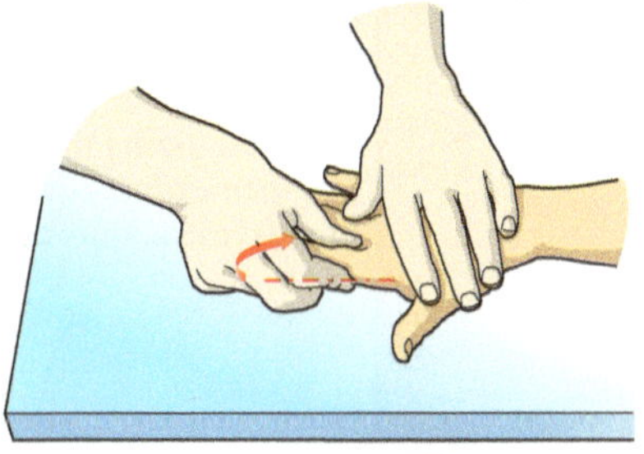 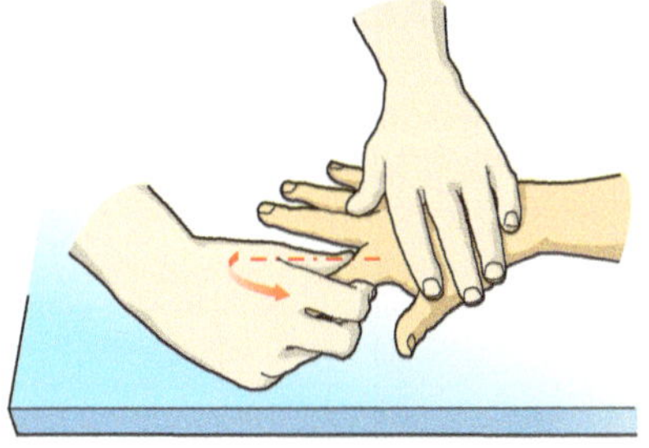

An alternative procedure consists of measuring the full opening of the hand, including the interdigital space of the thumb, measuring the abduction of the digits and the extension of the thumb in centimeters. A sheet of paper is placed under the hand of the patient after stabilizing the wrist and the metacarpals. The patient opens the fingers and the examiner traces the outline of the hand. The hand of the patient is lifted and a ruler used to measure the distance between the tips of the fingers, including the distance between the index finger and thumb.

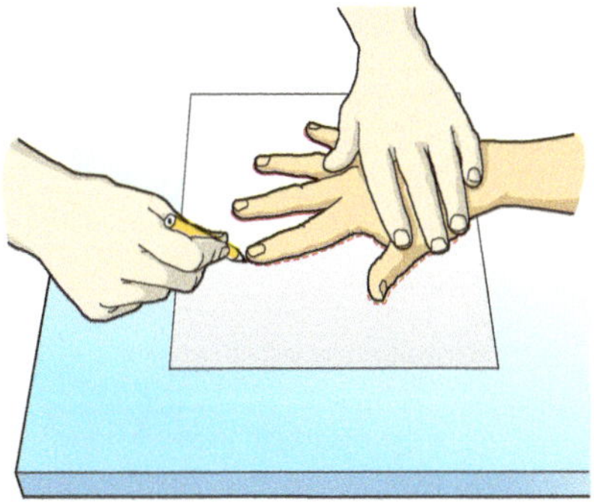

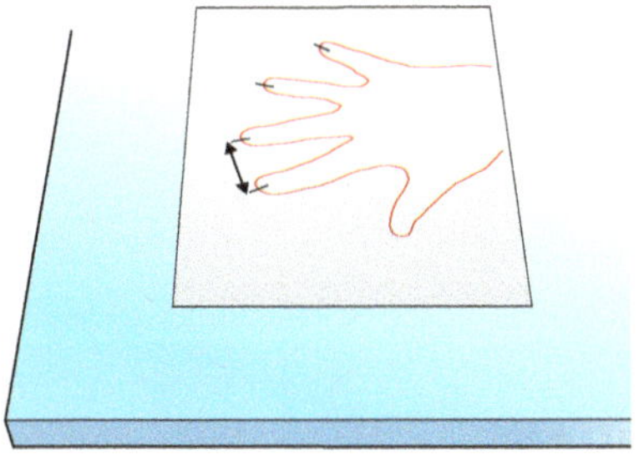

Interphalangeal flexion-extension of the 2nd, 3rd, 4th and 5th digits

Starting position	Seated position, with the forearm and fingers in a neutral position, resting on the examination table
Movement	After stabilizing the proximal phalanx, the examiner flexes and then extends the middle phalanx of each digit to the limit of movement allowed (100° or more and 0°, respectively); after stabilizing the middle phalanx, the examiner flexes and then extends the distal phalanx of each digit to the limit of movement allowed (70° and 0° or more, respectively) 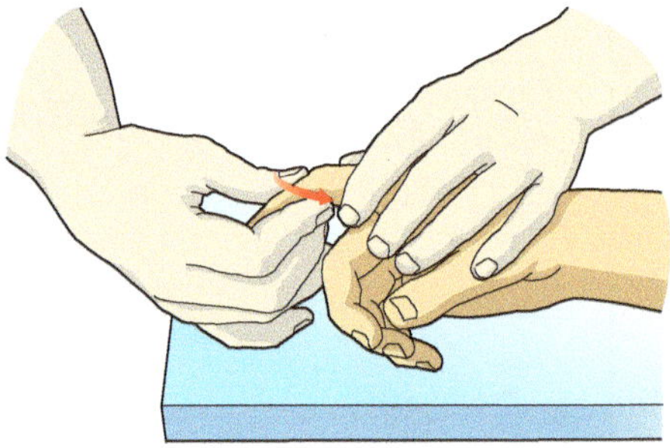 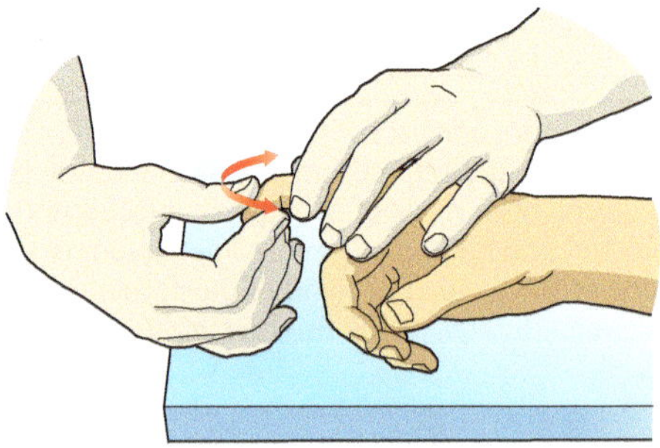

(Active) metacarpophalangeal and interphalangeal flexion of the 2nd, 3rd, 4th and 5th digits

When assessing a functional deficit of the hand (especially when gripping), it is necessary to make a linear measurement of the flexion of the fingers.

Starting position	Seated position with the forearm supine and resting on the examination table
Movement	Active flexion by the patient of the interphalangeal joints, maintaining the metacarpophalangeal joints extended. The examiner measures with a ruler the distance between the fingertip of the 3rd digit and the distal palmar crease. 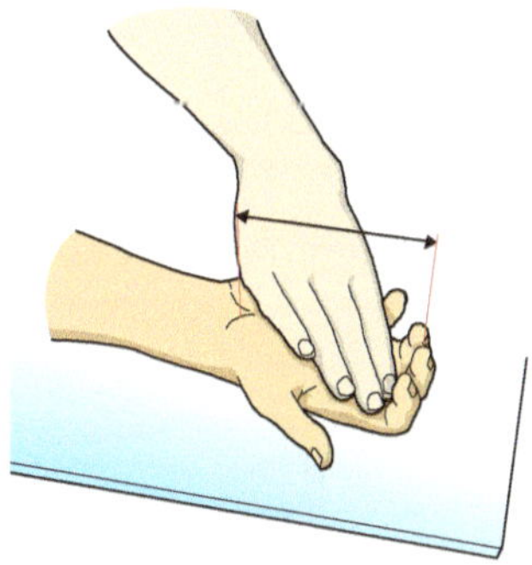 Active flexion by the patient of the metacarpophalangeal and interphalangeal joints. The examiner measures with a ruler the distance between the fingertip and the distal palmar crease 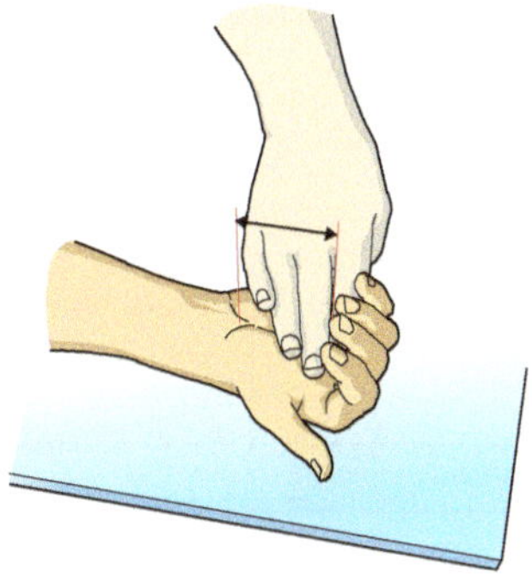

Carpometacarpal flexion-extension of the thumb (between the trapezium and the first metacarpal)

Starting position	Seated position with the forearm resting on the examination table in an intermediate position between pronation and supination and the fingers in anatomical position (thumb in contact with the second metacarpal and the proximal phalanx of the index finger)
Movement	After holding the first metacarpal, the examiner moves it in the ulnar direction, across the palm of the hand, up to the limit of movement allowed (15°) and then in the radial direction, away from the palm of the hand, up to the limit of movement allowed (40°) 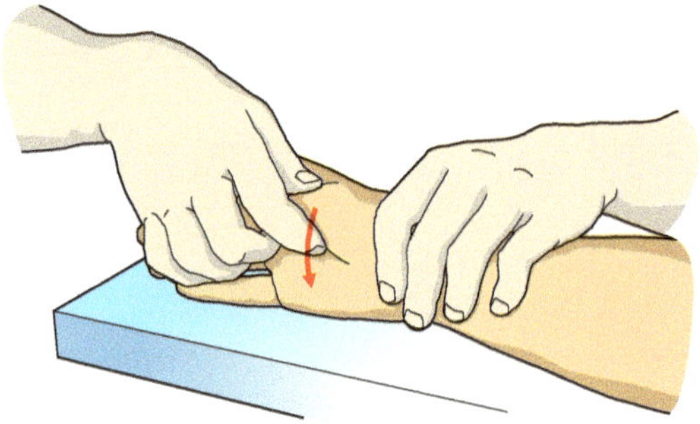 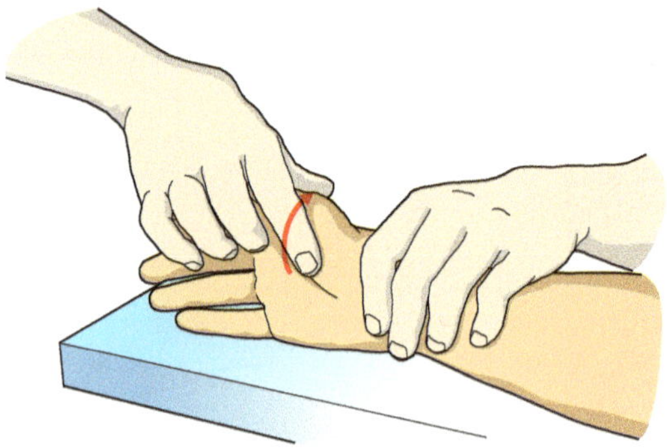

Metacarpophalangeal and interphalangeal flexion-extension of the thumb

Starting position	Seated position with the forearm resting on the examination table in an intermediate position between pronation and supination and the thumb extended
Movement	After stabilizing the first metacarpal, the examiner moves the proximal phalanx of the thumb in the ulnar direction over the palm of the hand up to the limit of movement allowed (45-60°) and then in the radial direction, back to the starting position. 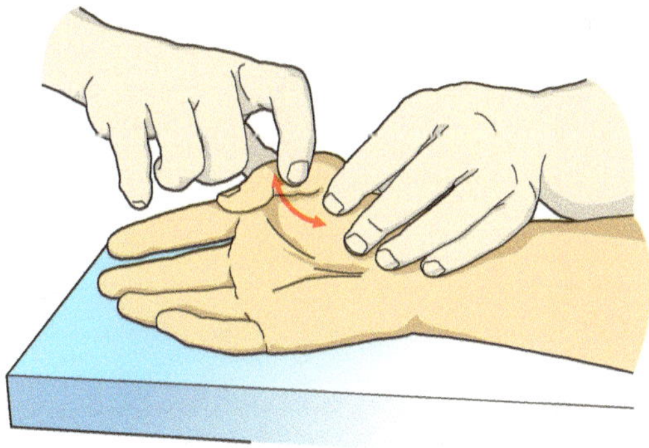 After stabilizing the proximal phalanx of the thumb, the examiner moves the distal phalanx in the ulnar direction over the palm of the hand up to the limit of movement allowed (80-90°) and then in the radial direction, back to the starting position (beyond 0° of extension there is an active hyperextension of 5°-10° and a passive hyperextension of 30°) 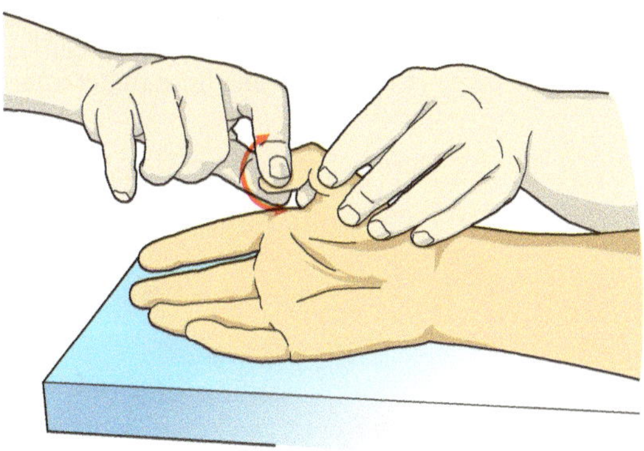

Carpometacarpal abduction and adduction of the thumb

Starting position	Seated position with the forearm resting on the examination table in an intermediate position between pronation and supination and the fingers in anatomical position (thumb in contact with the second metacarpal and the proximal phalanx of the 2nd digit)
Movement	After stabilizing the second metacarpal, the examiner moves the first metacarpal away from the second metacarpal in a direction perpendicular to the plane of the palm of the hand up to the limit of movement allowed (70° passively and 40-45° actively). Abduction is performed between 20 and 30° 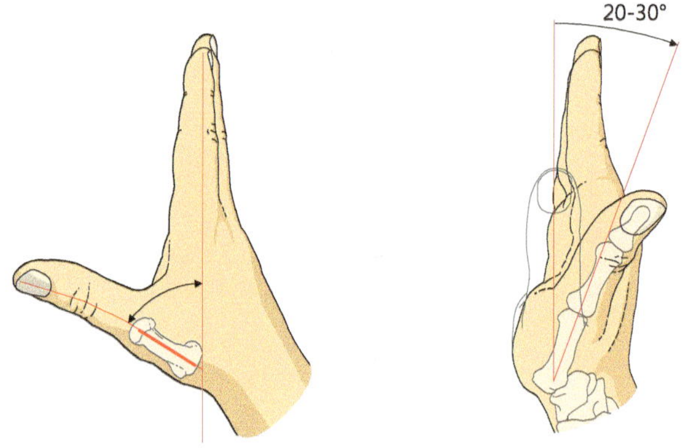

Opposition of the thumb

When the opposition movement of the thumb to the little finger is performed in its full amplitude, contact between the pulps of the two fingers is usually possible. The assessment of a deficit of the opposition movement of the thumb can be obtained by measuring the distance between the pulps of the thumb and little finger after their maximum approach.

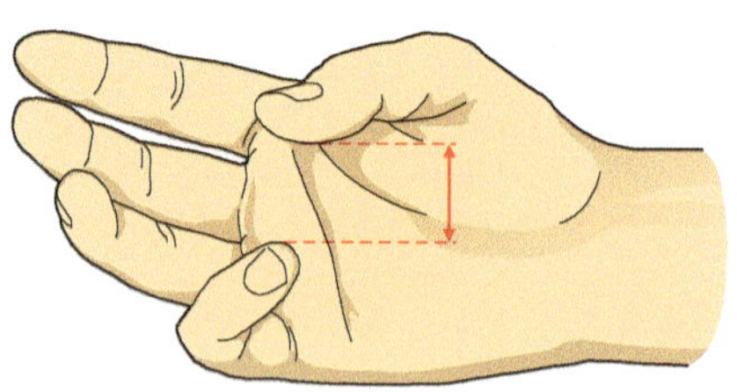

Functional aspects of the joints of the wrist and hand

Functions of the wrist:
- optimizes the function of the hand for touching, grasping and manipulating objects, positioning it in the space in relation to the forearm
- controls the length-tension relationship of the extrinsic muscles of the hand both through its own movements and in static position.

In terms of activities of daily living, the most important movements of the wrist are represented by:
- extension of the wrist and hand
- ulnar abduction of the wrist and hand.

Activities of daily living and movements of the wrist

Authors	Number of daily activities evaluated	Amplitude of wrist movements
Brumfield and Champoux	15	10° flexion 35° extension
Ryu et al.	31	54° flexion 60° extension 17° radial abduction 40° ulnar abduction
Palmer et al.	52	5° flexion 30° extension 10° radial abduction 15° ulnar abduction

Activities of daily living related to eating (for example, drinking from a glass, using a fork, spoon or knife)

Wrist joint range variations range from 3° of flexion to 35° of extension and from 20° of ulnar abduction to 5° of radial abduction.

125 activities of daily living were evaluated (not including work or leisure activities). These activities were performed with wrist joint mobility reduced to 5° of flexion, 6° of extension, 7° of radial abduction and 6° of ulnar abduction. It was found that 123 activities could be completed and observed how even a marked loss of wrist joint mobility could allow most activities of daily living to be fully performed.

Functions of the hand:
- grasping and manipulating objects (prehension function) (see section "Prehension and grip functions", page 432)
- receiving information from the surrounding environment.

Activities of daily living and amplitude of the flexion movements of the digits

Flexion	Amplitude
Metacarpophalangeal of the thumb	10°-32°
Metacarpophalangeal of the 2nd, 3rd, 4th and 5th digits	33°-73°
Proximal interphalangeal of the thumb	2°-43°
Proximal interphalangeal of the 2nd, 3rd, 4th and 5th digits	36°-86°
Distal interphalangeal of the digits	20°-61°

Arches of the hand

The arches of the hand can be observed by holding the forearm in supination and resting the hand on the examination table.

The **carpal arch**, covered by the flexor retinaculum (transverse carpal ligament), keeps the flexor muscles of the last four fingers close to the wrist joint, reducing their capacity to flex the hand and reinforcing the synergistic action of the carpal flexor and extensor muscles in the power grip of the hand. When the hand is relaxed, the fingers are slightly bent, delimiting a bowl-shaped concavity. When grasping or manipulating objects, the palmar concavity

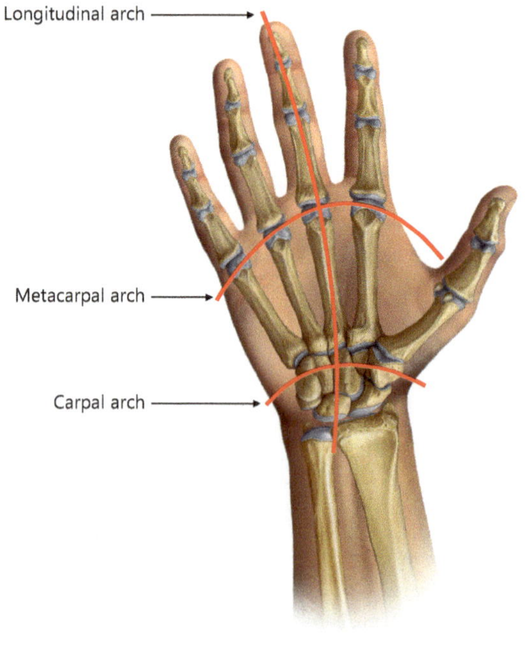

Arches of the hand.

becomes deeper and more concave. When the hand is completely open, the palm flattens. The concavity and flattening of the palm of the hand depend on the mobility of the metacarpals and the phalanges of the 1st, 4th and 5th digits. These bones flex and rotate, moving towards the center of the palm of the hand so that the pulps of the thumb and of the other fingers tend to meet. This movement occurs at the metacarpophalangeal joints (metacarpal arch). The mobile group of metacarpals and phalanges at the periphery of the hand (longitudinal arches) moves around the fixed metacarpals of the 2nd and 3rd digits.

Arch	**Location**	**Support element**	**Mobility**
Carpal	Proximal and distal carpal rows	Capitate	Fixed
Metacarpal	At the level of the metacarpal heads	Head of the third metacarpal	Mobile
Longitudinal	Carpal bones and each of the five rays (metacarpal + phalanges of each finger)	Metacarpophalangeal joints	Mobile, except the phalanges of the 2nd digit and of the second and third metacarpals

Muscles of the wrist and hand

Muscle	Action	Origin	Insertion	Innervation
Flexor carpi radialis	Flexion and radial abduction of the hand (with contribution to the pronation of the elbow)	Common origin of the flexor muscles from the medial epicondyle of the humerus	Volar surface of the base of the 2nd metacarpal and the base of the 3rd metacarpal	Median nerve [C6, C7]
Palmaris longus	Flexion of the hand and anchoring of the fascia and the skin of the palm of the hand (with contribution to the flexion and pronation of the elbow)	Common origin of the flexor muscles from the medial epicondyle of the humerus	Distal palmar surface of the flexor retinaculum; palmar aponeurosis; skin and fascia of the palm of the hand located distally and in the interdigital spaces	Median nerve [C7, C8]
Flexor carpi ulnaris	Flexion and ulnar abduction of the hand and wrist	*Humeral head*: common origin of the flexor muscles from the medial epicondyle of the humerus *Ulnar head*; medial border of the olecranon and upper two-thirds of the posterior border of the ulna	*Both heads*: pisiform; hamate (pisohamate ligament), base of the 5th metacarpal (pisometacarpal ligament) and transverse carpal ligament	Ulnar nerve [C7, C8, T1]
Extensor carpi radialis longus	Extension and radial abduction of the hand (with contribution to the flexion of the elbow)	Lower third of the lateral supraepicondylar ridge of the humerus; common origin of the extensor muscles from the lateral epicondyle of the humerus	Dorsal surface of the base of the 2nd metacarpal	Radial nerve [C6, C7]

(*continued*)

Muscles of the wrist and hand (*continued*)

Muscle	Action	Origin	Insertion	Innervation
Extensor carpi radialis brevis	Extension and radial abduction of the hand (with contribution to the flexion of the elbow)	Common origin of the extensor muscles from the lateral epicondyle of the humerus; radial collateral ligament of the elbow joint	Dorsal surface of the base of the 3rd metacarpal	Posterior interosseous nerve, branch of the radial nerve [C7, C8]
Extensor carpi ulnaris	Extension and ulnar abduction of the hand	Common origin of the extensor muscles from the lateral epicondyle of the humerus; posterior border of the ulna	Tubercle on the ulnar surface of the base of the 5th metacarpal	Posterior interosseous nerve, branch of the radial nerve [C7, C8]
Flexor digitorum superficialis	Flexion of the proximal and middle phalanges of the digits	*Humeroulnar head*: common origin of the flexor muscles from the medial epicondyle of the humerus, ulnar collateral ligament and medial surface of the coronoid process of the ulna *Radial head*: anterior border of the radius, from the radial tuberosity to the insertion of the pronator teres	Anterior surface of the middle phalanges of the 2nd, 3rd, 4th and 5th digits	Median nerve [C8, T1]

(*continued*)

9

Muscles of the wrist and hand (*continued*)

Muscle	Action	Origin	Insertion	Innervation
Flexor digitorum profundus	Interphalangeal flexion of the digits (especially of the distal phalanges)	Upper three-quarters of the anterior and medial surface of the ulna; medial surface of the coronoid process; upper three-quarters of the posterior border of the ulna; anterior surface of the medial half of the interosseous membrane	Volar surface of the bases of the distal phalanges of the 2nd, 3rd, 4th and 5th digits	*Lateral part of the muscle*: anterior interosseous nerve, branch of the median nerve [C7, C8] *Medial part of the muscle*: ulnar nerve [C7, C8, T1]
Extensor digitorum	Extension and abduction of the digits (with contribution to the extension and adduction of the wrist)	Common origin of the extensor muscles from the lateral epicondyle of the humerus	Dorsal surface of the bases of the middle and distal phalanges of the 2nd, 3rd, 4th and 5th digits	Posterior interosseous nerve, branch of the radial nerve [C7, C8]
Extensor indicis	Extension of the index finger (with contribution to the extension of the wrist)	Posterior surface of the ulna distal to the origin of the extensor pollicis longus; posterior surface of the interosseous membrane	Joins the ulnar side of the tendon for the index finger of the extensor digitorum at the head of the 2nd metacarpal	Posterior interosseous nerve, branch of the radial nerve [C7, C8]
Extensor digiti minimi	Extension of the little finger (with contribution to the extension and adduction of the wrist)	Common origin of the extensor muscles from the lateral epicondyle of the humerus	Dorsal digital expansion* of the 5th digit	Posterior interosseous nerve, branch of the radial nerve [C7, C8]

(*continued*)

Muscles of the wrist and hand (*continued*)

Muscle	Action	Origin	Insertion	Innervation
Interossei				
Dorsal	(Radial) abduction of the index finger and adduction (ulnar abduction) of the ring and little fingers (separation from the middle finger). Flexion of the proximal phalanges and extension of the middle and distal phalanges of the last four fingers	*First dorsal interosseous*: adjacent surfaces of the 1st and 2nd metacarpals *Second dorsal interosseous*: adjacent surfaces of the 2nd and 3rd metacarpals *Third dorsal interosseous*: adjacent surfaces of the 3rd and 4th metacarpals *Fourth dorsal interosseous*: adjacent surfaces of the 4th and 5th metacarpals	Common insertion to the dorsal digital expansions* of the index, middle and ring fingers. The *first dorsal interosseous*: on the radial side of the base of the proximal phalanx of the index finger; the *second* and *third* respectively on the radial side and on the ulnar side of the base of the proximal phalanx of the middle finger; the *fourth*: on the ulnar side of the base of the proximal phalanx of the ring finger	Deep branch of the ulnar nerve [C8, T1]
Palmar	(Radial) abduction of the little and ring fingers (bringing closer to the middle finger) and ulnar abduction (adduction) of the index finger (bringing closer to the middle finger). Flexion of the proximal phalanges and extension of the middle and distal phalanges of the index, ring and little fingers	*First palmar interosseous* (not always present): ulnar side of the base of the 1st metacarpal *Second palmar interosseous*: ulnar side of the volar surface of the 2nd metacarpal *Third palmar interosseous*: radial side of the volar surface of the 4th metacarpal *Fourth palmar interosseous*: radial side of the volar surface of the 5th metacarpal	Common insertion to the dorsal digital expansions* of the thumb, index, ring and little fingers. The first palmar interosseous also inserts on the proximal phalanx of the thumb and on the sesamoid bone located on the ulnar side of the base of the proximal phalanx of the thumb, the fourth palmar interosseous also inserts on the radial side of the base of the proximal phalanx of the little finger	Deep branch of the ulnar nerve [C8, T1]

(*continued*)

Muscles of the wrist and hand (*continued*)

Muscle	Action	Origin	Insertion	Innervation
Lumbricals				
	Flexion of the proximal phalanges and extension of the middle and distal phalanges of the last four fingers	Tendons of the flexor digitorum profundus: - *first and second lumbricals*: radial sides and volar surfaces of the tendons that insert at the distal phalanges of the 2nd and 3rd fingers - *third lumbrical*: adjacent sides of the tendons that insert at the distal phalanges of the 3rd and 4th fingers - *fourth lumbrical*: adjacent sides of the tendons that insert at the distal phalanges of the 4th and 5th fingers	Radial border of the dorsal digital expansion* of the corresponding fingers (index, middle, ring and little fingers)	The first and second lumbricals are innervated by the median nerve [C8, T1], the third and fourth by the deep branch of the ulnar nerve [C8, T1]. The third is often innervated by the median nerve [C8, T1], instead of the ulnar nerve. Sometimes, the first and second are innervated by the deep branch of the ulnar nerve [C8, T1], instead of the median nerve
Little finger				
Abductor digiti minimi	Abduction of the little finger (with contribution to the flexion of the proximal phalanx of the thumb)	Pisiform; pisohamate ligament; tendon of flexor carpi ulnaris	Ulnar face of the base of the proximal phalanx of the little finger; dorsal digital expansion of the little finger	Deep branch of the ulnar nerve [C8, T1]
Opponens digiti minimi	Opposition of the little finger (flexion and internal rotation of the 5th metacarpal)	Hamate; flexor retinaculum	Ulnar surface and adjacent volar surface of the 5th metacarpal	Deep branch of the ulnar nerve [C8, T1]

(continued)

Muscles of the wrist and hand *(continued)*

Muscle	Action	Origin	Insertion	Innervation
Little finger				
Flexor digiti minimi brevis	Flexion of the proximal phalanx of the little finger	Hamate; flexor retinaculum	Ulnar surface of the base of the proximal phalanx of the little finger	Deep branch of the ulnar nerve [C8, T1]
Thumb				
Flexor pollicis longus	Flexion of the first metacarpal and of the proximal and distal phalanges of the thumb (with contribution to the flexion and radial abduction of the wrist)	Anterior surface of the radius between the radial tuberosity and the pronator quadratus; anterior surface of the lateral half of the interosseous membrane; lateral surface of the coronoid process of the ulna	Volar surface of the base of the distal phalanx of the thumb	Anterior interosseous nerve, branch of the median nerve [C7, C8]
Flexor pollicis brevis	Flexion of the proximal phalanx of the thumb and of the first metacarpal (movement is made upwards, forwards and medially)	*Superficial head*: flexor retinaculum (transverse carpal ligament) and tubercle of the trapezium *Deep head*: capitate, trapezoid and palmar intercarpal ligaments	Radial side of the base of the proximal phalanx of the thumb	The superficial head is innervated by the median nerve [C8, T1], the deep head by the deep branch of the ulnar nerve [C8, T1]
Extensor pollicis longus	Extension of the thumb (with contribution to the extension of the wrist)	Middle third of the posterolateral surface of the ulna and posterior surface of the interosseous membrane	Dorsal surface of the base of the distal phalanx of the thumb	Posterior interosseous nerve, branch of the radial nerve [C7, C8]
Extensor pollicis brevis	Extension and adduction of the proximal phalanx of the thumb	Posterior surface of the radius below the abductor pollicis longus and the posterior surface of the interosseous membrane	Dorsal surface of the base of the proximal phalanx of the thumb	Posterior interosseous nerve, branch of the radial nerve [C7, C8]

(continued)

Muscles of the wrist and hand (*continued*)

Muscle	Action	Origin	Insertion	Innervation
Thumb Abductor pollicis longus	Radial abduction of the 1st metacarpal (with contribution to the supination of the elbow and to the flexion and radial abduction of the wrist)	Posterior surface of the ulnar diaphysis distally to the insertion of the anconeus; posterior surface of the radial diaphysis distally to the insertion of the supinator; posterior surface of the interosseous membrane	Trapezium and radial surface of the base of the 1st metacarpal	Posterior interosseous nerve, branch of the radial nerve [C7, C8]
Abductor pollicis brevis	Radial abduction of the proximal phalanx of the thumb and the 1st metacarpal (movement is made outwards, forwards and upwards)	Flexor retinaculum (transverse carpal ligament); tubercles of the scaphoid and trapezium; tendon of the abductor pollicis longus	Radial surface of the base of the proximal phalanx of the thumb; dorsal digital expansion* of the thumb	Median nerve [C8, T1]
Adductor pollicis	Adduction and flexion of the proximal phalanx of the thumb and the 1st metacarpal	*Oblique head*: capitate and volar surfaces of the bases of the 2nd and 3rd metacarpals *Transverse head*: distal two-thirds of the volar surface of the diaphysis of the 3rd metacarpal	Ulnar surface of the base of the proximal phalanx of the thumb; dorsal digital expansion* of the thumb	Deep branch of the ulnar nerve [C8, T1]
Opponens pollicis	Opposition of the thumb (abduction, flexion and internal rotation of the 1st metacarpal)	Flexor retinaculum (transverse carpal ligament); tubercle of the trapezium	Lateral surface and lateral face of the volar surface of the 1st metacarpal	Median nerve [C8, T1]

* Prolongation of the dorsal fascia of the hand onto the dorsal surface of the fingers (dorsal digital expansion of the extensor digitorum).

Topographical classification of the muscles of the wrist and hand

Anterior muscles of the forearm:
- flexor pollicis longus
- flexor digitorum profundus
- flexor carpi radialis (also acts on the elbow; see Chapter 8 "Elbow")
- flexor digitorum superficialis
- flexor carpi ulnaris
- palmaris longus (also acts on the elbow; see Chapter 8 "Elbow")

Lateral muscles of the forearm:
- extensor carpi radialis brevis (also acts on the elbow; see Chapter 8 "Elbow")
- extensor carpi radialis longus (also acts on the elbow; see Chapter 8 "Elbow")

Posterior muscles of the forearm:
- abductor pollicis longus
- extensor pollicis brevis (also acts on the elbow; see Chapter 8 "Elbow")
- extensor digitorum
- extensor pollicis longus (also acts on the elbow; see Chapter 8 "Elbow")
- extensor indicis
- extensor digiti minimi
- extensor carpi ulnaris.

All the muscles acting on the wrist are arranged obliquely in relation to the axis of wrist motion (flexion-extension and radial-ulnar abduction) and none of them is exactly on the frontal or sagittal plane. As such, the action of these muscles on the wrist are associated with secondary actions that are neutralized by other muscles.

Some muscles have a dual action on the wrist:
- flexor carpi ulnaris – palmar flexion and ulnar abduction of the hand
- flexor pollicis longus – palmar flexion and radial abduction of the hand
- flexor carpi radialis – palmar flexion and radial abduction of the hand
- abductor pollicis longus – palmar flexion and radial abduction of the hand
- extensor digitorum – dorsal flexion and ulnar abduction of the hand
- extensor digiti minimi – dorsal flexion and ulnar abduction of the hand
- extensor carpi radialis longus – dorsal flexion and radial abduction of the hand
- extensor carpi radialis brevis – dorsal flexion and radial abduction of the hand
- extensor pollicis longus – dorsal flexion and radial abduction of the hand.

Action of the muscles in the movements of the wrist

Palmar flexor muscles of the hand (from greatest to least muscular force)

- Flexor digitorum superficialis
- Flexor digitorum profundus
- Flexor carpi ulnaris
- Flexor pollicis longus
- Flexor carpi radialis
- Abductor pollicis longus
- Palmaris longus

Flexor digitorum superficialis

Action at the finger level → flexion of the proximal and middle phalanges.

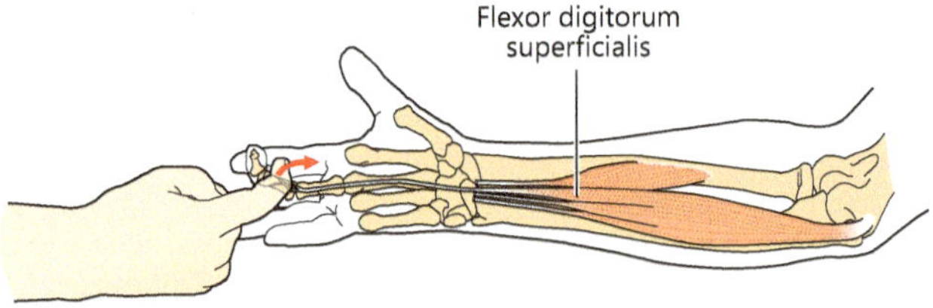

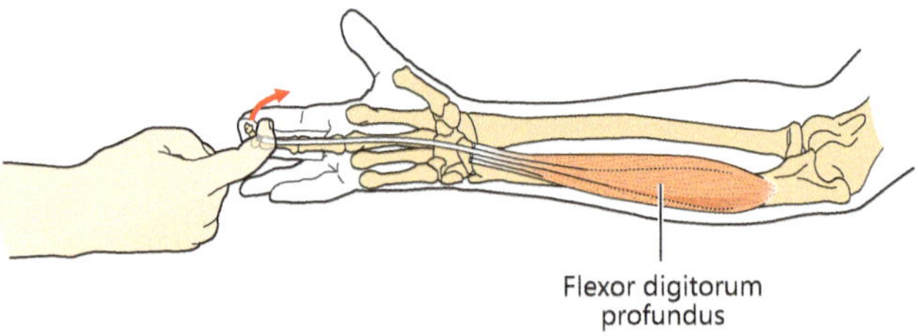

Flexor digitorum profundus

Action at the finger level → flexion of the proximal, middle and distal phalanges.

Flexor carpi ulnaris

It is also an abductor of the hand.

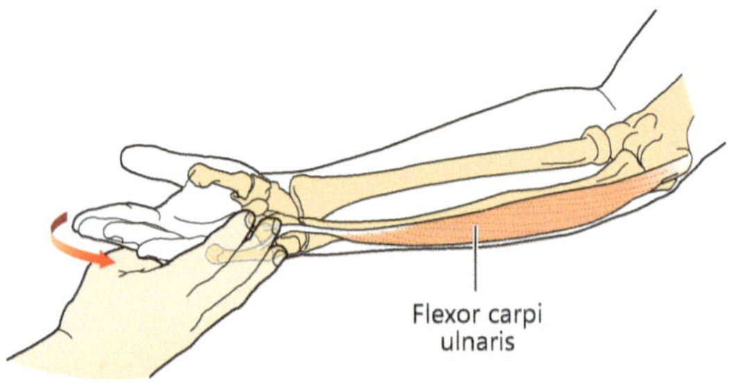

Flexor pollicis longus

It is also an abductor of the hand.

Action at the finger level → flexion of the distal and proximal phalanges of the thumb (in temporal order) and of the 1st metacarpal.

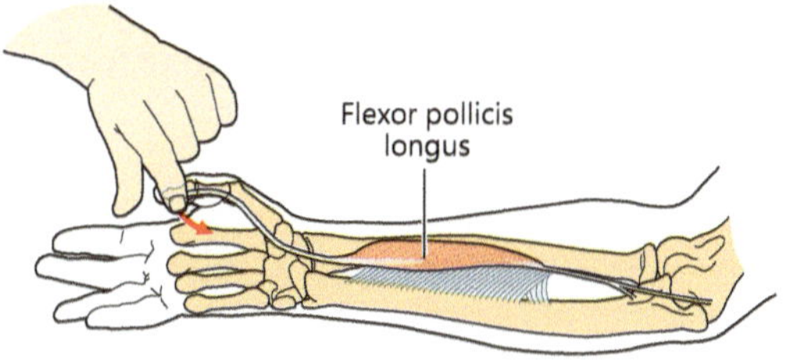

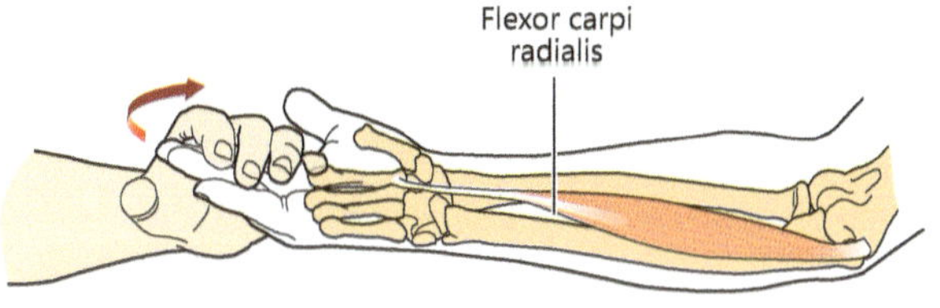

Flexor carpi radialis

It is also an abductor of the hand.

Abductor pollicis longus

It is also an abductor of the hand.

Action at the finger level → abduction of the 1st metacarpal.

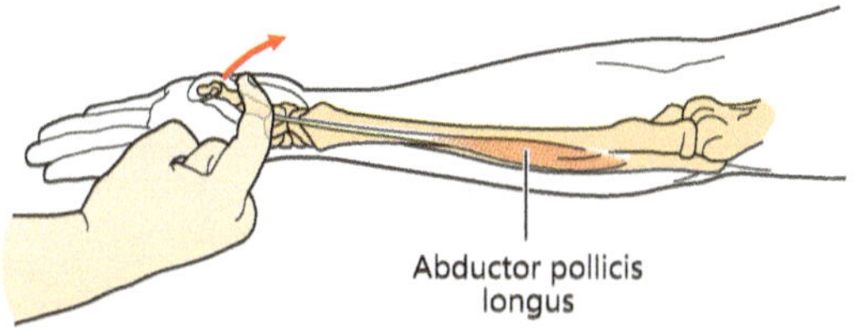

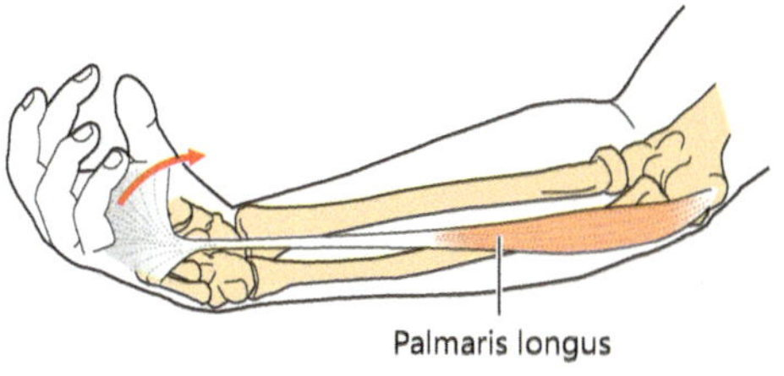

Palmaris longus

It also stretches the palmar aponeurosis.

Dorsal flexor muscles of the hand (from greatest to least muscular force)

- Extensor digitorum
- Extensor carpi radialis longus
- Extensor carpi radialis brevis
- Extensor indicis
- Extensor pollicis longus
- Extensor digiti minimi

Extensor digitorum

It is also an abductor of the hand.

Action at the finger level → extension and abduction of the fingers.

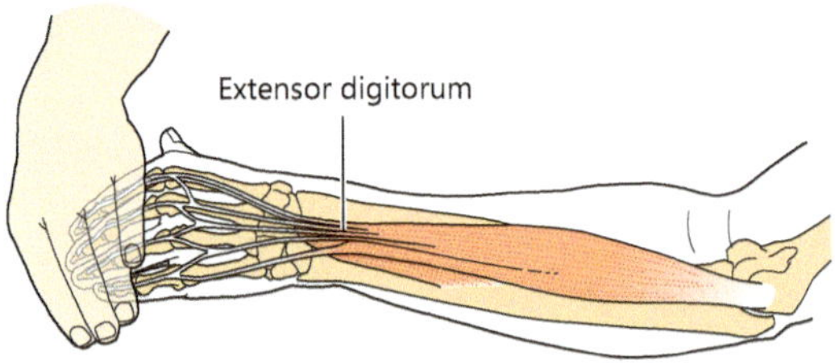

Extensor carpi radialis longus

It is also an abductor of the hand.

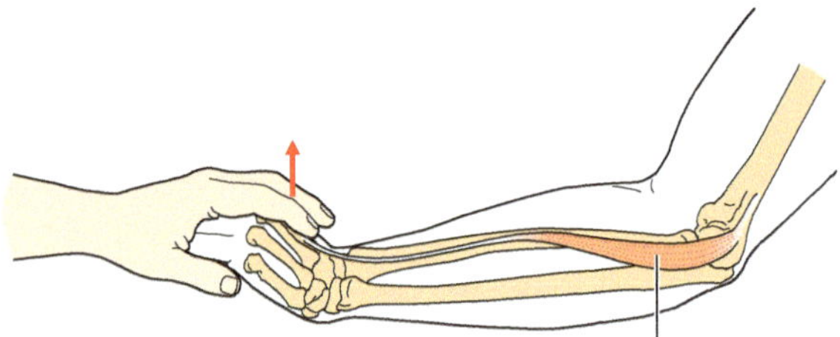

Extensor carpi radialis brevis

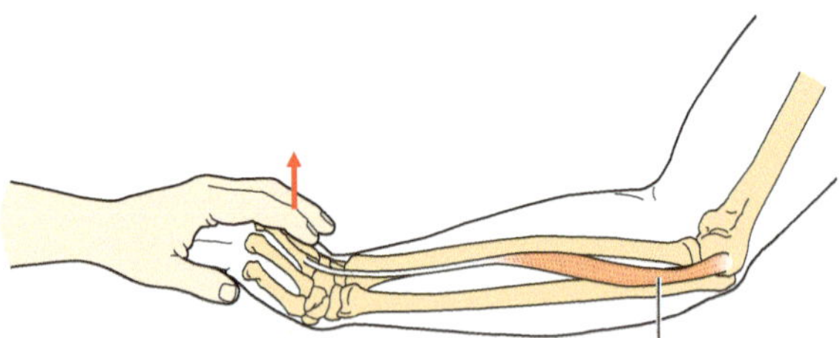

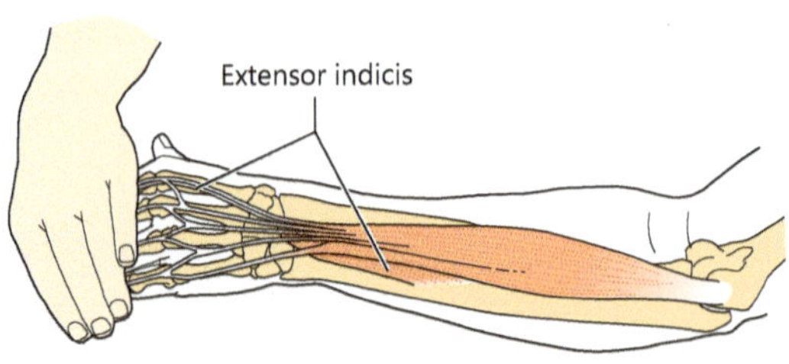

Extensor indicis

Action at the finger level → extension of the index finger.

Extensor pollicis longus

Action at the finger level → extension of the thumb.

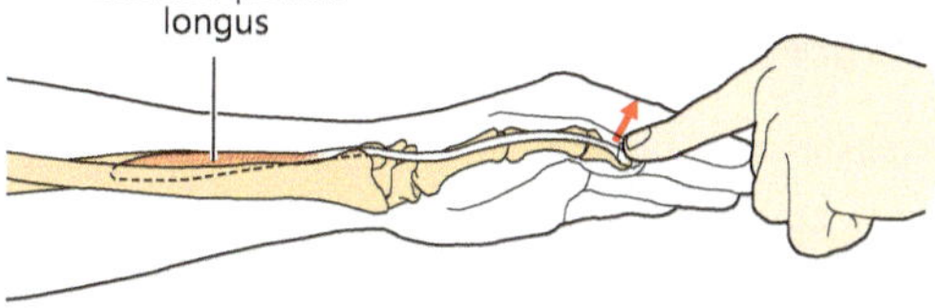

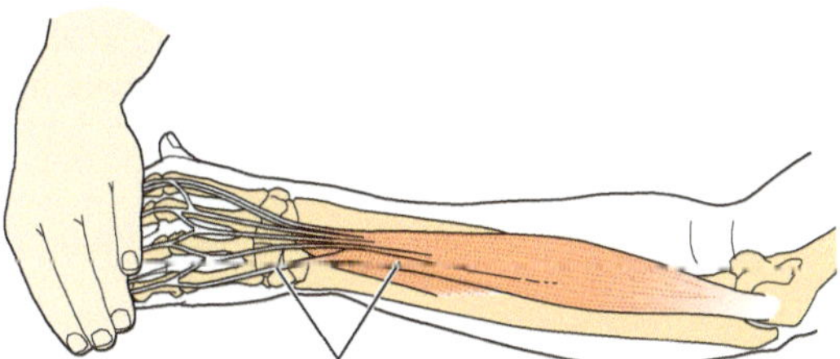

Extensor digiti minimi

It is also an adductor of the hand.
Action at the finger level → extension of the little finger.

Radial abductor muscles of the hand (from greatest to least muscular force)

- Extensor carpi radialis longus (see "Dorsal flexor muscles of the hand", page 408)
- Abductor pollicis longus (see "Palmar flexor muscles of the hand", page 407)
- Extensor pollicis longus (see "Dorsal flexor muscles of the hand", page 409)
- Flexor carpi radialis (see "Palmar flexor muscles of the hand", page 407)
- Flexor pollicis longus (see "Palmar flexor muscles of the hand", page 407)
- Extensor pollicis brevis.

Extensor pollicis brevis

Action at the finger level → extension and abduction of the thumb.

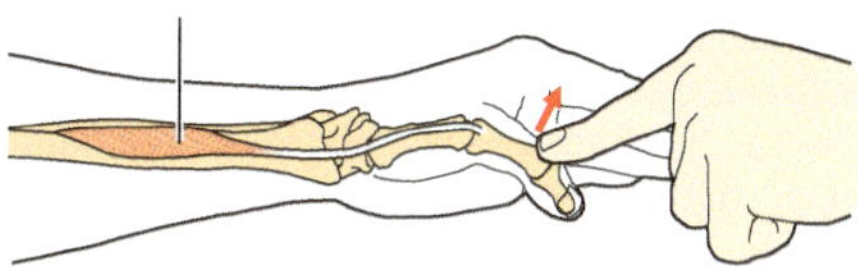

Ulnar abductor muscles of the hand (from greatest to least muscular force)

- Extensor carpi ulnaris
- Flexor carpi ulnaris (see "Palmar flexor muscles of the hand", page 406)
- Extensor digitorum (see "Dorsal flexor muscles of the hand", page 408)
- Extensor digiti minimi (see "Dorsal flexor muscles of the hand", page 409)

Extensor carpi ulnaris

It is defined as such because it is responsible for an extensor action (dorsal flexion) at the wrist joint and a flexor action (palmar flexion) at the midcarpal joint that cancel each other out.

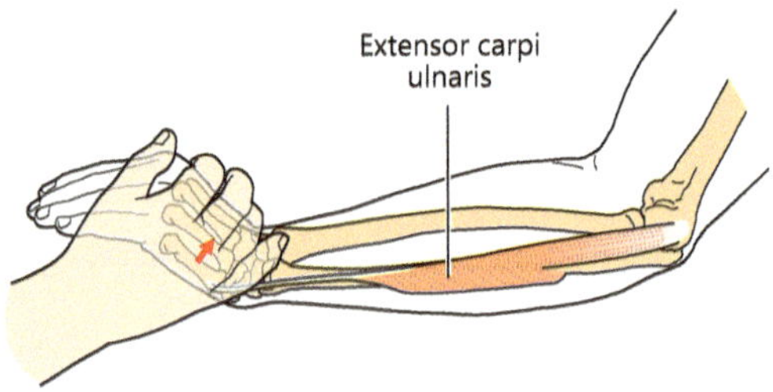

Action of the muscles in the movements of the hand

The muscles acting on the joints of the hand (especially on the carpometacarpal, intermetacarpal, metacarpophalangeal and interphalangeal joints) are divided into:
- extrinsic – originate at the level of the arm or forearm and insert at the level of the hand
- intrinsic – originate and insert at the level of the hand.

Extrinsic muscles of the hand

- Flexor digitorum superficialis (see "Palmar flexor muscles of the hand", page 406)
- Flexor digitorum profundus (see "Palmar flexor muscles of the hand", page 406)
- Flexor pollicis longus (see "Palmar flexor muscles of the hand", page 407)
- Extensor digitorum (see "Dorsal flexor muscles of the hand", page 408)
- Extensor indicis (see "Dorsal flexor muscles of the hand", page 408)
- Extensor digiti minimi (see "Dorsal flexor muscles of the hand", page 409)
- Extensor pollicis longus (see "Dorsal flexor muscles of the hand", page 409)
- Extensor pollicis brevis (see "Radial abductor muscles of the hand", page 409)
- Abductor pollicis longus (see "Palmar flexor muscles of the hand", page 407)

Intrinsic muscles of the hand

- Of the thenar eminence
- Of the hypothenar eminence
- Lumbricals
- Interossei:
  - palmar
  - dorsal.

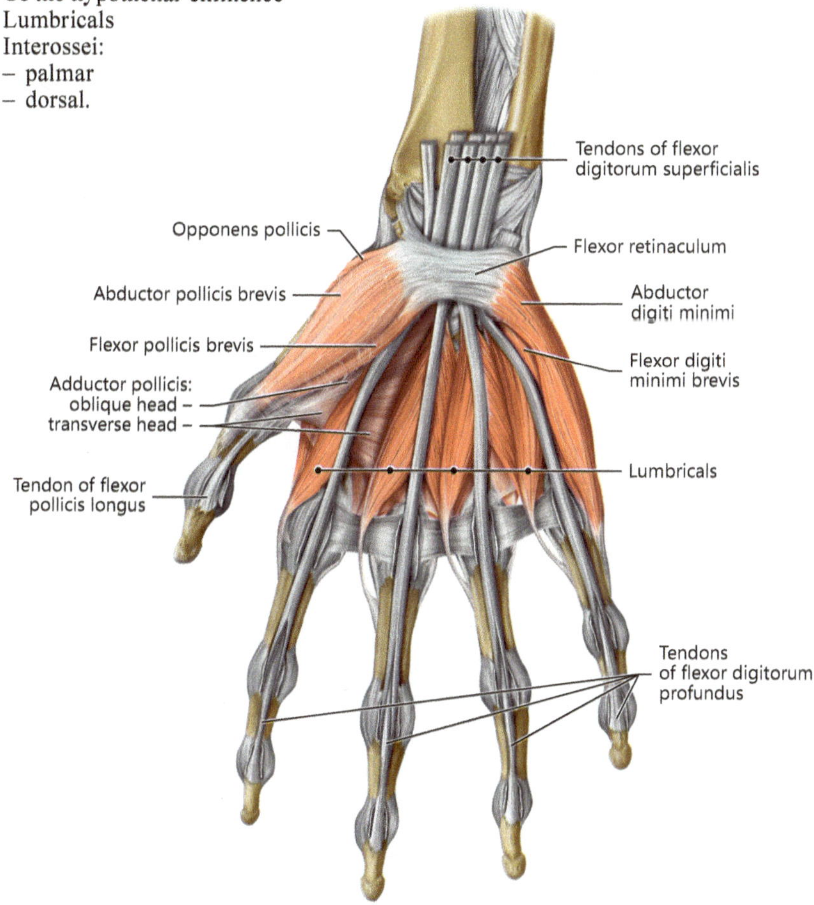

Intrinsic muscles of the hand.

Muscles of the thenar eminence

They are defined as such because they form a bulge on the palm of the hand, laterally and in continuity with the thumb. They allow the opposition movements of the thumb.

- Flexor pollicis brevis
- Abductor pollicis brevis
- Adductor pollicis
- Opponens pollicis.

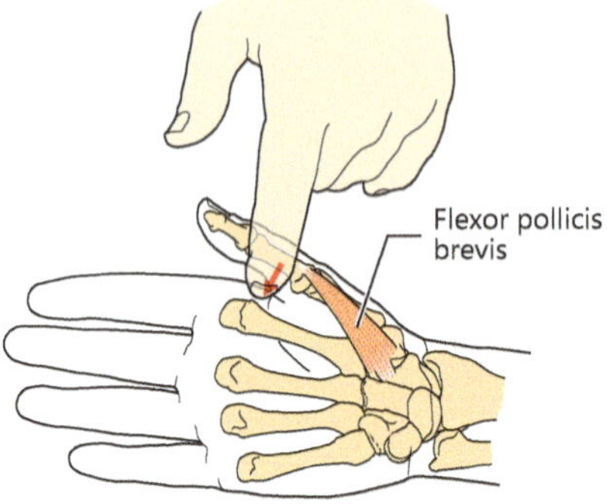

Flexor pollicis brevis

Flexion and adduction of the proximal phalanx of the thumb and the 1st metacarpal, bringing the thumb upwards, forwards and medially, in an intermediate position between flexion and adduction.

Abductor pollicis brevis

Abduction of the proximal phalanx of the thumb and the 1st metacarpal (which rotates internally), bringing the thumb outwards, forwards and upwards (the movement occurs principally on the sagittal plane), in position of flexion.

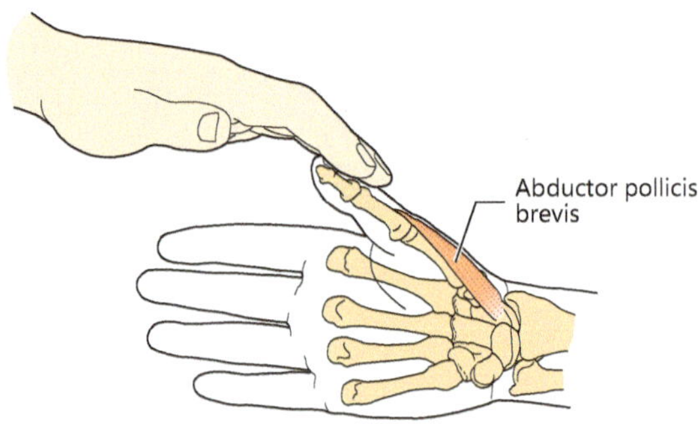

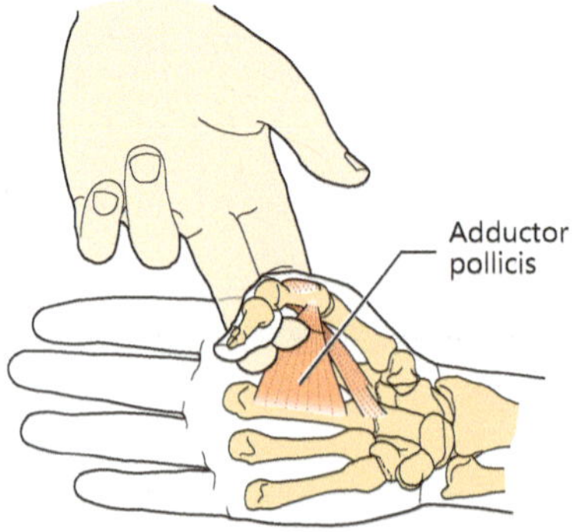

Adductor pollicis

Adduction and flexion of the proximal phalanx of the thumb and the 1st metacarpal, bringing the thumb forwards and inwards, contributing to the opposition movement of the thumb.

Opponens pollicis

Movement of the 1st metacarpal forwards and upwards and then inwards and backwards, in position of flexion-adduction or circumduction, through which the distal phalanx of the thumb opposes the other fingers.

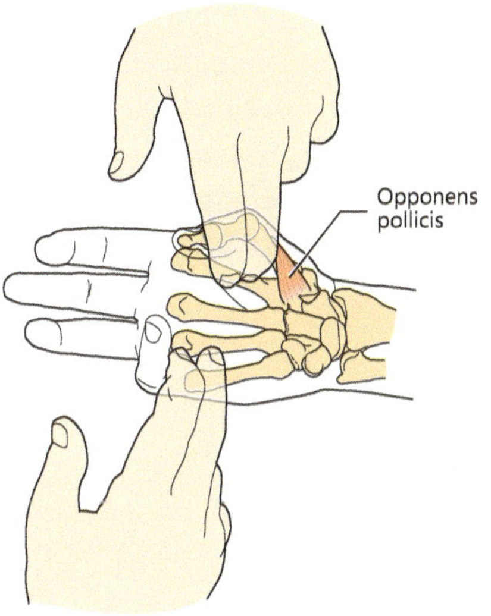

Muscles of the hypothenar eminence

They are defined as such because they form a bulge on the palm of the hand in medial and proximal location. They allow the opposition movements of the thumb.

- Abductor digiti minimi
- Flexor digiti minimi brevis
- Opponens digiti minimi

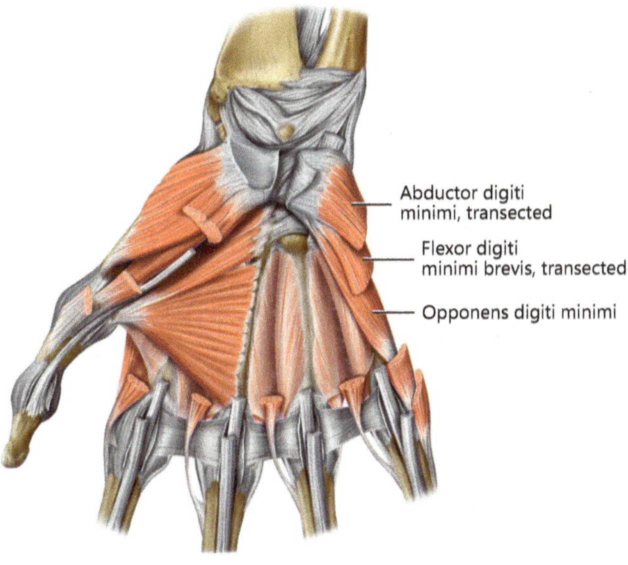

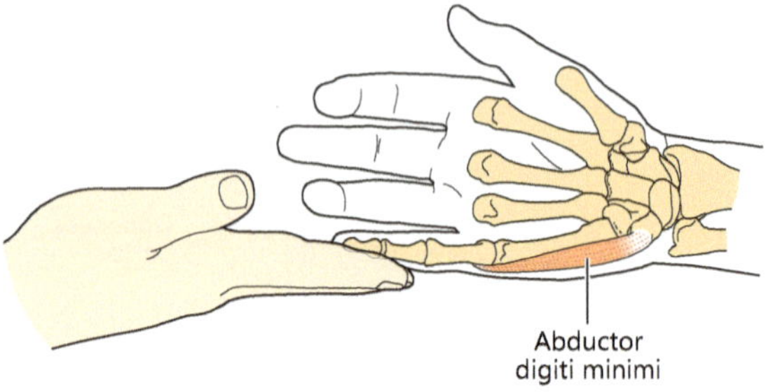

Abductor digiti minimi

Abduction in the ulnar direction and flexion of the proximal phalanx of the little finger.

Flexor digiti minimi brevis

Flexion of the proximal phalanx of the little finger, contributing to the opposition movement of the little finger to the thumb.

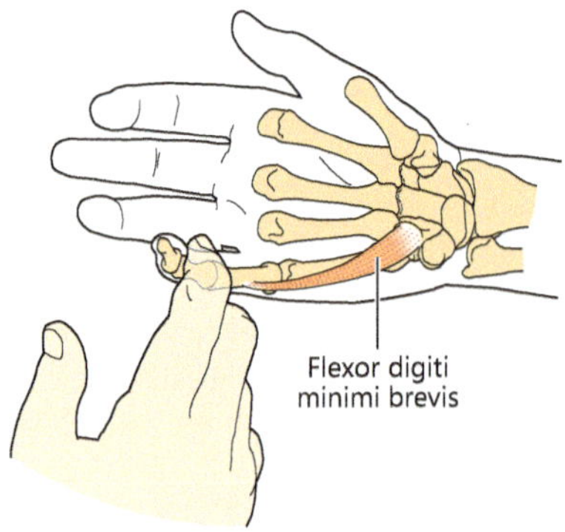

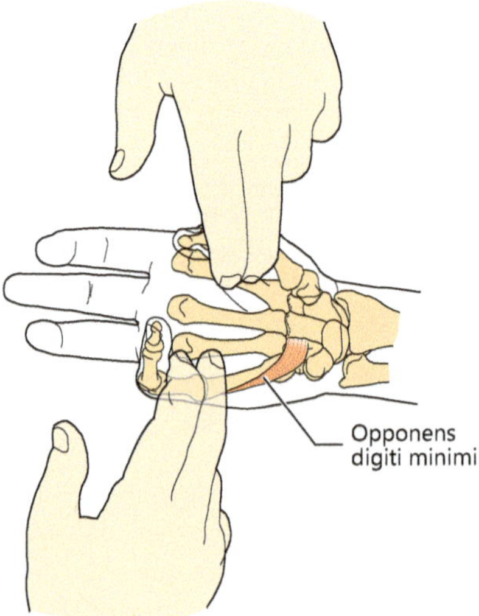

Opponens digiti minimi

Flexion and radial rotation of the 5th metacarpal, contributing to the opposition movement of the little finger to the thumb.

Lumbricals

Four in number, they flex the proximal phalanx and extend the middle and distal phalanges of the last four fingers.

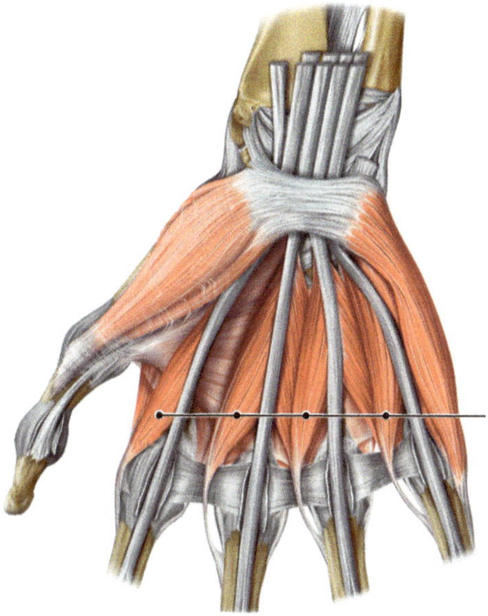

Interossei

- Palmar. Three or four in number:
  - bring the index, ring and little fingers towards the middle finger (adduction of the fingers)
  - flex the proximal phalanx and extend the middle and distal phalanges of the index, ring and little fingers.

- Dorsal. Four in number:
  - separate the index and ring fingers from the middle finger (abduction of the fingers)
  - abduct the middle finger in ulnar or radial direction
  - flex the proximal phalanx and extend the middle and distal phalanges of the last four fingers.

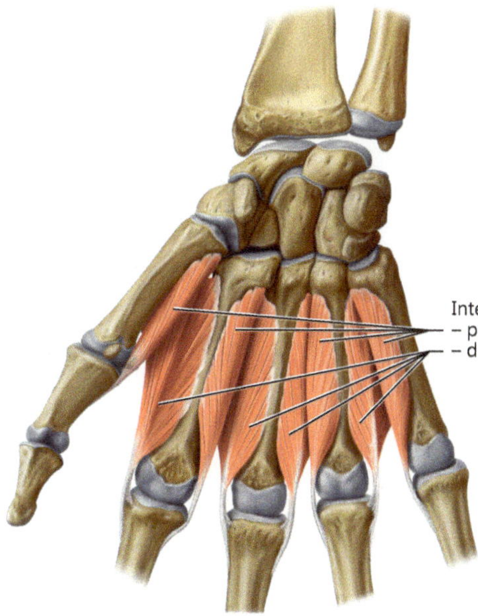

Assessment of the length of muscle fibers

Flexor digitorum superficialis, flexor digitorum profundus, flexor digiti minimi brevis and palmaris longus

Starting position	Supine or seated position with the forearm extended, supinated and fingers extended
Movement	Keeping the fingers extended, the hand is extended (dorsally flexed) up to the limit of movement allowed, thus stretching the fibers of the flexor muscles of the last four fingers. If the fibers are shortened, the extension movement of the hand will be reduced proportionally to the degree of reduction of the muscle length 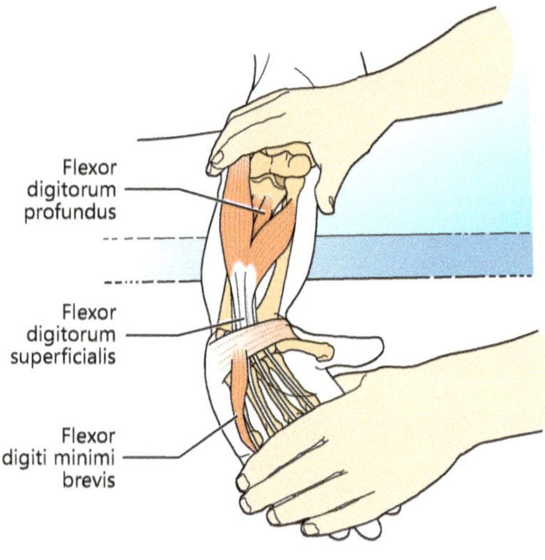

Extensor digitorum, extensor indicis and extensor digiti minimi

Starting position	Supine or seated position with the forearm extended, pronated and fingers flexed
Movement	The hand is flexed (palmar flexion) up to the limit of movement allowed, thus fully stretching the fibers of the extensor muscles of the last four fingers. If the fibers are shortened, the flexion movement of the hand will be reduced proportionally to the degree of reduction of the muscle length

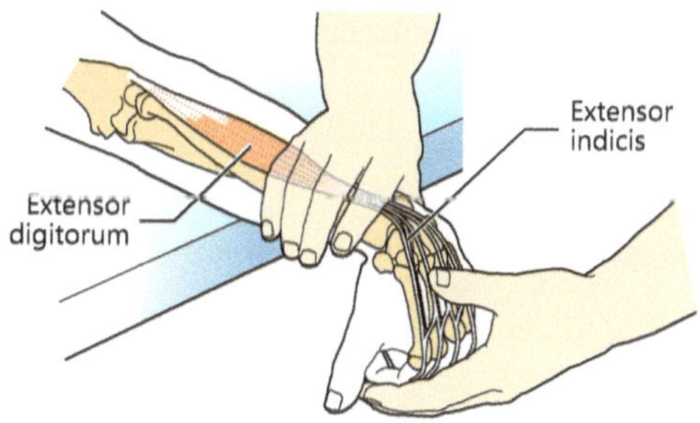

Lumbricals

Starting position	Seated or supine position with the forearm flexed and in an intermediate or supine position, the hand extended and the middle and distal phalanges flexed
Movement	Additional flexion of the middle and distal phalanges and simultaneous extension of the proximal phalanges up to the limit of movement allowed, thus fully stretching the fibers of the lumbricals. If the fibers are shortened, the extension movement of the proximal phalanges will be reduced proportionally to the degree of reduction of the muscle length

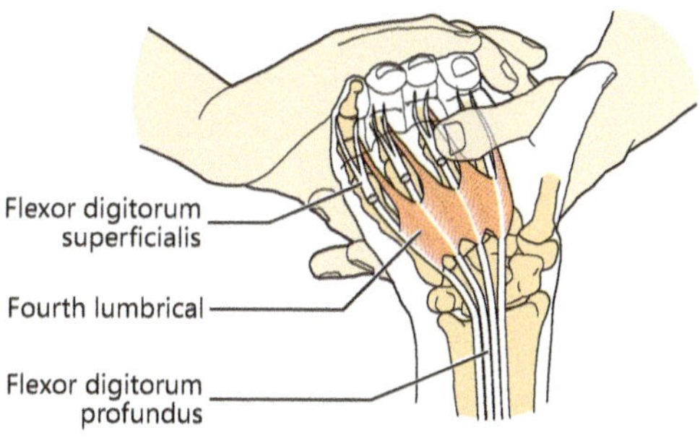

9

Assessment of the muscular force

Flexion and radial abduction of the wrist

Flexor carpi radialis

Against gravity

Flexion and radial abduction of the hand in a seated position with the supinated forearm resting on the examination table, the hand flexed dorsally and abducted in the ulnar direction beyond the edge of the examination table, fingers relaxed and resistance applied distally to the wrist above the thenar eminence.

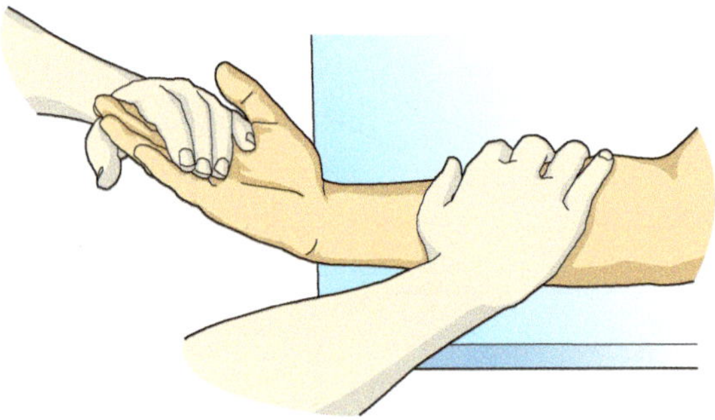

Without gravity

Flexion and radial abduction of the hand in a seated position with the forearm slightly pronated resting on the examination table, the hand flexed dorsally and abducted in the ulnar direction, resting on the examination table, with the fingers relaxed.

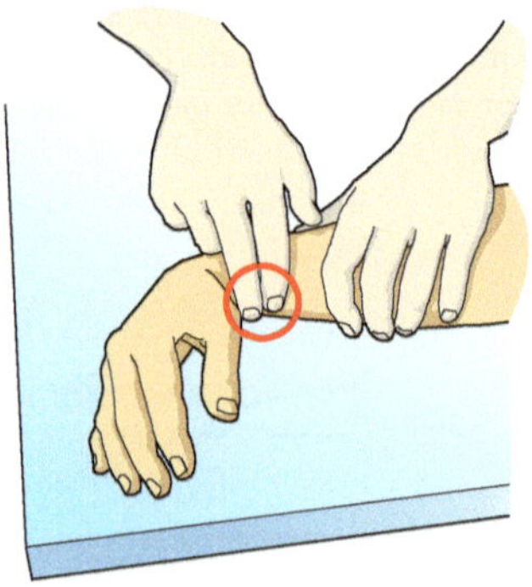

The flexor carpi radialis can be palpated on the anterolateral surface of the wrist in line with the second interdigital space, laterally to the palmaris longus.

Ulnar flexion and abduction of the wrist

Flexor carpi ulnaris

Against gravity

Flexion and ulnar abduction of the wrist in a seated position with the supinated forearm resting on the examination table, the hand flexed dorsally and abducted in the radial direction beyond the edge of the examination table, fingers relaxed and resistance applied above the hypothenar eminence.

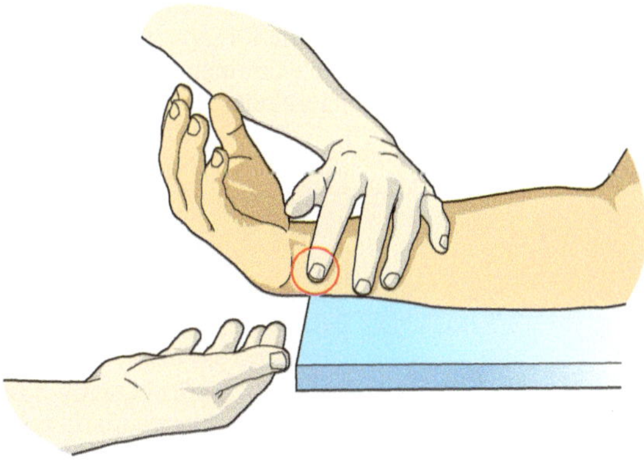

The flexor carpi ulnaris can be palpated on the anteromedial surface of the wrist, proximal to the pisiform.

Without gravity

Flexion and ulnar abduction of the hand in a seated position with the forearm slightly supinated resting on the examination table, the hand flexed dorsally and abducted in the radial direction, resting on the examination table, with the fingers relaxed.

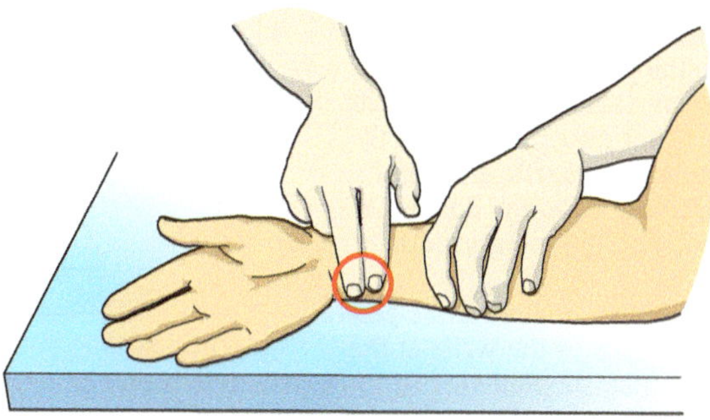

Flexion of the wrist

Flexor carpi radialis and flexor carpi ulnaris

Against gravity

Flexion of the wrist in a seated position with the supinated forearm resting on the examination table, the hand flexed dorsally beyond the edge of the examination table, fingers relaxed and resistance applied to the palm of the hand.

Without gravity

Flexion of the wrist in a seated position with the forearm in an intermediate position between pronation and supination, resting on the examination table, the hand flexed dorsally, resting on the examination table, and the fingers relaxed.

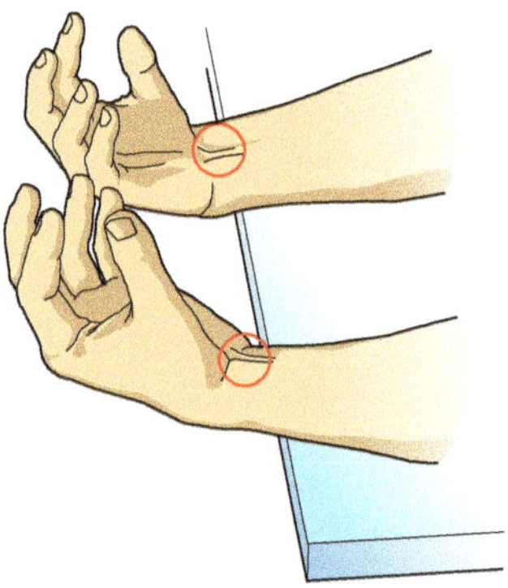

The palmaris longus is a weak flexor of the wrist whose muscle strength cannot be evaluated separately. It can be palpated on the midline of the anterior surface of the wrist during evaluation of the flexor carpi radialis and flexor carpi ulnaris. With the wrist and fingers flexed to accentuate the palmar concavity, the tendon of the palmaris longus protrudes visibly on the anterior surface of the wrist.

Extension (dorsal flexion) and radial abduction of the wrist

Extensor carpi radialis longus and extensor carpi radialis brevis

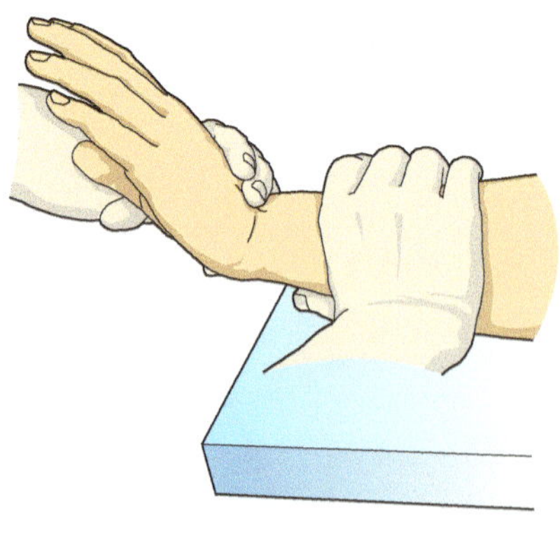

Against gravity

Extension and radial abduction of the wrist in a seated position with the pronated forearm resting on the examination table, the hand flexed and abducted in the ulnar direction beyond the edge of the examination table, fingers slightly flexed and resistance applied to the dorsum of the hand, above the 2nd and 3rd metacarpals.

The extensor carpi radialis longus can be palpated on the dorsal surface of the wrist at the base of the 2nd metacarpal; the extensor carpi radialis brevis can be palpated on the dorsal surface of the wrist at the base of the 3rd metacarpal.

Without gravity

Extension and radial abduction of the wrist in a seated position with the forearm slightly supinated resting on the examination table, the hand flexed and abducted in the ulnar direction, resting on the examination table, with the fingers slightly flexed.

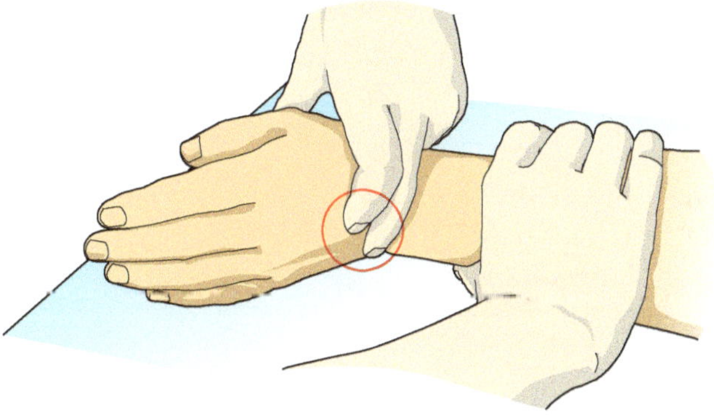

Extension and ulnar abduction of the wrist

Extensor carpi ulnaris

Against gravity

Extension and ulnar abduction of the wrist in a seated position with the pronated forearm resting on the examination table, the hand flexed and abducted in the radial direction beyond the edge of the examination table, fingers slightly flexed and resistance applied to the dorsum of the hand, above the 4th and 5th metacarpals.

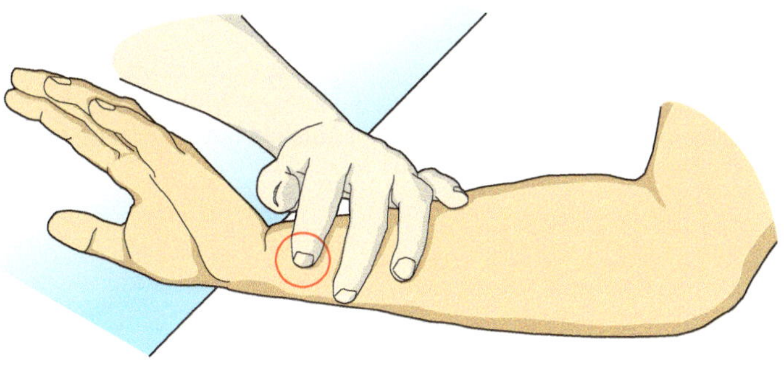

The extensor carpi ulnaris can be palpated on the dorsal surface of the wrist, proximal to the 5th metacarpal and distal to the radial styloid process.

Without gravity

Extension and ulnar abduction of the wrist in a seated position with the forearm slightly pronated resting on the examination table, the hand flexed and abducted in the radial direction, resting on the examination table, with the fingers slightly flexed.

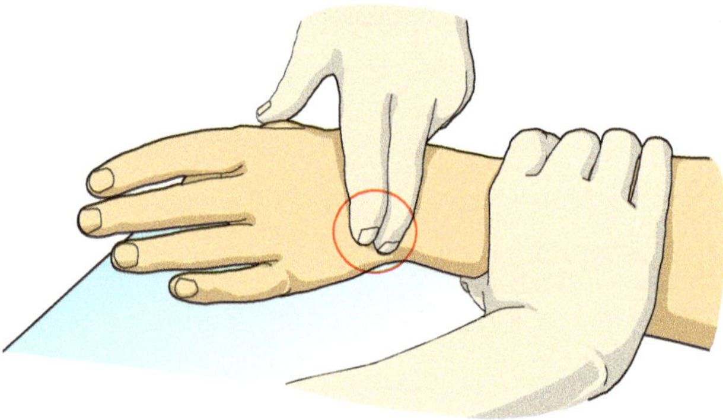

Extension of the wrist

Extensor carpi radialis longus, extensor carpi radialis brevis and extensor carpi ulnaris

Against gravity

Extension of the wrist in a seated position with the pronated forearm resting on the examination table, the hand flexed beyond the edge of the examination table, the fingers relaxed and resistance applied to the dorsum of the hand above the metacarpus.

Without gravity

Extension of the hand in a seated position with the forearm in an intermediate position between pronation and supination resting on the examination table, the hand flexed resting on the examination table, with the fingers slightly relaxed.

Metacarpophalangeal extension of the fingers

Extensor digitorum, extensor indicis and extensor digiti minimi

Extension of the proximal phalanges of the last four fingers in a seated position with the pronated forearm resting on the examination table, the hand beyond the edge of the examination table, the fingers flexed and resistance applied to the dorsal surface of the proximal phalanx of each finger.

The tendon of the extensor digitorum can be palpated on the dorsum of the hand proximal to each metacarpal head, the tendon of the extensor indicis medially to the tendon of the extensor digitorum for the index finger, the tendon of the extensor digiti minimi laterally to the tendon of the extensor digitorum for the little finger.

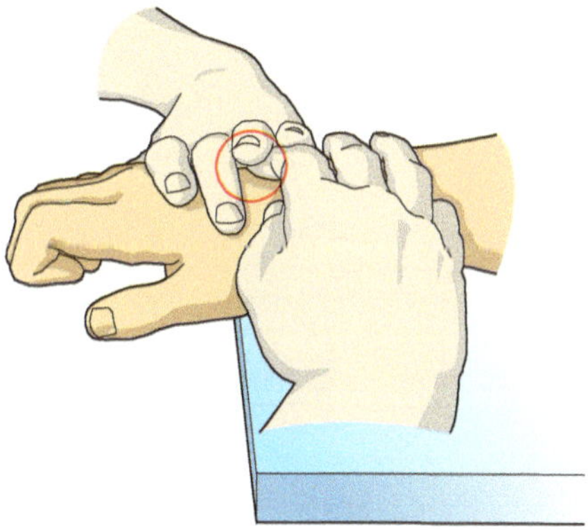

Metacarpophalangeal abduction of the fingers

Dorsal interossei and abductor digiti minimi

Dorsal interossei

Abduction of the index finger in the direction of the thumb, of the middle finger in the direction of the index finger and then of the ring finger, and of the ring finger in the direction of the little finger in a seated position with the pronated forearm resting on the examination table, the hand resting on the examination table, the fingers extended and adducted and resistance applied against the proximal phalanx of the finger examined.

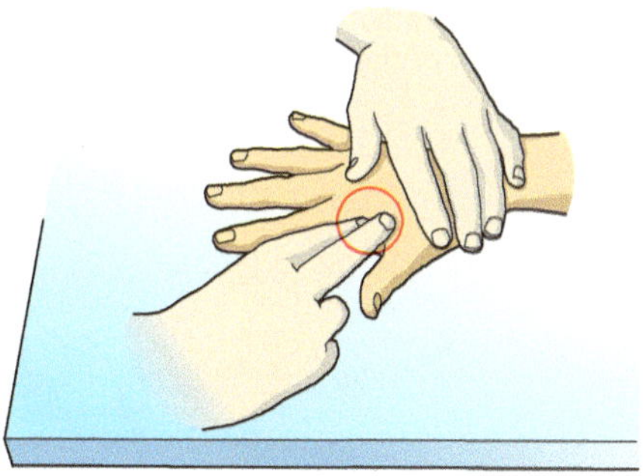

Of the dorsal interossei, only the first one can be palpated on the radial surface of the 2nd metacarpal.

Abductor digiti minimi

Abduction of the little finger in a seated position with the supinated forearm resting on the examination table, the hand resting on the examination table, the fingers extended and adducted and resistance applied against the proximal phalanx of the little finger.

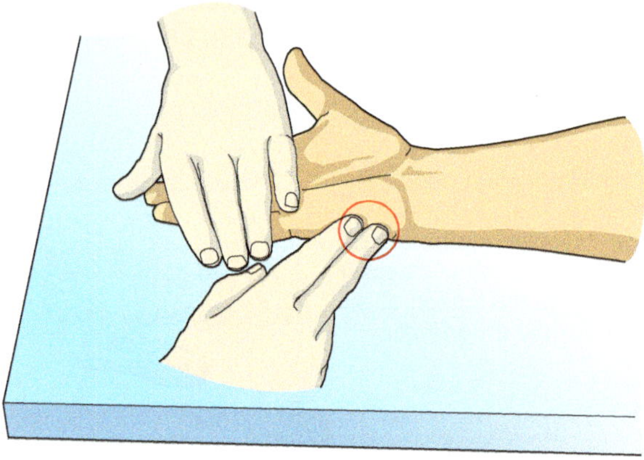

The abductor digiti minimi can be palpated on the ulnar surface of the 5th metacarpal.

Metacarpophalangeal adduction of the fingers

Palmar interossei

Adduction of the index, ring and little fingers in the direction of the middle finger in a seated position with the supinated forearm resting on the examination table, the hand resting on the examination table, the fingers abducted and resistance applied against the proximal phalanx of the finger under examination.

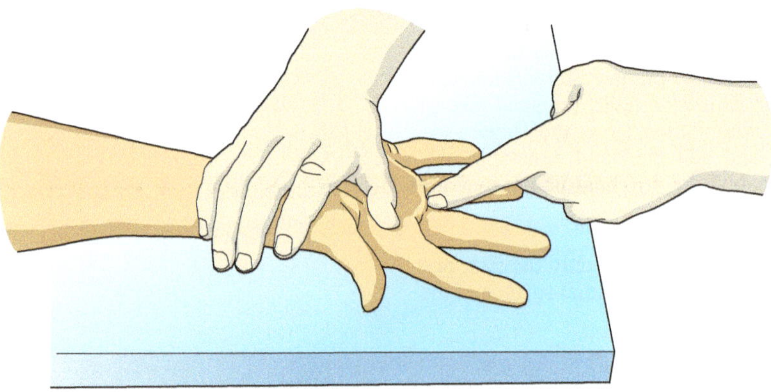

The palmar interossei cannot be palpated.

Metacarpophalangeal flexion and interphalangeal extension of the fingers

Lumbricals

Flexion of the proximal phalanges and extension of the middle and distal phalanges in a seated position with the forearm supinated or in an intermediate position resting on the examination table, the hand resting on the examination table, the proximal phalanges extended and adducted, the middle and distal phalanges slightly flexed and resistance applied to the palmar (volar) surface of the proximal phalanges and on the dorsal surface of the middle phalanges.

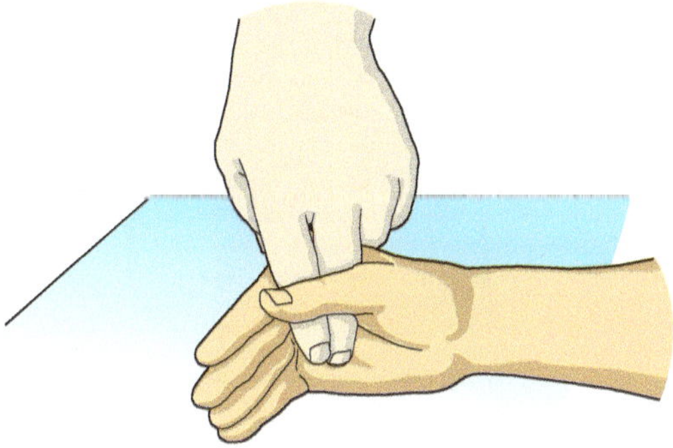

The lumbricals cannot be palpated.

Metacarpophalangeal flexion of the little finger

Flexor digiti minimi brevis

Flexion of the proximal phalanx of the little finger in a seated position with the supinated forearm resting on the examination table, the hand resting on the examination table, the phalanges extended and resistance applied to the palmar (volar) surface of the proximal phalanx of the little finger.

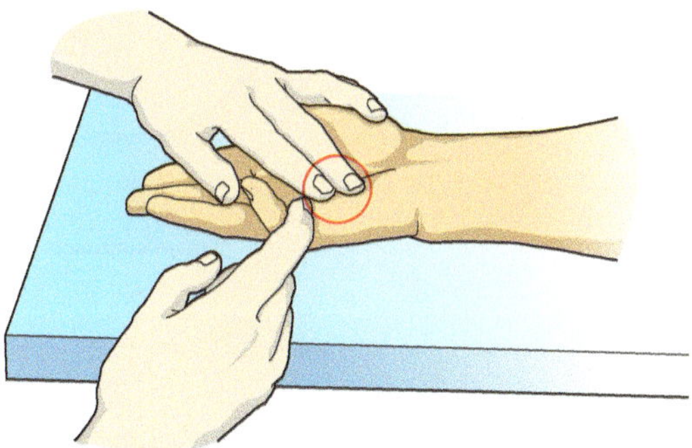

The flexor digiti minimi brevis can be palpated on the hypothenar eminence, medially to the abductor digiti minimi.

Interphalangeal flexion proximal to the fingers

Flexor digitorum superficialis

Flexion of the middle phalanx of each finger, maintaining the distal phalanx extended, in a seated position with the supinated forearm resting on the examination table, the hand resting on the examination table, the fingers extended and resistance applied to the palmar (volar) surface of the middle phalanx.

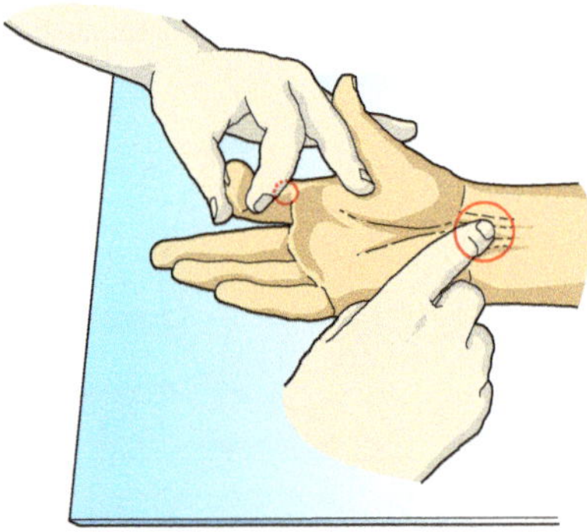

The flexor digitorum superficialis can be palpated on the palmar (volar) surface of the wrist, between the tendons of the palmaris longus and flexor carpi ulnaris, or on the proximal phalanx.

Distal interphalangeal flexion of the fingers

Flexor digitorum profundus

Flexion of the distal phalanx of each finger, in a seated position with the supinated forearm resting on the examination table, the hand resting on the examination table, the finger to be examinated extended and resistance applied to the palmar (volar) surface of the distal phalanx.

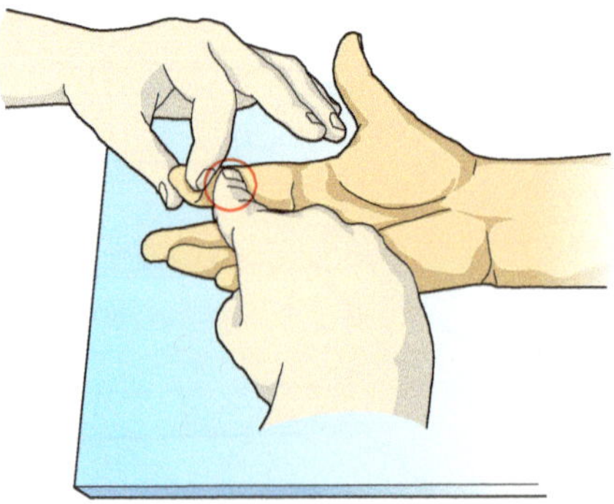

The flexor digitorum profundus can be palpated on the palmar (volar) surface of the middle phalanx.

Interphalangeal flexion of the thumb

Flexor pollicis longus

Flexion of the distal phalanx in a seated position with the supinated forearm resting on the examination table, the hand resting on the examination table, the thumb extended and resistance applied to the palmar (volar) surface of the distal phalanx.

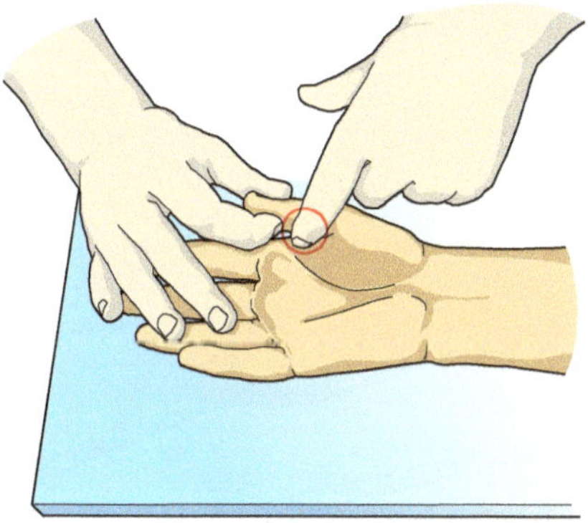

The flexor pollicis longus can be palpated on the palmar (volar) surface of the proximal phalanx.

Metacarpophalangeal flexion of the thumb

Flexor pollicis brevis

Flexion of the proximal phalanx, maintaining the distal phalanx extended, in a seated position with the supinated forearm resting on the examination table, the hand resting on the examination table, the thumb extended and adducted and resistance applied to the palmar (volar) surface of the proximal phalanx.

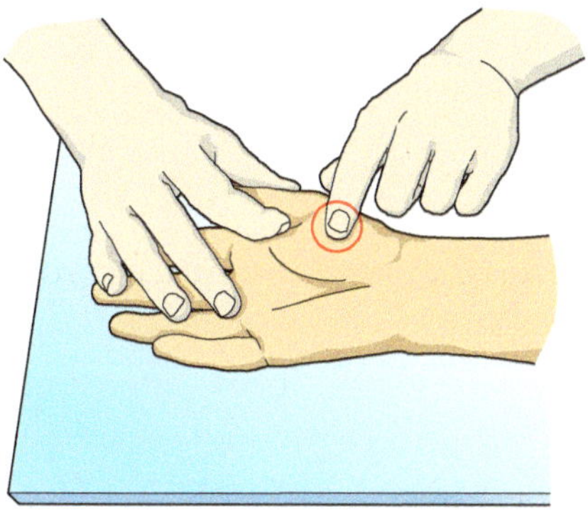

The flexor pollicis brevis can be palpated proximal to the metacarpophalangeal joint, at the center of the thenar eminence, medially to the abductor pollicis brevis.

Interphalangeal extension of the thumb

Extensor pollicis longus

Extension of the distal phalanx in a seated position with the forearm in the intermediate position or slightly pronated resting on the examination table, the hand resting on the examination table, the thumb adducted with the proximal phalanx extended and the distal phalanx flexed, and resistance applied to the dorsal surface of the distal phalanx.

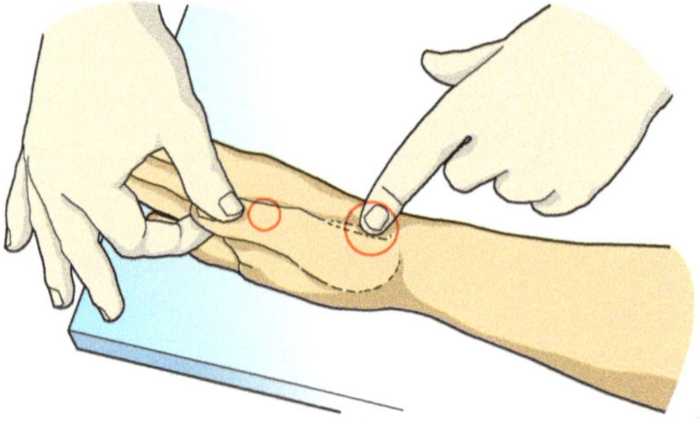

The extensor pollicis longus can be palpated on the dorsal surface of the proximal phalanx or on the ulnar margin of the anatomical snuffbox.

> The anatomical snuffbox is the depression observed laterally on the dorsum of the carpus, when the thumb is extended and abducted, between the skin crease of the tendon of the extensor pollicis longus and the crease of the tendon of the extensor pollicis brevis. In ancient times, this depression was used to place a pinch of tobacco and then smell it; hence the name of this anatomical formation.

Metacarpophalangeal extension of the thumb

Extensor pollicis brevis

Extension of the proximal phalanx, maintaining the distal phalanx slightly flexed, in a seated position with the forearm in the intermediate position or slightly pronated resting on the examination table, the hand resting on the examination table, the proximal and distal phalanges of the thumb flexed and resistance applied to the dorsal surface of the proximal phalanx.

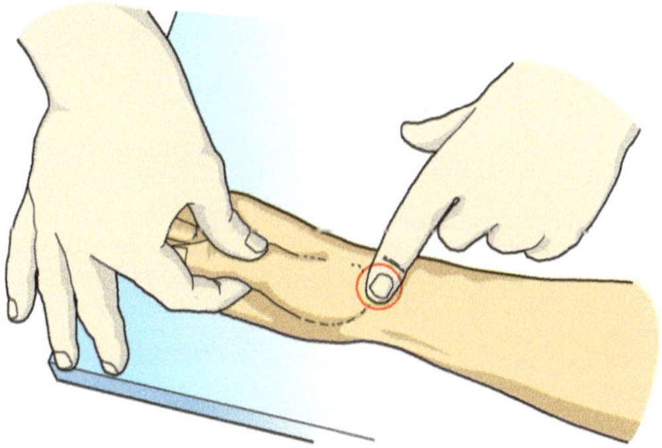

The extensor pollicis brevis can be palpated on the dorsoradial surface of the wrist at the base of the 1st metacarpal. Its tendon forms the radial margin of the anatomical snuffbox.

Radial abduction of the thumb

Abductor pollicis longus

Abduction of the thumb in the radial direction, forming a 45° angle between the thumb and index finger, in a seated position with the supinated forearm resting on the examination table, the hand resting on the examination table, the thumb adducted against the palmar (volar) surface of the index finger and resistance applied to the lateral surface of the 1st metacarpal.

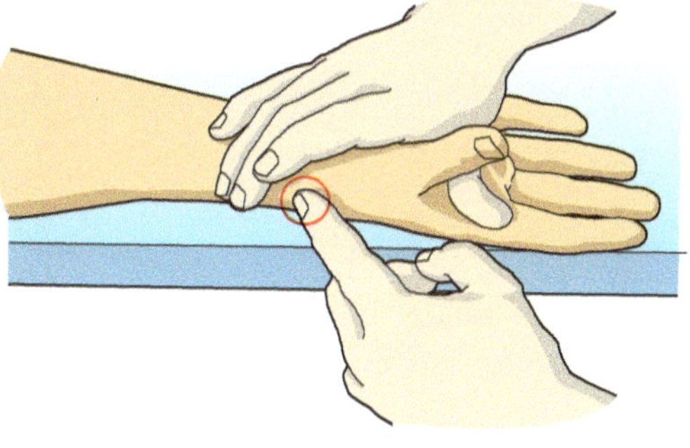

The abductor pollicis longus can be palpated on the lateral surface of the wrist at the base of the 1st metacarpal and on the radial side of the extensor pollicis brevis.

Palmar abduction of the thumb

Abductor pollicis brevis

Abduction of the thumb, forming a 90° angle between the thumb and index finger, in a seated position with the supinated forearm resting on the examination table, the hand resting on the examination table, the thumb adducted against the palmar (volar) surface of the index finger and resistance applied to the lateral surface of the proximal phalanx of the thumb.

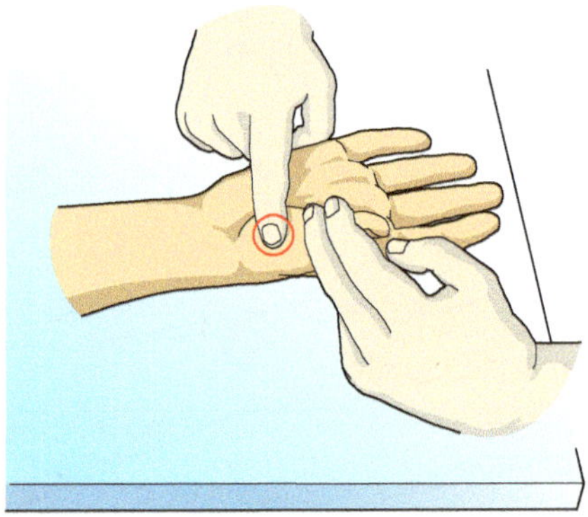

The abductor pollicis brevis can be palpated on the lateral surface of the 1st metacarpal.

Adduction of the thumb

Adductor pollicis

Adduction of the thumb, maintaining the proximal and distal phalanges flexed, in a seated position with the supinated forearm resting on the examination table, the hand resting on the examination table, the fingers extended and resistance applied to the medial surface of the proximal phalanx of the thumb.

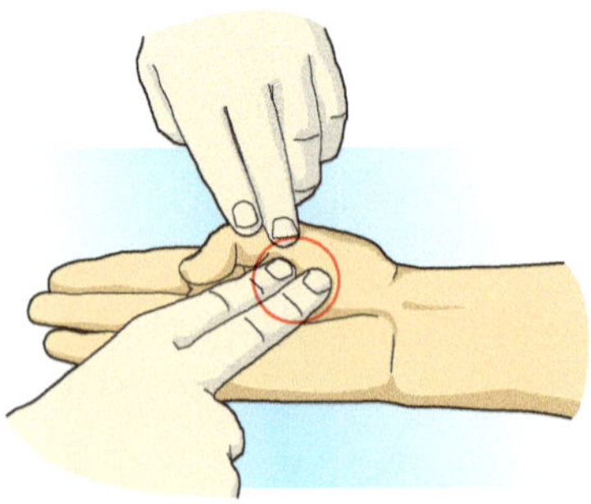

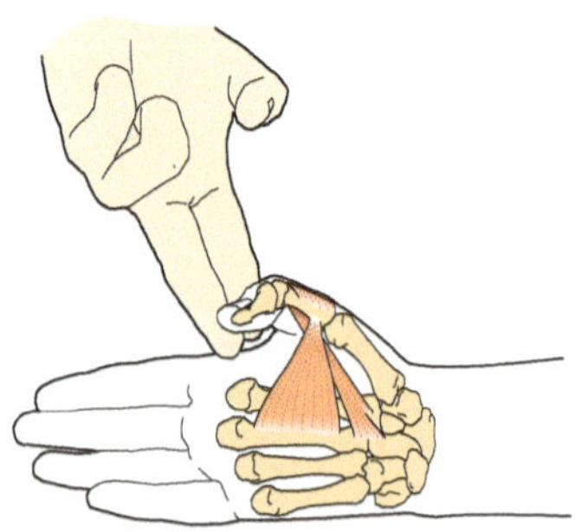

The adductor pollicis can be palpated on the palmar (volar) surface of the hand between the 1st and 2nd metacarpals.

Opposition of the thumb to the little finger

Opponens pollicis and opponens digiti minimi

Flexion and internal rotation of the 1st metacarpal in the direction of the little finger and flexion and rotation of the little finger in the direction of the thumb up to the contact between the pulps of the two fingers, keeping the distal phalanges extended, in a seated position with the supinated forearm resting on the examination table, the hand resting on the examination table, the last four fingers extended and the thumb extended and abducted in the palmar direction, then adducted (since vice versa the opposition of the thumb is not possible).

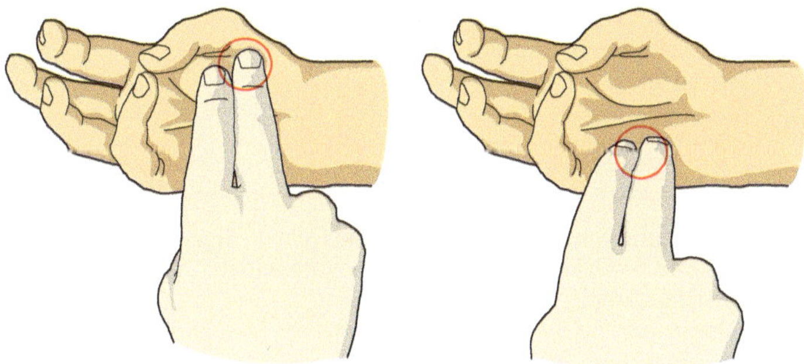

The opponens pollicis can be palpated laterally to the abductor pollicis brevis on the radial surface of the body of the 1st metacarpal; the opponens digiti minimi can be palpated on the palmar (volar) surface of the body of the 5th metacarpal.

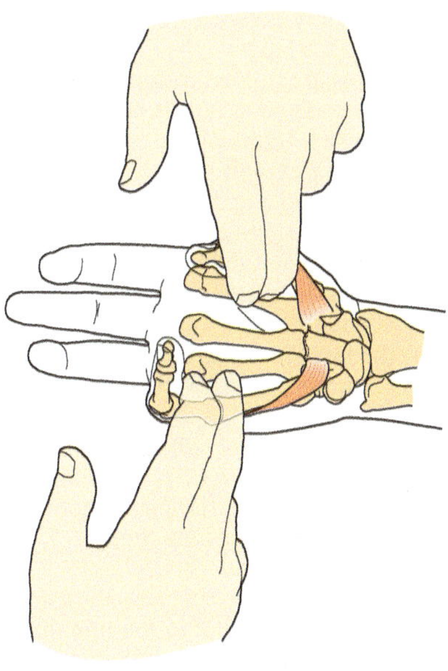

Prehension and grip functions

Prehension

The total of functions brought into play when an object is grasped with the hands. These include:
- intentionality
- continuous sensory control
- gripping mechanism.

Grip

Mechanical manual component of prehension.
Grip can be classified as:
- power grip
- precision grip and fine manipulation.

Power grip

The object is grasped tightly in a vice formed by the flexed fingers and the palm of the hand, to which extra pressure produced by the thumb may be added.
Four phases are distinguished:
- opening of the hand
- placement of the fingers
- digits approaching the object
- gripping.

Opening of the hand

- The hand is positioned in relation to the physical characteristics of the object (full hand opening is not required during daily activities such as personal care, while it may be necessary during leisure or work activities)
- The flexion of the wrist facilitates the full extension of the fingers, which is necessary to fully open the hand and grip large objects (in this position, the tip of the thumb is at the level of the proximal interphalangeal joints of the other fingers)
- If the dimensions of the open hand exceed those of the object, the proximal phalanges remain fully extended, while the middle and distal phalanges are flexed to some extent, so that the gripping surfaces of the fingers coincide with the object
- The opening phase is dynamic, characterized by concentric contractile muscular activity:
  - the active opening is performed thanks to the synergistic action of the flexor muscles of the hand and extensors of the fingers:
    - the extensor muscles of the last four fingers extend the proximal phalanges and have a secondary extensor action on the hand (their integrity is essential to the active opening of the fingers)
    - the flexor muscles of the hand contract synergistically, keeping the hand in neutral or flexed position
- The larger the object to be grasped, the greater the abduction movements of the last four fingers and radial abduction and extension of the thumb.

Placement of the fingers

- The choice of finger position is made parallel to the opening phase of the hand and the desired position is achieved through the metacarpophalangeal and interphalangeal joints.

- The extensor muscles of the fingers are essential to be able to extend the proximal phalanges
- The lumbricals are essential to be able to reach the required gripping position
- The interossei replace the lumbricals when the grip requires ulnar abduction of one or more metacarpophalangeal joints.

Digits approaching the object

- The movement pattern that characterizes this phase comprises:
  - extension of the hand
  - flexion of the thumb and other fingers
  - adduction of the fingers
- The extension of the wrist facilitates the full flexion of the last four fingers when they grip the object (once the object has been reached, the fingers are generally flexed at the same time, so that the palm of the hand comes into contact with the object)
- The flexor digitorum profundus is essential in order to freely close the hand
- The extensor carpi muscles fix the joint, neutralizing the flexion caused by the flexor digitorum profundus and flexor digitorum superficialis
- The muscles of the thenar eminence, when the thumb is also involved, are active to bring the finger closer to the object and take it to its final position of adduction and/or opposition
- The position of the hand and the activity of the muscles are influenced by the shape of the object to be held.

Gripping

- This last phase, of power or stabilization (static phase), is characterized by isometric muscle contraction
- It has three characteristics:
  - the wrist is maintained in neutral position or in extension
  - the fingers are maintained in flexion and abduction or adduction
  - the palmar (volar) surfaces of the fingers and certain areas of the palm of the hand exert strong pressure on the object
- The thumb may or may not be involved in gripping (in the latter case it may be a hook grip or digital-palmar opposition) – flexed and adducted when it must apply force; flexed and abducted when requiring precision
- The shape, size and/or weight of the object influence the degree of finger flexion, the palmar contact area and the position of the thumb (when holding cylinders of different sizes, the angle of the distal interphalangeal joints remains constant and the fingers adapt to the dimensions of each cylinder by changing the joint angles at the metacarpophalangeal and proximal interphalangeal joints; as the diameter of the cylindrical object increases, the total gripping force decreases)
- The ability of the last two ulnar fingers to flex and rotate at the carpometacarpal joints and to flex more than 90° in correspondence with the metacarpophalangeal joints contributes to the digital-palmar contact of the ulnar part of the hand
- The muscles of the hypothenar eminence, especially the flexor digiti minimi brevis and abductor digiti minimi, contract by flexing the 5th metacarpal and the proximal phalanx of the little finger, and the abductor digiti minimi also rotates the 5th metacarpal (by contracting, these muscles provide force to the grip, which also requires the participation of the flexor carpi ulnaris, in order to increase the contractions of the flexor digiti minimi brevis and abductor digiti minimi through the common insertion of these muscles in the pisiform)
- The ring and the little fingers can only generate 70% of the force developed by the index and middle fingers, meaning that the radial fingers are primarily responsible for the power

- If more force is needed in the grip, the hand is abducted in the ulnar direction (in this position the greatest degree of force can be obtained at the level of the phalanges)
- The extrinsic flexor muscles of the hand provide the greatest force to the grip; both the flexor digitorum profundus and flexor digitorum superficialis contribute to the power of the grip and the work of the latter increases as force requirement increases
- The major work of the intrinsic muscles of the hand is done by the interosseous muscles that abduct or adduct the proximal phalanges by aligning the fingers with the object, allowing the extrinsic flexor muscles of the hand to contribute to the power of the grip by flexing the proximal phalanges
- If the power grip involves the adduction and flexion of the thumb, the muscle power is provided by the isometric contraction of the adductor pollicis and flexor pollicis longus, while the flexor pollicis brevis contributes to the stability of the grip
- There are three types of power grip:
  - hooked grip (or digital-palmar opposition) – does not require the use of the thumb; for example: holding the handle of a suitcase
  - full hand palmar grip – the thumb in far from, near or above the other fingers depending on the size of the object; for example: holding a glass in the hand
  - vice grip – the last four fingers press one side of the object and the thumb presses on the opposite side; for example: holding a book in the hand.

Precision grip and fine manipulation

The object is held between the volar surface of one or more fingers with the thumb in opposition, stabilized and kept still in order to be moved via the actions of the proximal part of the upper limb.
The object may be manipulated while it is held in the hand (**fine manipulation** or **precision dexterity**).
In the precision grip and fine manipulation, three phases are recognized:
- opening of the hand
- placement of the fingers
- movement of the fingers towards the object.

However, the last phase is different: in precision grip it corresponds to static grip of the object, in fine manipulation to manipulation of the object.

Opening of the hand

- The amplitude of the opening and the number of fingers used depend on the size of the object and its use
- The position of the hand varies according to the location and use of the object and the task to be performed
- Due to the great variability of ways in which an object can be gripped or manipulated, the magnitude of movement and muscle activity is much greater than in power grips (even in case of similar movement patterns, more refined motor control is required due to the greater precision required).

Placement of the fingers

- The placement of the fingers in relation to the object is verified at the same time as the opening phase of the hand, thanks to the numerous positions allowed by the metacarpophalangeal and interphalangeal joints (in precision grip and fine manipulation, the thumb is almost always involved and in opposition, making contact with the pulp of another finger or more fingers).

Movements of the fingers towards the object

- The hand may be extended or remain flexed, while the proximal phalanges are flexed (generally the proximal phalanges of the index, middle and ring fingers are flexed, while that of the little finger may be flexed or extended according to functional needs – the little finger is flexed when pressing an object or the other fingers, and extended when an object is held or manipulated with the other fingers, providing tactile information or helping to stabilize the hand on the action surface)
- There is no abduction of the hand
- The abduction or adduction of one or more fingers may be added to the flexion of the proximal phalanges of the fingers
- The middle phalanges are flexed or extended (while flexion of the interphalangeal joints is needed for successive manipulation, their flexion or extension may be required for precision gripping)
- The distal phalanges may be flexed or extended
- The integrity of the flexor digitorum profundus is critical for the approach to the object in the pattern of flexion movement
- The activity of the lumbricals is essential for starting an approach in extension
- The approach of the thumb includes the movement of opposition (involving a sequential movement that comprises abduction, flexion and adduction of the 1st metacarpal with simultaneous rotation)
- The control by the thenar eminence is achieved with the opponens pollicis, flexor pollicis brevis, abductor pollicis brevis and adductor pollicis.

Precision grip

- There are four types of precision grip:
  - interdigital pinch (or laterolateral interdigital) grip – between the internal surface of the index finger and that of the middle finger (or also between the other fingers); for example: holding a pencil or a cigarette with the hand
  - grip by terminal opposition (superior pinch) – between two or three fingers; for example: picking a needle from the ground (between the thumb and index finger)
  - grip by subterminal opposition (superior pinch) – gripping between three or more fingers performed by the entire fingertip; for example: holding a small ball (between three fingers) or drinking from a glass (between five fingers)
  - grip by subterminolateral opposition (inferior grip or lateral pinch) – between the thumb and another finger (usually the index finger), characterized by the pressure exerted by the pulp of the thumb on the lateral surface of another finger; for example: using a key or holding the handle of a cup.

Fine manipulation (or precision dexterity)

- Manipulation of an object using the five fingers
- Mainly involves the two radial fingers and the thumb, while the two ulnar fingers may be involved in the manipulation and stabilization of the object
- The position of the five fingers is partially determined by the size and shape of the object, but the most important element is represented by the changes in the position of the object made by the hand.
- The static phase is very short and the pressure exerted on the object is light
- The hand can be extended or flexed
- It is carried out through concentric muscle contractions
- The muscles of the thenar eminence are involved – flexor pollicis brevis, opponens pol-

licis and abductor pollicis brevis (the latter contracts only when a force action against the index finger is required)

- The muscles of the hypothenar eminence are involved when the little finger is flexed or abducted (contraction of the abductor digiti minimi, opponens digiti minimi and flexor digiti minimi brevis).

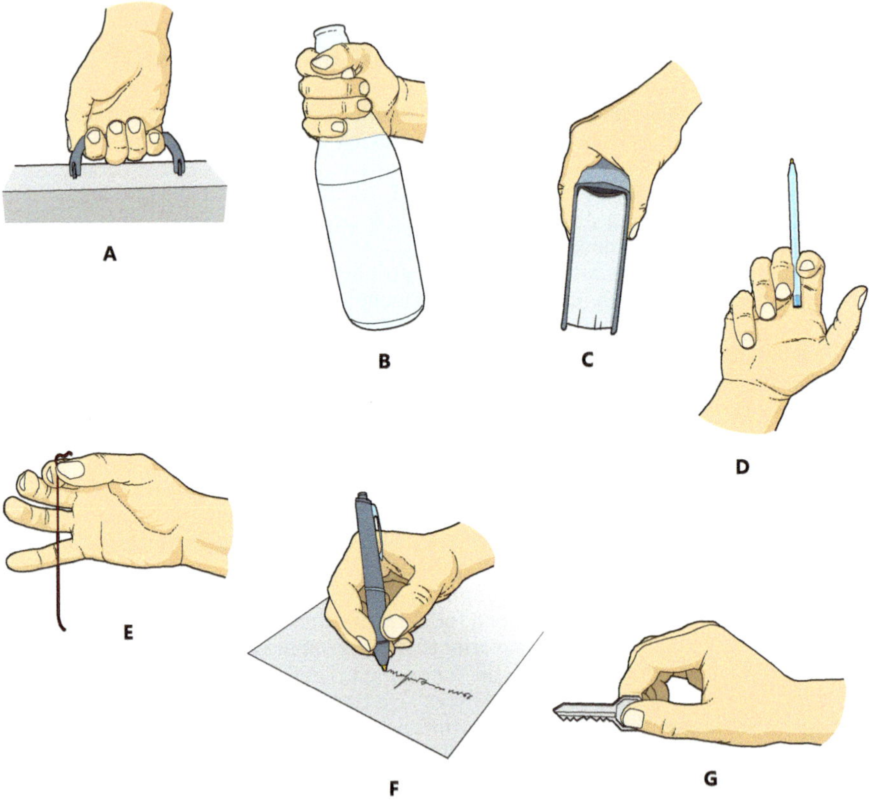

A, Hook grip (or by digital-palmar opposition); **B**, full hand palmar grip; **C**, vice grip; **D**, interdigital pinch grip (or laterolateral interdigital grip); **E**, superior pinch (or grip by terminal opposition); **F**, grip by subterminal opposition; **G**, inferior grip (or grip by subterminolateral opposition or lateral pinch).

Palpation of the wrist and hand

Proximal carpal row

To easily identify the carpal bones, start by locating the radial and ulnar styloid processes; the former is a robust protuberance on the distal extremity of the radius; the latter, more proximal than the former, is an obvious ulnar relief and distal to the head of the ulna. Proceeding with palpation in the distal direction, a slight depression can be appreciated, where the proximal carpal row is located.

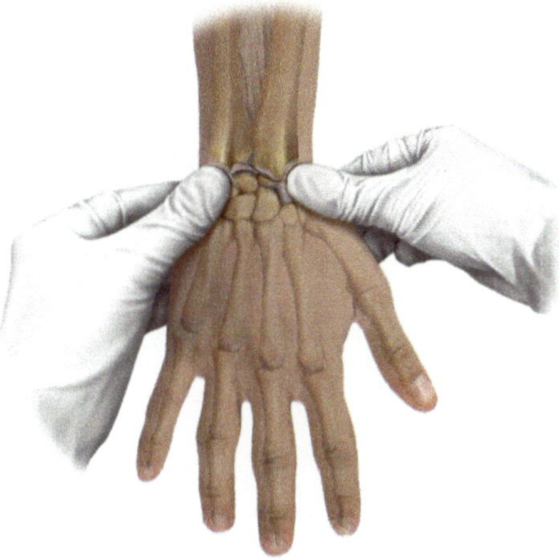

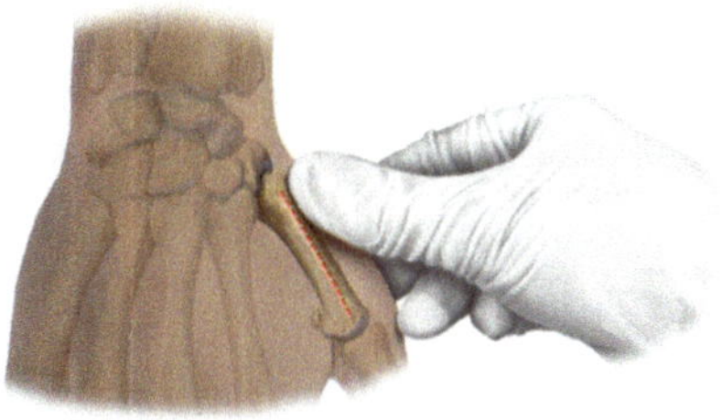

First metacarpal

Palpation starts from the distal extremity, easily evidenced by asking the patient to flex the thumb. From here, the palpating finger follows the shaft (body) of the first metacarpal to the base, the identification of which is made even easier by a passive circumduction of the thumb.

9

Second metacarpal

To identify the metacarpophalangeal joints, the patient is asked to flex the fingers and wrist. On the dorsal side of the hand, about 1 cm from the wrist crease, some protuberances corresponding to the base of the metacarpals can be palpated. The base of the second metacarpal can also be easily identified by starting palpation from its head, an obvious bony relief on the dorsum of the hand, at the metacarpophalangeal joint.

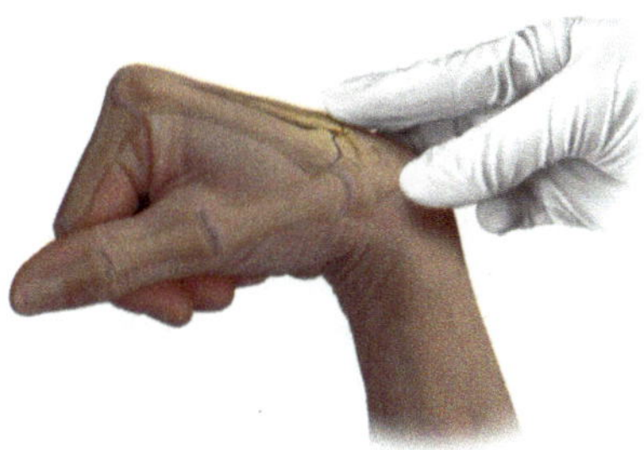

Pisiform

The base of the palm is explored on the ulnar side, looking for the small roundness of the pisiform. When passively flexing the wrist, it may oscillate from side to side, while extending the wrist will render it immobile, due to the tension created by the tendon of the flexor carpi ulnaris.

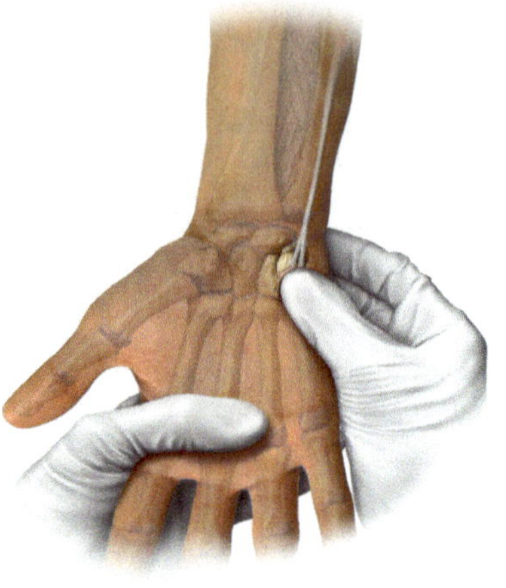

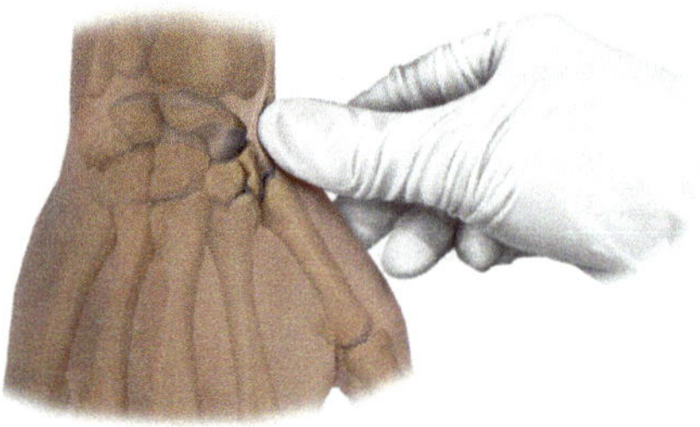

Trapezium

From the radial styloid process, move distally reaching first the scaphoid and then the trapezium, recognizable by the presence, on the palmar surface, of the protrusion of the tubercle of the trapezium. To verify that the trapezium has not been passed, the patient is asked to slowly perform some flexion-extensions of the thumb: if we are already at the base of the first metacarpal, the movement of the bone should be clearly perceived.

Scaphoid

From the radial styloid process, continue distally with the thumb until it reaches the depression where the scaphoid is lodged. The ulnar deviation of the wrist causes the scaphoid to press against the palpating finger. On the palmar surface, the tubercle of the scaphoid can be appreciated.

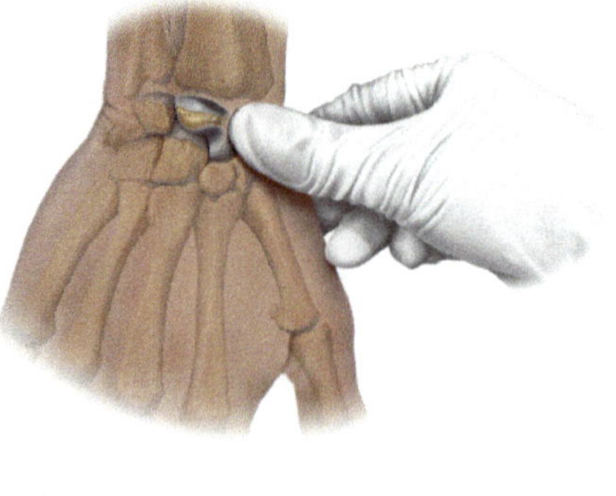

Hook of the hamate

The flat surface of the body of the hamate is palpable over the dorsal side of the hand, where the bases of the fourth and fifth metacarpals articulate. The hook of the hamate is palpable over the palmar surface, starting at the pisiform and proceeding along an imaginary line pointing towards the index finger.

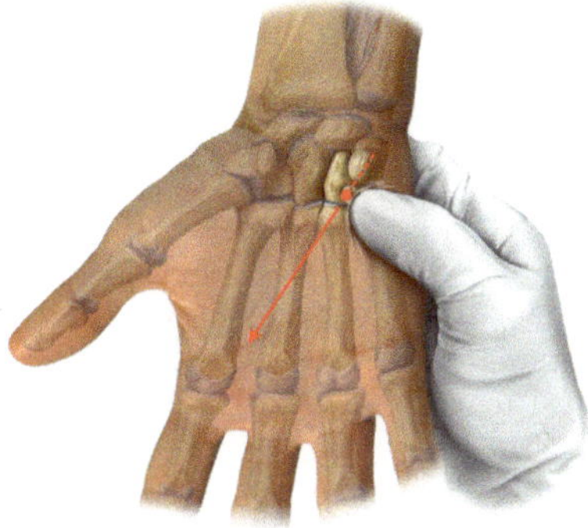

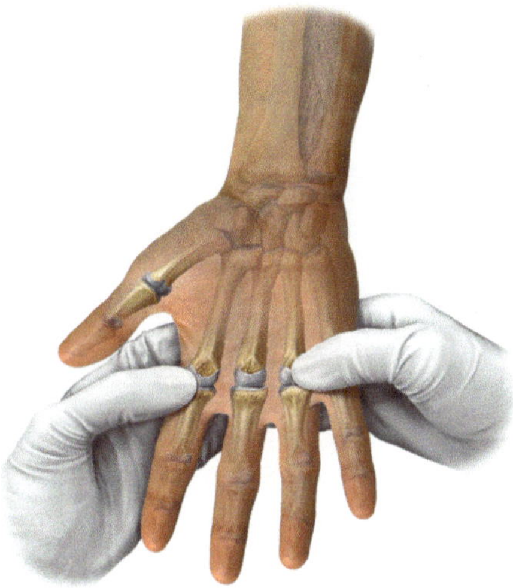

Metacarpophalangeal joints

They are easily identified by palpation because they protrude on the dorsal surface of the hand in the flexion movement of the fingers. Once one of these joints has been identified on the dorsal side, it is possible to distinguish the head of the metacarpal from the base of the proximal phalanx also on the palmar side.

Flexor retinaculum (transverse carpal ligament)

Holding the patient's hand in the supine position, the palpating thumb is placed in the center of the wrist crease. From here proceed distally for approximately 1 cm, until sliding into the carpal tunnel, where the tendons of the flexor muscles and the median nerve pass.

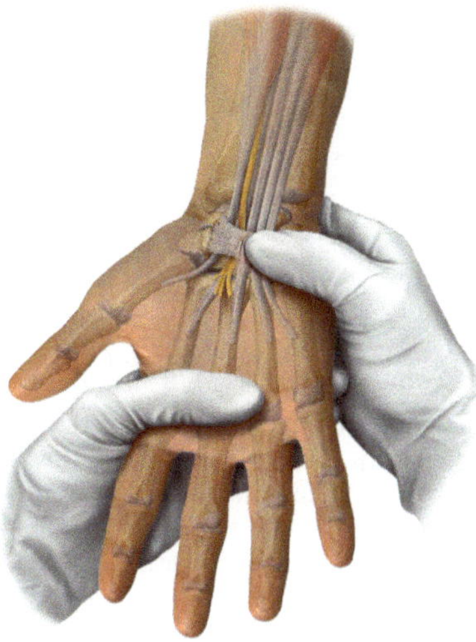

Tendon of the flexor pollicis longus

The muscle belly extends into the anterior region of the forearm, deep to the flexor carpi muscles and is therefore not palpable. The distal tendon crosses the carpal tunnel before reaching the base of the distal phalanx of the first finger and can be appreciated by asking the patient to flex the finger against resistance.

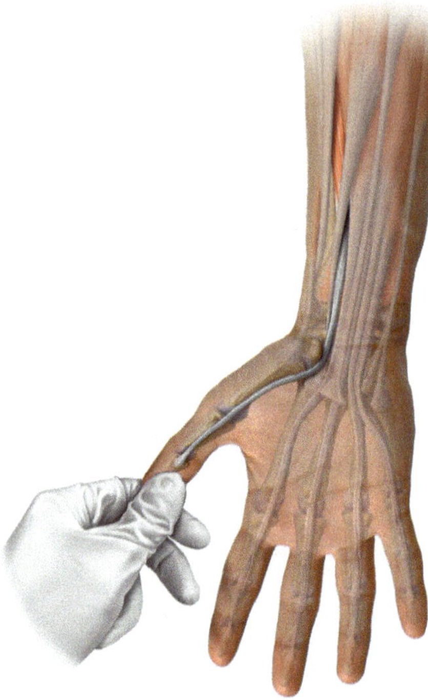

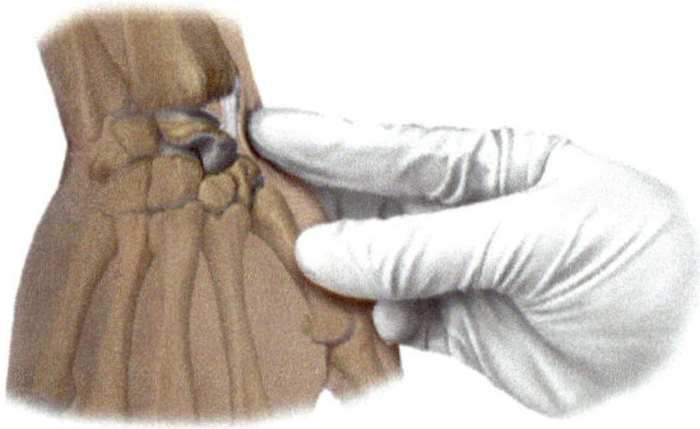

Radial collateral ligament of the wrist

Palpation is performed with the patient's forearm in pronation, his hand in the examiner's hand. A point is located between the radial styloid process and the scaphoid and palpated by asking the patient to deviate the wrist in the ulnar direction. During this movement, the tendon is tensed, facilitating palpation.

Ulnar collateral ligament of the wrist

Holding the patient's forearm in the supine position, palpation begins by locating a point between the ulnar styloid process and, distally, the triquetrum. Bringing the wrist in radial deviation, the tension of the ulnar collateral ligament of the wrist can be felt.

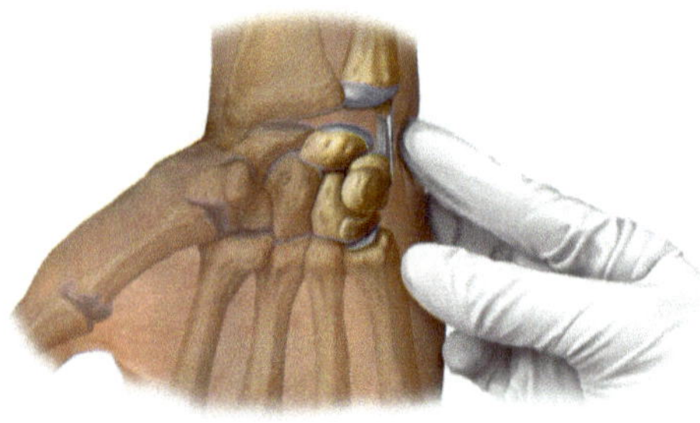

Anatomical landmarks on the surface of the wrist and hand

1	Ulnar styloid process: bony prominence on the posteromedial surface of the forearm, at the distal extremity of the ulna
2	Radial styloid process: bony prominence on the lateral surface of the forearm, at the distal extremity of the radius
3	Metacarpals [I-V]: the bases and shafts (bodies) are palpable between the tendons of the extensor muscles on the dorsal surface of the wrist and hand, while the bony prominences at the base of the fingers are formed by the heads
4	Capitate: in a small proximal concavity at the base of the 3rd metacarpal
5	Pisiform: medial bone of the proximal carpal row, proximal to the base of the hypothenar eminence
6	Interdigital space of the thumb: skin fold between the 1st finger and the hand
7	Distal palm crease: transverse sulcus running laterally from the medial border of the palm of the hand to the interdigital space between the 2nd and 3rd fingers
8	Proximal palmar crease: transverse sulcus traveling medially from the palm of the hand to the hypothenar eminence
9	Thenar eminence: muscular prominence on the palm of the hand at the base of the thumb, bounded medially and distally by the longitudinal palmar sulcus
10	Hypothenar eminence: muscular prominence on the medial side of the base of the palm of the hand

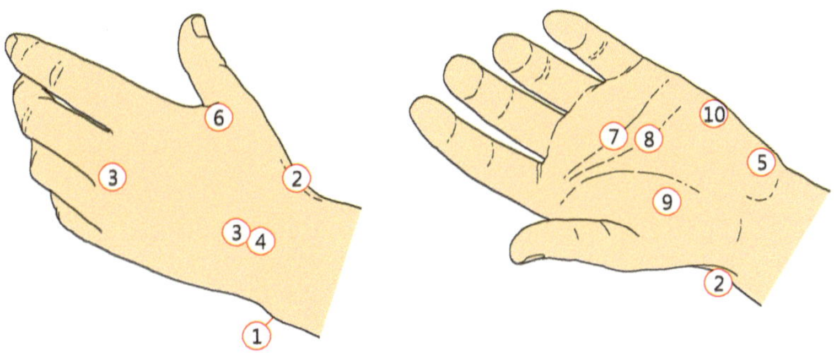

Pelvis

Also called pelvic girdle, it is formed:

- laterally: by the two hip bones (joined anteriorly through the pubic symphysis)
- in the center: by the sacrum (joined to the two hip bones through the sacroiliac joints) and the coccyx.

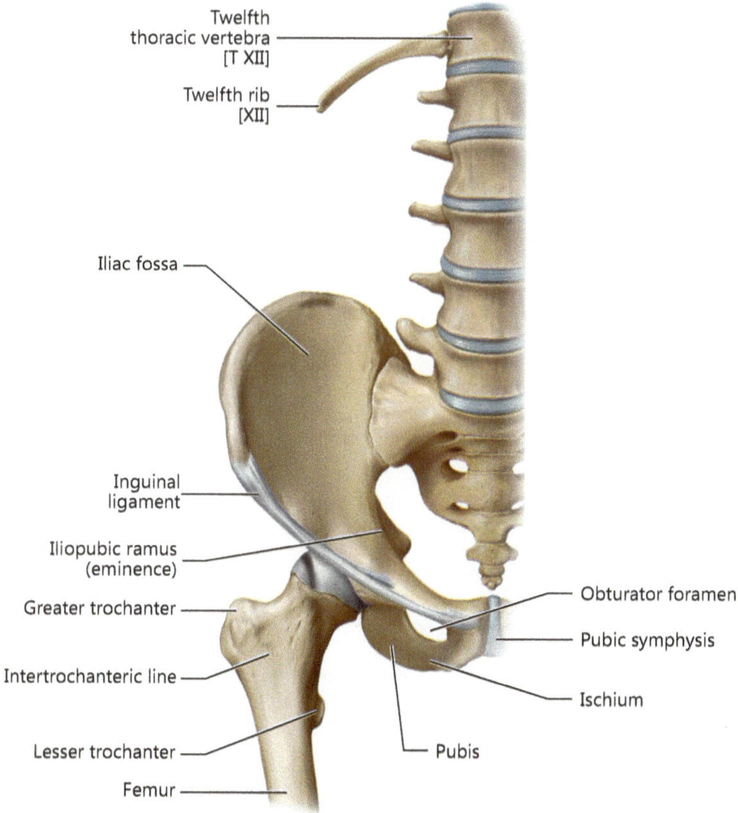

Anterior view of the pelvis.

The hip bone is joined to the femur through the coxofemoral joint (hip joint).

Hip bone

It derives from the fusion of three distinct bony parts separated by cartilage during fetal life and childhood:

- ilium
- ischium
- pubis.

Morphology

Two surfaces, external and internal, and four borders, anterior, superior, posterior and inferior.

The external surface

- In the center → the acetabulum
- Superior to the acetabulum → the gluteal surface
- Inferior to the acetabulum → the obturator foramen.

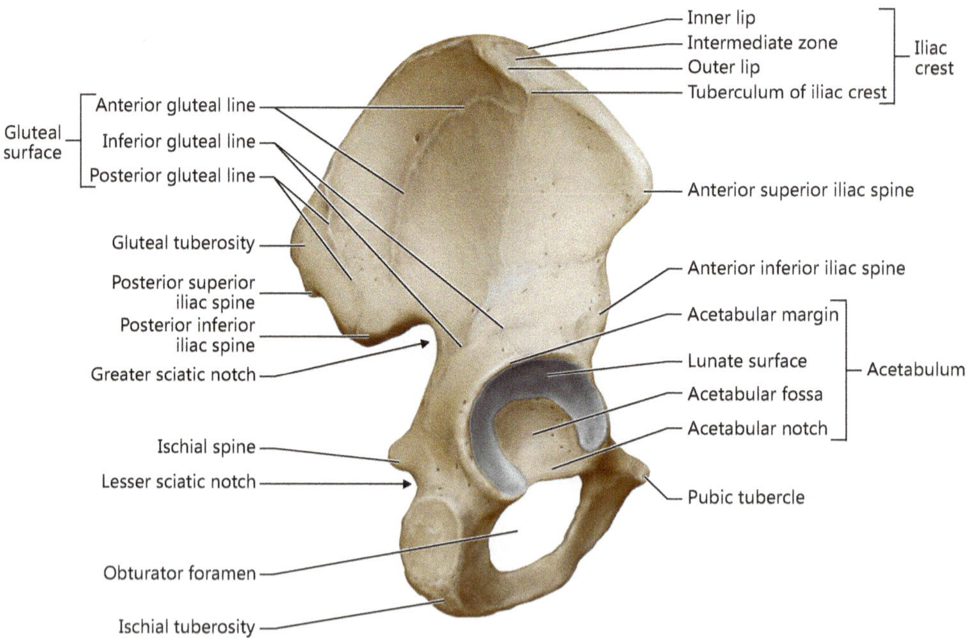

External view of the right hip bone. On the surface of the iliac part, the reliefs formed by the gluteal lines are observed. The meeting point of the ilium, ischium, and pubis is in the acetabular fossa.

The internal surface

- Divided into two parts by → the arcuate line
- Superior to the arcuate line → the iliac fossa
- Behind the arcuate line → the auricular surface
- Behind the auricular surface → the iliac tuberosity
- Inferior to the arcuate line → a flat surface corresponding externally to the acetabulum.

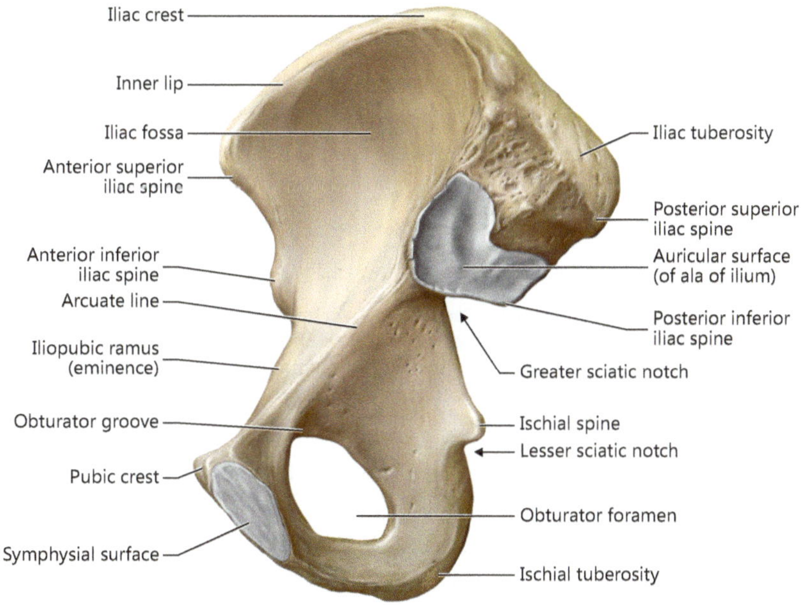

Internal view of the right hip bone. The arcuate line marks the limit between the iliac part of the hip bone that is part of the abdomen and the ischial and pubic portions that are part of the walls of the lesser pelvis.

Borders
- Anterior (from top to bottom):
  - anterior superior iliac spine
  - anterior inferior iliac spine
  - iliopubic ramus (eminence)
  - pectineal surface with pecten pubis (pectineal line)
  - pubic tubercle
- Posterior (from top to bottom):
  - posterior superior iliac spine
  - posterior inferior iliac spine
  - greater sciatic notch
  - ischial spine
  - lesser sciatic notch
  - ischial tuberosity
- Superior → iliac crest (delimited by two lips – outer and inner)
- Inferior → from the ischial tuberosity to the surface of the pubic symphysis.

Sacrum

It is the continuation of the lumbar segment of the vertebral column through the lumbosacral joint (between the body of the 5th lumbar vertebra and the base of the sacrum, and between the articular processes of the 5th lumbar vertebra and the 1st sacral vertebra) and joins the coccyx through the sacrococcygeal joint.

Morphology

Base upward, apex downward, and anterior, posterior and lateral surfaces.

Base
- Oval L-shaped central surface with greater transverse diameter → it articulates with the body of the 5th lumbar vertebra
- Angle with the 5th lumbar vertebra (convex anteriorly) → promontory of the sacrum
- Behind the articular surface for the 5th lumbar vertebra → superior orifice of the sacral canal
- Laterally to the superior orifice of the sacral canal → superior articular processes
- Laterally to the articular surface for the 5th lumbar vertebra → alae (wings) of the sacrum

Apex
- Elliptical articular surface for the base of the coccyx

Anterior surface
- Four transverse ridges (synostosis between the bodies of the primitive sacral vertebrae)
- Laterally to the line of synostosis → anterior (or ventral) sacral foramina (four pairs, in communication with the sacral canal)

Posterior surface
- On the midline → median sacral crest
- Inferiorly to the median sacral crest → sacral hiatus (posterior opening of the sacral canal)
- Laterally to the median sacral crest → posterior (dorsal) sacral foramina

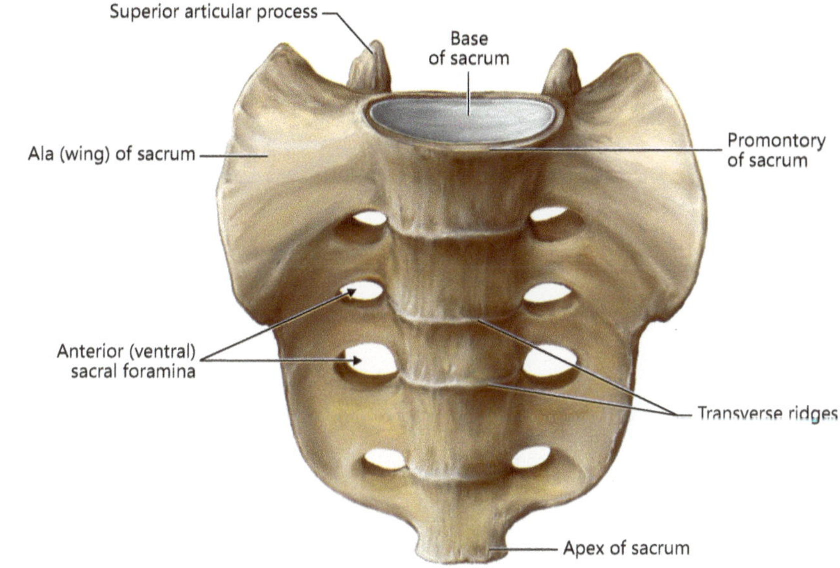

Anterior surface of the sacrum. The upper part of the bone is broadened into the wings; a number of transverse ridges in the middle mark the welding between the primitive bone metamers.

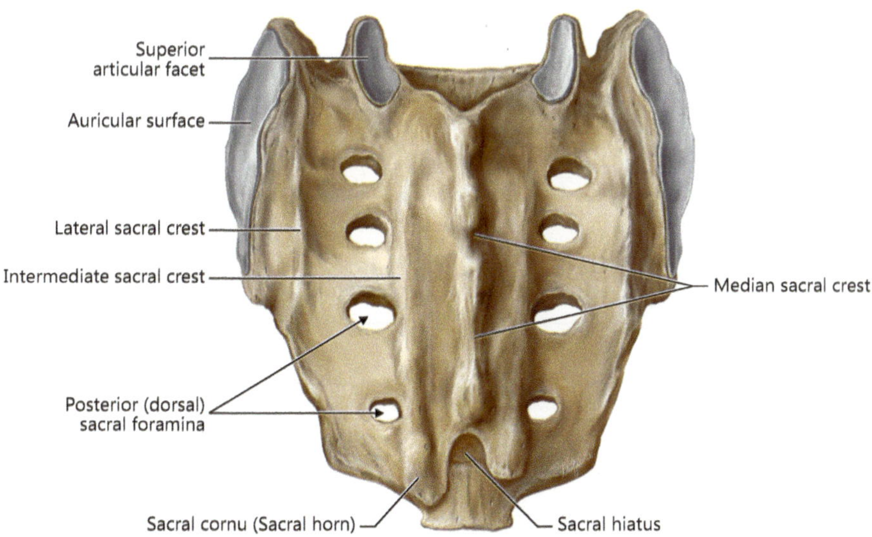

Posterior surface of the sacrum. The bone surface appears prominent in the center of the median sacral crest and rough laterally where it gives insertion to numerous muscles.

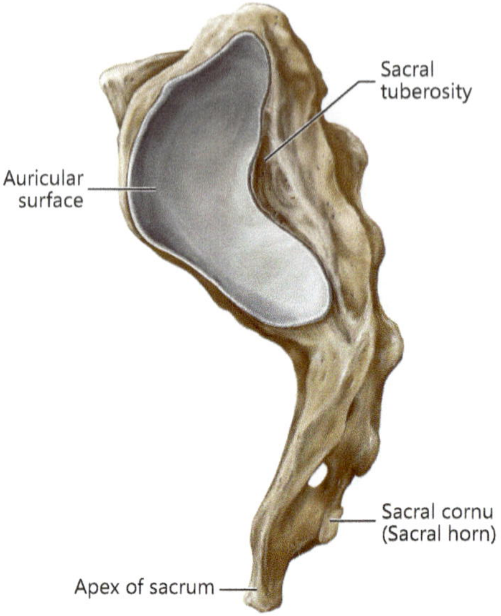

- Laterally to the posterior (or dorsal) sacral foramina → lateral sacral crests with tubercles

Lateral surface
- Superiorly → auricular surface
- Posteriorly to the auricular surface → the sacral tuberosity.

Left lateral surface of the sacrum. This surface broadens towards the top into the auricular surface; the prominence of the sacral tuberosity is behind this articular surface.

Coccyx

Base upward, tip downward, anterior and posterior surfaces and lateral borders.
Base → articulates with the apex of the sacrum.

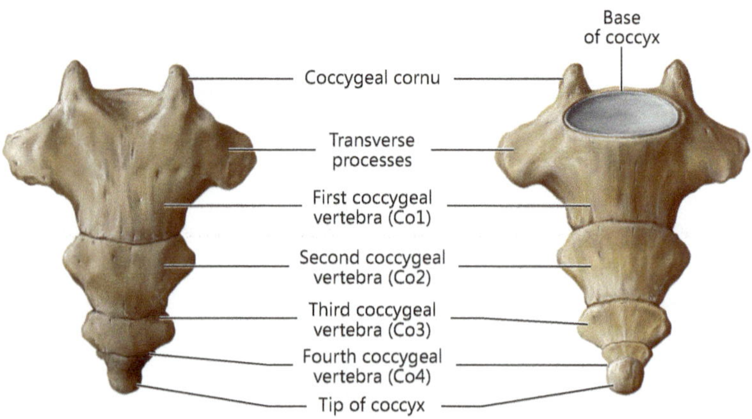

Posterior surface (**A**) and anterior surface (**B**) of the coccyx. The vestiges of the primitive bone segments can be observed.

Diameters of the pelvis

Pelvic inlet

- True conjugate:
  - distance between the promontory of the sacrum and the superior border of the pubic symphysis (approximately 11 cm)
- Diagonal conjugate:
  - distance between the promontory of the sacrum and the inferior border of the pubic symphysis (approximately 13 cm)
- Oblique diameter:
  - distance between the sacroiliac joint of one side and the iliopubic ramus (eminence) of the opposite side (approximately 12 cm)
- Transverse diameter (maximum):
  - distance between the most lateral points of the arcuate lines of each side (approximately 13 cm).

Pelvic outlet

- Anteroposterior diameter:
  - distance between the tip of the coccyx and the superior border of the pubic symphysis (approximately 9 cm)
- Transverse diameter:
  - distance between the ischial tuberosity of one side and that of the opposite side (approximately 11 cm).

Note: During labor, the conditions of ligamentous relaxation allow as increase in the width of the pelvic outlet of 3-4 cm.

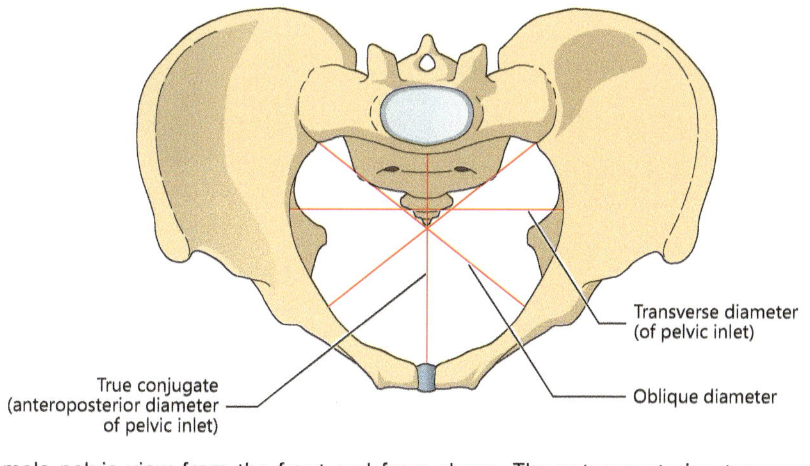

Female pelvis view from the front and from above. The anteroposterior, transverse and oblique diameters have been delineated in the pelvic inlet.

Superior extremity and shaft (body) of the femur

In the femur, which forms the skeleton of the thigh, a shaft (body) and two extremities, superior and inferior, can be distinguished.

Superior extremity

Head of the femur:
- spherical shape
- articular facet

Anatomical neck:
- its axis is aligned with that of the head
- it forms an angle of 130° with the axis of the shaft (body)

Greater trochanter:
- at the base of the anatomical neck, laterally and upward

Lesser trochanter:
- at the base of the anatomical neck, medially and downward

Intertrochanteric crest:
- joins the two trochanters

Trochanteric fossa:
- at the base of the greater trochanter, medially

Surgical neck:
- just below the lesser trochanter
- marks the boundary between the diaphysis and the epiphysis.

Shaft (body) of the femur

Three surfaces – anterior, posteromedial and posterolateral – and three borders – medial, lateral and posterior.
- Linea aspera (posterior border):
  - in the lower part gives rise to two branches that are directed to the condyles (bulky oval masses located in the inferior extremity of the femur), in the upper part gives rise to three branches represented (lateromedially) by:
    - the lateral lip of the linea aspera
    - the pectineal line
    - the medical lip of the linea aspera
- Popliteal triangle:
  - triangle between the branches of the lower division of the linea aspera.

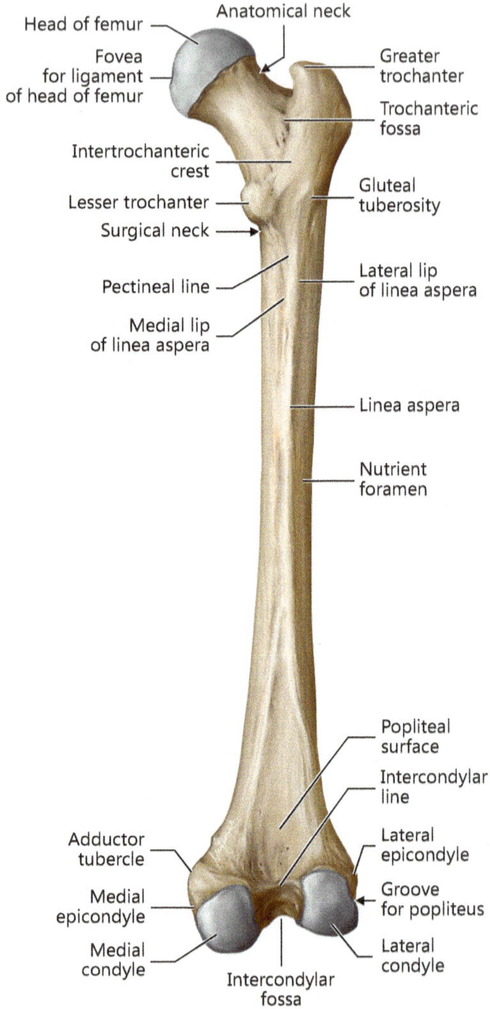

Posterior surface of the right femur.

Joints of the pelvis

- Sacroiliac joint
- Pubic symphysis
- Lumbosacral joint
- Sacrococcygeal joint
- Coxofemoral joint (hip joint)

Sacroiliac joint

Type of joint	Amphiarthrosis
Articular surfaces	Auricular surface of the sacrum: • with predominant irregularities and prominences • concave mainly in the center • convex inferiorly Auricular surface of the hip bone: • irregular • wider and shorter • prevalence of convexity only partially in concordance with the corresponding concavities of the auricular facet of the sacrum
Movements	The conformation of the auricular facets limits the possibility of reciprocal sliding between the two bones Minimal movements cushion the stresses on the vertebral column and coxofemoral joints (and also during birth) 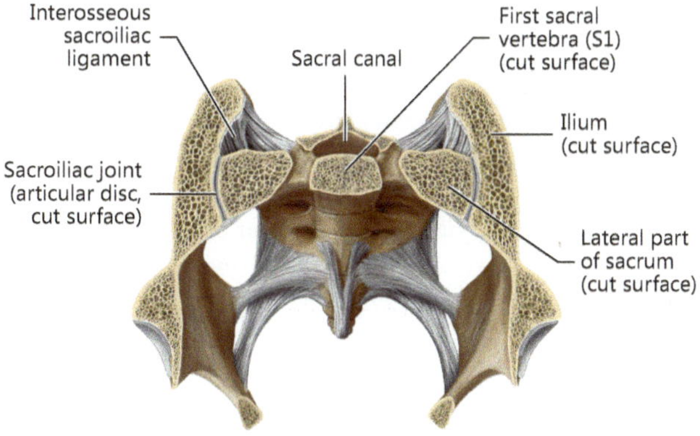 Transverse section passing through the first sacral segment showing the relationships between the sacrum and the hip bones at the level of the sacroiliac joints.

Pubic symphysis

Type of joint	Symphysis
Articular surfaces	Surfaces of the pubic symphysis: • oval shape • located at the junction points between the superior and inferior branches of the pubis • covered by fibrous cartilage and joined by hyaline cartilage and connective tissue (interpubic disc)
Movements	Reduced motility: • cushioning stresses of the lower limbs • during labor, the laxity of the interpubic disc, produced by hormonal variations and increased by the imbibition of serous fluid, facilitates fetal transit 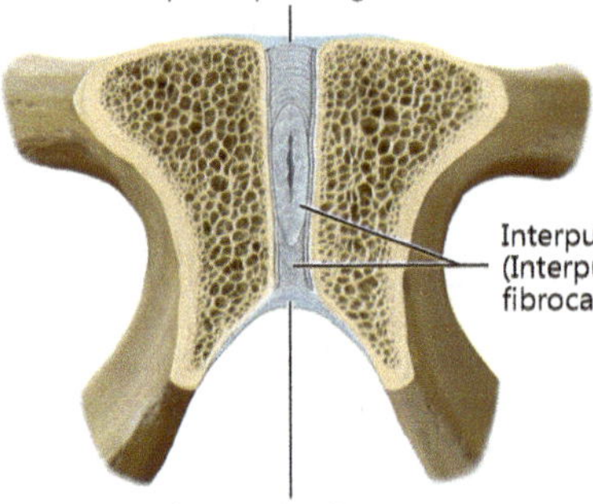

Lumbosacral joint

Type of joint	Synchondrosis (intervertebral joint) and plane joint (zygapophysial joint)
Articular surfaces	Intervertebral joint: • inferior surface of the 5th lumbar vertebra • oval surface in the center of the base of the sacrum • between the articular surfaces is the intervertebral disc: – reduced disc height – greater asymmetry between the anterior and posterior disc height in relation to the other vertebrae Zygapophysial joint: • posteroinferior articular surfaces of the 5th lumbar vertebra • superior articular processes of the 1st sacral vertebra

The 5th lumbar vertebra is the one with the largest transverse diameter among all the vertebrae. This characteristic, together with those of the intervertebral disc, makes it more mobile. The movements are of sliding at the level of the articular processes and of the disc in the body of the 5th lumbar vertebra and at the base of the sacrum.

Sacrococcygeal joint

Type of joint	Amphiarthrosis (presence of the "articular disc" between the two surfaces as interosseous ligament)
Articular surfaces	Convex sacral surface Concave coccygeal surface
Movements	Modest degree of flexion-extension (retropulsion of the coccyx) during labor and defecation (increase of the anteroposterior diameter of the pelvic outlet)

Coxofemoral joint (hip joint)

Type of joint	Ball and socket (spheroidal) joint
Articular surfaces	Acetabulum: • cavity consisting of a semilunar articular surface that: – is enlarged outward by a fibrocartilaginous contour (acetabular labrum) and surrounds the acetabular fossa (spherical in shape) • head of the femur (approximately two thirds of a sphere with a diameter of 40-50 cm) The acetabulum covers approximately two thirds of the head of the femur. While standing, it is directed upward, forward and medially, while the axis of the acetabulum is directed downward, forward and laterally, therefore, there is no concordance between the articular surfaces and much of the anterior surface of the head of the femur remains uncovered. On the other hand, there is concordance between the articular surfaces in the flexion, abduction and external rotation movements of the thigh and in the quadruped position.
Movements	All possible movements (6) in the frontal, sagittal and transverse planes (3 degrees of freedom): flexion-extension, abduction-adduction, external and internal rotation; to these the circumduction movement, derived from all the movements around the three rotation axes, is added

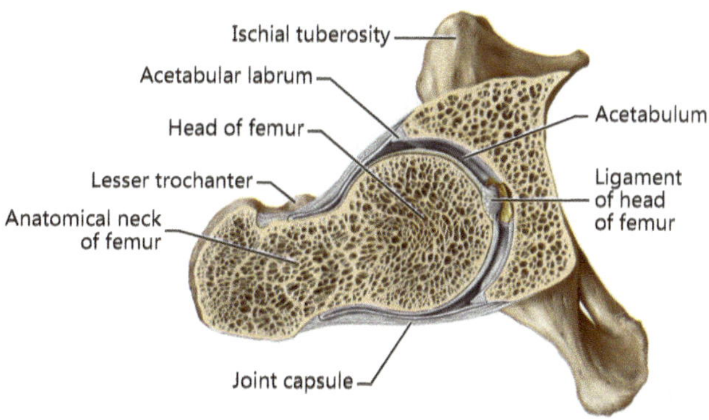

Ligaments of the joints of the pelvis

Sacroiliac joint

Direct ligaments:

- sacroiliac:
  - anterior
    - superior – between the anterior surface of the sacrum and the iliac crest
    - inferior – between the anterior surface of the sacrum and the greater sciatic notch
  - posterior – between the last tubercles of the lateral sacral crest and the posterior superior iliac spine
  - interosseous – between the posterior surface of the sacrum and the iliac part of the hip bone.

> The interosseous ligaments run in a horizontal plane between the posterior surface of the sacrum and the anterior part of the ilium and represent the rotation axis around which the movements of the sacrum occur.

Indirect ligaments:

- iliolumbar – between the transverse processes of the 4th and 5th lumbar vertebrae and the iliac crest
- sacrotuberous – between the posterior surface of the sacrum and the ischial tuberosity
- sacrospinous – between the lateral surface of the sacrum and the ischial spine.

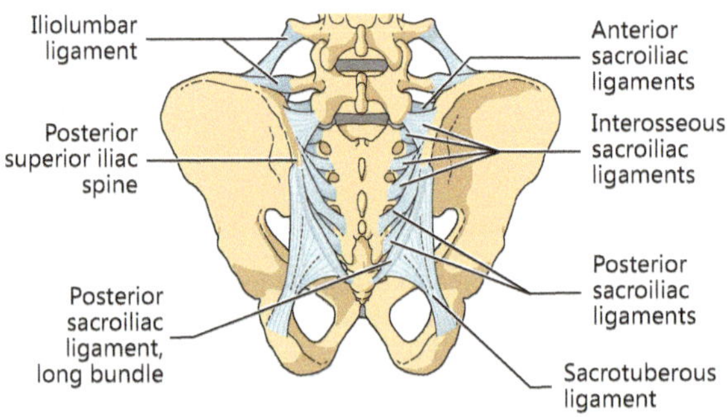

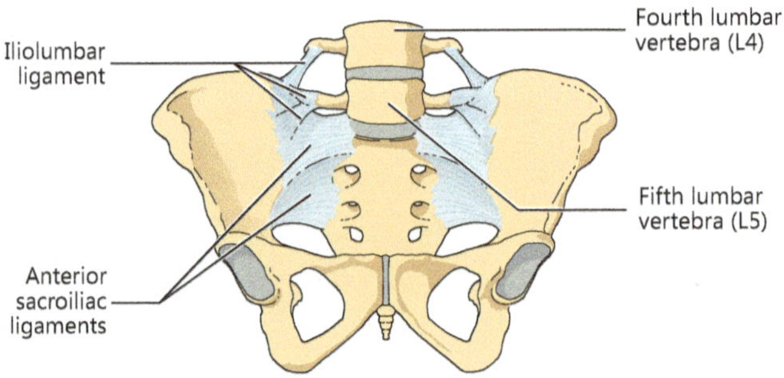

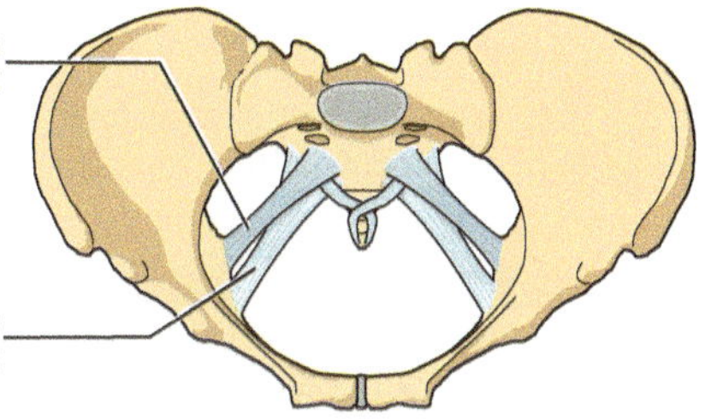

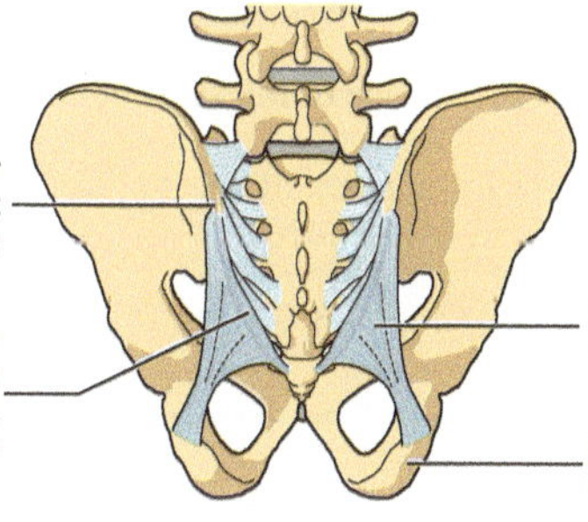

Function of these ligaments:

- to reinforce the joint capsule
- to hold the sacrum to the alae (wings) of the ilium (iliac crests and fossae).

Pubic symphysis

Ligaments:

- superior pubic – between the two pubic tubercles
- inferior (or arcuate) pubic – delimits the subpubic angle.

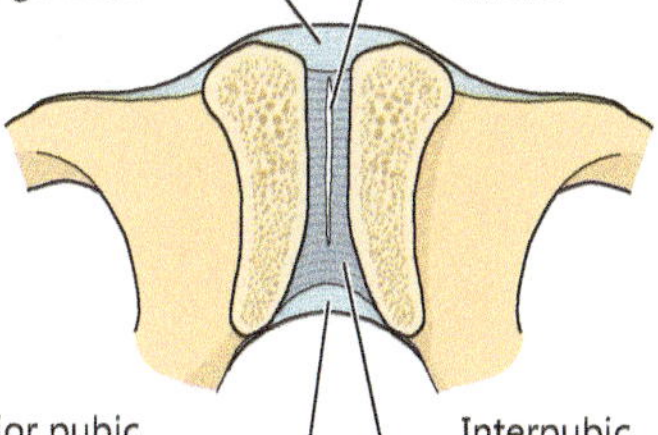

Function:

- stabilization of the joint.

Lumbosacral joint

(For the ligaments of the lumbosacral joint, see section "Ligaments of the vertebral column" in Chapter 5 "Vertebral column and movements of the trunk").

Sacrococcygeal joint

Sacrococcygeal ligaments:
- anterior – between the anterior surface of the sacrum inferiorly and the tip of the coccyx
- lateral:
  - external – between the lateral sacral crest inferiorly and the transverse process of the coccyx
  - middle – between the posterior surface of the sacrum and the transverse process of the coccyx
  - internal – between the posterior surface of the sacrum medially to the lateral sacral crest and the transverse process of the coccyx
- posterior:
  - superficial bundle – between the lateral sacral crest and the posterior surface of the coccyx
  - deep bundle – between the bodies of the last sacral segment and the first coccygeal segment.

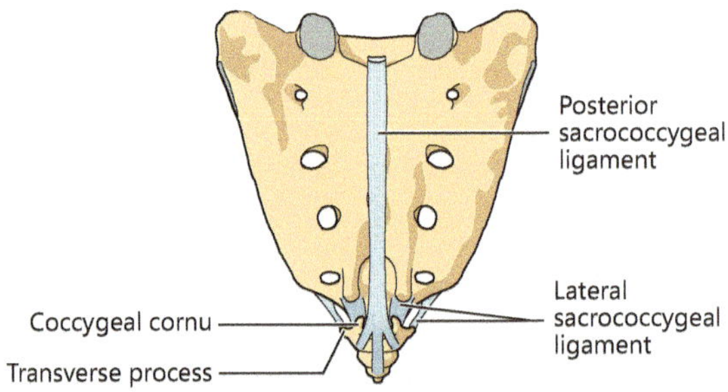

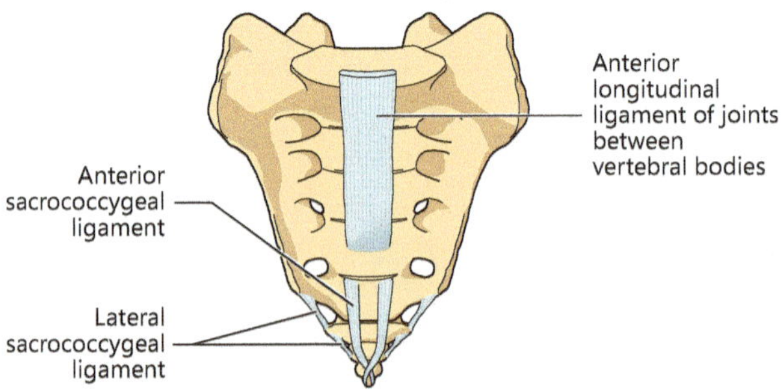

Function:
- stabilization of the joint.

Coxofemoral joint (hip joint)

Joint capsule:
- insertion on the hip bone – acetabular labrum and laterally on the hip bone
- insertion on the femur:
  - anteriorly → on the intertrochanteric line
  - posteriorly → laterally on the intertrochanteric crest (1-2 cm from it)

Ligaments:
- intracapsular:
  - of the head of the femur – between the acetabular fossa and the fovea for the ligament of the head of the femur
- extracapsular:
  - iliofemoral (or Bertin's ligament) – between the anterior inferior iliac spine and the intertrochanteric line (shaped like an "inverted Y", with two bundles directed towards the femur)
  - ischiofemoral – between the ischial side of the acetabular labrum and the trochanteric fossa (triangular in shape)
  - pubofemoral – between the superior pubic ramus anteriorly and the joint capsule anteromedially
  - bundle of the zona orbicularis – from the common origin with that of the ischiofemoral ligament, posteriorly from the acetabular labrum, it wraps the joint capsule under the iliofemoral, ischiofemoral and pubofemoral ligaments (with which it is connected).

> The extracapsular ligaments are longitudinal reinforcing ligaments of the capsule, which form thickening.

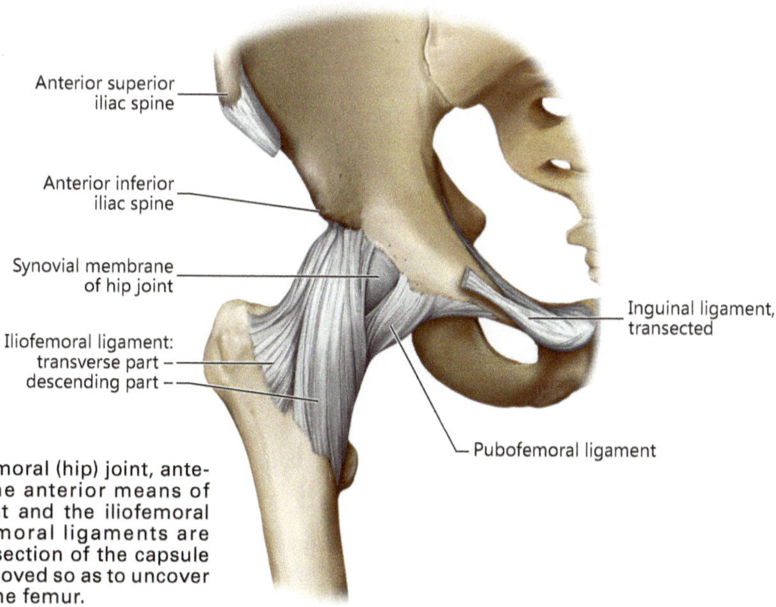

Right coxofemoral (hip) joint, anterior view. The anterior means of reinforcement and the iliofemoral and pubofemoral ligaments are observed; a section of the capsule has been removed so as to uncover the head of the femur.

10

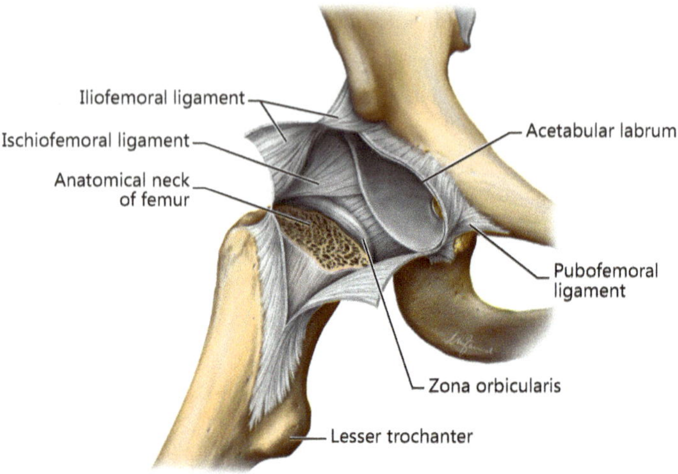

Right coxofemoral (hip) joint. After the anterior opening of the capsule and the resection of the head of the femur, the means of reinforcement, the ischiofemoral and pubofemoral ligaments, as well as the zona orbicularis can be observed.

Functions of the coxofemoral joint ligaments

- ligament of the head of the femur → stabilizes the head of the femur
- iliofemoral ligament:
  - mainly limits the extension of the hip (and in general also the other movements of the thigh, except flexion)
  - limits (with reverse traction) an excessive retroversion of the pelvis during erect position
  - prevents, together with the gluteal muscles, the fall of the pelvis towards the oscillation side (lower limb suspended from the ground) while walking, limiting the moving of the body's center of gravity in this direction

> The iliofemoral ligament is the strongest ligament in the human body, resisting a traction of 350 kg and, together with the other ligaments and the capsule of the coxofemoral joint, a traction of 500 kg.

- ischiofemoral ligament → mainly limits the internal rotation of the hip and its adduction when it is flexed
- pubofemoral ligament → limits the abduction of the hip and weakly its external rotation and extension.

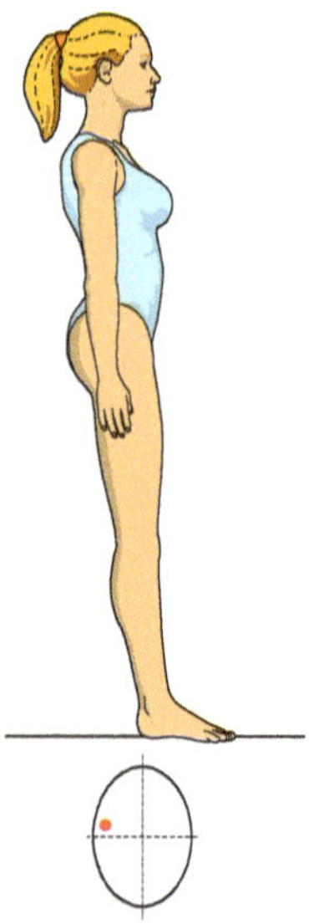

In the erect position, if the body's center of gravity falls behind the transverse axis that joins the centers of the femoral heads (bicondylar or coxofemoral axis), it accentuates the retroversion of the pelvis which, if not limited, would cause the trunk to fall posteriorly.

Movements of the pelvis

Anteversion (nutation or flexion of the pelvis)

Definition: rotation movement of the sacrum around the axis represented by the interosseous sacroiliac ligament (axial ligament), through which the base of the sacrum moves forward and downward and the tip of the coccyx moves backward and upward.

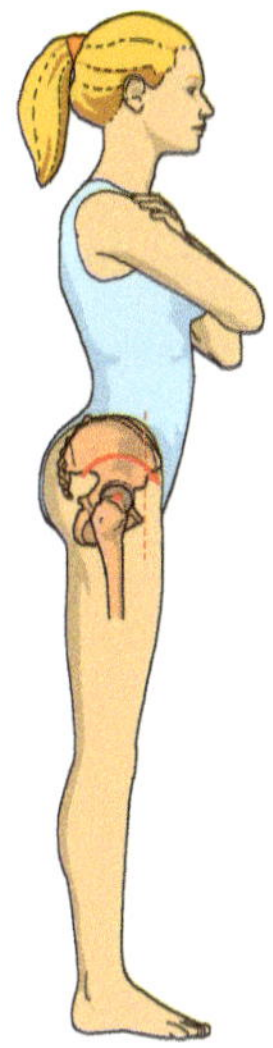

The movements of the sacrum, when occurring simultaneously with the movements of the two hip bones, result in a **forward rotation** of the entire pelvis, in the sagittal plane which, in this case, occurs around a transverse axis passing through the coxofemoral joints.

The forward rotation of the entire pelvis (anteversion) is accompanied by flexion of the trunk when a maximum joint amplitude of the flexion movement of the vertebral column is required. This movement pattern is called **lumbo-pelvic rhythm**.

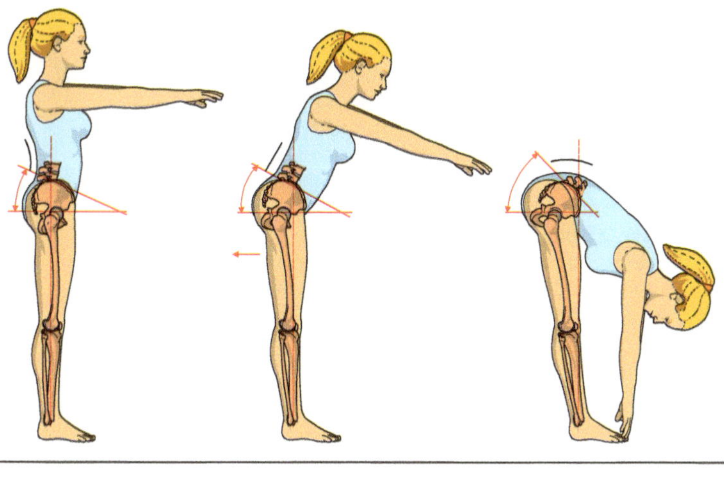

Retroversion (counternutation or extension of the pelvis)

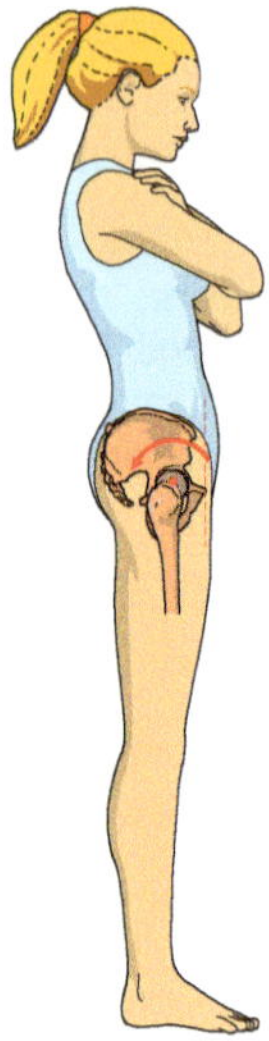

Definition: movement opposite to anteversion, through which the base of the sacrum moves backward and upward and the tip of the coccyx moves forward and upward, with the entire pelvis rotating backward.

Normoversion of the pelvis

The pelvis is subjected to stress from:

- the trunk and upper limbs – especially from the vertebral column
- the lower limbs

which modify the position (statokinetics) of the pelvis in relation to the motor action. These statokinetic variations of the pelvis generate direct thrusts to the other body segments, improving their kinetics.

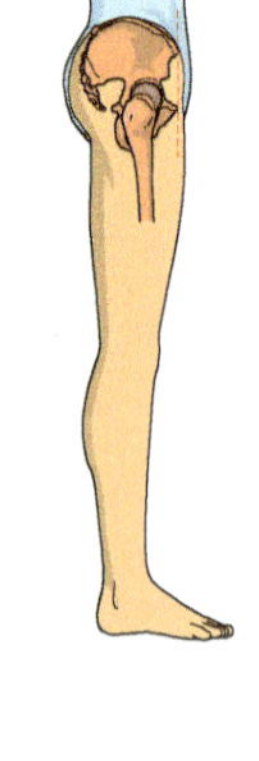

In orthostatism, the load of the vertebral column is applied to the promontory of the sacrum and the resultant of this force is directed obliquely downward and forward, breaking down into two forces that, through the sacroiliac joints, are discharged on the femoral heads. As a consequence, there is a modest anteversion of the sacrum (forward and downward displacement) with forward rotation of the pelvis, which is however balanced by the force from the ground to the feet and from the feet to the femoral heads and acetabula, causing a modest retroversion of the sacrum (forward and downward displacement) with backward rotation of the pelvis, due to the anterior position of this force with respect to the pelvis.

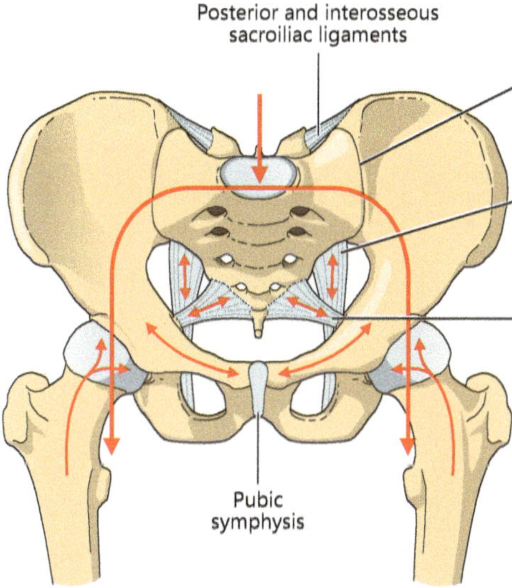

Frontal view of the pelvis. Load distribution on the pelvis and lower limbs (downward arrows). Response to ground pressure (upward arrows). The arrows with opposite directions indicate the pressure exerted by traction or thrust forces on the ligaments and bones.

Other movements of the pelvis

Lateral inclination of the pelvis (around a sagittal axis) – with slope to the right or left.

Rotation (around a longitudinal axis)

- Of the complete pelvis:
  - to the left
  - to the right
- Internal of the right hemipelvis and external of the left hemipelvis
- External of the right hemipelvis and internal of the left hemipelvis

Translation of the pelvis – anterior, posterior or lateral.

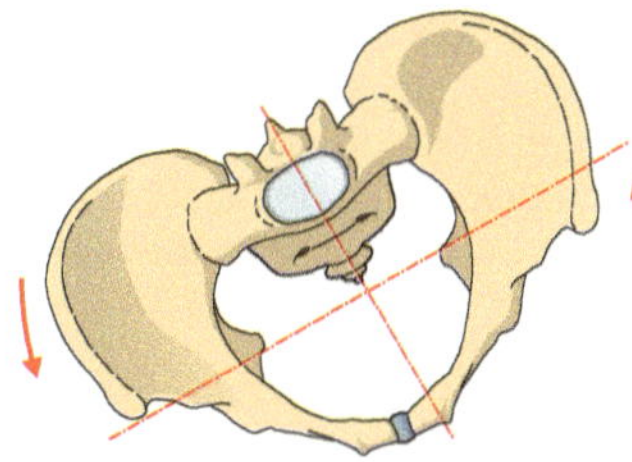
A

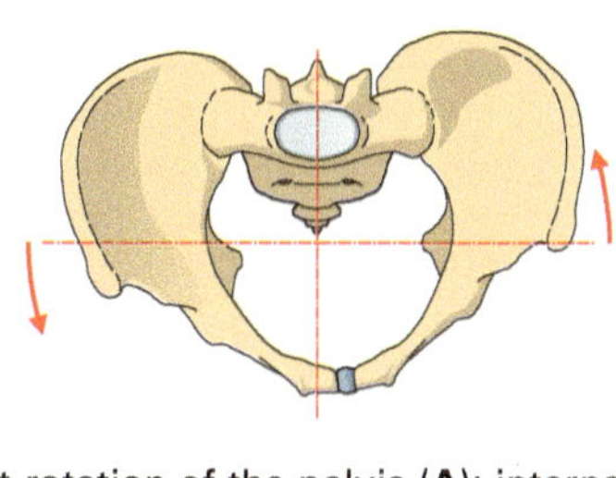
B

Left rotation of the pelvis (**A**); internal rotation of the right hemipelvis and external rotation of the left hemipelvis (**B**).

Functional aspects

- The movements of the pelvis:
  - can result from stresses transmitted to the pelvis by other body segments (secondary movements)
  - can be produced by the insertion in the pelvis of muscles that originate in the thorax, in the vertebral column or by the inversion of the origin in the pelvis (which becomes insertion) of muscles that insert in the bones of the thigh and leg (thus creating external fixed points) (primary movements)
- The pelvis, as a whole, is almost completely rigid, with the sacroiliac joint, sacrococcygeal joint and pubic symphysis being very rigid and the lumbosacral and, obviously, coxofemoral joints being more mobile
- Minor, mostly passive pelvic movements occur at the sacroiliac joint, sacrococcygeal joint and pubic symphysis and larger, partially active movements occur at the lumbosacral and coxofemoral joints
- The movements of the pelvis are largely involuntary (secondary movements) and mainly occur while standing and walking:
  - in the erect position, these are postural variations produced by movements of the vertebral column and lower limbs
  - while walking, the forward, backward and lateral movement of the lower limb causes retroversion, anteversion, lateral inclination and rotation of both hemipelvises
- The movements of the sacroiliac joints and pubic symphysis occur mainly during walking and upright standing in single-leg support (downward sliding of the pubic symphysis on the oscillation side)
- If the sacrum, due to the great stiffness of the joint and its equally very tense ligaments, were not a single unit with the ilium bones, there would be an obvious displacement of the sacrum downward and forward, largely depriving the hip bones of the thrust of the lateral bones and, therefore, also significantly reducing the load on the femoral heads
- The pathophysiological elements underlying an easy sacrum mobility are a laxity of the ligaments blocking flexion-extension (anteversion-retroversion or nutation-counternutation), a hypermobile sacroiliac joint or a laxity or a rupture of the connective structures of the pubic symphysis.

Movements of the hip

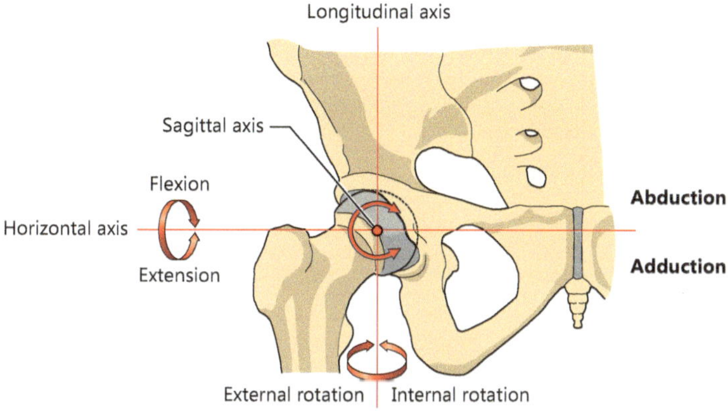

Flexion of the hip

- Occurs on the sagittal plane around a transverse or horizontal axis
- When upright standing and in the supine position it has an amplitude of:
  - 130°, with the knee flexed (actively performed)
  - 145°, with the knee flexed (passively performed)
  - 80-90°, with the knee extended (actively performed); the reduction in amplitude is due to the tension of the hamstring muscles (and the paravertebral muscles).

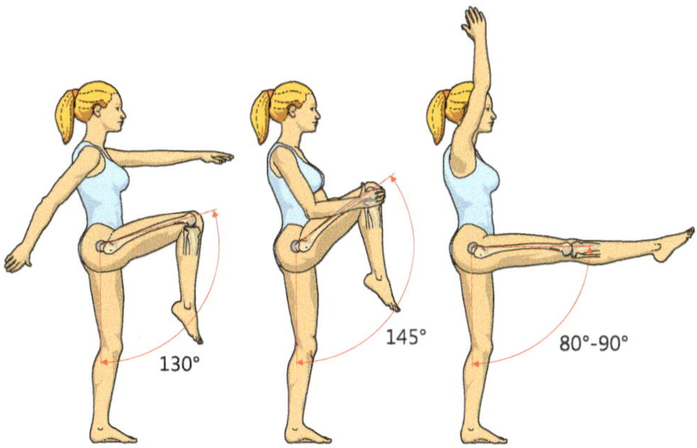

Limitations

- Tension of the hamstring muscle fibers
- Accentuation of lumbar lordosis.

In the supine position, flexion of the hip is facilitated by the straightening of the lumbar lordosis, which results in the retroversion of the pelvis. This is also favored by flexion of the knee.

Extension of the hip

- Occurs on the sagittal plane around the transverse or horizontal axis
- Amplitude of:
  - 10°, with the knee flexed (actively performed)
  - 25-30°, with the knee flexed (passively performed)
  - 10-20°, with the knee extended.

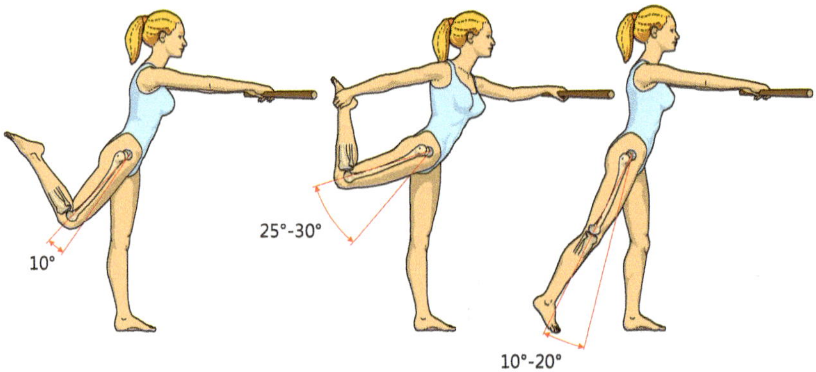

Limitations

- Ligaments:
  - iliofemoral
  - ischiofemoral
  - pubofemoral
- Joint capsule (anterior part)
- Tension of the fibers of the iliopsoas.

Extension movements of the hip with greater ampitude require compensatory movements, mainly pelvic anteversion and an accentuation of the lumbar lordosis.

Extension of the hip is facilitated by flexion of the contralateral thigh, as is evident from the sagittal split.

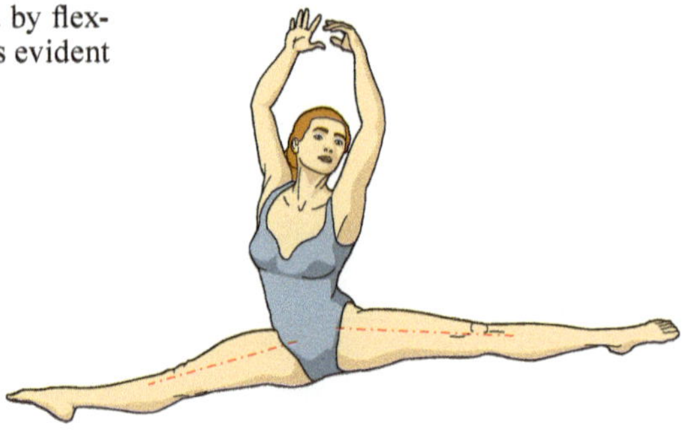

Abduction of the hip

- Occurs on the frontal plane around a sagittal axis
- Amplitude of:
  - 40-60°.

Limitations

- Ligaments:
  - iliofemoral
  - ischiofemoral
  - pubofemoral
- Joint capsule (inferior part)
- Tension of the fibers of the adductor muscles of the hip.

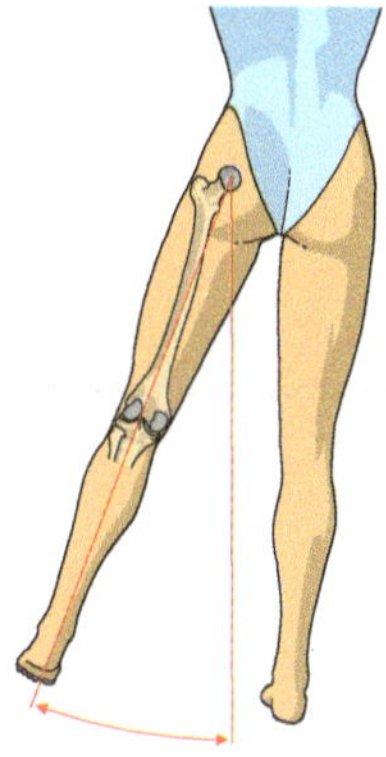

The abduction movement of the hip can reach values of 70° when the thigh is flexed at 60° and externally rotated, and 90° in bilateral abduction performed by gymnasts (front split). In the latter case, compensatory movements occur, represented by the anteversion of the pelvis and an accentuation of the lumbar lordosis, which reduce the tension of the ligaments of the hip (coxofemoral) joint.

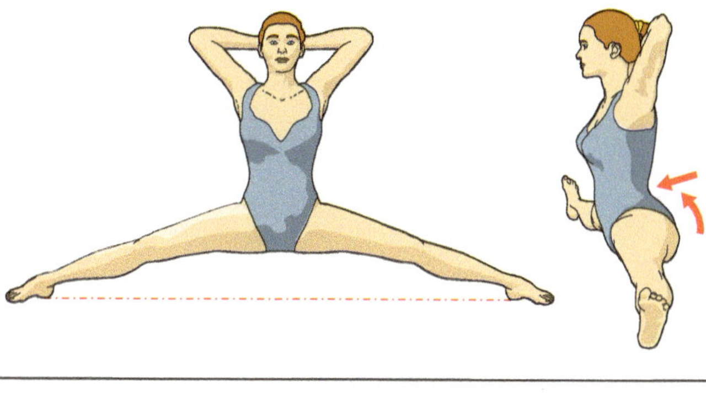

Adduction of the hip

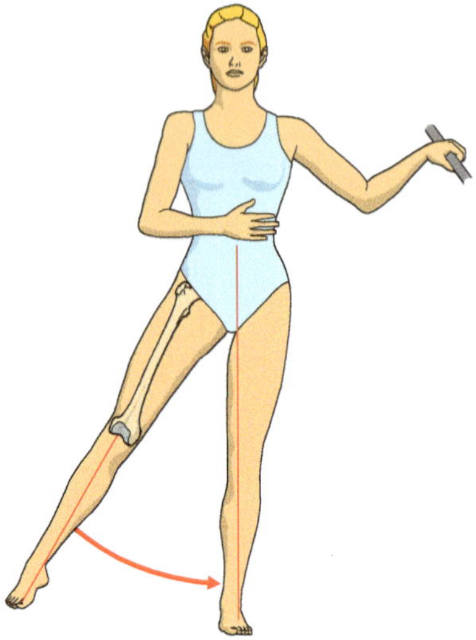

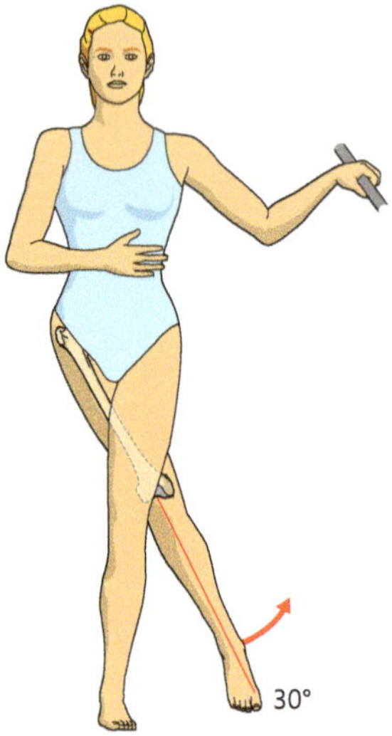

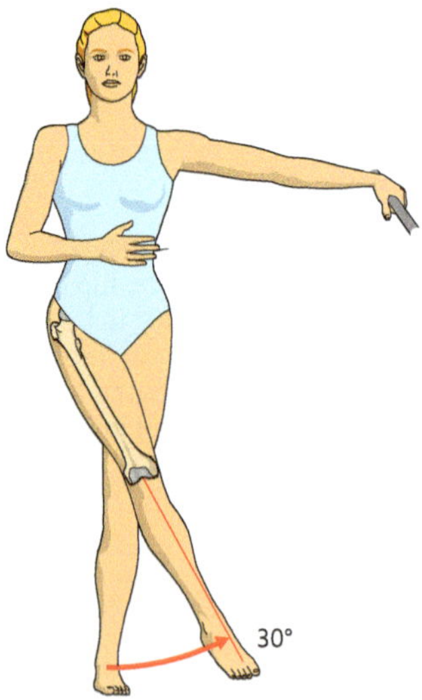

- Occurs on the frontal plane around a sagittal axis
- Relative:
  - return from any abduction position to the midline of symmetry
- Absolute:
  - is accompanied by a movement of:
    - flexion of the hip (forward movement of the contralateral limb)
    - extension of the hip (backward movement of the contralateral limb)
  - amplitude of: 30°.

Limitations

- Ligaments:
  - iliofemoral
  - ischiofemoral
- Joint capsule (superior part)
- Tension of the fibers of the abductor muscles of the hip.

A common example of a hip position during adduction is represented by the seated position with the legs crossed, in which the hip is also flexed and externally rotated (this is also the most unstable position of the hip joint).

External rotation (or supination) of the hip

- Occurs on the transverse plane around a longitudinal axis represented by the mechanical axis of the lower limb (a line that vertically connects the center of the femoral head with the centers of the base of the tibia and foot)
- From an intermediate position between external and internal rotation (neutral position)
- Amplitude of:
  - 30°, with the knee extended
    - in the upright position (including external rotation of the foot of 10-15°)
    - in the supine position (including external rotation of the foot of 10-15°)
  - 60°:
    - with the knee extended and hip flexed while slanding or in supine position
    - with the knee flexed (the greater amplitude of the rotation movement of the hip is due to the additional movements derived from the knee in flexion, a position in which all ligaments of the knee joint are released):
      - in the seated position
      - in the prone position.

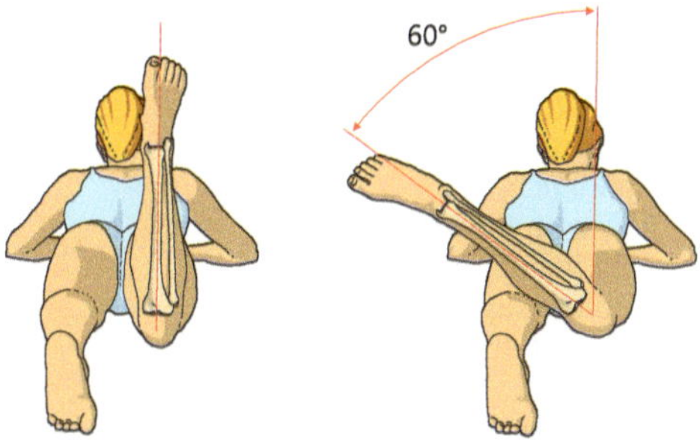

Limitations

- Ligaments:
  - iliofemoral
  - pubofemoral
- Joint capsule (anterior part)
- Tension of the fibers of the internal rotator muscles of the hip.

10

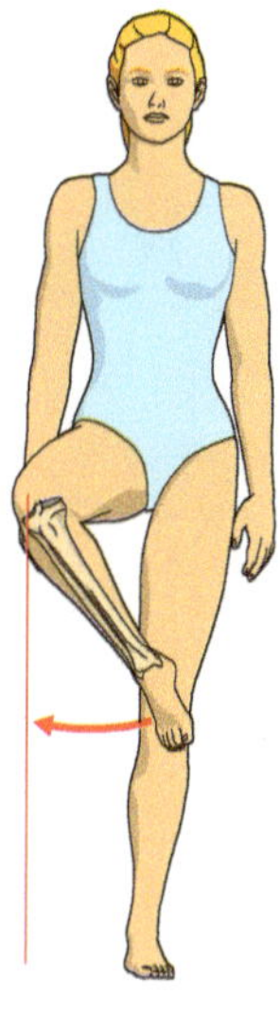

The range of motion of the external rotation of the hip is increased by the flexion of the knee, which may be combined with rotational movements.

Internal rotation (or pronation) of the hip

- Occurs on the transverse plane around the mechanical axis of the lower limb
- From an intermediate position between external and internal rotation (neutral position)
- Amplitude of:
  - 25°, with the knee extended:
    - in the upright position
    - in the supine position
  - 50°, with the knee extended and thigh flexed while standing or in the supine position
  - 30°, with the knee flexed:
    - in the seated position
    - in the prone position.

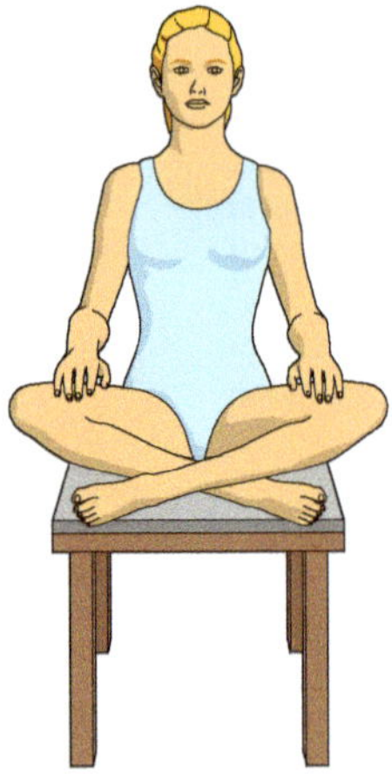

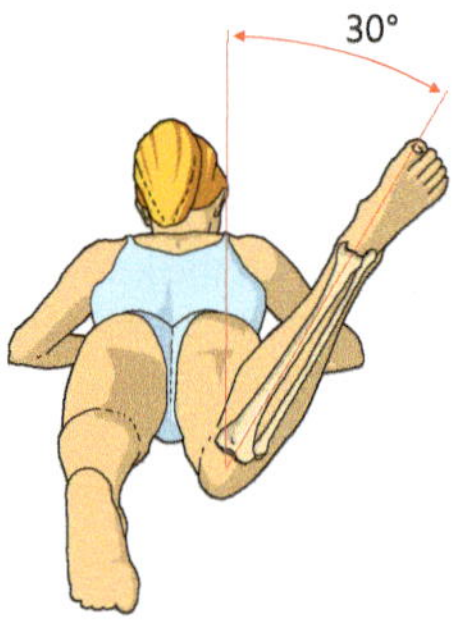

Limitations

- Ischiofemoral ligament
- Joint capsule (posterior part)
- Tension of the fibers of the external rotator muscles of the hip.

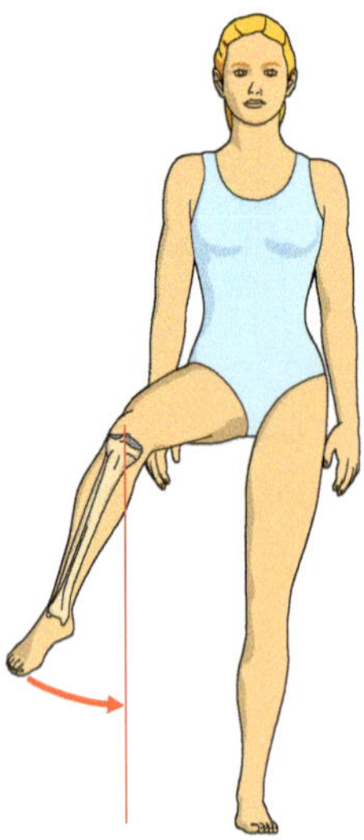

The range of motion of the internal rotation of the hip is increased by the flexion of the knee, which may be combined with rotational movements.

Circumduction of the hip

Definition: the set of the following movements:

- flexion – abduction – external rotation of the thigh
- internal rotation – adduction – extension of the thigh which follow one another around the three axes.

The representation of these successive movements is given by a cone with a vertex at the center of the head of the femur and base described by the different maximum amplitude of each movement.

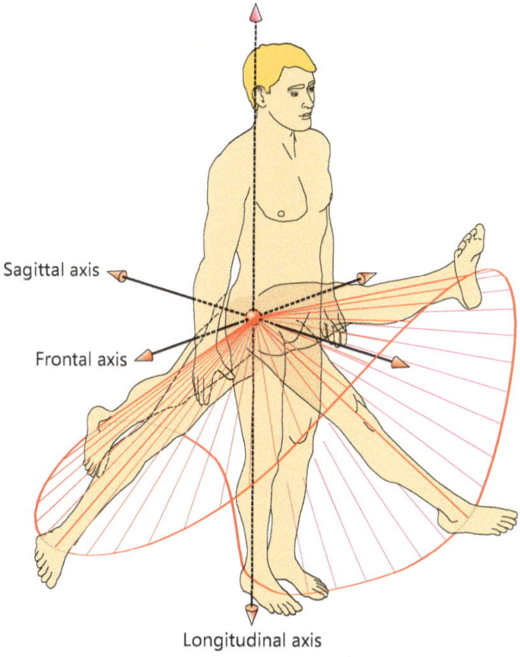

Stability of the hip joint

Angles and axes of the femur

Angle of inclination (cervical-diaphysial) – angle between the axis of the neck and the axis of the diaphysis of the femur, on the frontal plane:

→ 124°-127° (in adults)

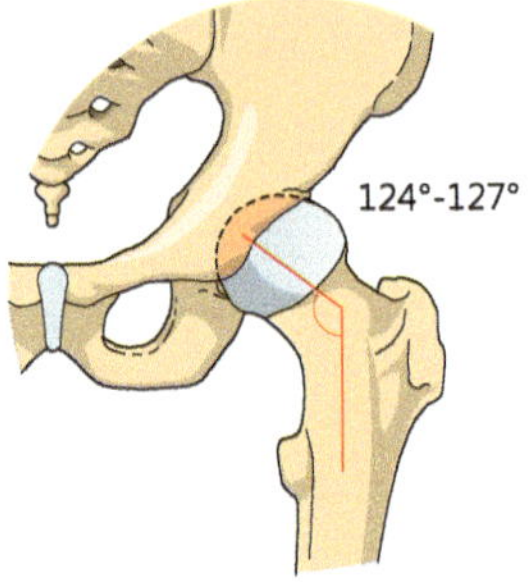

→ 140°-150° (in newborns and children)

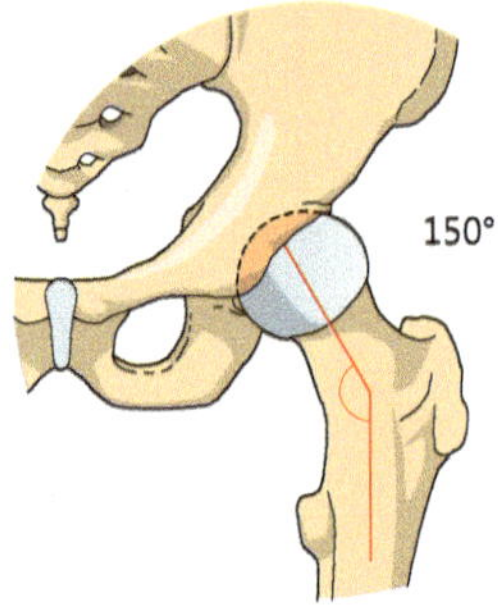

→ 120° (in the elderly)

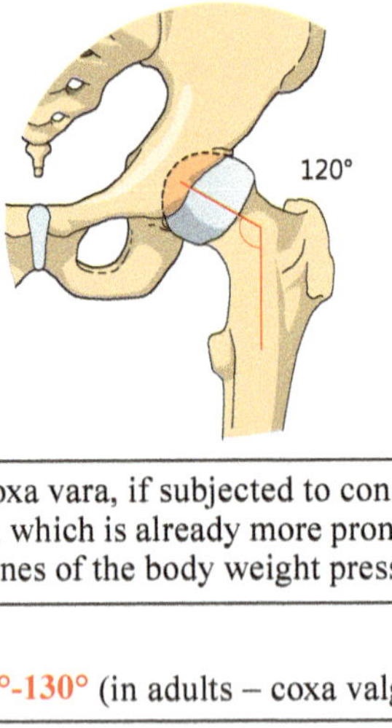

→ < 125° (in adults – coxa vara)

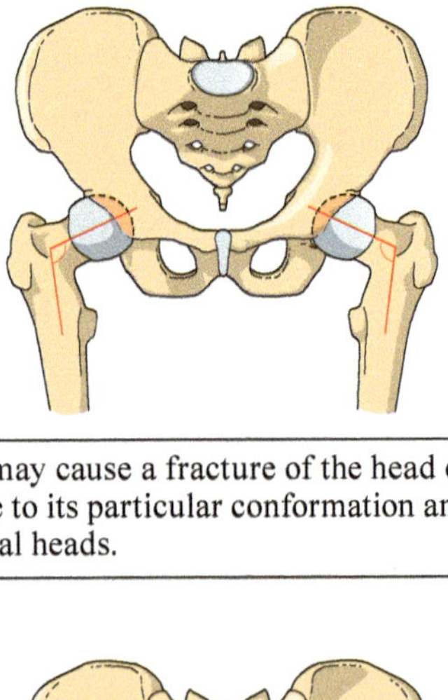

The coxa vara, if subjected to considerable stress, may cause a fracture of the head of the femur, which is already more prone to fractures due to its particular conformation and the load lines of the body weight pressing on the femoral heads.

→ 128°-130° (in adults – coxa valga)

The coxa valga facilitates the upward and outward sliding of the femoral head from the acetabular cavity and may be associated with a greater amplitude of thigh adduction motion, responsible in turn for increased trophism of the hip adductor muscles, leading to the establishment of a vicious circle that reduces the stability of the hip joint.

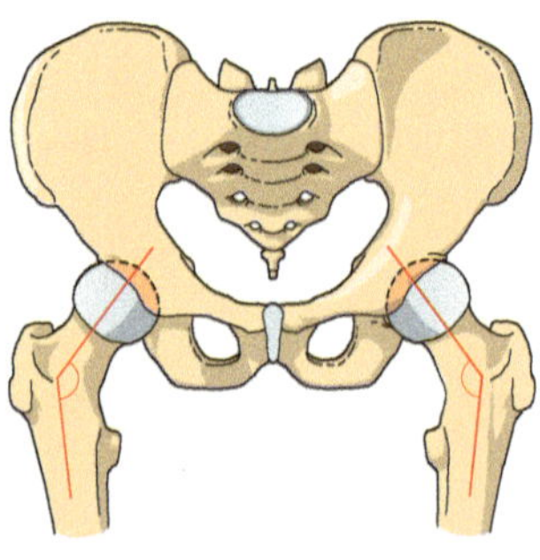

Angle of declination (anteversion or torsion) – angle between the axis of the neck and the line joining the condyles of the femur (condylar axis), on the horizontal plane:

→ 12°-15° (in adults)

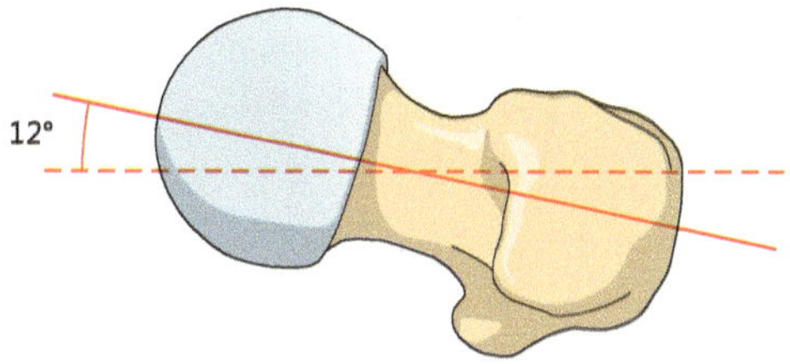

An excessive amplitude of this angle, so that the condylar axis is almost on the frontal plane, may facilitate the anterior dislocation of the femoral head, while its reduction may be a stabilizing element; the angle of declination facilitates the rotation of the thigh in flexion.

→ 30°-40° (in newborns and children)

Mechanical axis of the lower limb – line vertically joining the center of the femoral head with the center of the base of the tibia and with that of the foot.

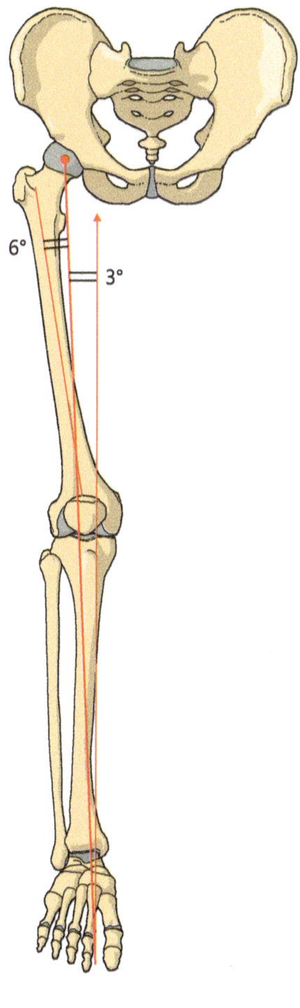

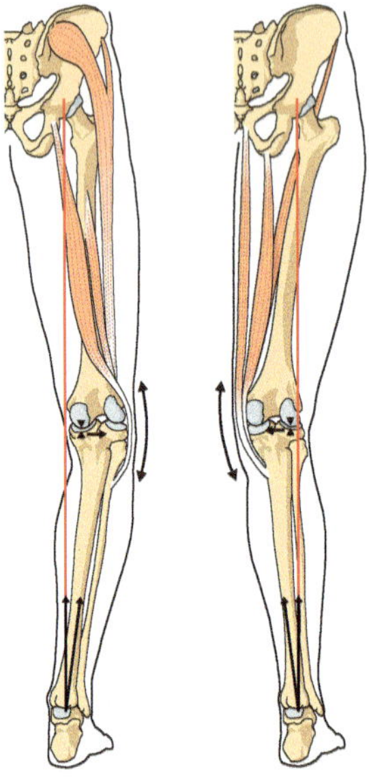

This axis does not coincide with the axis of the femoral diaphysis, nor with the vertical driven by the foot; instead, it coincides with the axis of the diaphysis of the tibia. Therefore, the amount of force transmitted to the tibia through the femoral diaphysis depends on its greater or lesser obliquity with respect to the mechanical axis, which in turn depends on the angle of inclination of the femur. In case of coxa valga, there will be a lesser obliquity of the femoral diaphysis, corresponding to a varus knee (**A**) and a load that acts medially on the tibia, with traction on the lateral articular surfaces of the knee and its displacement (in addition to the stretching of the external collateral ligaments). In case of coxa vara the opposite situation will occur (**B**).

Comparison between glenohumeral (shoulder) and hip joints

Both are ball and socket joints (with great mobility), but while the upper limb adds a load to the body, being suspended from the trunk, the lower limb, through the femoral heads, receives 80% of the body weight, so it is necessary a remarkable stability in the coxofemoral joints, without which the movements of the lower limbs would not be possible. The body weight stabilizes the surfaces of the coxofemoral joint and contributes, by opposing, to the force that is discharged upward from the ground on the lower limbs, which maintains, in static conditions, the upright position and, in dynamic conditions, ambulation.

Elements for stabilization of the hip joint

- Angle of inclination (if this angle decreases, the force – power – acting on the head of the femur would have a very wide lever arm [see neck], while the force – resistance – produced by the femoral diaphysis would have a very short lever arm; the angle of inclination reduces the difference between the two lever arms, reducing the power one and increasing the resistance one)

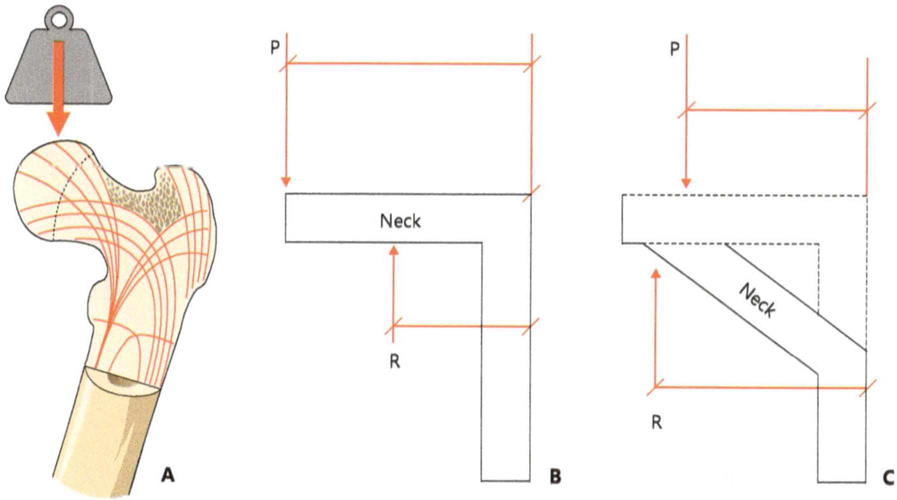

A, Schematic representation of the trabecular structure of the proximal segment of the femur, a fundamental support element. **B**, Schematic representation of the disadvantage of the resistance arm (R) with respect to the power arm (P) in a structure illustrating a horizontal femoral neck. **C**, In this case, the disadvantage is of the power arm due to the oblique structure of the neck and the greater weight of the distal segment.

10

- Trabecular structure of the superior extremity of the femur (perpendicular crossing of the bony trabeculae arranged on the frontal and sagittal planes, according to the lines of force that increase the resistance of the head and neck of the femur to pressure and tension)
- Load in upright position (stabilization of the femoral head)
- Joint capsule, ligaments and muscles
- Negative pressure between the head of the femur and the bottom of the acetabulum (air void that maintains the head firmly attached to the bottom of the cavity).

Assessment of the passive joint mobility of the hip

Flexion of the hip

Starting position	Supine, with the lower limb to be examinated in anatomical position (neutral position of hip and knee joints); the contralateral thigh may be flexed or extended
Movement	The examiner lifts the lower limb by holding the distal part of the femur posteriorly and, while stabilizing the pelvis with the other hand, applies a slight traction by moving the thigh forward with the knee flexed up to the limit of movement allowed (120-130°) 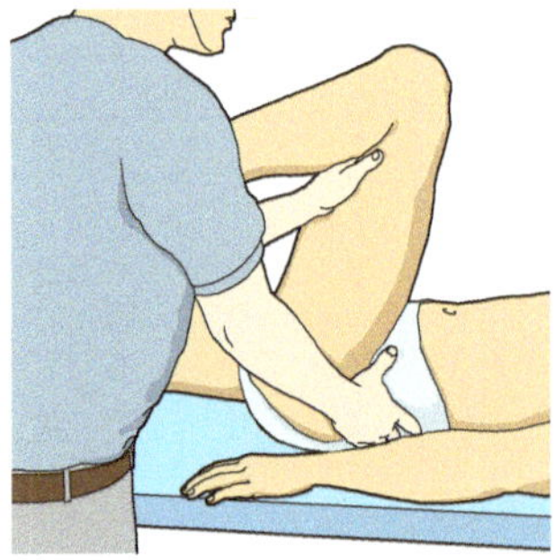

Extension of the hip

Starting position	Prone, with the lower limb in anatomical position
Movement	The examiner lifts the lower limb by holding the distal part of the femur anteriorly and, while stabilizing the pelvis with the other hand, applies a slight traction by moving the thigh upward with the knee extended up to the limit of movement allowed (15-30°) 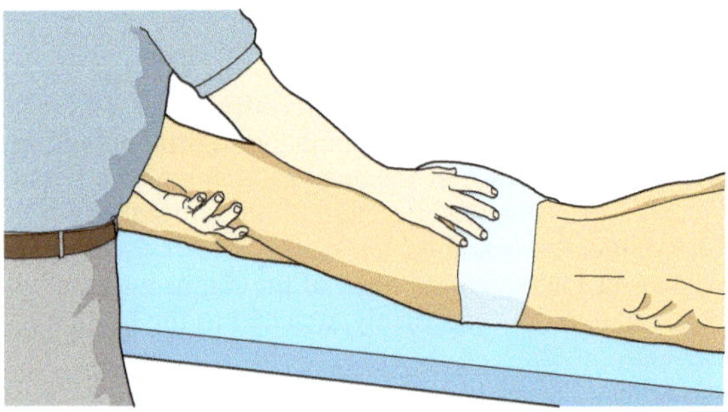

Abduction of the hip

Starting position	Supine, with the pelvis in a horizontal position (i.e., without unevenness or not tilted laterally) and the lower limbs in anatomical position
Movement	The examiner lifts the lower limb by holding the distal part of the femur medially and, while stabilizing the pelvis with the other hand, applies a slight traction by moving the thigh laterally up to the limit of movement allowed (45°, but can reach 60-70°) 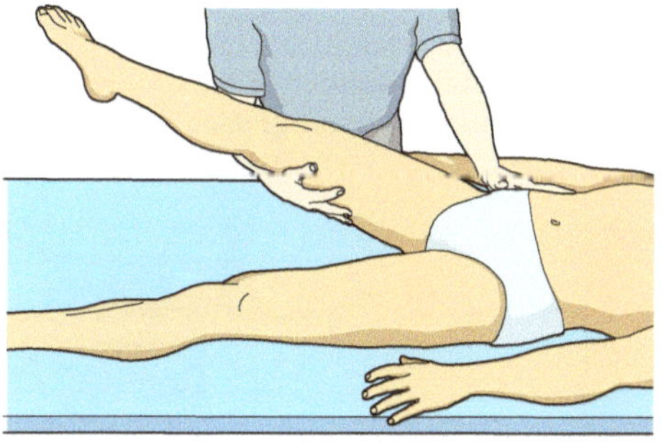

Adduction of the hip

Starting position	Supine, with the pelvis in a horizontal position and the lower limb to be examined in anatomical position; the contralateral thigh is abducted to allow full excursion of the adduction movement of the examined hip
Movement	The examiner lifts the lower limb by holding the distal part of the femur and, while stabilizing the pelvis with the other hand, applies a slight traction by moving the thigh medially up to the limit of movement allowed (30°) 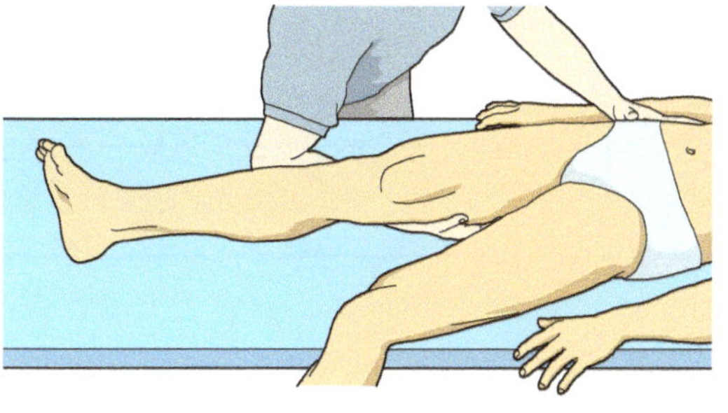

External and internal rotation of the hip

Starting position	Supine, with the thigh and the leg flexed at 90°
Movement	The examiner, after holding the distal part of the thigh with one hand and the distal part of the leg with the other hand, applies a slight traction by moving the thigh laterally and the leg medially up to the limit of the external rotation movement of the hip (45°) and then the thigh medially and the leg laterally up to the limit of the internal rotation movement of the hip (45°) **Note**: the external and internal rotation of the hip, without the addition of the knee rotations that these maneuvers determine, is never greater than 30° 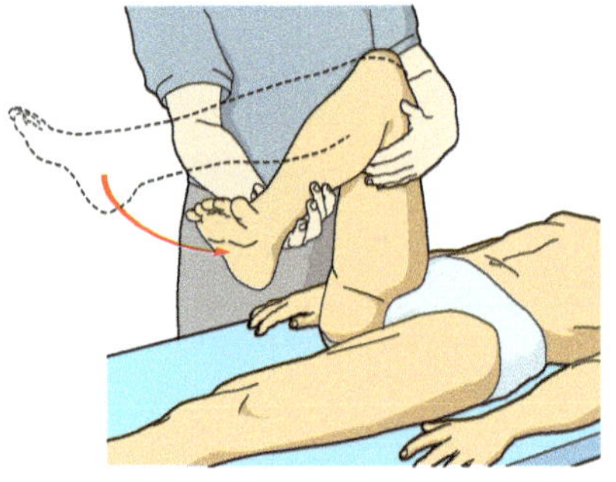 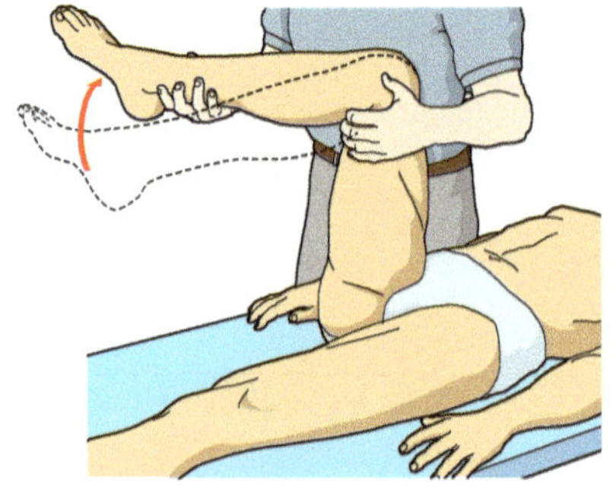

General analysis of the active joint mobility of the lower limb

Starting position	Supine position with the limbs in anatomical position
Movement	Extension of the toes and dorsiflexion of the foot, with the calcaneus being carried in correspondence with the contralateral hip 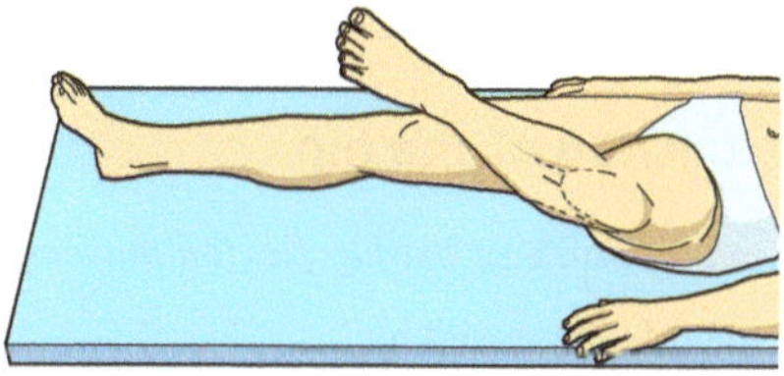
Assessment of the joint amplitude of active movements	• Flexion, abduction and external rotation of the hip • Flexion of the knee • Dorsiflexion of the ankle • Extension of the toes The level reached by the calcaneus can be used as a reference point during the assessment of the active mobility of the hip and knee joints

Starting position	Supine position with the limbs in anatomical position
Movement	Toe flexion, plantar flexion, knee extension, adduction, internal rotation and extension of the hip 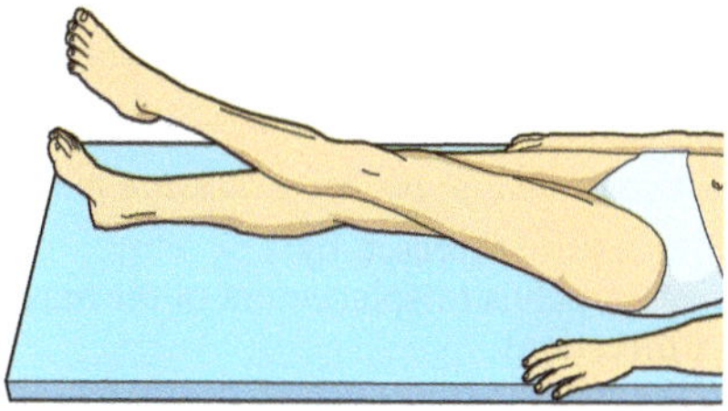
Assessment of the joint amplitude of active movements	• Adduction and internal rotation of the hip • Extension of the knee • Plantar flexion of the ankle • Flexion of the great toe

Functional aspects of the hip joint

Functions of the hip joint:
- transmission of forces between the supporting surface and the pelvis:
  - body weight support
  - fulcrum action during single-leg stance
- hip movements:
  - approaching and moving the limb away from the supporting surface
  - displacement of the lower limb in space
  - approach of the foot to the trunk.

Flexion and extension of the hip

Normal active joint amplitude of the hip flexion movement → **0°-120°**

Hip flexion movement is increased by:
- the retroversion of the pelvis (displacement of the anterior superior iliac spine in the superior and posterior direction)
- the flexion of the lumbar column.

Activities taht require a hip flexion between 110° and 120° are represented by:
- squatting to lift an object off the ground
- tying shoelaces with the foot on the ground
- sitting with the foot on the contralateral thigh
- getting up from a sitting position.

Activities that require a hip flexion of less than 90° are represented by:
- climbing stairs (mean value of 67°)
- walking down stairs (mean value of 36°)
- sitting in a chair
- putting on pants.

Sitting down from the upright position requires an average hip flexion of 104°, while the opposite action – standing up from a sitting position – requires an average hip flexion of 98° to 101°; approximately 84° of hip flexion is necessary to sit in a chair of normal height.

Normal active joint amplitude of the hip extension movement → **0°-30°**

Hip extension movement is increased by:
- the anteversion of the pelvis (displacement of the anterior superior iliac spine in the inferior and anterior direction)
- the extension of the lumbar column.

The upright position requires a hip extension of 0° or a few degrees, going up and down the stairs require a maximum extension of 1° or 2°.

Abduction and adduction of the hip

Normal active joint amplitude of the hip abduction movement → 0°-45°

Most daily life activities do not require full mobility of the hip in abduction and many can be performed within an abduction range of 0-20°, such as squatting to lift an object off the ground or sitting with one foot on the contralateral thigh; however, getting on a bicycle may require a full range of the hip abduction movement.

Normal active joint amplitude of the hip adduction movement → 0°-30°

Hip adduction in daily life activities is exemplified by sitting with legs crossed and standing in single-leg stance; in this case the supported limb is in adduction due to the contralateral inclination (unevenness) of the pelvis.

External and internal rotation of the hip

Normal active joint amplitude of the hip external rotation movement → 0°-45°

In daily life activities, extreme degrees of rotational mobility are rarely reached and, in most of them, only a 0-20° amplitude of the external rotational movement of the hip is required. Examples where this movement is used are represented by getting on a bicycle and sitting in a chair with the foot on the contralateral thigh in order to tie shoelaces.

Normal active joint amplitude of the hip internal rotation movement → 0°-45°

An example of a functional activity that requires a 20° hip internal rotation is represented by squatting to lift an object off the ground.

Muscles of the hip

Muscle	Action	Origin	Insertion	Innervation
Psoas major	Flexion of the hip; adduction of the hip; external rotation of the hip (with inverted insertions ipsilaterally flexes the vertebral column from T12 to L5)	Anterior surface of the transverse processes of all lumbar vertebrae; lateral surface of the body and intervertebral disc of T12 and of all lumbar vertebrae	Lesser trochanter of the femur	Branches of the lumbar plexus (mainly L1, L2, with some contribution of L3)
Iliacus	Flexion of the hip, adduction of the hip; external rotation of the hip	Upper two-thirds of the iliac fossa and inner lip of the iliac crest; anterior sacroiliac and iliolumbar ligaments; upper part of the lateral surface of the sacrum	Lateral surface of the tendon of the psoas major; lesser trochanter of the femur	Branches of the lumbar plexus [L2, L3] and femoral nerve
Sartorius	Flexion, abduction and external rotation of the hip; flexion and internal rotation of the knee (with inverted insertions it facilitates the anteversion of the pelvis)	Anterior superior iliac spine and the upper half of the underlying notch	Upper part of the medial surface of the tibia (in front of the gracilis and semitendinosus)	Femoral nerve [L2, L3]
Obturator internus	External rotation of the hip (and abduction of the hip from a seated position with the knee extended)	Internal surface of inferior pubic and ischial rami and superior pubic ramus; internal surface of the obturator membrane; above and behind the obturator foramen to the superior part of the greater sciatic foramen	Anterior groove of the medial surface of the greater trochanter of the femur, above and in front of the trochanteric fossa (after passing through the lesser sciatic foramen)	Nerve to the internal obturator [L5, S1]

(*continued*)

Muscles of the hip *(continued)*

Muscle	Action	Origin	Insertion	Innervation
Gemellus superior	External rotation of the hip	Posterior surface of the ischial spine	Medial surface of the greater trochanter together with the obturator internus	Nerve to the obturator internus [L5, S1, S2]
Gemellus inferior	External rotation of the hip	Superior surface of the ischial tuberosity	Medial surface of the greater trochanter together with the obturator internus	Nerve to the quadratus femoris [L4, L5, S1]
Obturator externus	External rotation of the hip; adduction of the hip	Superior and inferior pubic rami and inferior ischial ramus; middle two-thirds of the external surface of the obturator membrane; medial part of the obturator foramen	Trochanteric fossa	Posterior branch of the obturator nerve [L3, L4]
Quadratus femoris	External rotation of the hip; adduction of the hip	Upper part of the external surface of the ischial tuberosity	Intertrochanteric crest	Nerve to the quadratus femoris [L5, S1]
Pectineus	Flexion of the hip; adduction of the hip	Pecten pubis (pectineal line of the pubis) between the iliopubic ramus and the pubic tubercle	Line between the lesser trochanter of the femur and the linea aspera	Femoral nerve [L2, L3]
Adductor longus	Adduction of the hip; external rotation and flexion of the hip	Anterior part of the pubis in the angle between the pubic crest and the pubic symphysis	Medial third of the linea aspera of the femur	Obturator nerve [L1-L4]
Abductor brevis	Adduction of the hip; external rotation and flexion of the hip	External surface of the inferior pubic ramus between the gracilis and obturator externus	Line between the lesser trochanter and the linea aspera; upper part of the linea aspera	Obturator nerve [L2-L4]

(continued)

Muscles of the hip *(continued)*

Muscle	Action	Origin	Insertion	Innervation
Gracilis	Adduction of the hip (with knee extended); internal rotation of the hip; flexion of the hip; flexion of the knee	Lower half of the body of the pubis; inferior pubic and ischial rami	Upper part of the medial surface of the tibia (between the sartorius and the semitendinosus)	Obturator nerve [L2-L4]
Adductor magnus	Adduction of the hip; extension of the hip; external rotation of the hip (and internal rotation from position of external rotation and flexion)	External surface of the inferior pubic ramus adjacent to the ischium; external surface of the inferior ischial ramus; inferolateral surface of the ischial tuberosity	Medial margin of the gluteal tuberosity of the femur; medial lip of the linea aspera; medial supracondylar line; adductor tubercle	Obturator nerve and tibial nerve [L3-L5]
Piriformis	External rotation of the hip (from position of extension); abduction of the hip (from position of flexion)	Anterior surface of the sacrum between the second and fourth sacral foramina and gluteal surface of the ilium adjacent to the posterior inferior iliac spine	Medial surface of the superior margin of the greater trochanter of the femur (after passing through the greater sciatic foramen)	Nerve to the piriformis [L5, S1, S2]
Gluteus maximus	Extension and external rotation of the hip (with inverted insertion carries the pelvis in retroversion); abduction of the hip (with the upper fibers); adduction of the hip (with the lower fibers)	Posterior gluteal line of the ilium and iliac crest above and behind the posterior gluteal line; erector spinae aponeurosis; posterior surface of the inferior part of the sacrum and lateral surface of the coccyx; sacrotuberous ligament	Iliotibial tract and gluteal tuberosity	Inferior gluteal nerve [L5, S1, S2]

(continued)

Muscles of the hip *(continued)*

Muscle	Action	Origin	Insertion	Innervation
Tensor fasciae latae	Flexion, abduction and internal rotation of the hip (flexion of the knee through the iliotibial tract)	Anterior surface of the outer lip of the iliac crest; external surface and notch below the anterior superior iliac spine; deep surface of the fascia lata	Iliotibial tract	Superior gluteal nerve [L4, L5, S1]
Gluteus medius	Abduction of the hip and external rotation and extension of the hip (with posterior fibers); flexion and internal flexion of the hip (with anterior fibers)	External surface of the ilium between the iliac crest and the posterior gluteal line, superiorly, and anterior gluteal line, inferiorly	External surface of the greater trochanter	Superior gluteal nerve [L4, L5, S1]
Gluteus minimus	Same movements as the gluteus medius	External surface of the ilium between the anterior and inferior gluteal lines and the margin of the greater sciatic notch	Anterolateral surface of the greater trochanter of the femur	Superior gluteal nerve [L4, L5, S1]
Adductor minimus	Adduction and external rotation of the hip	Inferior pubic ramus **Note**: according to some authors, it is part of the adductor magnus	Medial lip of the linea aspera, posteriorly	Obturator nerve [L2]

(For origin, insertion and action of the semimembranosus, semitendinosus and biceps femoris, see Chapter 11 "Knee").

Topographical classification of the muscles of the hip

Posterior muscles of the hip

- Superficial:
  - gluteus maximus (the most superficial and the widest)
  - gluteus medius
  - gluteus minimus
  - tensor fasciae latae (the most lateral)
  - biceps femoris
  - semitendinosus (the most medial together with the semimembranosus)
  - semimembranosus (the most medial together with the semitendinosus)
- Deep:
  - piriformis (less deep)
  - obturator internus (less deep)
  - obturator externus
  - gemellus superior
  - gemellus inferior
  - quadratus femoris (less deep).

Anterior muscles of the hip

- Iliopsoas (psoas major and iliacus)
- Psoas minor
- Rectus femoris
- Sartorius
- Pectineus

Medial muscles of the hip (from lateral to medial)

- Adductor magnus
- Adductor brevis
- Adductor longus
- Gracilis.

Action of the muscles in the movements of the hip

Flexion of the hip

Flexor muscles of the hip (from greatest to least muscular force)

- Iliopsoas
- Rectus femoris
- Sartorius
- Tensor fasciae latae
- Pectineus
- Adductor longus
- Adductor brevis
- Gracilis
- Gluteus medius: anterior fibers
- Gluteus minimus: anterior fibers

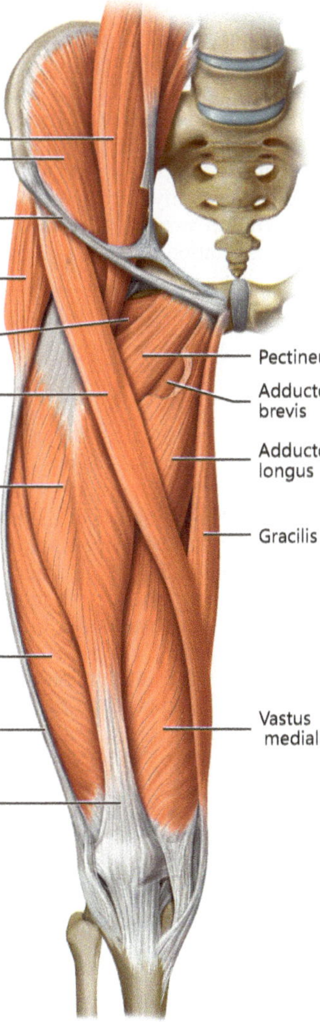

Superficial plane of the anterior muscles of the right thigh.

Action of the flexor muscles of the thigh

Iliopsoas

- Main flexor muscle of the hip
- Adducts and rotates the hip externally
- Inclines the vertebral column laterally (with fixed point on the distal insertion)
- Flexes the trunk forward by action of both muscles (with fixed point on the distal insertion)
- Favors the stability of the hip joint (together with the iliofemoral ligament)
- Acts constantly during walking (with maximum work of the iliacus during the oscillation phase of walking).

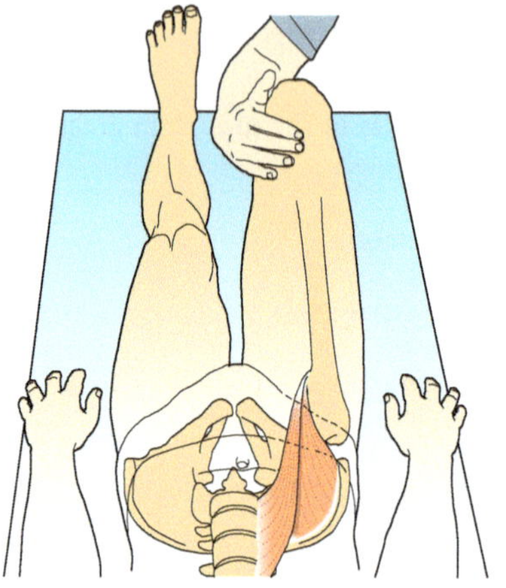

Rectus femoris

- Second flexor muscle of the hip
- Extends the knee (together with the vastus medialis, vastus lateralis and vastus intermedius muscles, with which it constitutes the quadriceps femoris)
- Facilitates the anteversion of the pelvis (with fixed point on the tibia).

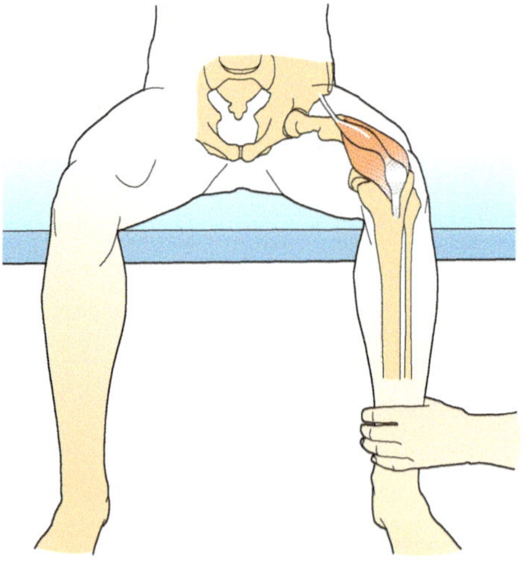

Sartorius

- Third flexor muscle of the hip
- Abducts and rotates the hip externally
- Facilitates the anteversion of the pelvis (contraction of both muscles with fixed point on the tibia)
- Flexion and internal rotation of the knee.

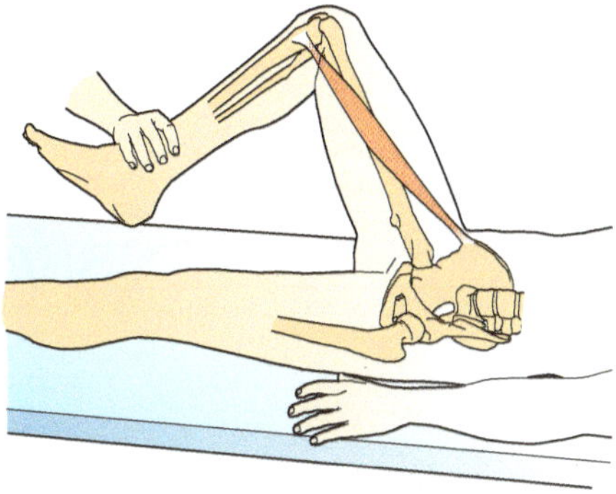

Tensor fasciae latae

- Flexion, abduction and internal rotation of the hip
- Flexion of the knee and external rotation of the flexed knee.

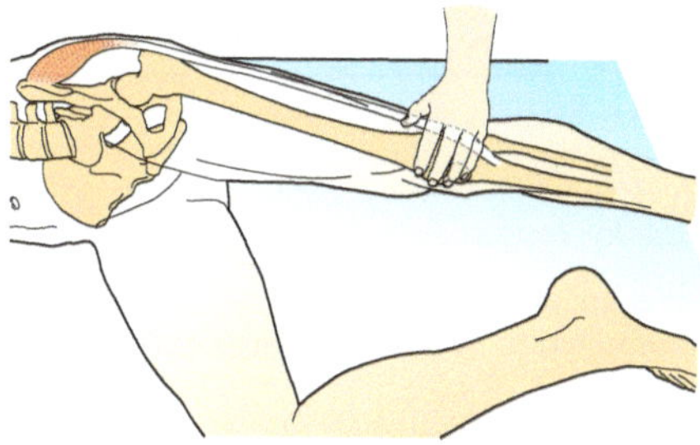

Pectineus

- Flexion and adduction of the hip.

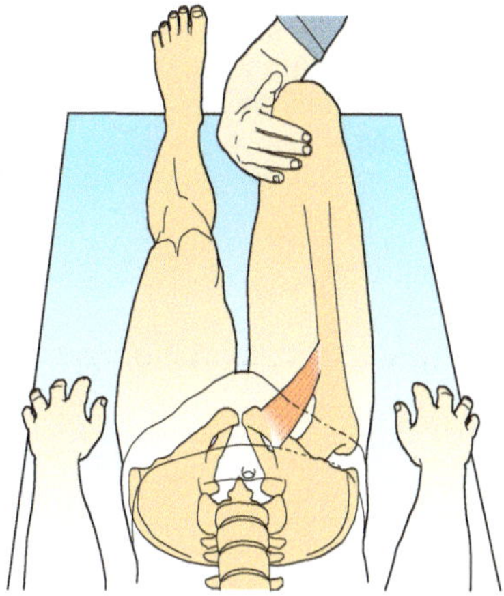

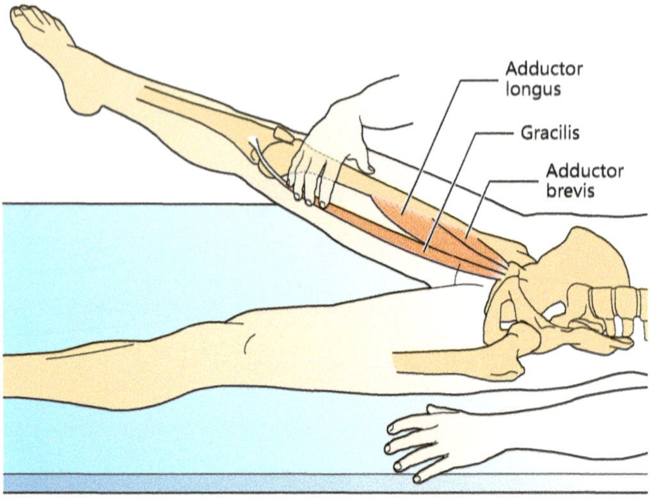

Adductor longus

- Weak flexor of the hip
- Main action of adduction and external rotation of the hip.

Adductor brevis

- Weak flexor of the hip
- Main action of adduction and external rotation of the hip.

Gracilis

- Weak flexor of the hip
- Adduction of the hip when the knee is extended
- Internal rotation of the hip
- Flexion of the knee.

Extension of the hip

Extensor muscles of the hip (from greatest to least muscular force)

- Gluteus maximus
- Gluteus medius
- Gluteus minimus
- Semimembranosus
- Semitendinosus
- Adductor magnus
- Biceps femoris (long head)

The gluteus medius is located deeply and anteriorly to the gluteus maximus; the gluteus minimus is between the gluteus medius, the ala (wing) of the ilium and the hip joint.

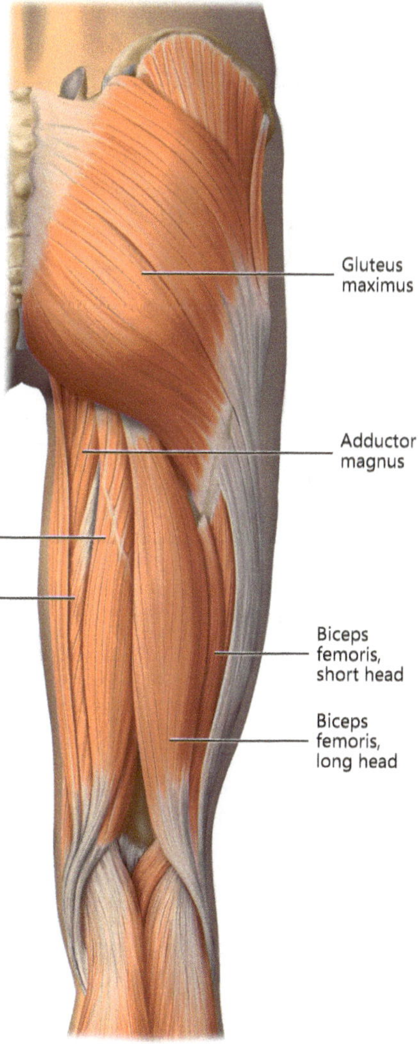

Posterior view of the external and posteromedial muscles of the hip.

Action of the extensor muscles of the hip

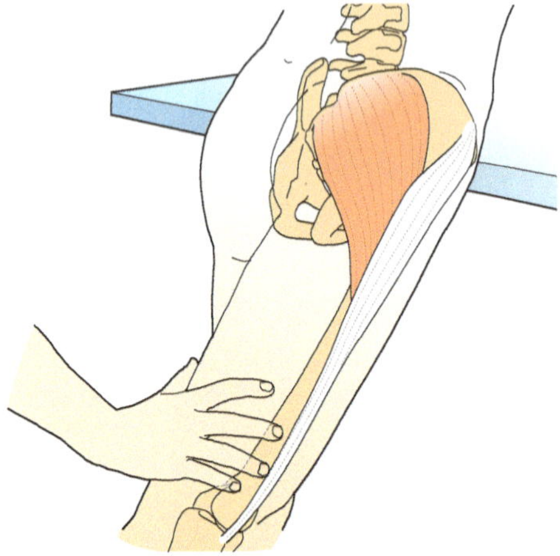

Gluteus maximus

- Main action of extension and external rotation of the hip → its extensor action is greater when the thigh is flexed between 45 and 90°
- It is both abductor (insertion of the fibers to the iliotibial tract) and adductor of the thigh (insertion of the fibers to the gluteal tuberosity of the femur)
- Retroversion of the pelvis (action of both muscles with a fixed distal point).

The gluteus maximus is mainly involved in activities such as rising from a seat, walking uphill, climbing stairs, and its action is very often used in sports (cycling, starting blocks in racing).

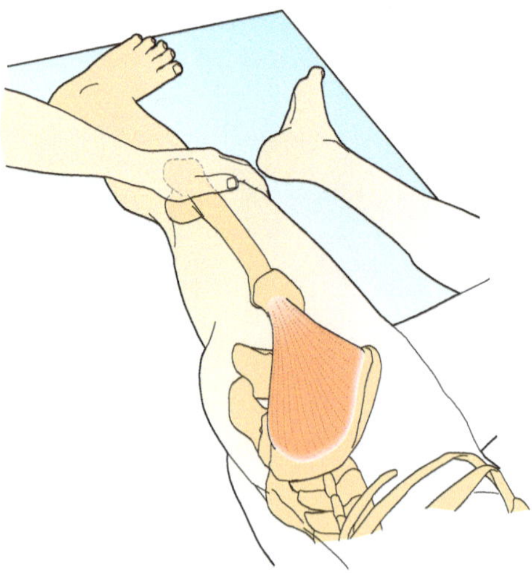

Gluteus medius

- Extension and external rotation of the hip (posterior fibers)
- Flexion and internal rotation of the hip (anterior fibers)
- Main action of abduction of the hip.

Gluteus minimus

- Extension of the hip (posterior fibers)
- Flexion of the hip (anterior fibers)
- Main action of abduction of the hip.

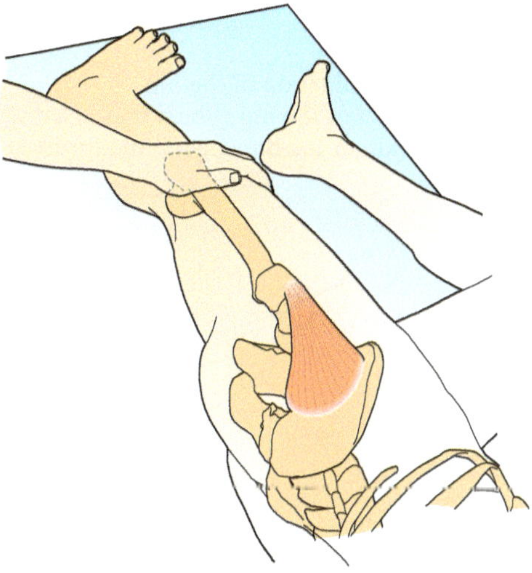

Semimembranosus

- Extension of the hip
- Main action of flexion and internal rotation of the knee.

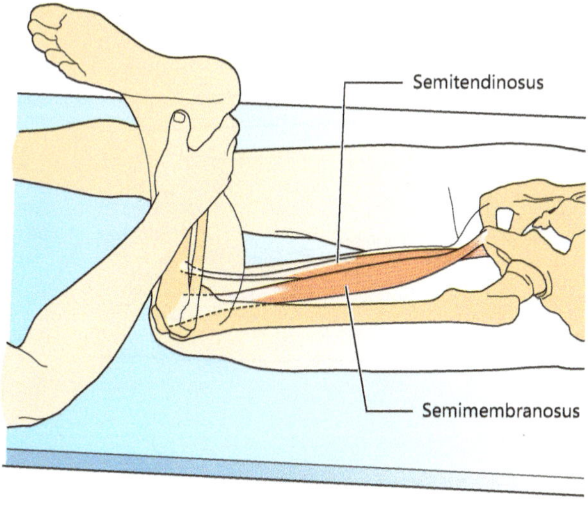

Semitendinosus

- Extension of the hip
- Main action of flexion and internal rotation of the knee.

Adductor magnus

- Extension of the hip
- Main action of adduction of the hip
- External rotation of the hip (fibers that insert at the linea aspera)
- Internal rotation of the hip (fibers that insert at the adductor tubercle) rotated externally and flexed.

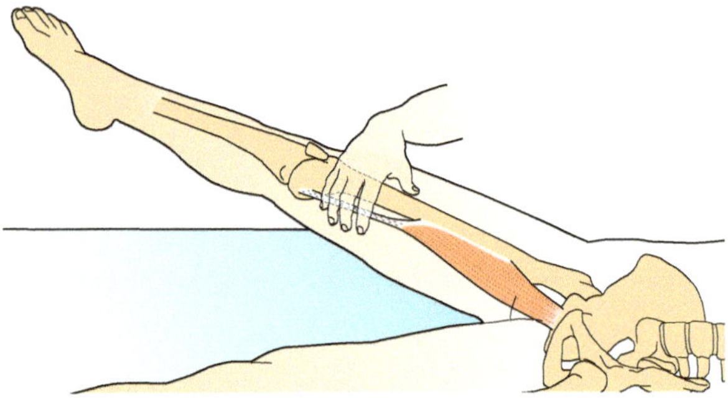

Biceps femoris (long head)

- Extension of the thigh
- Flexion and external rotation of the knee.

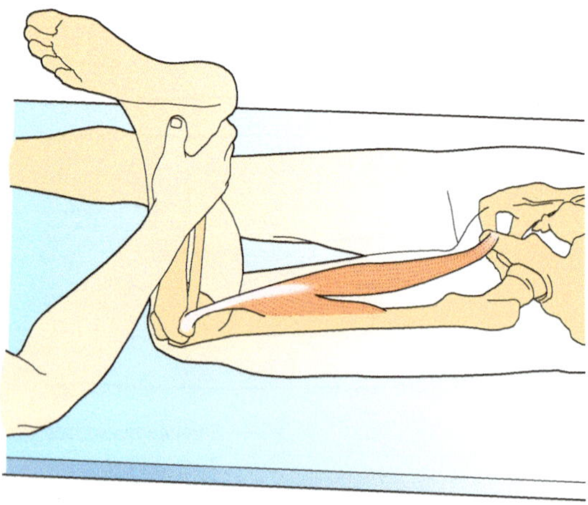

Abduction of the hip

Abductor muscles of the hip (from greatest to least muscular force)

- Gluteus medius (see section "Extension of the hip", page 489)
- Tensor fasciae latae (see section "Flexion of the hip", page 485)
- Gluteus maximus (see section "Extension of the hip", page 489)
- Gluteus minimus (see section "Extension of the hip", page 489)
- Piriformis
- Obturator internus
- Sartorius (see section "Flexion of the hip", page 485)

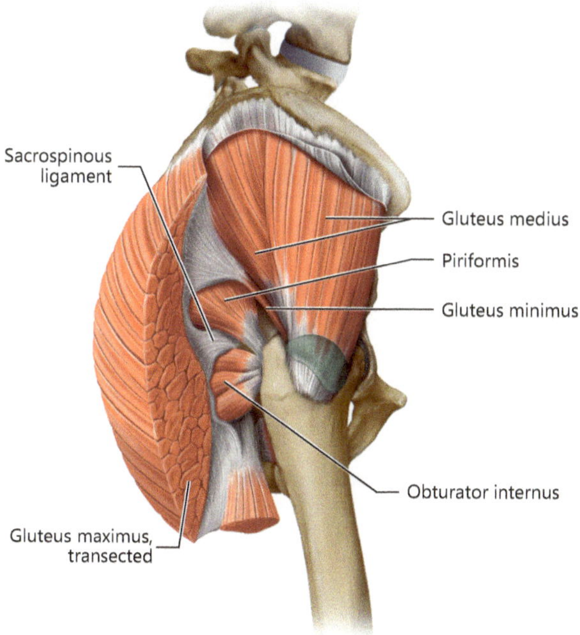

External muscles of the right hip in lateral projection after removal of the gluteus maximus and the tensor fasciae latae.

Action of the abductor muscles of the hip

Piriformis

- Abduction of the flexed hip
- External rotation of the extended hip.

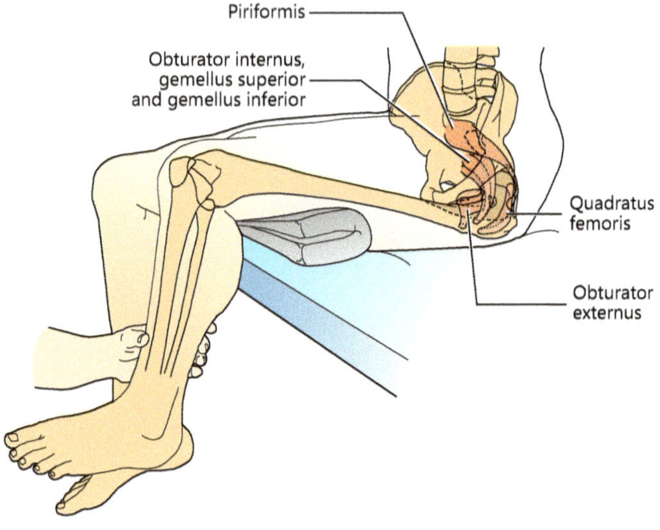

Obturator internus

- Abduction of the hip in a seated (flexed) position with the knee extended
- Main action of external rotation of the hip.

Adduction of the hip

Adductor muscles of the hip (from greatest to least muscular force)

- Adductor magnus (see section "Extension of the hip", page 489)
- Adductor longus (see section "Flexion of the hip", page 485)
- Adductor minimus (originates from the inferior pubic ramus, inserts on the medial lip of the linea aspera of the femur and is innervated by the obturator nerve; also considered the superior part of the adductor magnus (see "Adductor magnus", page 492)
- Adductor brevis (see section "Flexion of the hip", page 485)
- Gluteus maximus (see "Extension of the hip", page 489)
- Gracilis (see section "Flexion of the hip", page 485)
- Pectineus (see section "Flexion of the hip", page 485)
- Quadratus femoris
- Obturator externus.

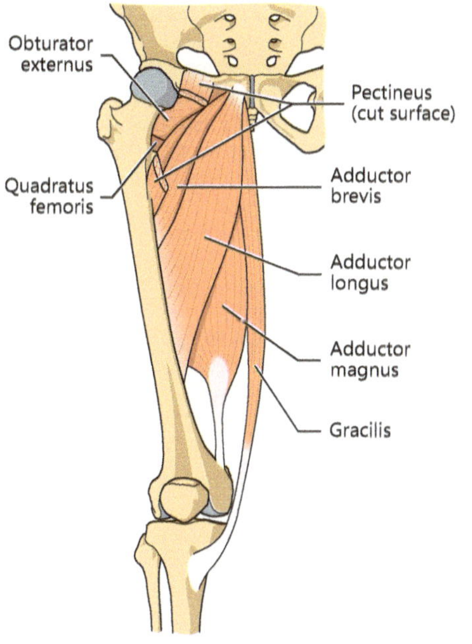

Action of the adductor muscles of the hip

Quadratus femoris

- Weak adductor
- Main action of external rotation of the hip
- Facilitates the retroversion of the pelvis (contraction of both muscles).

Obturator externus

- Weak adductor
- Main action of external rotation of the hip.

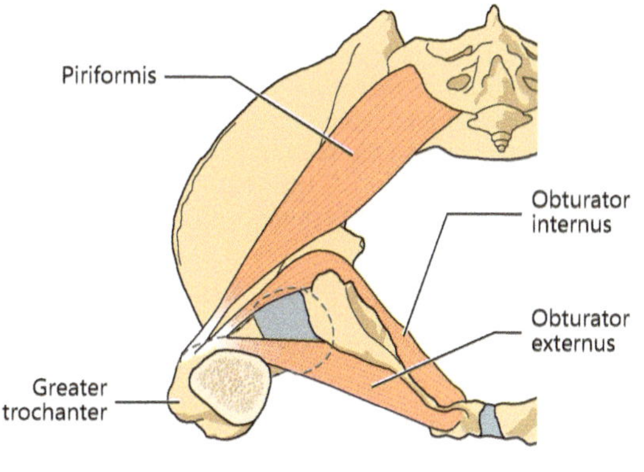

External rotation of the hip

External rotator muscles of the hip (from greatest to least muscular force)

- Gluteus maximus (see section "Extension of the hip", page 489)
- Quadratus femoris (see section "Adduction of the hip", page 495)
- Obturator internus (see section "Abduction of the hip", page 493)
- Gluteus medius (see section "Extension of the hip", page 489)
- Gluteus minimus (see section "Extension of the hip", page 489)
- Iliopsoas (see section "Flexion of the hip", page 485)
- Obturator externus (see section "Adduction of the hip", page 495)
- Adductor longus (see section "Flexion of the hip", page 485)
- Adductor brevis (see section "Flexion of the hip", page 485)
- Adductor magnus (see section "Extension of the hip", page 489)
- Piriformis (see section "Abduction of the hip", page 493)
- Sartorius (see the "Flexion of the hip", page 485)
- Gemellus:
  - superior (single action of external rotation of the hip)
  - inferior (single action of external rotation of the hip)
- Biceps femoris (see section "Extension of the hip", page 489)

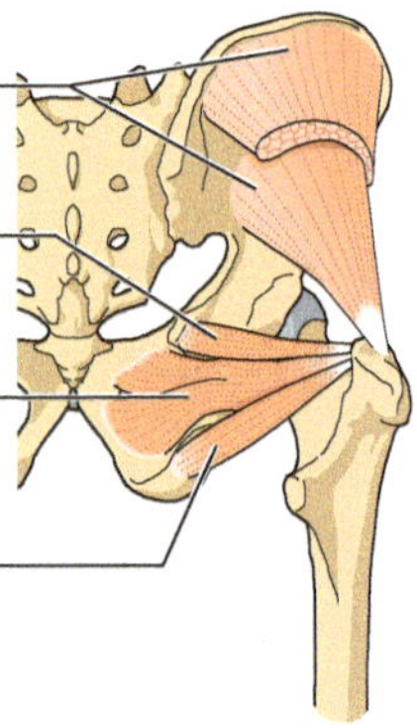

Internal rotation of the hip

Internal rotator muscles of the hip

- Gluteus medius (see section "Extension of the hip", page 489)
- Gluteus minimus (see section "Extension of the hip", page 489)
- Tensor fasciae latae (see section "Flexion of the hip", page 485)
- Adductor magnus (see section "Extension of the hip", page 489)
- Pectineus (see section "Flexion of the hip", page 485)
- Gracilis (see section "Flexion of the hip", page 485).

Assessment of the length of muscle fibers

Hamstring or ischiocrural muscles

Semitendinosus, semimembranosus and biceps femoris (long head) – so called because of their origin in the ischial tuberosity and their tibial insertion.

Starting position	Supine, with the lower limbs in anatomical position
Movement	Flexion of the hip up to the limit of movement allowed while keeping the knee extended, after stabilizing the pelvis and preventing its rotation by securing the contralateral thigh with a band. The fibers of the ischiocrural muscles will thus be completely stretched

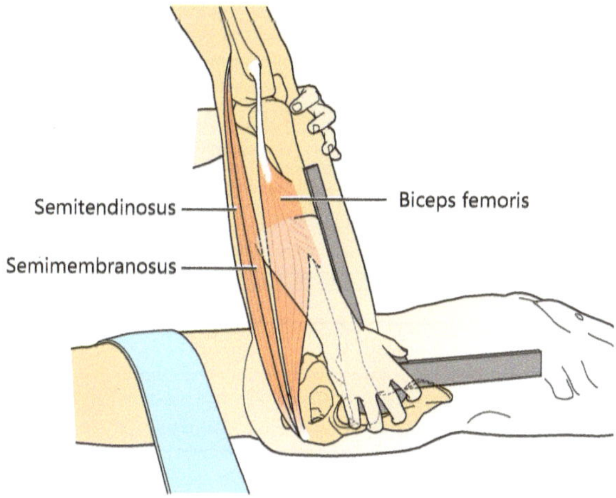

The normal joint mobility of the flexed hip associated with the hamstring muscles stretch is approximately 80°. A decrease in this value during the lifting movement from the supine position of the limb in the upright position in a normal subject is usually due to a deficit in the extension of the hamstring muscles.

Adductor muscles of the hip

Adductor longus, adductor brevis, adductor magnus, pectineus and gracilis.

Starting position	Supine, with the lower limbs in anatomical position; the patient holds on to the edges of the examination table and the unexamined lower limb remains extended.
Movement	Abduction of the hip, after stabilizing the pelvis, up to the limit of movement allowed. The fibers of the adductor muscles of the thigh will thus be completely stretched 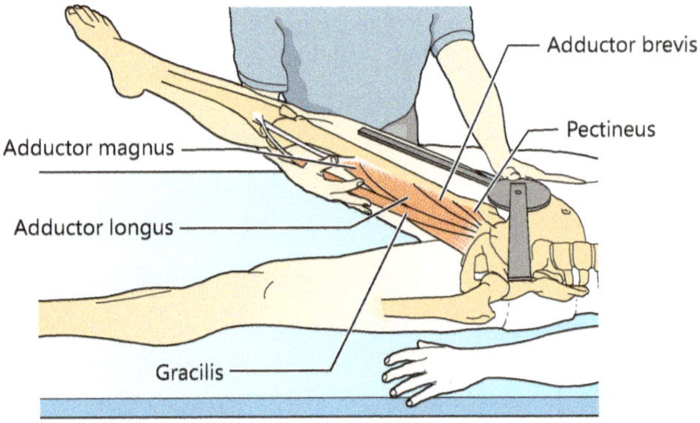

In case of retraction (shortening) of the fibers of the adductor muscles of the hip, the abduction of the hip will be limited proportionally to the reduction of the muscle length.

Flexor muscles of the hip (Thomas test)

Iliopsoas.

Starting position	Supine, with the patient with both hands placed on the knees, keeping the thighs and legs flexed, flattening the lumbar segment of the vertebral column
Movement	The limb to be examined is dropped onto the examination table and the examiner applies light pressure on the anterior surface of the thigh up to the limit of movement allowed, while the other hand stabilizes the pelvis 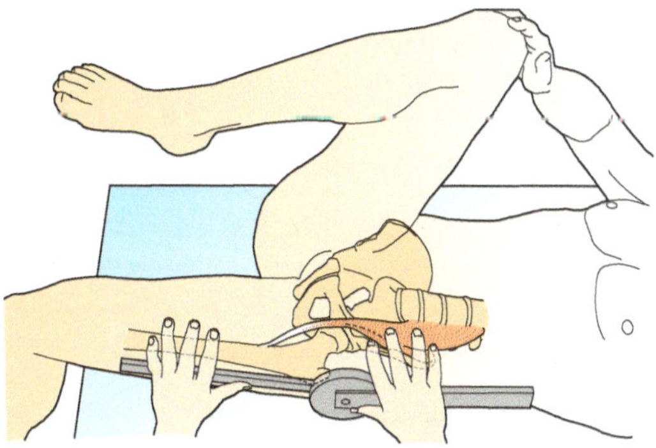

In case of shortening of the fibers of the iliopsoas, the angle formed by the midaxillary line with the longitudinal axis of the femur will indicate the degree of contracture (posture) of the hip in flexion. An increase in lumbar lordosis may mask hip contracture in flexion, but a knee extension deficit may be equally responsible.

Tensor fasciae latae

Iliotibial tract (Ober test).

Starting position	In lateral decubitus on the unexamined side, with the patient holding the hip and knee of the unexamined limb flexed with one hand
Movement	The examiner abducts and extends the hip, in neutral rotation and with the knee flexed 90°, positioning behind and against the patient's buttocks, to maintain the lateral decubitus position, and stabilizing the pelvis with one hand. In this way, the iliotibial tract is stretched above the greater trochanter of the femur. The limb is then dropped onto the examination table, accompanied by the examiner's hand which exerts light pressure on the lateral surface of the thigh up to the limit of movement allowed

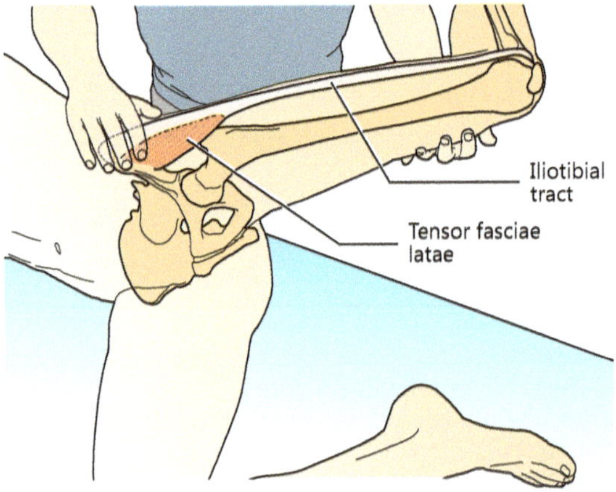

In case of shortening of the fibers of the tensor fasciae latae, the hip will remain abducted. The stiffening of the tensor fasciae latae may be masked by a lateral inclination of the pelvis on the examined side, accompanied by a contralateral inclination of the trunk.

Assessment of the muscular force

Flexion of the hip

Iliopsoas

Against gravity

Flexion of the hip through the entire range of joint motion from the seated position, with the knee flexed off the examination table and foot not in support, allowed instead to the contralateral one, while the examiner stabilizes the pelvis by placing one hand on the iliac crest of the examined side; or from the supine position, with the thigh and leg of the examined limb in anatomical position and the unexamined limb flexed. The examiner applies resistance to the anterior surface of the thigh.

The iliacus and the psoas major are not easily palpable.

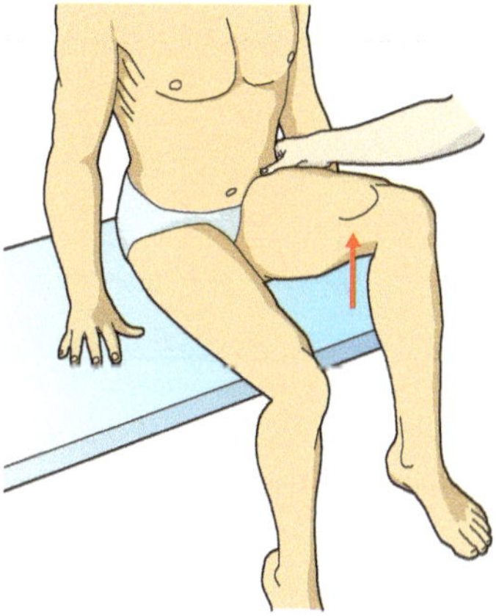

Without gravity

Flexion of the hip through the entire range of joint motion from the lateral decubitus position on the unexamined side, with the patient's hand holding the unexamined hip and knee in maximum flexion and the examiner standing next to the patient, maintaining the lateral decubitus position and holding the examined limb, with the hip extended and the knee flexed to reduce the tension of the hamstring muscles, while stabilizing the pelvis with the other hand.

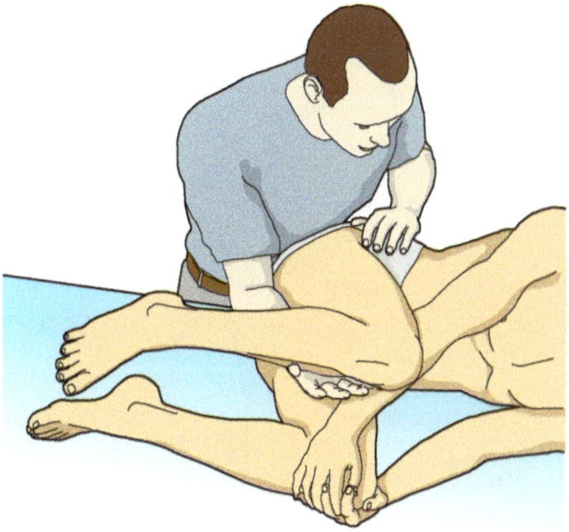

Flexion, abduction and external rotation of the hip with knee flexed

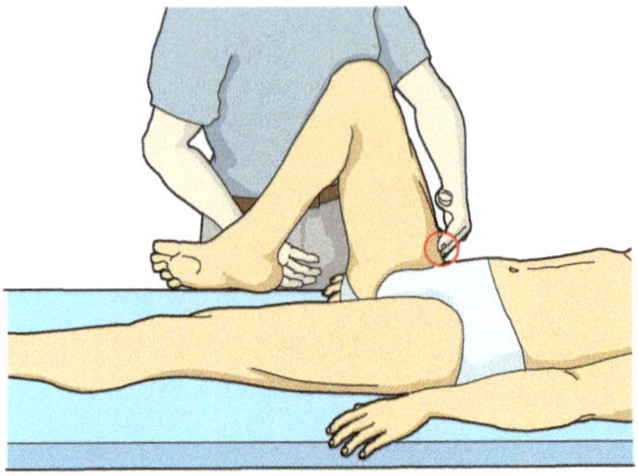

Sartorius

Against gravity

Flexion, abduction and external rotation of the hip with simultaneous flexion of the leg from the supine position with the lower limbs in anatomical position and the resistance applied to the anterolateral surface of the thigh, just above the knee, and on the posterior surface of the leg, just above the ankle.

The sartorius can be palpated on the anterior surface of the thigh, medially to the tensor fasciae latae.

Extension of the hip

Gluteus maximus, biceps femoris, semitendinosus and semimembranosus

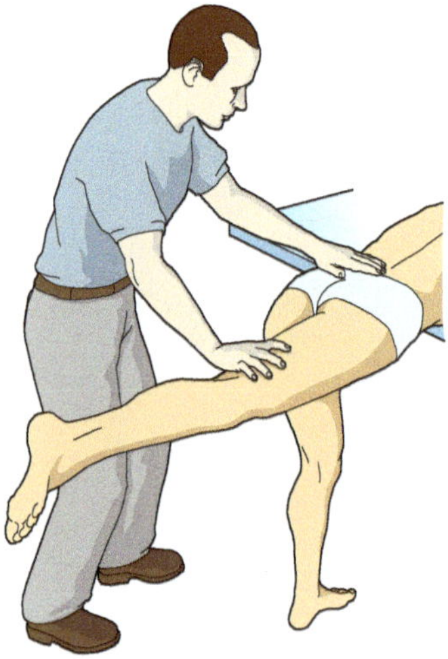

Against gravity

Extension of the hip by keeping the knee extended (and the external rotation of the hip, to obtain the maximum contraction of the gluteus maximus) from the orthostatic position with the trunk flexed and the thorax resting on the examination table, the unexamined limb brought forward so that the hip and knee are flexed, the hip of the examined limb flexed and the knee extended, with the examiner fixing the pelvis and applying resistance to the posterior surface of the thigh, just above the knee.

The gluteus maximus can be palpated medially at its insertion on the gluteal tuberosity or near its origin on the gluteal surface of the ilium.

The extension of the hip with the knee flexed actively shortens the hamstring muscles (decreasing the effectiveness of the contraction), so this method of examination is used to isolate the gluteus maximus.

Without gravity

Extension of the hip through the entire extension amplitude of the knee (in case of contraction of the rectus femoris) from the lateral decubitus position on the unexamined side with the hip and knee maintained in maximum flexion by the patient (to prevent the extension of the lumbar segment of the vertebral column) and the hip and knee of the examined limb flexed by the examiner.

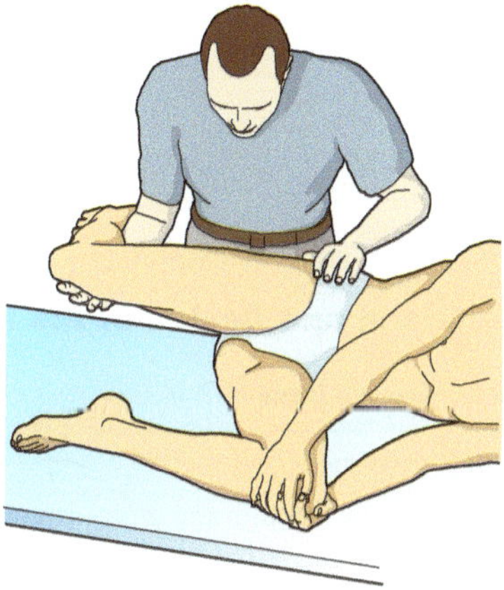

Abduction of the hip

Gluteus medius and gluteus minimus

Against gravity

Hip abduction through the entire range of joint motion from the lateral decubitus position on the unexamined side, with the patient holding the hip and knee of the unexamined limb in flexion and the hip of the examined limb in slight extension and neutral rotation and the examiner positioned behind the patient's buttocks to maintain the lateral decubitus, with one hand on the iliac crest to fix the pelvis and the other hand applying resistance to the lateral surface of the thigh, just above the knee.

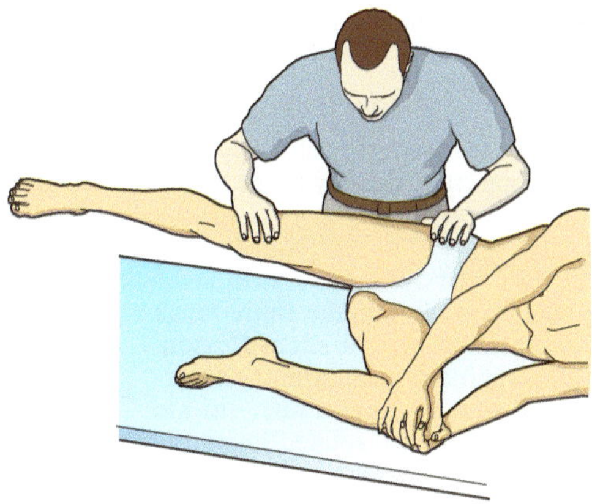

The gluteus medius can be palpated just distally to the lateral margin of the iliac crest or proximally to the greater trochanter of the femur, while the gluteus minimus, located deeply to the gluteus medius, cannot be palpated.

Without gravity

Hip abduction through the entire range of joint motion from the supine position with the lower limb in anatomical position held by the examiner.

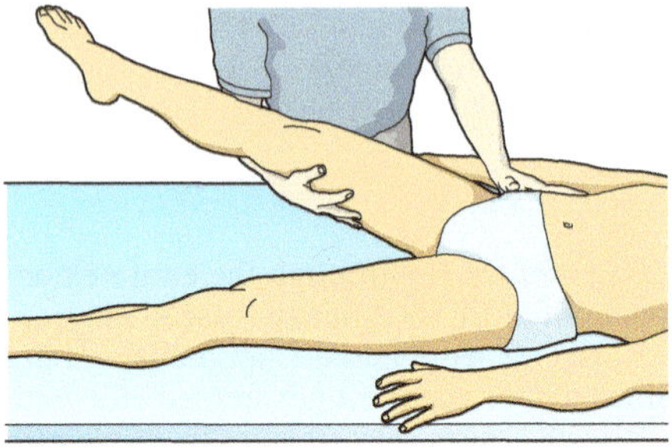

Abduction and flexion of the hip

Tensor fasciae latae

Against gravity

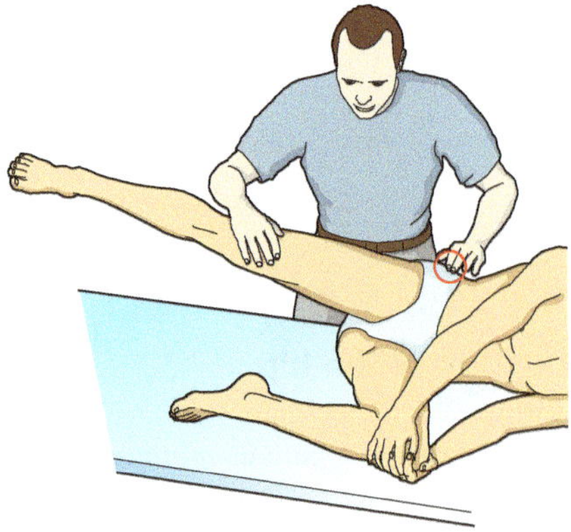

Hip abduction through the entire range of joint motion, with a slight flexion, from the lateral decubitus position on the unexamined side, with the patient holding the hip and knee of the unexamined limb in maximum flexion and the hip of the examined limb flexed at 10-20° and rotated internally, the knee extended and the pelvis in retroversion, and the examiner positioned behind the patient's buttocks, maintaining the lateral decubitus, stabilizing the pelvis with one hand on the iliac crest and applying resistance with the other hand to the anterolateral surface of the thigh, just above the knee.

The tensor fasciae latae can be palpated laterally to the superior part of the sartorius or on the iliotibial tract, distally to the greater trochanter of the femur.

Without gravity

Hip abduction through the entire range of joint motion, with a slight flexion, from the supine position with the examined limb held by the examiner, the hip flexed at 10-20° and rotated internally and the knee extended.

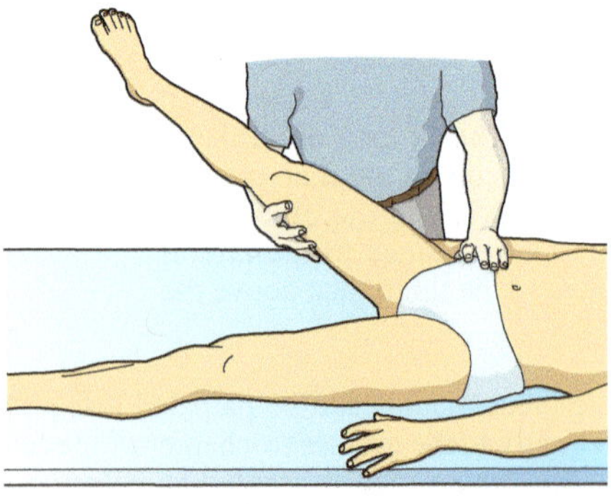

Weakness of the abductor muscles of the hip

The main action of the abductor muscles of the hip is to maintain the pelvis in a horizontal position (avoiding its lateral inclination) during the unilateral foot support during gait (when one limb swings forward while the contralateral one is in contact with the ground). In the upright position, with the foot raised off the ground, the weight of the head, upper limbs, trunk and lower limb raised causes the pelvis to tilt towards the unsupported side, which is then neutralized by the contraction of the abductor muscles of the hip of the supported limb. In case of weakness of these muscles, the pelvis will tend to fall on the opposite side. The deficit of these muscles is evidenced by the Trendelenburg test.

The Trendelenburg Test

- The patient is in upright position on the limb to be examinated
- The thigh and leg of the unsupported contralateral limb are in flexion (the foot is raised off the ground)
- The examiner, located behind the patient, observes the posture of the trunk and pelvis

Negative Trendelenburg test

- The superior posterior iliac spines are at the same level (efficiency of the abductor muscles of the thigh).

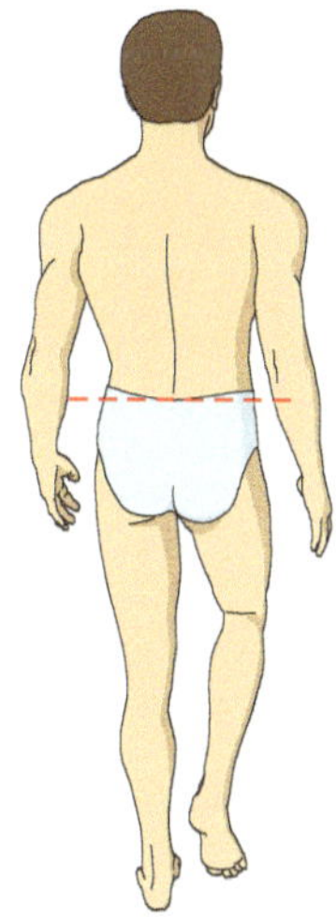

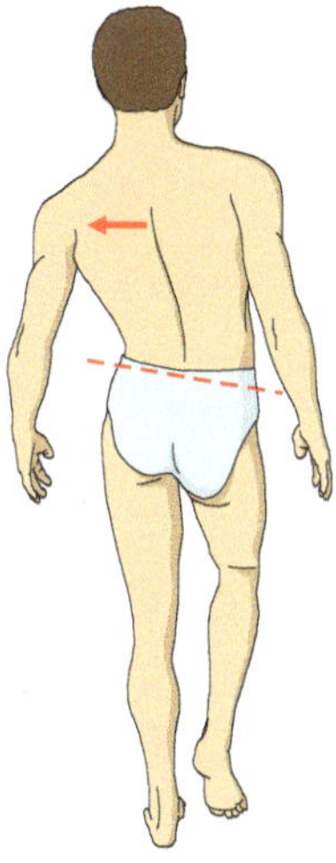

Positive Trendelenburg Test

- The posterior superior iliac spines are not at the same level – the pelvis is tilted towards the unsupported side (weakness of the abductor muscles of the hip)
- Tilting of the trunk on the supporting side (where the muscle deficit is located) – compensation mechanism for the muscle deficit.

Adduction of the hip

Adductor longus, adductor brevis, adductor magnus, pectineus and gracilis

Against resistance and without gravity

Hip adduction, until touching the contralateral limb, starting from the supine position with the examined limb held by the examiner (no gravity), hip abducted at 40°, in neutral rotation and extended, knee extended and the contralateral lower limb in anatomical position; the examiner applies resistance to the medial surface of the thigh, just above the knee.

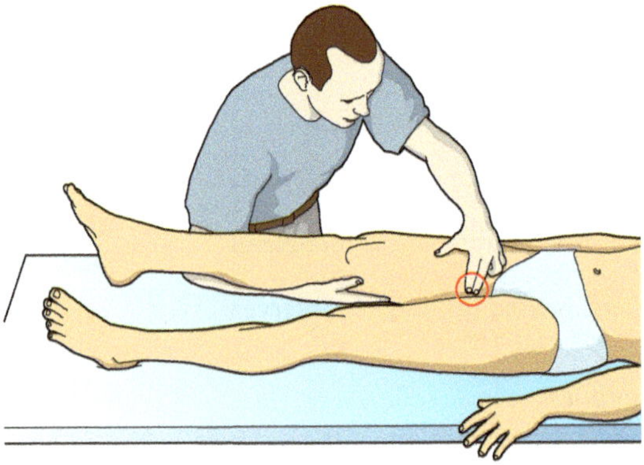

The adductor muscle group is palpated on the medial surface of the thigh in the proximal region.

External rotation of the hip

Piriformis, obturator externus, gemellus superior, quadratus femoris, gemellus inferior and obturator internus

Against gravity

External rotation of the hip through the entire range of joint motion from the seated position, with the hip flexed at 90°, in neutral rotation, and with the center of the patella aligned with the anterior superior iliac spine, with one hand of the examiner placed on the anterolateral surface of the lower part of the thigh, to prevent abduction and flexion, while with the other hand applies resistance to the medial surface of the lower part of the leg, just above the ankle.

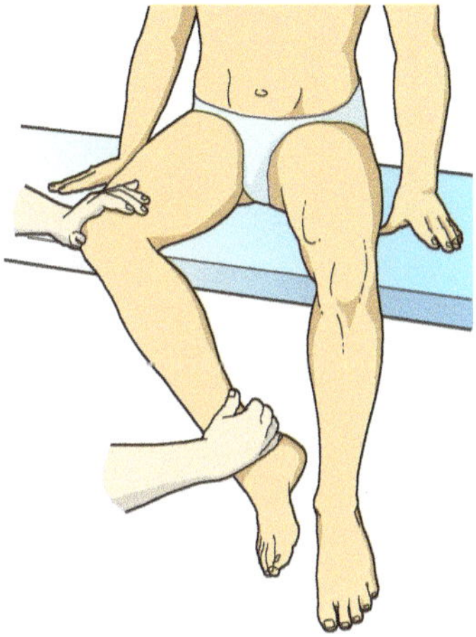

The external rotator muscles are located deeps enough to be palpated.

Without gravity

External rotation of the hip from the supine position with the hip flexed at 90°, in neutral rotation, and the knee of the examined limb flexed and held by the examiner.

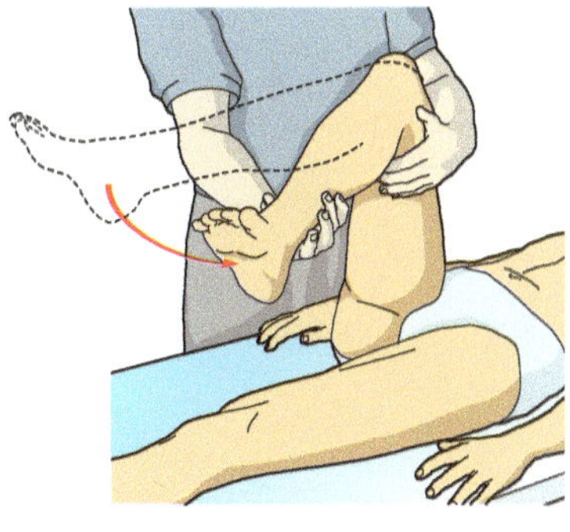

Internal rotation of the hip

Gluteus medius, gluteus minimus and tensor fasciae latae

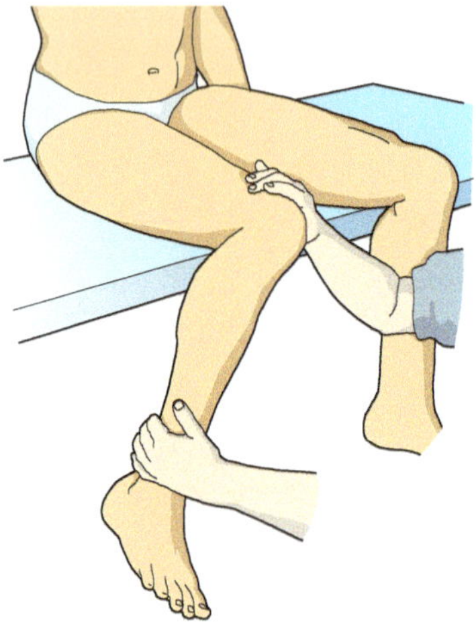

Against gravity

Internal rotation of the hip through the entire range of joint motion, from the seated position with the hip flexed at 90° and in neutral rotation, the center of the patella aligned with the anterior superior iliac spine, the unexamined limb abducted with the foot supported and the hand of the examiner on the medial surface of the lower part of the examined thigh, to avoid adduction, while with the other hand applies resistance to the lateral surface of the lower part of the leg, just above the ankle.

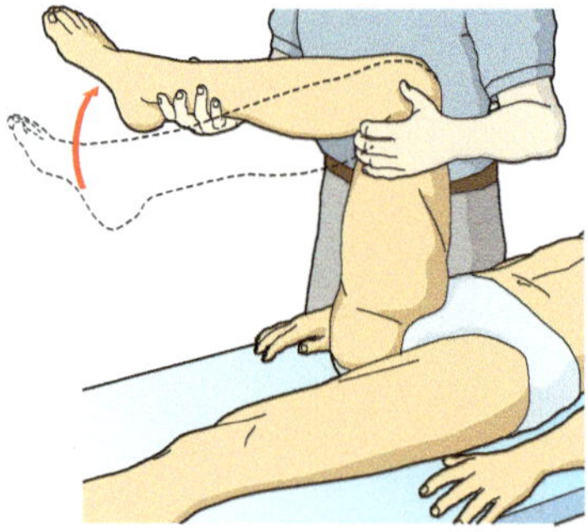

Without gravity

Internal rotation of the hip through the entire range of joint motion, from the supine position with the hip flexed at 90°, in neutral rotation, and the knee of the examined limb flexed and supported by the examiner.

Functional aspects of the muscles of the hip

Flexion of the hip

- The contraction of the flexor muscles of the hip is exemplified by activities such as:
  - putting on pants
  - climbing a ladder
  - going up the stairs
  - getting in or out of the bathtub
- The flexor muscles of the hip contract along with the muscles of the abdomen to lift the trunk when moving from a supine to a seated position
- The iliopsoas:
  - is the only flexor muscle capable of flexing the hip beyond 90° in a seated position, for example in activities such as:
    - sitting with the lower limbs crossed
    - bringing the foot onto the contralateral thigh in the seated position
    - putting on socks
  - controls the movements of the trunk and the pelvis when leaning backwards in a seated position to look over the shoulder
  - lowers the trunk when lying supine from a seated position
- The adductor muscles contribute to the flexion of the hip when it is extended
- The gracilis flexes the hip especially in the initial phase of movement and when the knee is extended and not flexed
- The intervention of the adductor muscles and the gracilis in the flexion of the hip is exemplified by activities such as:
  - kicking a ball
  - swimming with fins
- The intervention of the sartorius as a flexor, abductor and external rotator muscle of the hip and as a flexor of the knee is exemplified by the action of bringing a foot onto the contralateral thigh in a seated position.

Extension of the hip

- The contribution of the extensor muscles of the hip to daily life activities is partly determined by the position of the hip and the force required for its extension
- The position of the knee between 0 and 90° of flexion does not affect the extension of the thigh
- The action of the extensor muscles of the hip is exemplified by activities in which the body is lifted, such as:
  - getting up from a seated position
  - going up the stairs
  - jumping
- The extensor muscles of the hip:
  - contract during lifting activities carried out with the hips and knees flexed
  - control the anteversion of the pelvis when one flexes forwards in a seated or standing position
  - produce the retropulsion of the pelvis when sitting or getting up
  - are active in the thrust phase when skating
- The hamstring or ischiocrural muscles (semimembranosus, semitendinosus and the long head of the biceps femoris):
  - start the extension of the hip
  - extend the hip during the upright position

- The gluteus maximus:
  - contracts when the thigh is moved from anatomical position in hyperextension or when the extension is carried out against resistance
  - contracts when bending forward, for example to change gears while driving or to look into a low drawer
  - extends the hip during the upright position in case of increased resistance
- The adductor magnus extends the hip when it is flexed between 0 and 90°.

Abduction of the hip

- The main function of the abductor muscles of the hip is to keep the pelvis in a horizontal position in single-leg support
- When the foot is lifted from the ground, the pelvis, not supported on the side of oscillation, tends to drop due to the weight of the head, upper limbs, trunk, and lifted lower limb, which makes it rotate around the head of the femur of the supporting limb
- The abductor muscles of the hip of the supporting side, contracting with inverted origin and insertion, drag down the iliac crest of the same side, causing the rotation of the pelvis around the head of the femur and elevating the unsupported side
- The action of maintaining the pelvis in a horizontal position during single-leg support by the hip abductor muscles occurs while walking, running or when kicking a ball
- During the single-leg support phase, the contraction of the abductor muscles of the hip may not be necessary to keep the pelvis in a horizontal position, if the weight of the trunk is shifted onto the supporting leg in such a way that the center of gravity of the head, arms and trunk passes through the hip joint on the supporting side
- The abductor muscles of the hip can contract bilaterally in activities that require the abduction of the non-supporting lower limb, such as when mounting a bicycle
- The upper fibers of the gluteus maximus contribute to the hip abduction when an increase in strength is required.

Adduction of the hip

- The action of the hip adductor muscles is exemplified by activities such as:
  - climbing a rope
  - kicking a ball, crossing the body anteriorly with the foot
  - horseback riding
- In many activities, the adductor muscles of the hip act primarily as postural muscles rather than as agonists of the adduction movement.

Internal rotation of the hip

- The internal rotator muscles are active during walking or when, in the upright position, rotation is carried out on one foot
- The semimembranosus and semitendinosus rotate the thigh internally when it is extended.

External rotation of the hip

- The piriformis and obturator internus work more effectively as external rotators of the hip when the hip is extended, and are less effective when the hip is flexed
- The gluteus maximus and biceps femoris also rotate the hip externally when it is extended
- Activities that require the contraction of the external rotator muscles are exemplified by:
  - mounting a bicycle
  - sitting, bringing the foot onto the contralateral thigh in order to tie the shoelaces.

Palpation of the pelvis and hip

Iliolumbar ligament

The patient is in the prone position. The examiner identifies the rounded protrusion of the spinous process of L5, located on the sacrum. From here, the examiner moves laterally about 5 cm to find the transverse process of the same vertebra. It then continues laterally, following the course of the iliolumbar ligament. The palpation is performed transversally to the course of the ligament, in a condition of total relaxation of the patient.

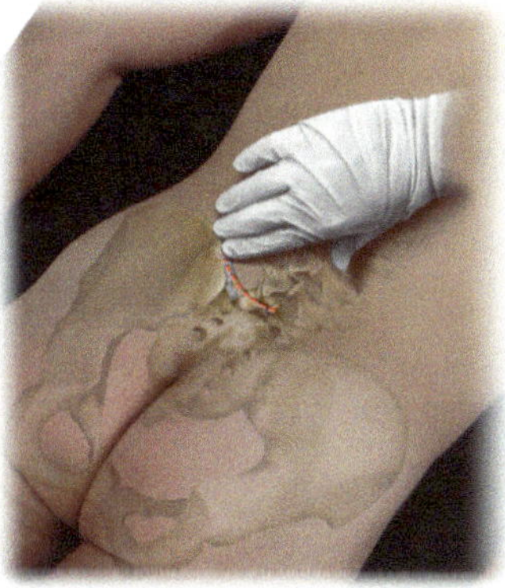

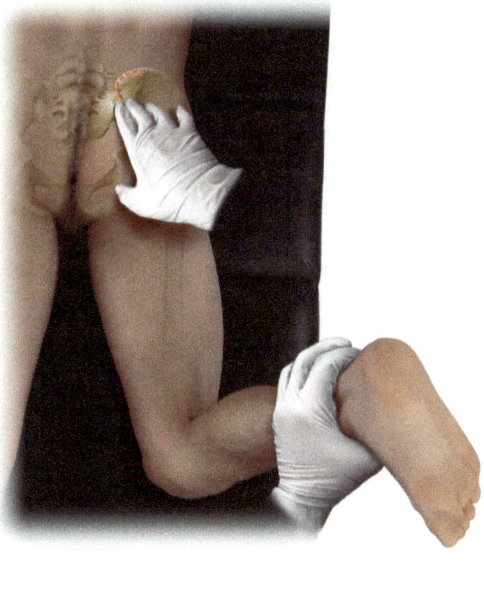

Sacroiliac joint

The patient is in the prone position. The examiner begins palpation from the posterior superior iliac spine, then moves slightly medially and caudally to appreciate a depression between the hip bone and the sacrum. With one hand on the joint, the examiner flexes the patient's knee to 90° and performs a passive internal rotation of the hip to feel the movement at the joint level under the palpating hand.

Iliac crest

The patient is in the upright position. The examiner identifies the anterior superior iliac spine by resting his hands on the patient's flanks with the thumbs backward and the other fingers forward. The examiner then slides his fingers along the borders of the iliac crests which first go up and then, posteriorly, back down again until ending with the posterior superior iliac spine.

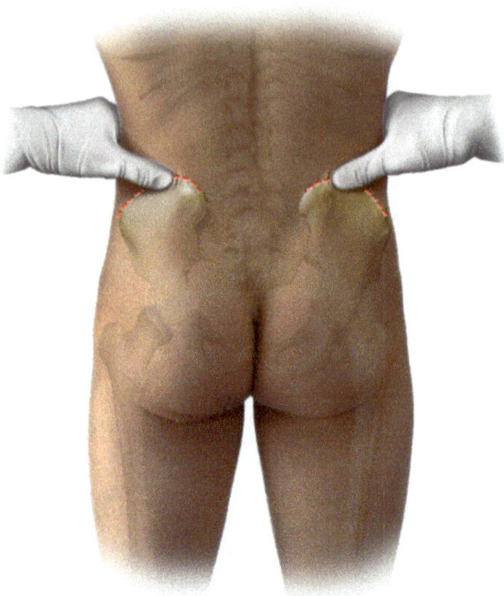

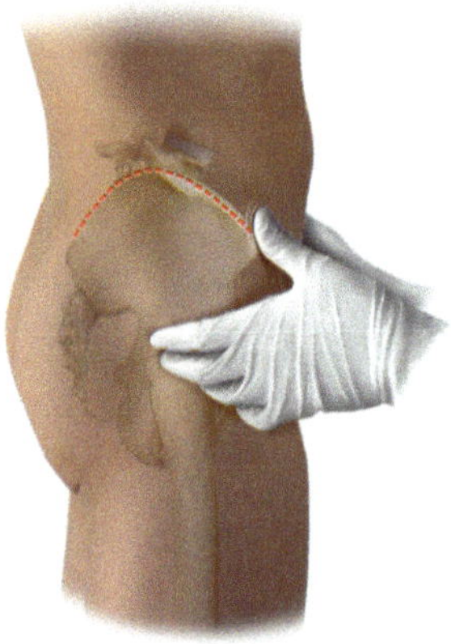

Anterior superior iliac spine

The patient is standing. The examiner rests the thumbs on the highest part of the iliac crests, then slides them forward and downward until the anterior superior iliac spines are encountered. From the anterior superior iliac spines, palpation can continue backward over the iliac crest to the posterior superior iliac spine or move medially with a 30° downward tilt to explore the inguinal ligament.

Median sacral crest

The patient is in the prone position. The examiner begins palpation from the posterior superior iliac spines and moving in a medial direction. The surface of the sacrum is easily recognizable thanks to the protrusions on the median crest, which can be followed in a caudal direction up to the apex of the sacrum.

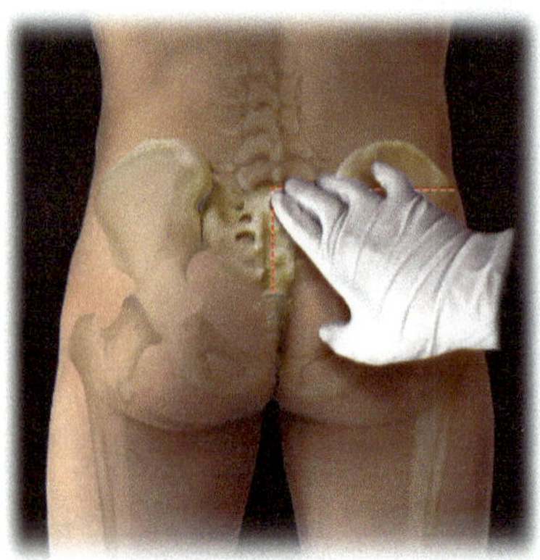

Sacrum

The patient is in the prone position. The examiner rests his fingers on the two posterior superior iliac spines and explores between these structures looking for the surface of the sacrum. Once the bony surface has been identified, the examiner slides his fingers laterally and then caudally to the coccyx.

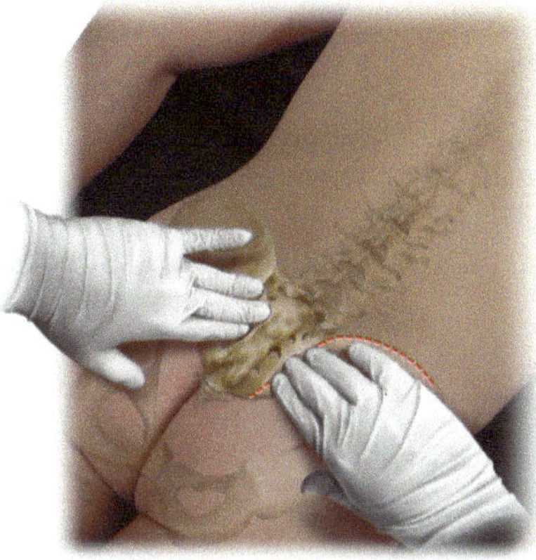

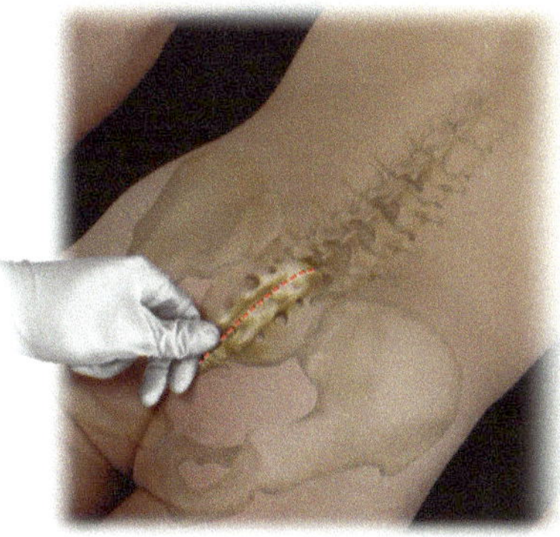

Coccyx

The patient is in prone position. The examiner follows the median sacral crest in a caudal direction, up to the gluteal fold, at the upper extremity of which the irregular surface of the coccyx can be identified.

Ischial tuberosity

The patient is in prone position. The hand rests on the upper third of the thigh and gradually ascends in a proximal direction: the most obvious bony prominence in the lower and medial part of the pelvis is the ischial tuberosity.

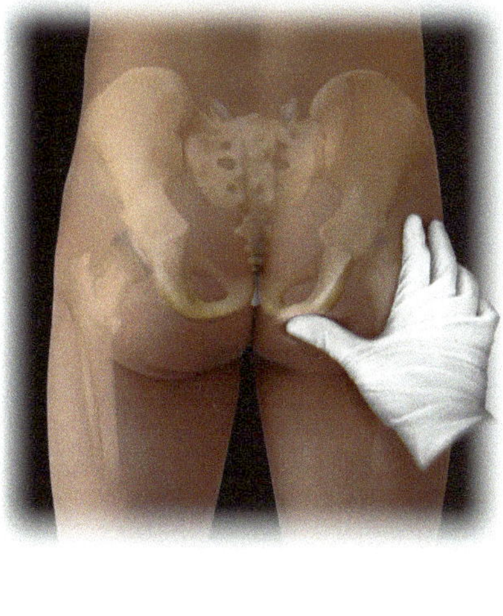

Inferior pubic ramus

The patient is in the supine position; resting the palm of the hand on the umbilicus with the fingers directed caudally, the pubic crest (the only horizontal bone in this region) is found. Moving over the lateral portion of the pubic crest, proceed caudally by sliding over the inferior pubic ramus.

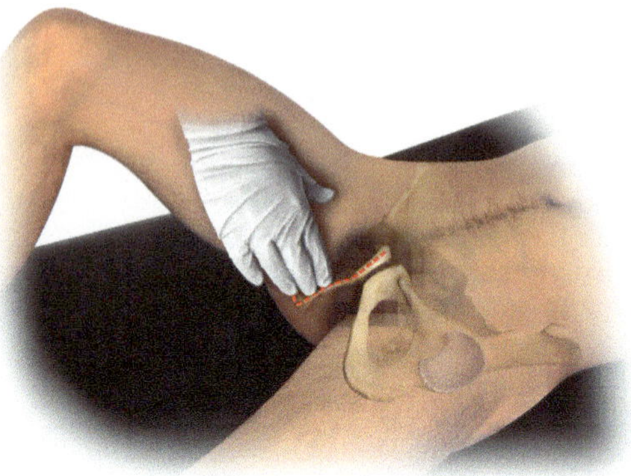

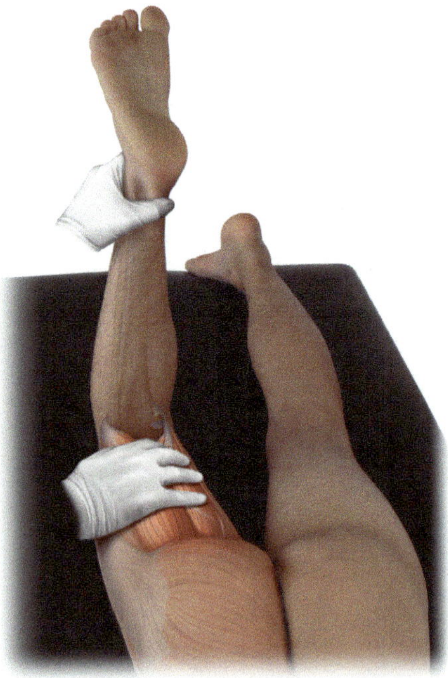

Hamstring or ischiocrural muscles

The patient is in the prone position. The hand is placed on the posterior region of the thigh and the patient is asked to flex the knee against resistance to tense the muscles: the biceps femoris is the most lateral, while medially the semitendinosus and semimembranosus are found, the latter in a deeper position. Continuing palpation of the muscle bellies in the proximal direction, the ischial tuberosity is reached. Here the enthesis is palpated, possibly painful.

Anatomical landmarks on the surface of the pelvis and hip

1	Iliac crest: convex bony margin representing the superior border of the ilium; the highest part of the iliac crest is at the level of the space between the spinous processes of L4 and L5
2	Anterior superior iliac spine: rounded bony prominence on the anterior extremity of the iliac crest
3	Iliac tuberosity: approximately 5 cm above and lateral to the anterior superior iliac spine, along the lateral border of the iliac crest
4	Posterior superior iliac spine: rounded bony prominence on the posterior extremity of the iliac crest, palpable through the skin at the base of the dimples above the buttocks; the posterior superior iliac spines are at the level of the spinous process of S2
5	Ischial tuberosity: when the hip is in passive flexion, this large bony prominence is located laterally to the midline of the body just above the gluteal fold – the deep transverse sulcus between the buttocks and the posterior surface of the thigh
6	Greater trochanter of the femur: when the tip of the thumb is placed on the lateral border of the iliac crest, the tip of the middle finger, pointing distally on the lateral surface of the thigh, rests on the superior border of the greater trochanter
7	Adductor tubercle: medial prominence on the inferior extremity of the femur behind and above the medial epicondyle
8	Lateral epicondyle of the femur: a bony prominence on the lateral condyle of the femur
9	Patella: large, triangular-shaped sesamoid bone on the anterior surface of the knee, with proximal base and distal apex

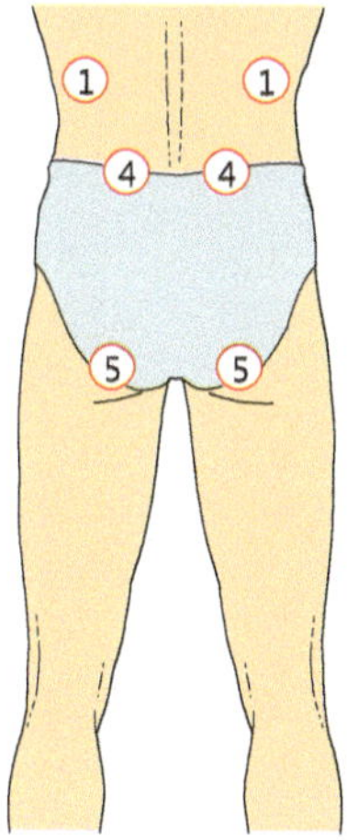

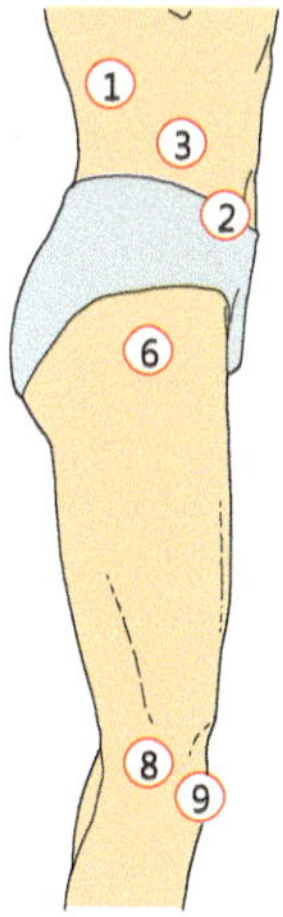

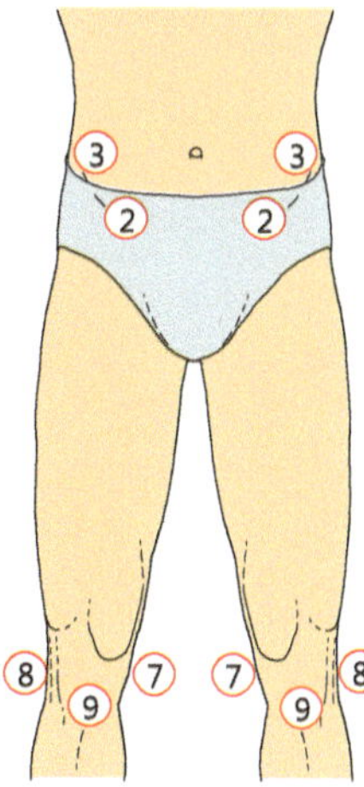

Inferior extremity of the femur

- Articular surface for the tibia and patella:
  - patellar surface (inferiorly and anteriorly) – it has two oblique sides with a central depression (trochlea)
  - intercondylar fossa (inferiorly and posteriorly) – posterior continuation of the depression of the patellar surface
- Medial and lateral condyles – masses, which are directed posteriorly and laterally, in which continue the two sides of the trochlea – articulate with the tibial condyles
- Medial and lateral epicondyles – lateral prominences on the medial and lateral condyles
- Adductor tubercle – posteriorly and superiorly to the medial epicondyle (insertion of the adductor magnus)

(For the superior extremity and shaft (body) of the femur, see Chapter 10 "Hip and pelvis").

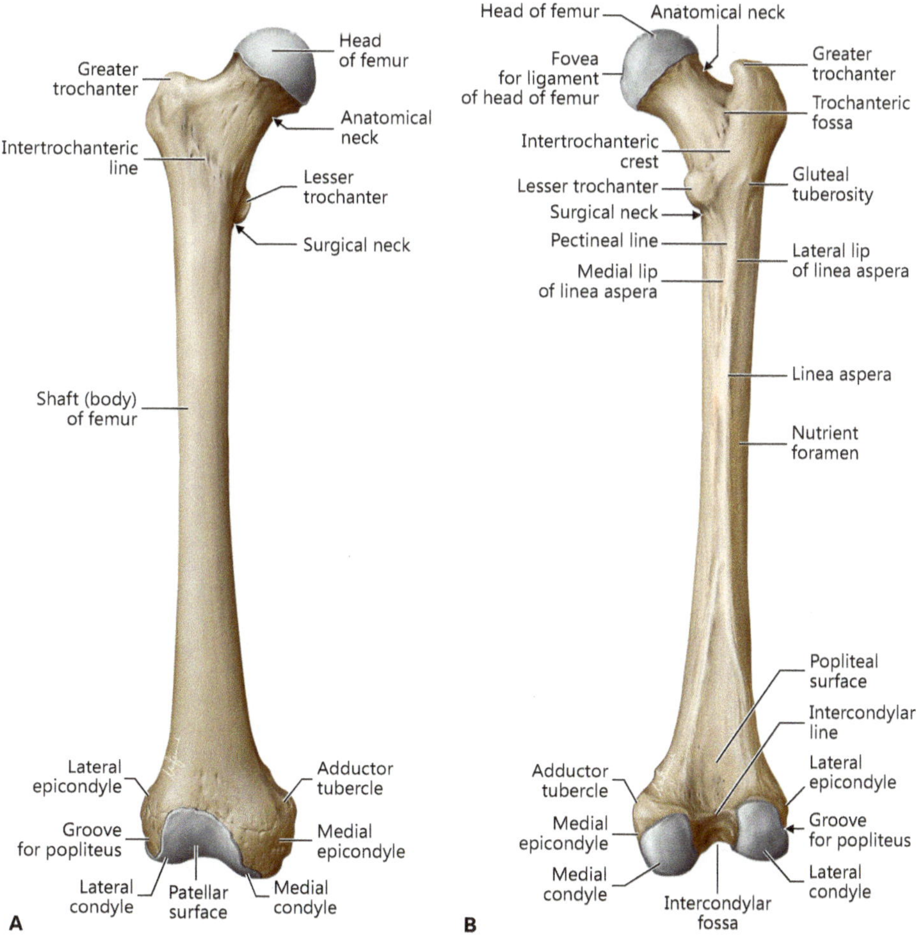

Anterior (**A**) and posterior (**B**) surfaces of the right femur.

11

Patella

- Sesamoid bone in the thickness of the insertion tendon of the quadriceps femoris
- Triangular shape (two faces, two borders, proximal base and distal apex):
  - anterior surface – cutaneous
  - posterior surface – articular:
    - superior part corresponding to the femur (vertical crest opposing the depression of the trochlea and two articular facets – lateral and medial – in relation to the patellar surface of the femur)
    - inferior part corresponding to the anterior fat pad of the knee
  - base – insertion of the tendon of the quadriceps femoris
  - apex – originates the patellar ligament.

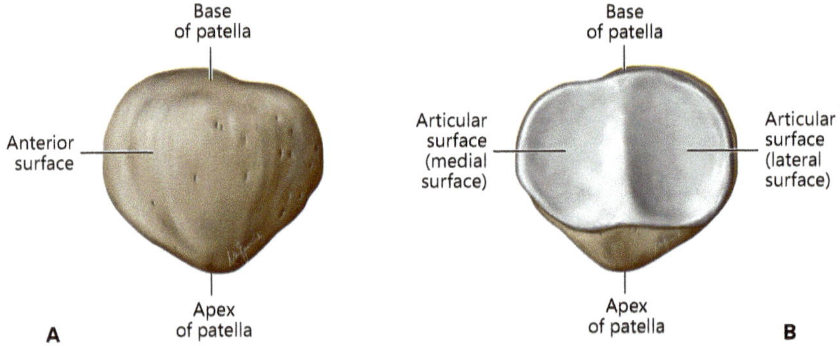

Anterior (**A**) and posterior (**B**) surfaces of the right patella.

Superior extremity and shaft (body) of the tibia

Superior extremity

- Medial and lateral tibial condyles:
  - the superior surface of each condyle (glenoid cavity) articulates with the corresponding condyle of the femur
  - glenoid cavities of the condyles – supported by the heads, of which the external one has the fibular articular facet
  - tibial tuberosity – anterior prominence on which the condyles converge
- Intercondylar eminence (relief formed by the medial and lateral intercondylar tubercles directed anteroposteriorly) between the two glenoid cavities of the condyles
- Intercondylar areas (anterior and posterior) – anteriorly and posteriorly to the intercondylar eminence – insertion of the cruciate ligaments

(For the inferior extremity of the tibia, see Chapter 12 "Ankle and foot").

Shaft (body)

- Triangular prism shape (three surfaces and three borders):
  - medial surface – corresponds to the integuments
  - lateral surface – origin or proximal attachment of the tibialis anterior
  - posterior surface – the superior part is crossed by a rough crest directed downward and medially: oblique line (soleal line)
  - anterior border – ends inferiorly at the medial malleolus
  - medial border – poorly accentuated
  - lateral border (interosseous) – gives insertion to the interosseous membrane.

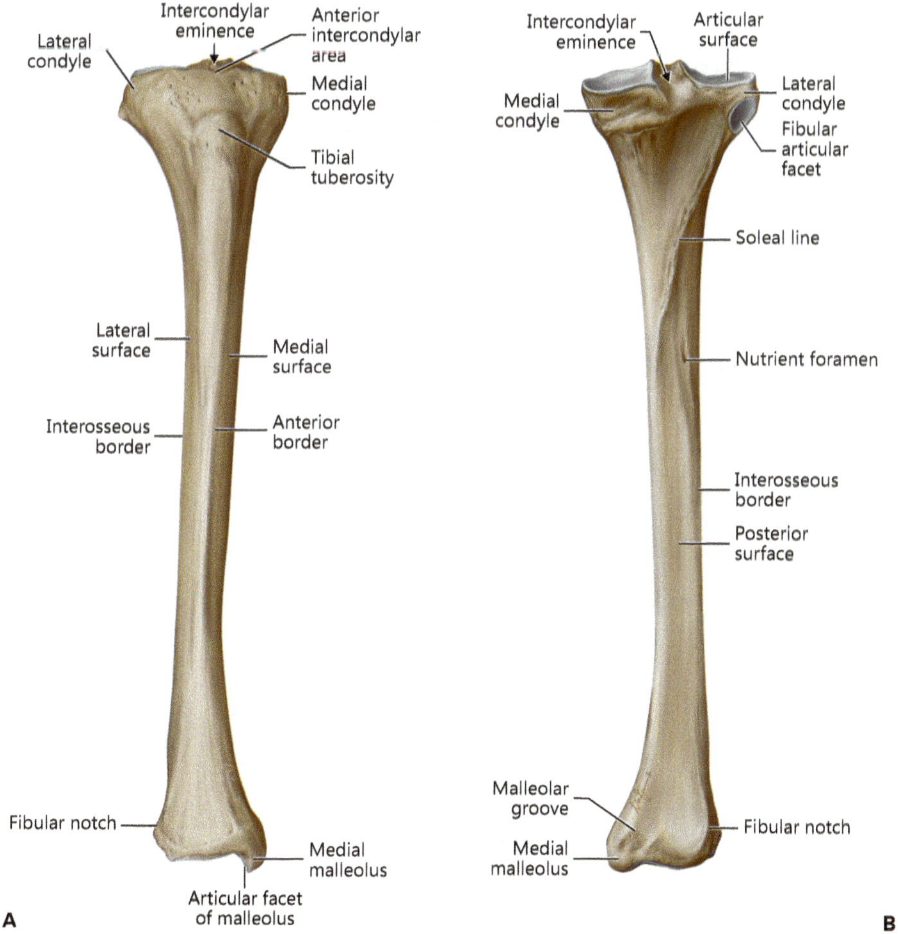

Anterior (**A**) and posterior (**B**) surfaces of the right tibia.

Superior extremity and shaft (body) of the fibula

Superior extremity (head)

- Tibial articular facet (upward and medially)
- Apex of the head of the fibula – lateral prominence in which the biceps femoris is inserted

(For the inferior extremity of the fibula, see Chapter 12 "Ankle and foot").

Shaft (body)

- Triangular prism shape:
  - lateral surface – origen or proximal attachment of the lateral fibular muscles
  - medial surface – is crossed by a vertical relief (interosseous border) on which the interosseous membrane is inserted
  - posterior surface – presents the medial crest.

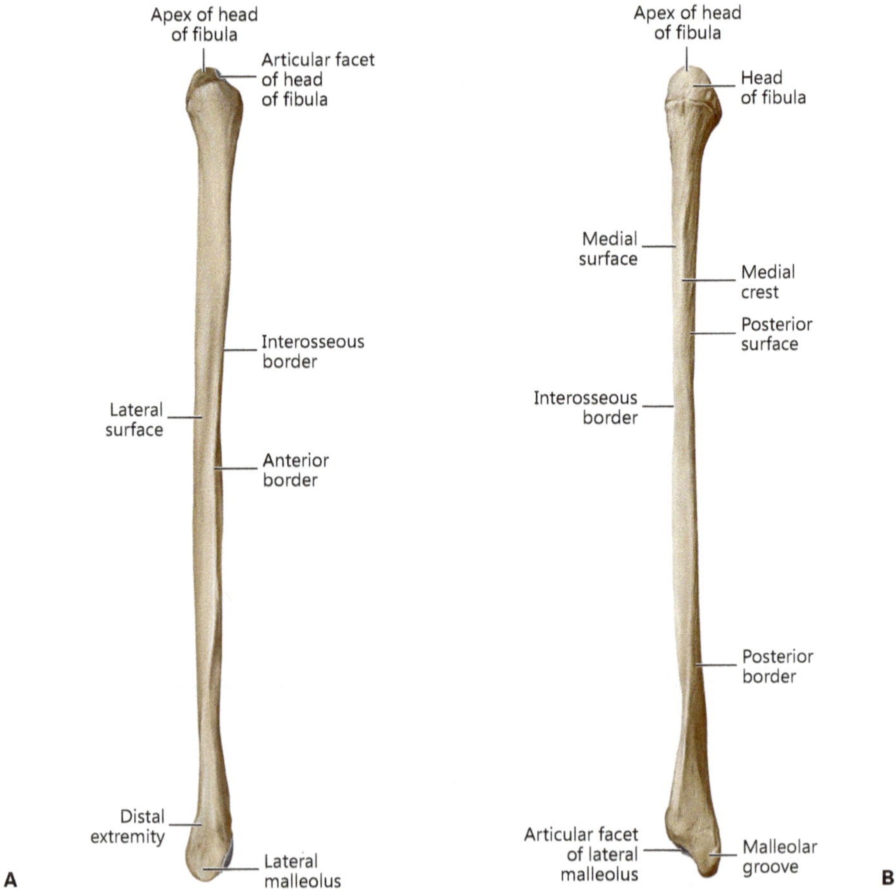

Anterior (**A**) and posterior (**B**) surfaces of the right fibula.

Knee joints

- Tibiofemoral joint
- Patellofemoral joint
- (Superior) tibiofibular joint

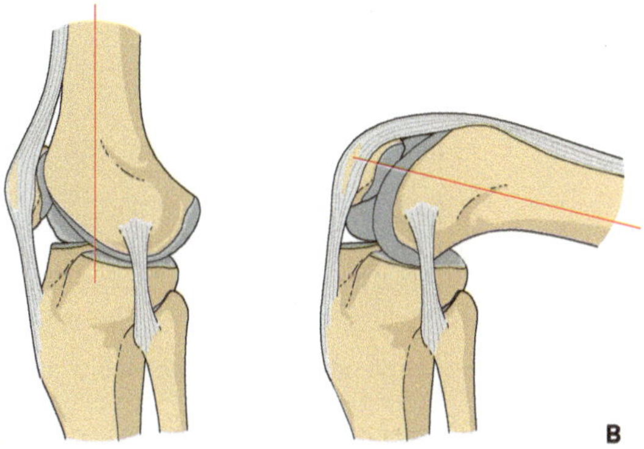

Right knee joint, lateral view: in extension (**A**) and in wide flexion position (**B**).

Tibiofemoral joint

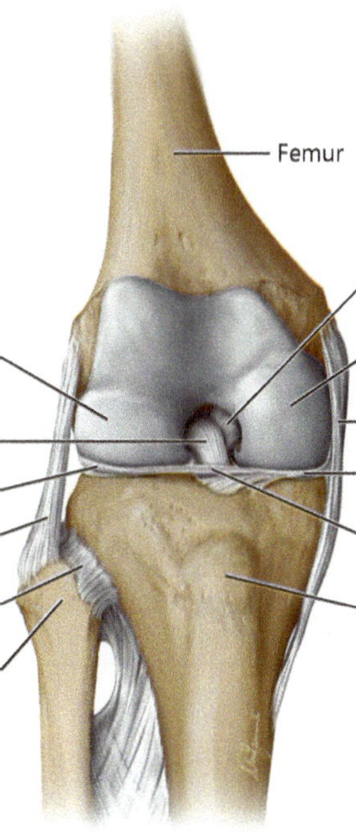

Right knee joint in slight flexion after removal of the joint capsule: anterior frontal view.

<table>
<tr><td>Type of joint</td><td>Hinge joint</td></tr>
<tr><td>Articular surfaces</td><td>Convex surfaces of the medial and lateral condyles of the femur

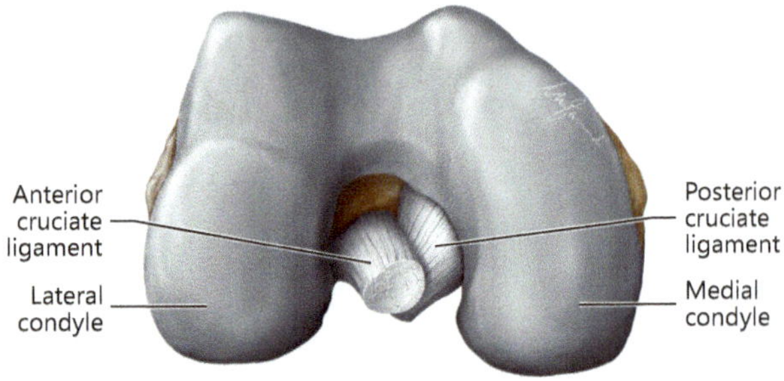

Glenoid cavities of the medial and lateral condyles of the tibia (the glenoid cavity of the medial condyle is flat and has an oval shape; that of the lateral condyle is slightly concave and has a round shape)

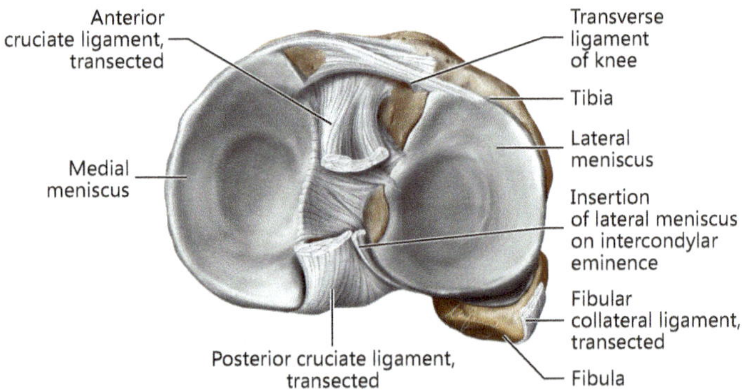

The articular surfaces are covered with hyaline cartilage and the menisci (connective tissue formations consisting of collagen fibers) are interposed between them (see section “Menisci of the tibiofemoral joint”, page 525)</td></tr>
<tr><td>Movements</td><td>In the frontal (flexion-extension) and transverse (rotation) planes (2 degrees of freedom)</td></tr>
</table>

Patellofemoral joint

<table>
<tr><td>Type of joint</td><td>Hinge joint</td></tr>
<tr><td>Articular surfaces</td><td>Posterior surface of the patella (wedge shape with rounded apex):
– medial and lateral articular surfaces separated by a vertical eminence

Patellar surface of the femur (generally concave shape)

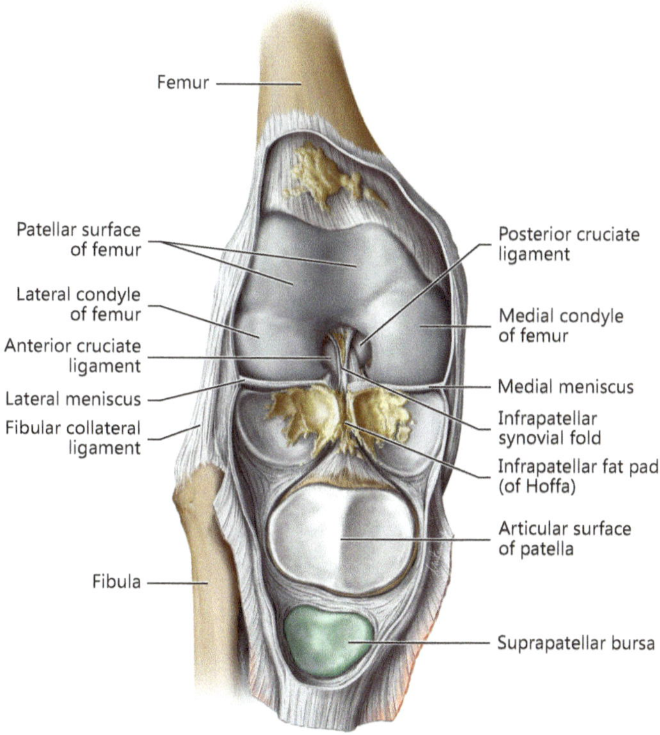
</td></tr>
<tr><td>Movements</td><td>In the frontal plane (flexion-extension) (one degree of freedom)</td></tr>
</table>

(Superior) tibiofibular joint

Type of joint	Amphiarthrosis
Articular surfaces	Articular surface for the tibia (on the superior extremity of the fibula) Articular surface for the fibula (on the superior extremity of the tibia) 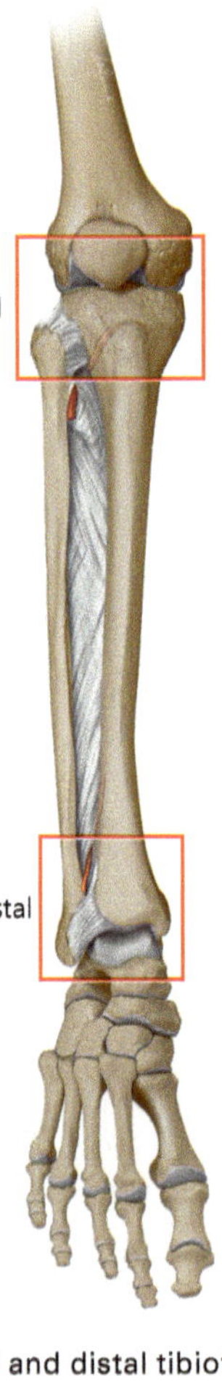 Proximal and distal tibiofibular joints.
Movements	Low mobility

The superior tibioperoneal joint is also called the "compensatory joint" because it acts as a cushion for the outward thrust stresses produced when the anterior articular surface of the talus, during major dorsiflexion of the foot, penetrates the anterior tibiofibular articular surface extending it. It is wrapped in a robust capsule and stabilized by the ligaments of the fibular head.

Menisci of the tibiofemoral joint

- Medial meniscus – in the shape of an "open C" (crescent-shaped)
- Lateral meniscus – in the shape of a "closed C"

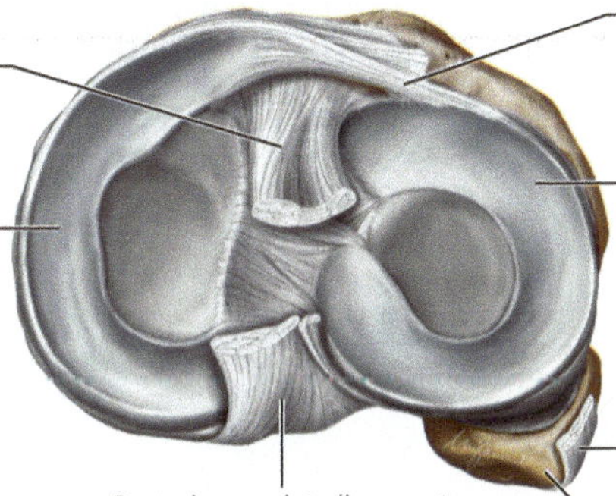

Right knee joint. Articular surface of the tibial condyles, seen from above; this surface is modified in its configuration due to the presence of menisci (medial and lateral) which attached at the intercondylar region of the tibia.

The two "C":
- are opposed to each other
- their extremities are called the anterior horn and the posterior horn

The menisci are fixed by the joint capsule, which is attached to them, and by ligaments:
- the medial meniscus is attached to the medial collateral ligament
- the anterior and posterior horns of the lateral meniscus are attached to the femur through the anterior and posterior meniscofemoral ligaments, located anteriorly and posteriorly, respectively, to the posterior cruciate ligament; the lateral meniscus is not attached to the lateral collateral ligament and this makes it more mobile than the medial meniscus
- both menisci attach anteriorly to the transverse ligament of the knee.

11

Function of the menisci:
- damping due to interposition between the articular surfaces
- increase of the contact surface with pressure distribution over a wider surface area

Movements of the menisci

Flexion of the knee (combined action of forward sliding and backward rotation of the femoral condyles on the tibial surfaces):

- **posterior** movement of the menisci (medial and lateral) (this is actually a deformation of the menisci, since they are fixed to the glenoid cavities of the tibial condyles through the anterior and posterior horns while the remaining part of the meniscus is free):
  - is facilitated by the semimembranosus and the posterior cruciate ligament (medial meniscus)
  - is facilitated by the popliteus (lateral meniscus)

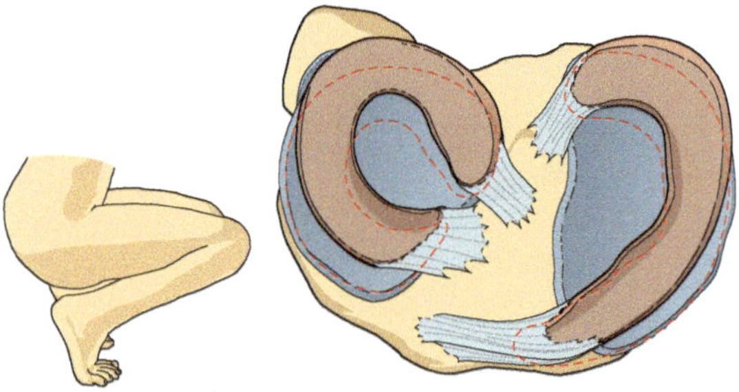

Extension of the knee (combined action of backward sliding and forward rotation of the femoral condyles on the tibial surfaces):

- **anterior** movement of the menisci (medial and lateral)
  - is facilitated by the alar ligaments of the patella (due to the forward movement of the patella itself)

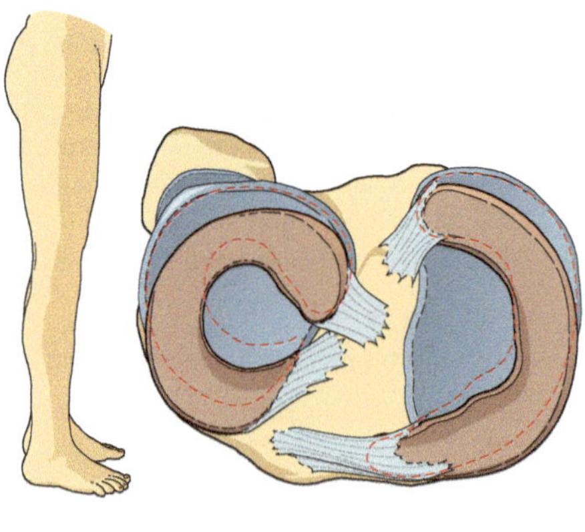

The movement of the menisci is due to the pressure exerted on them by the femoral condyles. During flexion-extension movements of the knee, the movement of the medial meniscus is approximately twice that of the lateral meniscus.

Internal rotation of the knee (external rotation of the tibia which corresponds to the internal rotation of the femoral condyles on the tibial surfaces)
- movement:
  - anterior movement of the lateral meniscus
  - posterior movement of the medial meniscus

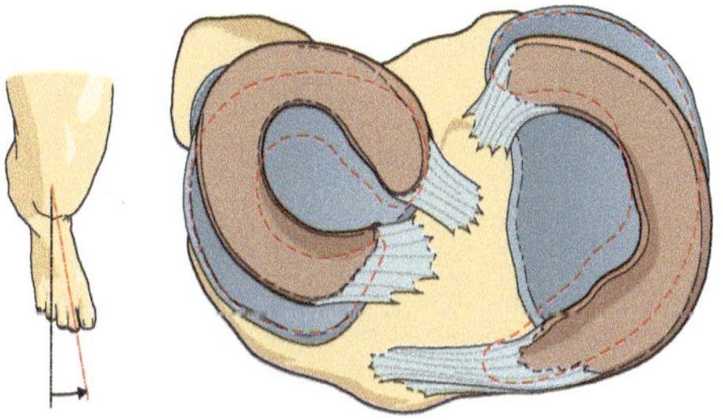

External rotation of the knee (internal rotation of the tibia which corresponds to the external rotation of the femoral condyles on the tibial surfaces)
- movement:
  - posterior movement of the lateral meniscus
  - anterior movement of the medial meniscus

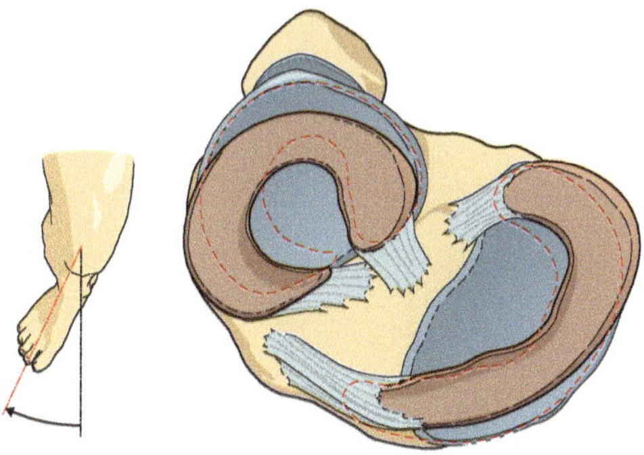

The medial meniscus, compared to the lateral meniscus, is more frequently affected by trauma from excessive external rotation concomitant with knee flexion or lateral thrusts of the knee in flexion. This increased fragility is due to the substantial immobility of the medial meniscus and the more intense traction exerted on it by the medial collateral ligament of the knee in rotation.

Ligaments of the knee

- Patellar ligament – between the inferior apex of the patella and the tibial tuberosity
- Alar ligaments (retinacula) of the patella:
  - lateral – between the patella and the surface of the tibia laterally to the tibial tuberosity
  - medial – between the patella and the surface of the tibia anteriorly to the medial collateral ligament

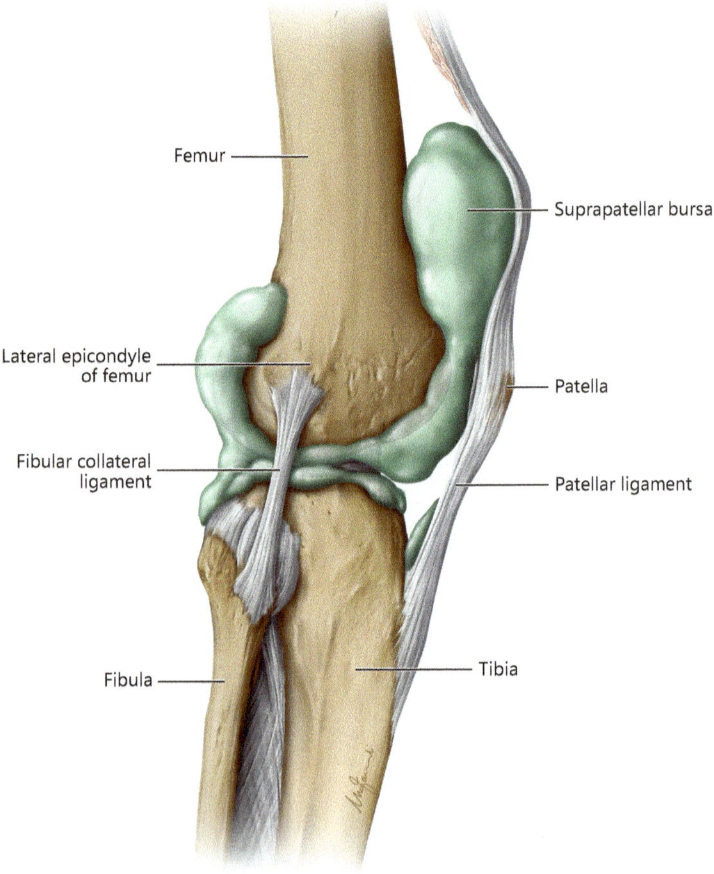

Right knee joint. The articular cavity has been stretched by the injection of a semisolid medium. The subsequent removal of the joint capsule makes it possible to obtain a mold of the cavity which expands mainly upward, to the back, and even to the front of the femur.

Function of the patellar ligament and the alar ligaments:
• fix the patella

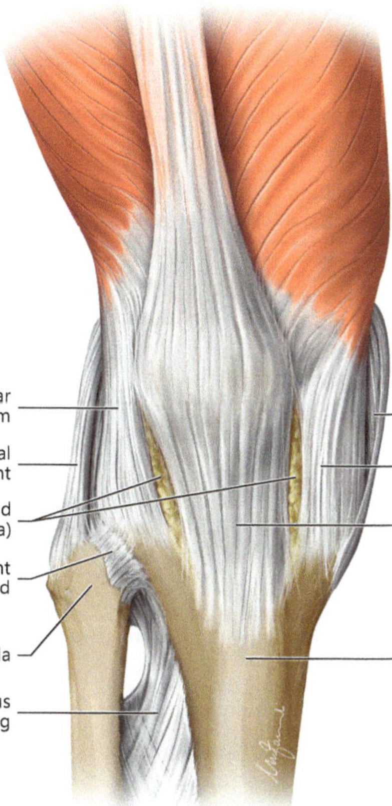

Right knee joint. The means of union of the joint are seen from the front.

- Fibular collateral ligament (lateral) – between the lateral epicondyle of the femur and the head of the fibula
- Tibial collateral ligament (medial) – between the medial epicondyle of the femur and the medial condyle of the tibia (runs in the joint capsule)

Function of the collateral ligaments:
- stabilize the knee in the frontal plane
- limit:
  - the extension of the knee
  - the rotation of the knee

- Oblique popliteal ligament – fibrous expansion of the tendon of the semimembranosus direct from the posteromedial surface of the tibia, upward and laterally, to the intercondylar fossa of the femur

Function of the oblique popliteal ligament:
• limits the extension of the knee

Arcuate popliteal ligament – between the head of the fibula and the joint capsule, where it is inserted in the form of an arch

Function of the arcuate popliteal ligament:
• fixes the fibula, together with the lateral collateral ligament

Cruciate ligaments

- Anterior cruciate ligament – between the inner surface of the lateral condyle of the femur and the anterior intercondylar area of the tibia
- Posterior cruciate ligament – between the inner surface of the medial condyle of the femur and the posterior intercondylar area of the tibia

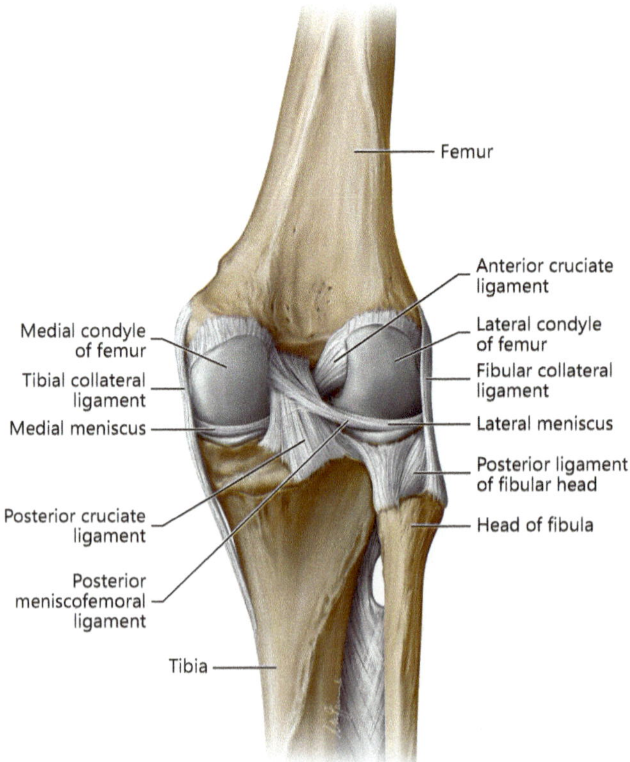

Right knee joint seen posteriorly. The removal of the joint capsule highlights the posterior contour of the menisci and some of the joint ligaments.

Function of the anterior cruciate ligament:
- stabilizes the knee anteroposteriorly
- limits:
- – anterior movement of the tibia on the femur
- – rotation of the knee

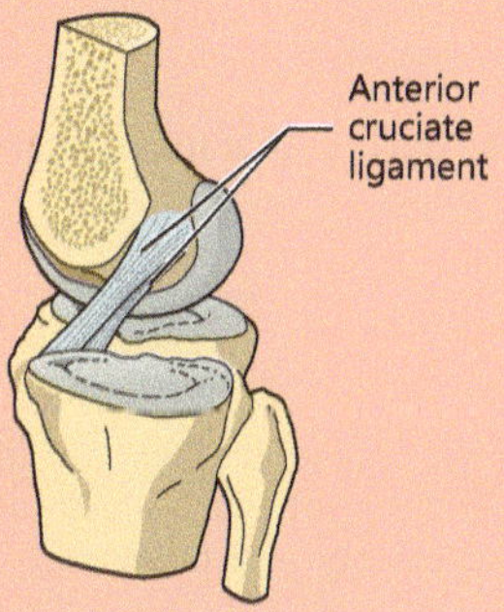

Right extended knee: medial view.

Function of the posterior cruciate ligament:
- stabilizes the knee anteroposteriorly
- limits:
- – posterior movement of the tibia on the femur
- – rotation of the knee

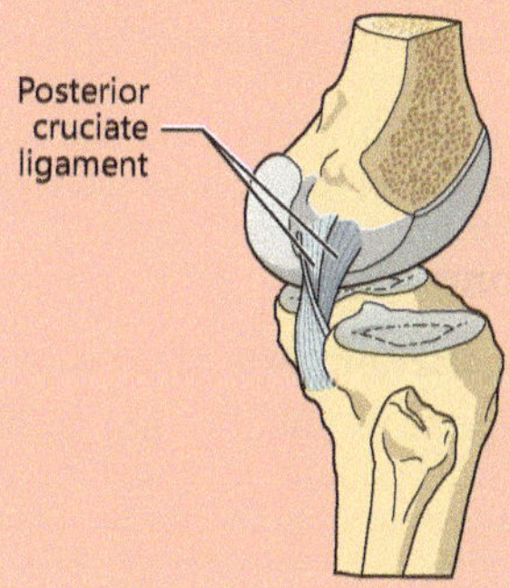

Right extended knee: lateral view.

The cruciate ligaments, passive factors, control the sliding and rotational movements of the femoral condyles on the tibial condyles that occur during flexion and extension of the knee. More precisely:

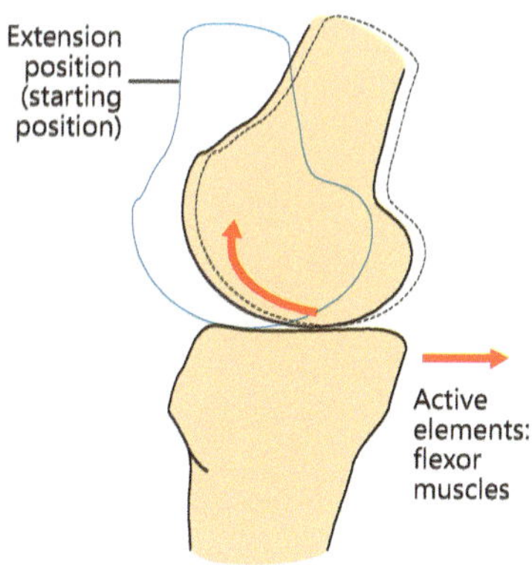

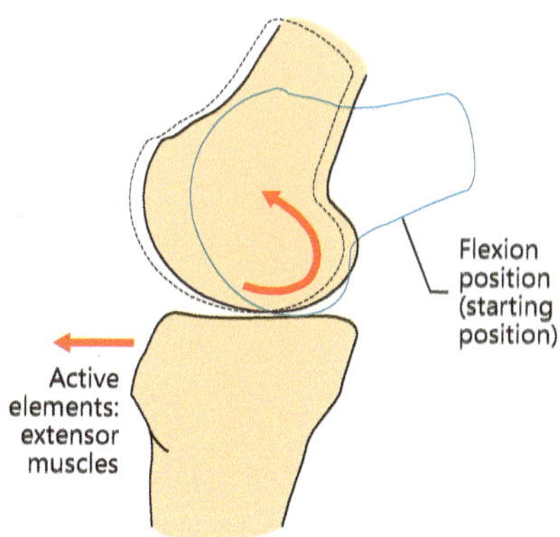

- during flexion there is a combined action of forward sliding and backward rotation of the lateral condyle of the femur – guided by the anterior cruciate ligament.
- during extension there is an opposite action (backward sliding and forward rotation of the medial condyle of the femur) – guided by the posterior cruciate ligament.

Capsule of the tibiofemoral joint

Characteristics:
- wide
- loose
- thin
- more robust posteriorly (thickening of the capsule where the gemellus muscles, which originate outside the joint, run)
- numerous reinforcing ligaments

Recesses (these are virtual cavities that open or close during joint movements):
- subquadricipital (suprapatellar) (anteriorly)
- lateral patellar (medially and laterally)
- posterior (posteriorly)

Anterior and posterior parts of the capsule

The cruciate ligaments (anterior and posterior) are intracapsular (they run inside the joint capsule), but extra-articular (they are inserted outside the joint capsule). In fact, their insertions are extra-articular at the level of the tibial (anteriorly and posteriorly) and femoral (inferiorly) insertions of the joint capsule.

Lateral part of the capsule

The popliteus is inserted inside the joint (within the capsule), laterally.

Medial part of the capsule

The tibial collateral ligament (medial) is intracapsular.

Infrapatellar fat pad (of Hoffa)

Situated behind the posteroinferior surface of the patella and the patellar ligament, in front of the femur and tibia.

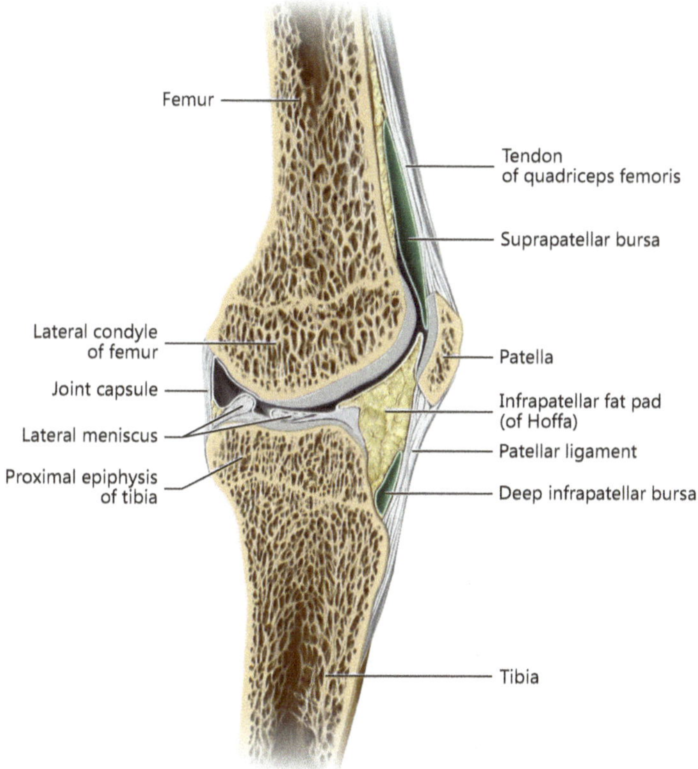

Right knee joint. The section has been done along a paramedian sagittal plane.

Serous or synovial bursae

- Suprapatellar – above the patella – communicates with the articular cavity
- Prepatellar – in front of the patella and below the tendon of the quadriceps femoris
- Infrapatellar – below the patella and below the tendon of the quadriceps femoris
- Of the semimembranosus – below the semimembranosus
- Subpopliteal recess – below the popliteus
- Subtendineous of the gastrocnemius – below its origin
- Subtendineous of the biceps femoris – below its insertion.

Movements of the patella

Flexion of the knee

Movement of the patella in a posteroinferior direction, upward, and anterosuperiorly, downward, from a vertical position corresponding to 0° of flexion to a horizontal position (posterior surface of the patella oriented downward and backward) in maximum flexion. This movement is equal to about twice the length of the patella and is made possible by the presence of the subquadricipital and lateral patellar capsular recesses.

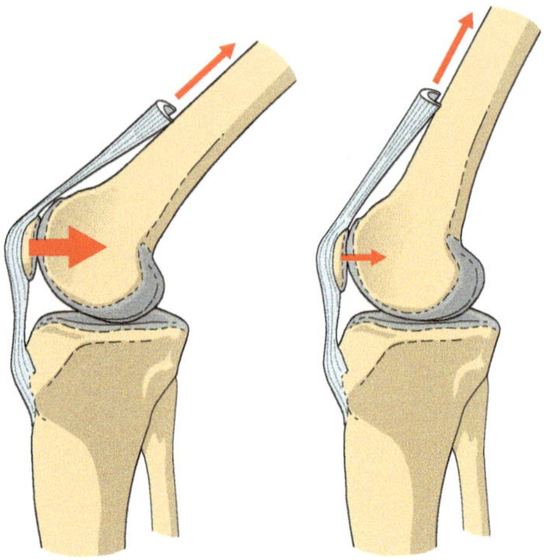

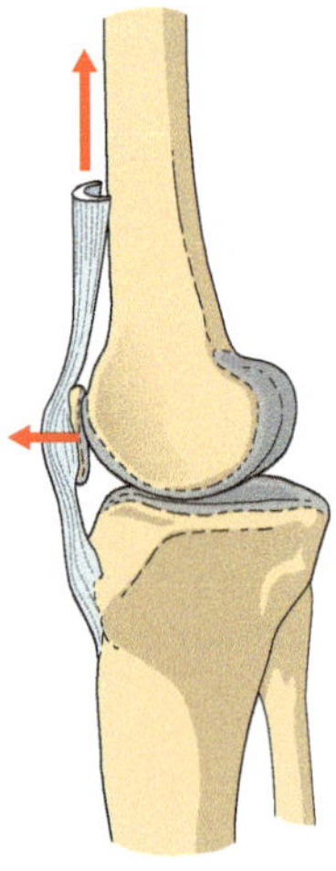

Extension of the knee

Vertical position of the patella.

Hyperextension of the knee

Movement of the patella in a lateral direction, to a small degree (due to a decreased tension of the fibers of the quadriceps femoris, within which tendon the patella is contained, and to an increased tension in the patellar ligament, which is a continuation of the tendon of the quadriceps femoris, with an increased external angle of the knee, which becomes equal to or greater than 180°).

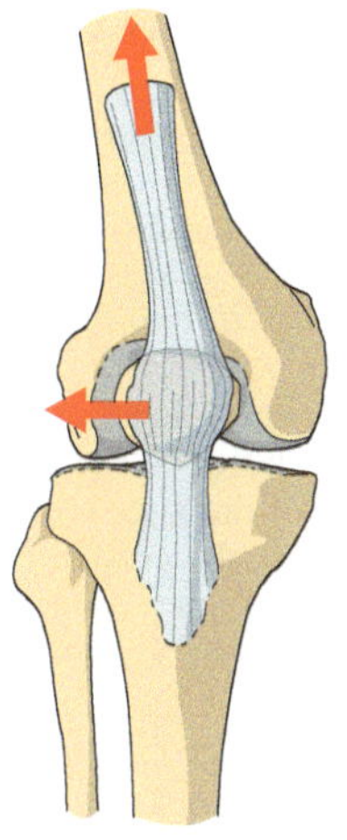

Internal rotation of the knee

Movement of the patella in a lateral direction produced by an increase in tension of the patellar ligament, caused by the external rotation of the thigh which accompanies the internal rotation of the leg.

External rotation of the knee

Movement of the patella in a medial direction produced by an increase in tension of the patellar ligament, caused by the internal rotation of the thigh which accompanies the external rotation of the leg.

Movements of the knee

Flexion of the knee

- Occurs in the sagittal plane around a frontal axis passing through the femoral condyles → this rotation axis is not orthogonal to the vertical axis of the ground (from the center of the foot) for two reasons:
  - the obliquity of the axis of the femoral diaphysis, which forms with the axis of the tibial diaphysis an open outward angle of 170°-175°
  - the obliquity of the mechanical axis of the lower limb (center of the femoral head – center of the knee – axis of the tibia – center of the foot), which forms with the vertical axis from the ground (which runs further inward) an angle of approximately 3°
- Approach of the posterior surfaces of the thigh and leg
- Reference position: lower limb in load or in decubitus with an angle of 180° between the thigh and the leg in the sagittal plane
- If the flexion of the knee occurs in the upright position from the fully extension position, a modest internal rotation of the knee (leg) is required in the initial phase
- Flexion
  - active:
    - **120°** when the hip is extended
    - **140°** when the hip is flexed (this greater amplitude is due to loss of tension of the hamstring muscles – semimembranosus, semitendinosus and biceps femoris –

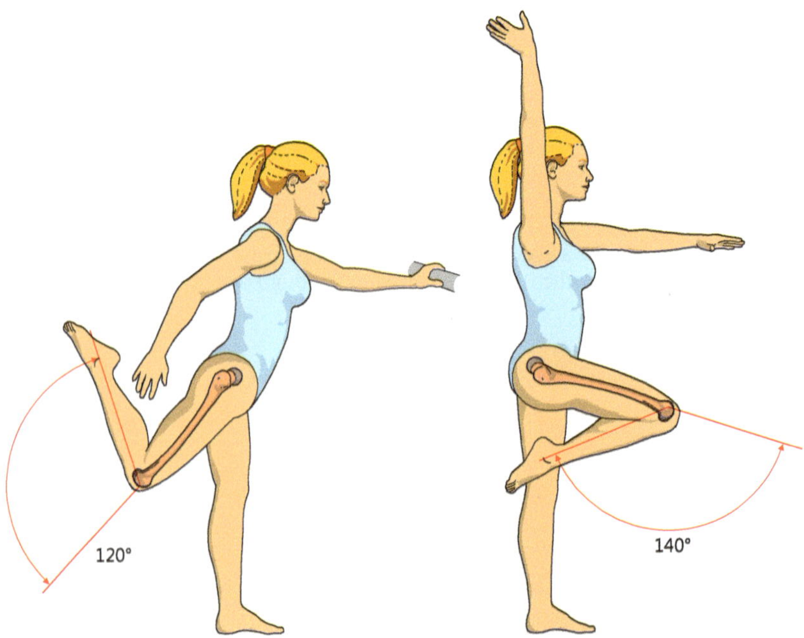

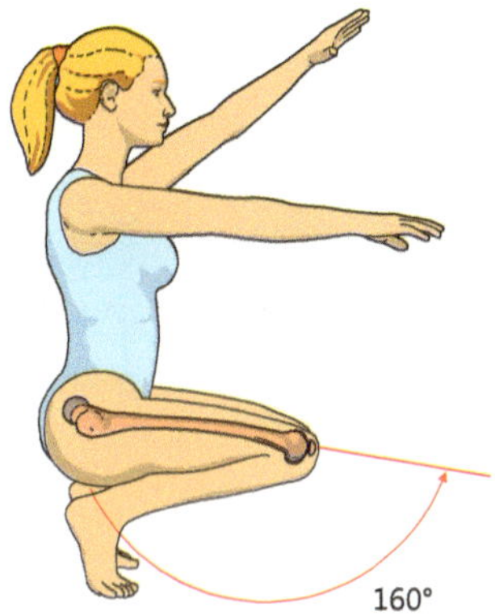

which, by being biarticular, in addition to flexing the knee also extend the hip)
  ◦ passive: **160°**.

Extension of the knee

- Equivalent to the reference position (0°)
- Relative:
  - full extension of the knee from any flexion position
- In the upright position, in order to obtain the full extension of the knee, a modest external rotation of the leg (internal of the hip) is necessary in the final phase which, by reducing the tension of the anterior cruciate ligament, allows the collateral ligaments of the knee to reach maximum tension.

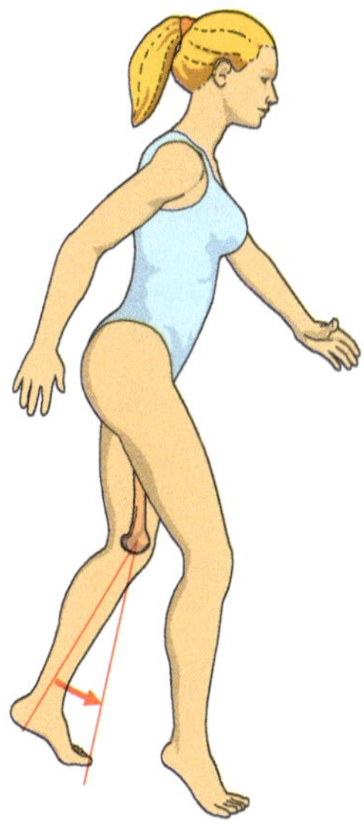

Hyperextension (absolute extension) of the knee

- Only in rare cases and usually in children

The flexion-extension movements of the knee are characterized by the sliding and rotation of the femoral condyles on the tibial surfaces. These movements of the humeral condyles are guided by the anterior and posterior cruciate ligaments (see section "Cruciate ligaments", page 530).

Rotation of the knee

- Only possible when the knee is flexed (when the knee is extended, the collateral ligaments are in maximum tension and stabilize the knee in the frontal plane, preventing lateral movements; the rotation of the extended knee is also prevented by the presence of the intercondylar eminence between the two glenoid cavities of the tibial condyles; therefore, only small passive abduction-adduction movements of the knee are possible: 2-3° when extended; 10-20° when flexed at 90°; the anterior and posterior cruciate ligaments, on the other hand, stabilize the knee anteroposteriorly, so that only slight slippage of the knee in the anteroposterior direction, equal to 2-3 mm, occur when the knee is flexed at 90°)
- Rotation of the tibia with respect to the femur
- The rotation occurs in the horizontal plane and the rotation axis (longitudinal) is located medially to the intercondylar eminence (this position is given by the orientations of the axis of the femoral diaphysis, mechanical axis of the lower limb and the vertical axis of the ground and the asymmetry of the condyles)
- Amplitude of the rotation movement (in sitting position with the lower limb in unloaded position, i.e., with the foot in support):
  - external: **40-50°**
  - internal: **20-30°**.

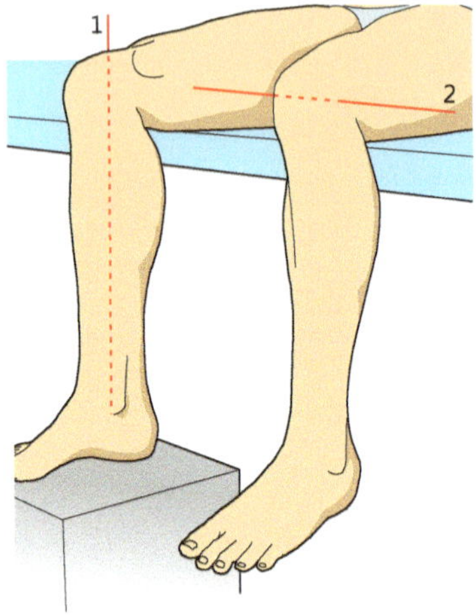

Axes of the knee joint: **1**, internal-external rotation of the tibia; **2**, flexion-extension.

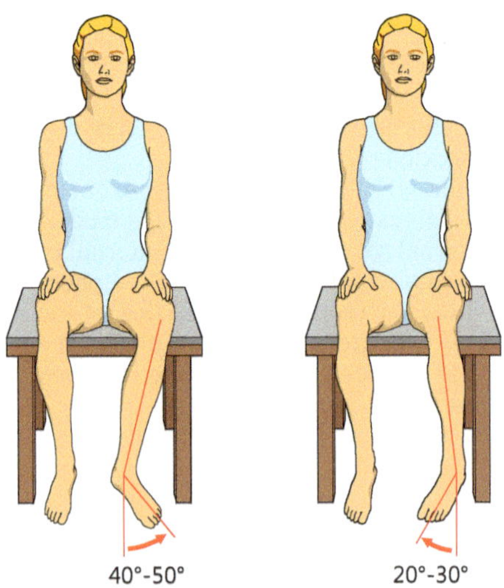

Assessment of the passive joint mobility of the knee

Flexion-extension of the knee

Starting position	Supine with the lower limbs in anatomical position (0° extension of the leg)
Movement	The examiner holds the lower leg with one hand and lifts it by moving it backwards (heel movement in the direction of the buttocks), flexing the knee (and hip) up to the limit of movement allowed (135°), while stabilizing the femur with the other hand 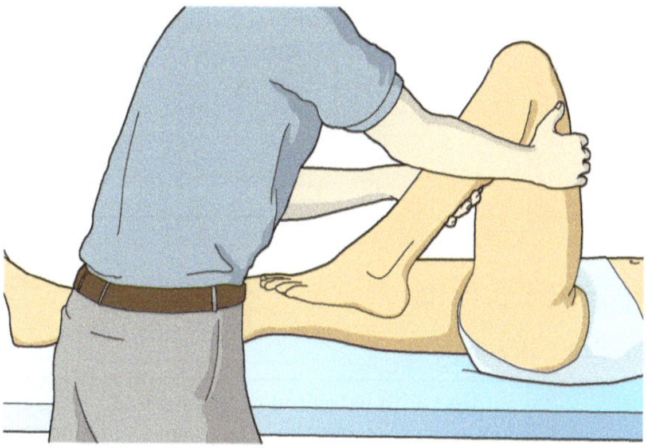 Return movement from the flexion position (extension of the knee and hip) 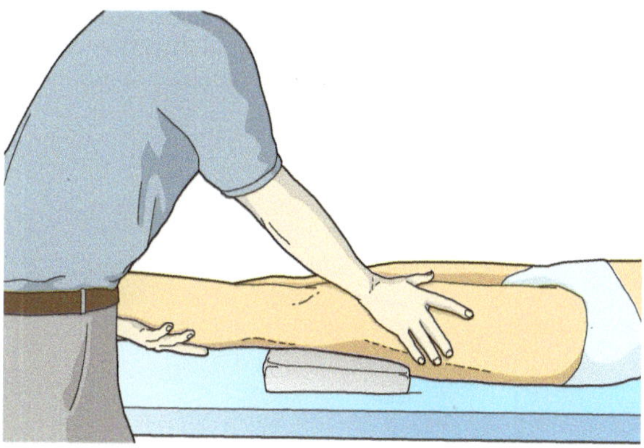

(continued)

(continued)	Elevation of the leg (forward movement in anatomical position) after reaching the 0° extension position (hyperextension of the knee with a variable amplitude from 0° to 10°) 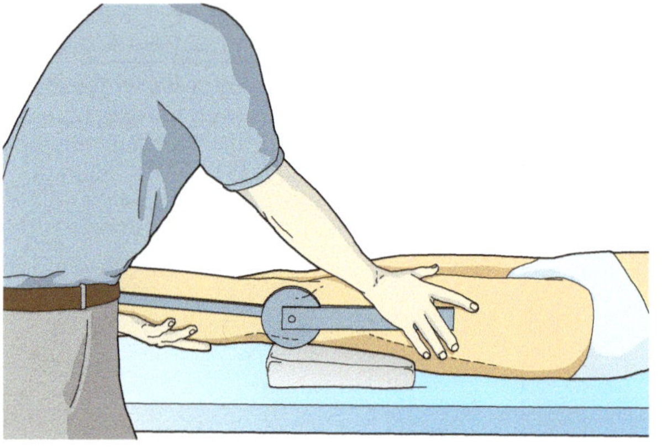

Mobility of the patella

Sliding in distal direction

Starting position	Supine with extended thigh and knee in slight flexion, achieved through the interposition of a support between the knee and the examination table
Movement	One hand of the examiner is applied against the base of the patella, with the forearm along the thigh, and the other is placed over the first so that both move the patella in distal direction up to the limit of movement allowed (vertical movement of 8 cm) (movement in the proximal direction compresses the patella against the femur and therefore should be avoided) 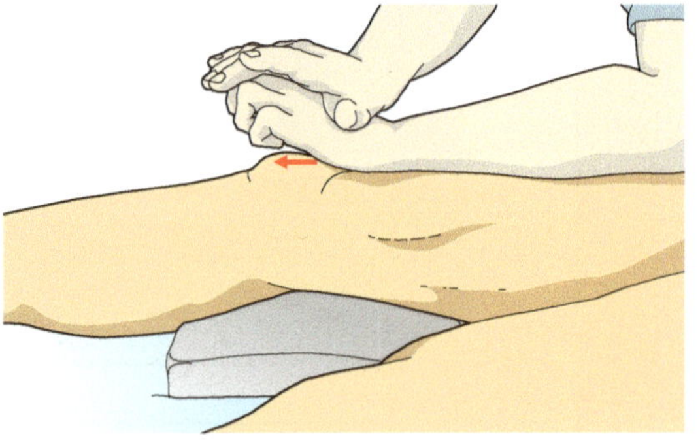

Sliding in mediolateral direction

Starting position	Supine with extended hip and knee in slight flexion, achieved through the interposition of a support between the knee and the examination table
Movement	With the thumbs on the lateral border of the patella and the tips of the index fingers on the medial border, the patella is moved medially with the thumbs (movement of 9.6 mm) and laterally by the index fingers (movement of 5.5 mm), while stabilizing the femur and tibia 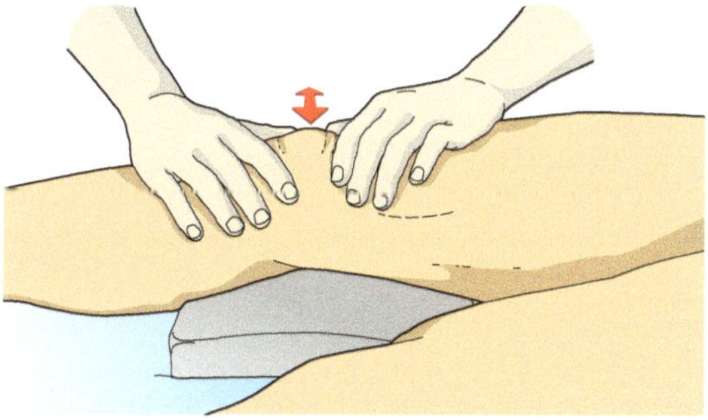

Rotation of the tibia

The measurement of the degrees of external and internal of rotation of the knee (leg) is unreliable, since it is difficult to define the starting position equivalent to 0° of the two individual movements. Therefore, an assessment is made of the total joint amplitude of the rotation movement of the leg, which is greater when the knee is flexed at 90°.

Starting position	Seated with the knee flexed at 90° and fully rotated internally
Movement	The examiner externally rotates the tibia to the entire range of joint motion (the total active joint mobility between internal and external rotation is on average 58°), stabilizing the femur with the other hand 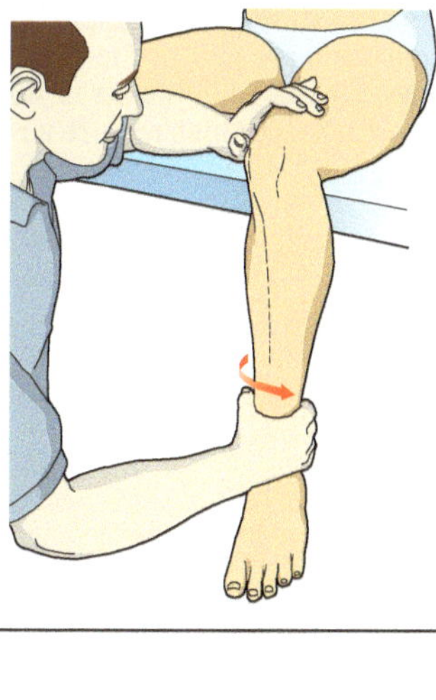

Functional aspects of the knee joint

Functions of the knee:
- supports the body weight
- shortens (flexion of the leg) or lengthens (extension of the leg) the lower limb
- the flexion of the knee with the foot resting on the ground brings the body closer to the ground
- the extension of the knee with the foot resting on the ground lifts the body
- when the foot is lifted off the ground, its spacial orientation is made possible by the flexion-extension and rotation of the knee
- when the foot is resting on the ground, the rotation of the knee allows twisting movements of the body
- during gait, the knee:
  - acts as a shock absorber
  - reduces the vertical movement of the body
  - by flexing, it shortens the lower limb, allowing the toes to get off the ground during the oscillation phase of the gait cycle.

Mobility of the knee:
- the normal active mobility of the knee ranges from 0° of extension to approximately 140° of flexion, but many functional activities require a flexion of the knee of less than 140°
- daily life activities that require a flexion of the knee up to approximately 117° can be exemplified as:
  - lifting an object from the ground
  - sitting in a chair
  - going up stairs (with a maximum flexion between 83° and 105° and a minimum between 1-2° and 15° in relation to the height of the steps)
  - going down stairs (with a maximum flexion between 86° and 107° and a minimum between 1-2° and 15° in relation to the height of the steps)
  - tying shoelaces
  - putting on socks
- normal daily activities do not require full extension of the knee:
  - the position of the knee in full extension (stable position) generally occurs in asymmetrical postures, for example, in the prolonged upright position when a lower limb supports a large part of the body weight or during powerful pushing movements such as those involved in the act of jumping
- many daily activities require a rotation of the knee (leg) of less than 25°.

Muscles of the knee

Muscle	Action	Origin	Insertion	Innervation
Popliteus	Flexion and internal rotation of the knee	Posterior surface of the lateral epicondyle of the femur	Posterior surface of the tibia, superiorly to the soleal line	Tibial nerve [L4, L5, S1]
Hamstring or ischiocrural				
Semimembranosus	Flexion of the knee and internal rotation of the flexed knee	Superolateral surface of the ischial tuberosity	Tubercle on the posterior surface of the medial condyle of the tibia	Sciatic nerve (tibial nerve) [L5, S1, S2]
Semitendinosus	Flexion of the knee and internal rotation of the flexed knee	Inferomedial sulcus on the superior surface of the ischial tuberosity	Proximal part of the medial surface of the tibia	Sciatic nerve (tibial nerve) [L5, S1, S2]
Biceps femoris	Flexion of the knee and external rotation of the flexed knee	*Long head*: inferomedial sulcus on the superior surface of the ischial tuberosity; inferior part of the sacrotuberous ligament	Head of the fibula; fascicle directed to the lateral condyle of the tibia; fascicle directed to the fibular collateral ligament	Sciatic nerve (tibial nerve [L5, S1, S2]
		Short head: lateral lip of the linea aspera and lateral supracondylar line		Sciatic nerve (common fibular nerve [L5, S1, S2]

(continued)

Muscles of the knee *(continued)*

Muscle	Action	Origin	Insertion	Innervation
Quadriceps femoris				
Vastus medialis	Extension of the knee; internal rotation of the knee from a position of external rotation and flexion)	Lower part of the intertrochanteric line (spiral line of the femur), medial lip of the linea aspera, proximal part of the medial supracondylar line, tendons of the adductor longus and adductor magnus, medial intermuscular septum of the thigh	Medial border of the patella, tibial tuberosity through the tendon of the quadriceps femoris	Femoral nerve [L2-L4]
Vastus lateralis	Extension of the knee; external rotation of the knee from a position of internal rotation and rotation)	Upper part of the intertrochanteric line (spiral line of the femur), anterior and inferior borders of the greater trochanter, tendon of the gluteus maximus, upper half of the lateral lip of the linea aspera	Lateral border and base of the patella, tibial tuberosity through the tendon of the quadriceps femoris	Femoral nerve [L2-L4]
Vastus intermedius	Extension of the knee	Upper two-thirds of the anterior and lateral surfaces of the shaft (body) of the femur	Base of the patella and tibial tuberosity through the tendon of the quadriceps femoris	Femoral nerve [L2-L4]
Rectus femoris	Flexion of the hip and extension of the knee	*Straight head*: anterior surface of the anterior inferior iliac spine *Reflected head*: supra-acetabular groove and capsule of the hip joint	Base of the patella and tibial tuberosity through the tendon of the quadriceps femoris	Femoral nerve [L2-L4]

Classification of the muscles of the knee

There are nine muscles that act on the knee:

- biceps femoris → flexor and external rotator of the knee → posterior muscle of the thigh
- tensor fasciae latae → external rotator of the knee → anterior muscle of the thigh
- popliteus → flexor and internal rotator of the knee → posterior muscle of the knee
- gastrocnemius (medial and lateral heads) (the gastrocnemius and soleus form the triceps surae) → flexor of the knee → posterior muscle of the leg
- sartorius → flexor and internal rotator of the knee → anterior muscle of the thigh
- gracilis → flexor and internal rotator of the knee → medial muscle of the thigh
- semimembranosus → flexor and internal rotator of the knee → posterior muscle of the thigh
- semitendinosus → flexor and internal rotator of the knee → posterior muscle of the thigh
- quadriceps femoris (rectus femoris, vastus medialis, vastus lateralis, vastus intermedius) → extensor of the knee → anterior muscle of the thigh.

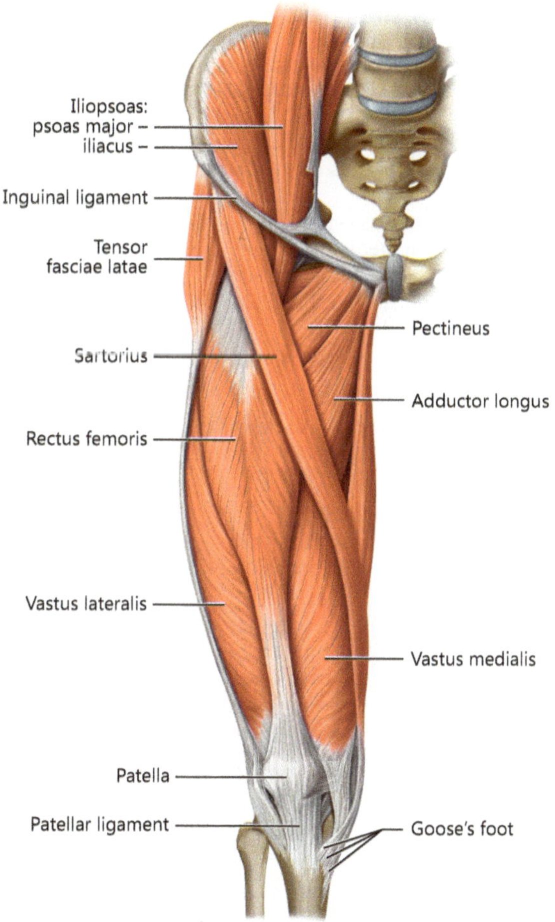

Anterolateral muscles of the right thigh, anterior view.

11

(For the classification of the muscles of the thigh, see Chapter 10 "Hip and pelvis").

(For the classification of the muscles of the leg, see Chapter 12 "Ankle and foot").

Action of the muscles in the movements of the knee

Flexion of the knee

Flexor muscles of the knee:
- biceps femoris (in lateroposterior position)
- sartorius (in medial position)
- semimembranosus (in medial position)
- semitendinosus (in medial position)
- gracilis (in medial position)
- popliteus (in posterior position)
- gastrocnemius (in posterior position).

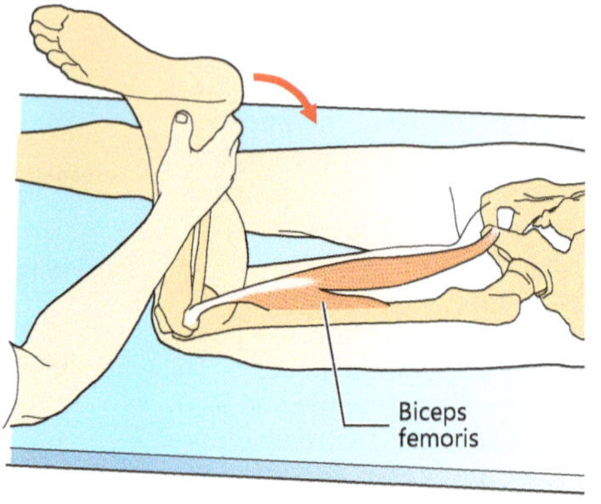

Action of the flexor muscles of the knee

Biceps femoris

- Flexion of the knee
- External rotation of the knee
- Participates in the extension of the hip (long head).

The biceps femoris, together with the semimembranosus and semitendinosus, forms the hamstring muscle group, also called ischiocrural muscles due to their origin from the ischial tuberosity and their tibial insertion.

They:
- extend the hip
- flex the knee
- rotate the knee
- participate in the retroversion of the pelvis

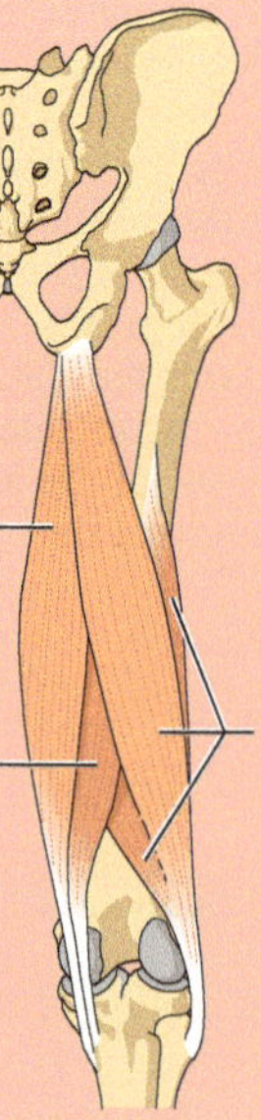

Sartorius

- Flexion of the knee (fifth in order of muscular force) and internal rotation of the knee
- Flexion of the hip (third in order of muscular force)
- Abduction of the hip
- External rotation of the hip.

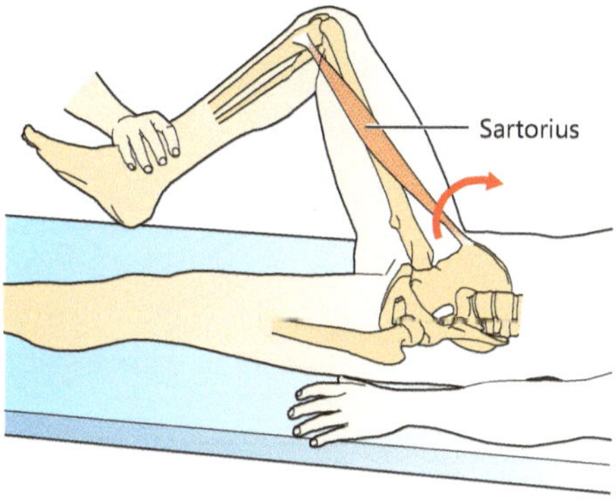

Semimembranosus

- Flexion of the knee
- Internal rotation of the knee
- Participates in the extension of the hip.

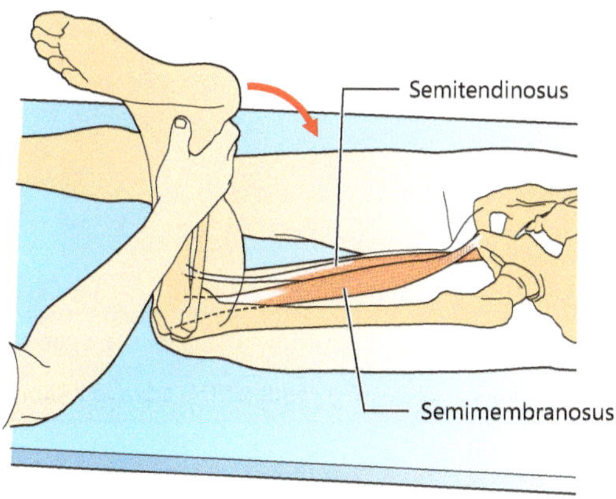

Semitendinosus

- Flexion of the knee
- Internal rotation of the knee
- Participates in the extension of the hip.

Gracilis

- Participates in the flexion and internal rotation of the knee
- Weak flexor of the hip
- Adduction and internal rotation of the hip when the knee is extended.

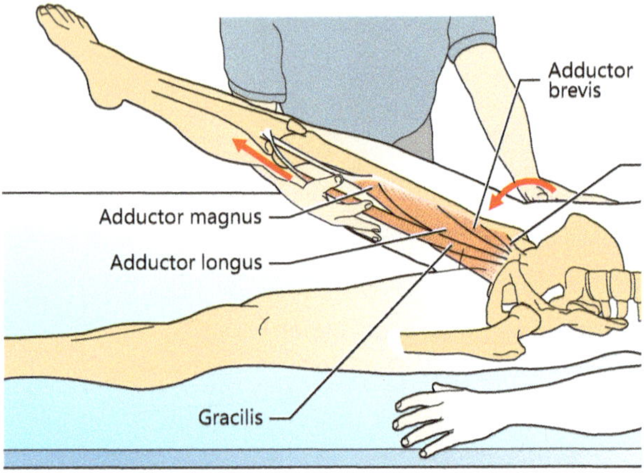

The insertion of the sartorius, gracilis and semitendinosus occurs through a common tendon called goose's foot due to its shape.

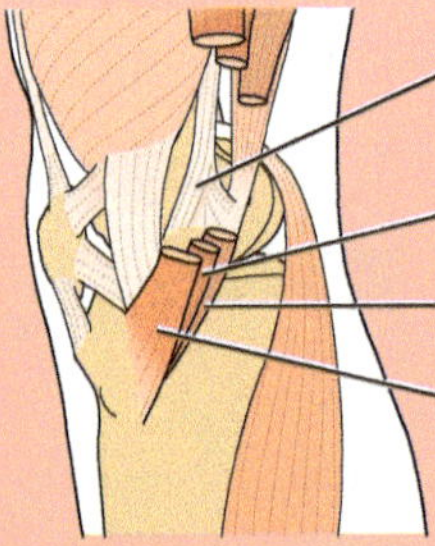

Right knee: medial view. The common insertion of the gracilis, semitendinosus and sartorius on the superior part of the medial surface of the tibia is seen.

Popliteus

- Flexion of the knee
- Internal rotation of the knee:
  – during the initial flexion of the knee, due to the course of its fibers directed from above to below and from the outside to the inside on the posterior surface of the leg (from the lateral condyle of the femur to the popliteal line on the posterior surface of the tibia), frees the knee (leg) from a potential external rotation; during this action, it stabilizes the knee on the sagittal and transverse planes, assisting the action of the posterior cruciate ligament and avoiding forward sliding of the femoral condyles.

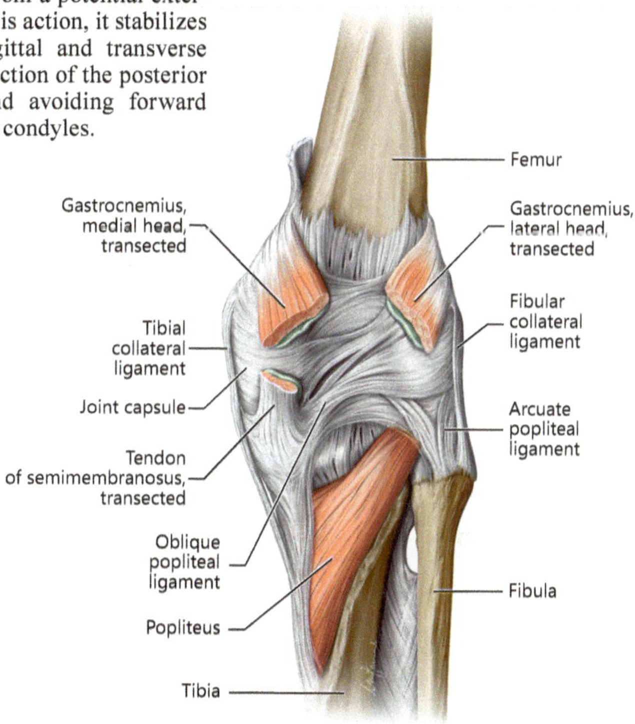

Right knee joint.

Gastrocnemius
(medial and lateral heads)

- Strong flexor of the knee, especially in the initial phase, when the knee is extended
- Stabilizes the knee in relation to the tibia (especially in the presence of wide extensor movements of the leg such as those made during running and jumping)
- Plantar flexion of the foot (together with the soleus, with which it forms the triceps surae).

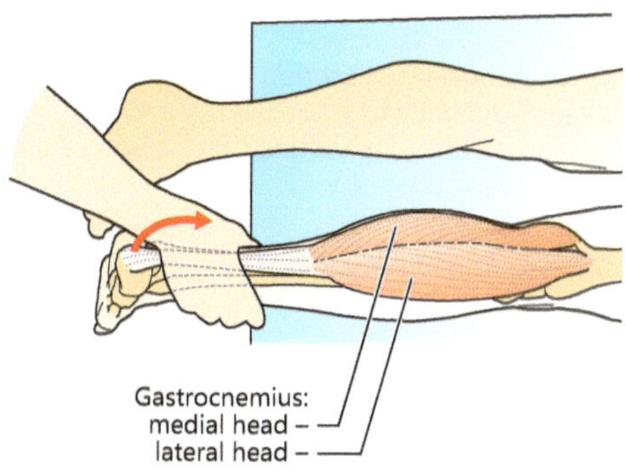

Extension of the knee

Quadriceps femoris

- Vastus lateralis
- Vastus intermedius
- Vastus medialis
- Rectus femoris.

- The only extensor muscle of the knee (the extensor action of some fibers of the tensor fasciae latae being negligible)
- Greater extensor work of the vastus medialis when the hip is flexed and the knee is rotated internally
- Greater extensor work of the vastus lateralis when the hip is flexed and the knee is rotated externally
- Greater force of the vastus medialis during extension against resistance
- Hip flexion action by the rectus femoris, more efficient when the leg is extended.

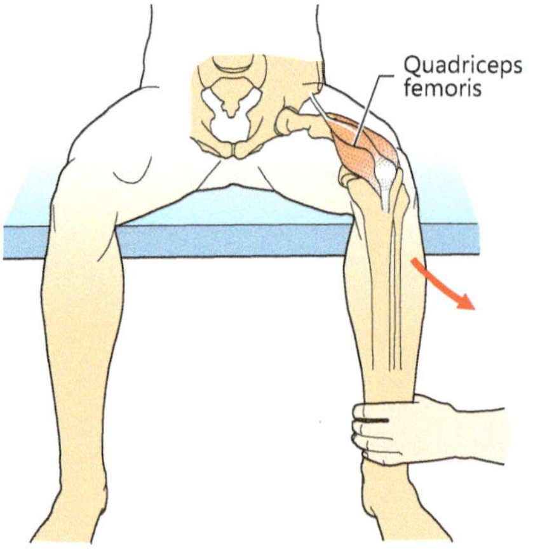

Overall, the work of the quadriceps femoris is more than three times greater than the work of the knee flexor muscles.

Some fibers of the vastus medialis, rectus femoris and vastus lateralis form the alar ligaments of the patella.

Rotation of the knee

External rotator muscles of the knee

- Biceps femoris (see section "Flexion of the knee", page 546)
- Tensor fasciae latae
- Vastus lateralis (see section "Extension of the knee", above)

Tensor fasciae latae

The tensor fasciae latae acts as an external rotator of the knee only when the knee is flexed.

Vastus lateralis

The vastus lateralis actually stabilizes an internal rotation position of the knee in flexion when returning from the flexed position to the extended position.

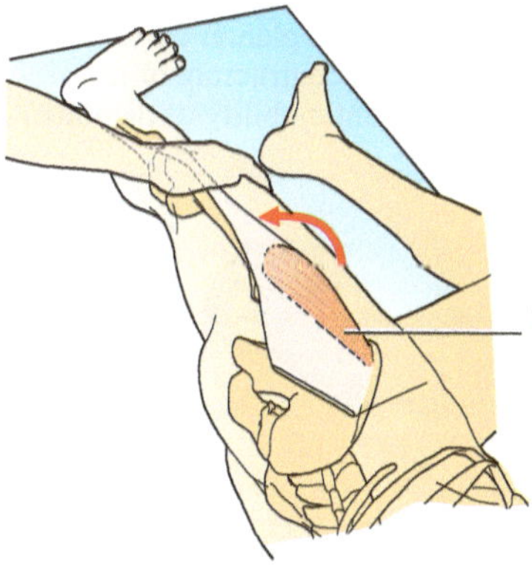

Internal rotator muscles of the knee (from greatest to least muscular force)

- Semimembranosus (see section "Flexion of the knee", page 546)
- Semitendinosus (see section "Flexion of the knee", page 546)
- Gracilis (see section "Flexion of the knee", page 546)
- Sartorius (see section "Flexion of the knee", page 546)
- Popliteus (see section "Flexion of the knee", page 546)

The work of the external rotator muscles of the knee is approximately equal to the work of the internal rotator muscles and much less than that of the extensor muscles of the knee (quadriceps femoris).

Assessment of the length of muscle fibers

Hamstring or ischiocrural muscles

Starting position	Seated, with the foot of the unexamined limb in support and the foot of the examined limb in plantar flexion
Movement	The examiner extends the knee with one hand up to the limit of movement allowed, so that the hamstring muscles are fully stretched, and with the other stabilizes the femur (the foot is maintained in plantar flexion during the execution of the test to prevent a contracture of the gastrocnemius in case of reduced joint mobility of the knee) 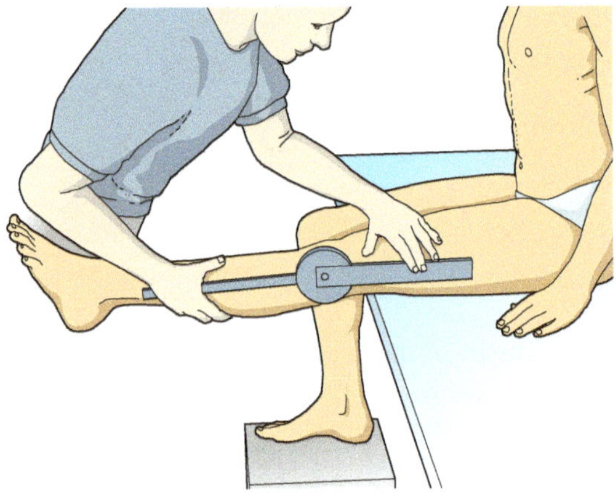

Rectus femoris

Starting position	Prone, with the lower limb extended
Movement	The examiner moves the lower leg in a posterior direction with one hand, bringing the heel close to the buttock, up to the limit of the flexion movement of the leg (in this position, the flexion of the knee may be limited by a shortening of the fibers of the rectus femoris), while the other hand stabilizes the femur 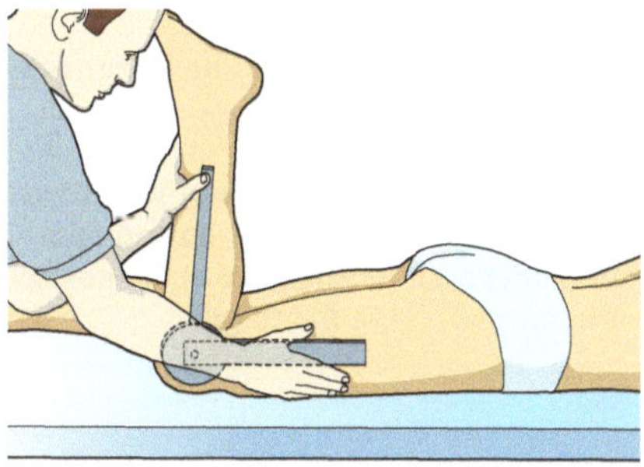
Alternative starting position	Supine near the end of the examination table, with the hips and knees flexed (the patient maintains the position by placing the hands on the knees)
Movement	The examiner keeps the knee flexed, while the leg is dropped onto the examination table, up to the limit of movement allowed, in order to fully stretch the fibers of the rectus femoris, while the other hand stabilizes the femur 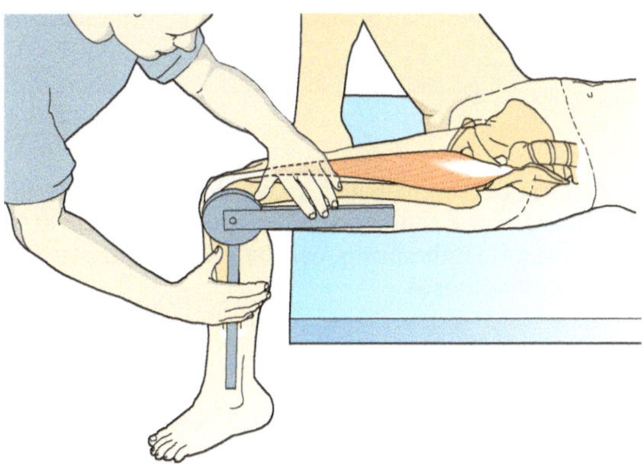

Assessment of the muscular force

Flexion of the knee

It is preferable to assess the force of the hamstring muscles as a whole (flexion of the knee in extension and in neutral rotation) and then that of the medial (semitendinosus and semimembranosus) and lateral (biceps femoris) hamstring muscles, isolating the former from the latter, and vice versa, placing the knee (leg), respectively, in internal and external rotation.

Biceps femoris, semitendinosus and semimembranosus

Against gravity

Flexion of the knee through the entire range of joint motion starting from the prone position with the knee extended and in neutral rotation and foot beyond the edge of the examination table, with the examiner applying resistance to the posterior surface of the leg with one hand and with the other hand stabilizing the thigh.

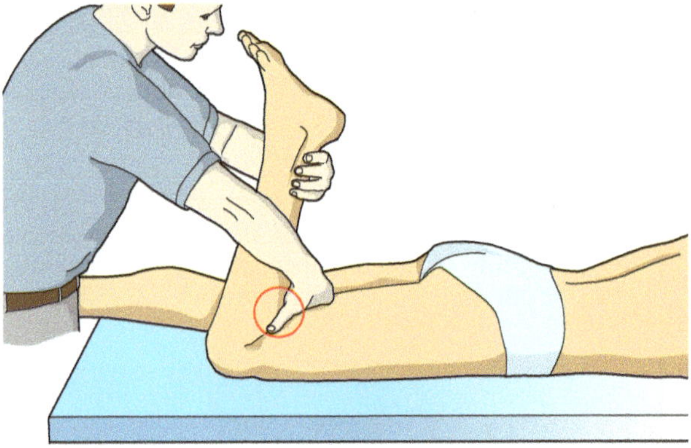

The biceps femoris can be palpated above the knee, at the lateral border of the popliteal fossa; the semitendinosus can be palpated above the knee, at the medial border of the popliteal fossa; the semimembranosus can be palpated above the knee, on both sides of the tendon of the semitendinosus.

In the prone position, the rectus femoris can limit the excursion of the knee in flexion. Moreover, in this position, it is not possible to perform a powerful flexion (against strong resistance) of the knee of more than 90° if the hip is fully extended (0°). In fact, beyond this limit, cramps generally appear in the hamstring muscles.

Isolation of the medial hamstring muscles – The semitendinosus and semimembranosus internally rotate the knee when it is flexed. In the prone position, with the knee flexed and in neutral rotation, this action is achieved by moving the heel towards the lateral surface of the ipsilateral buttock.

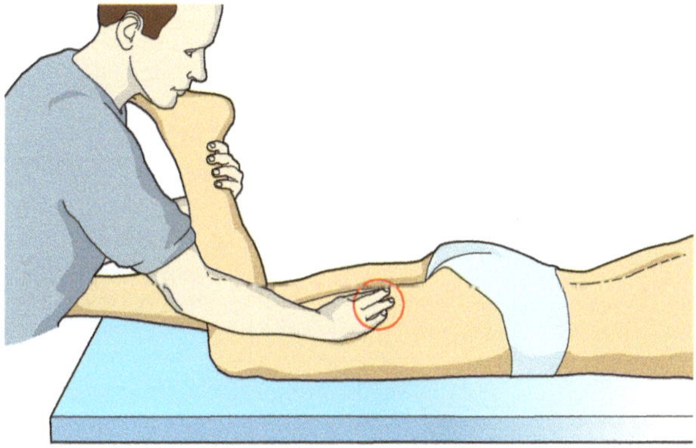

Isolation of the lateral hamstring muscles – The biceps femoris externally rotates the knee when it is flexed. In the prone position, with the knee flexed and in neutral rotation, this action is achieved by moving the heel towards the contralateral buttock.

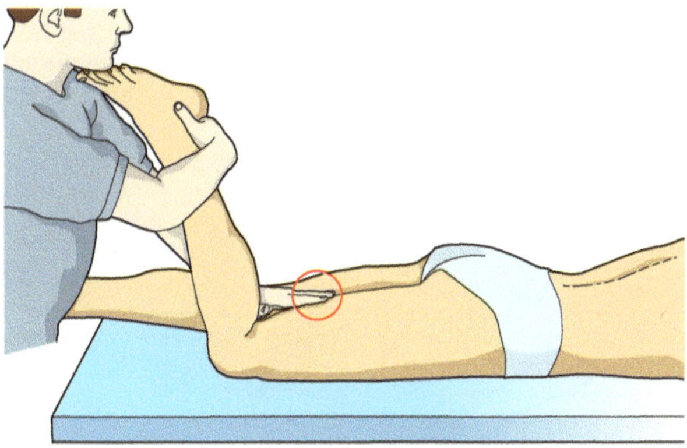

Without gravity

Flexion of the knee through the entire range of joint motion starting from the lateral decubitus position on the unexamined side, with the examiner holding the lower limb under examination with one hand, with the thigh in anatomical position and the knee extended, and with the other hand stabilizing the thigh.

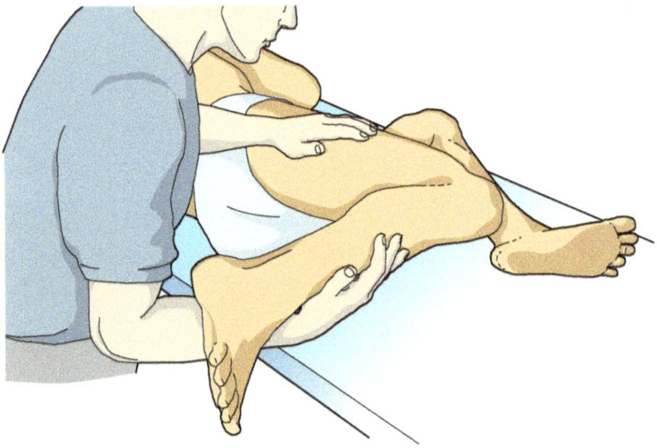

Extension of the knee

Rectus femoris, vastus intermedius, vastus lateralis and vastus medialis

Against gravity

Extension of the knee through the entire range of joint motion starting from the seated position with the knee flexed, with the examiner applying resistance to the anterior surface of the leg distally with one hand and stabilizing the thigh with the other hand.

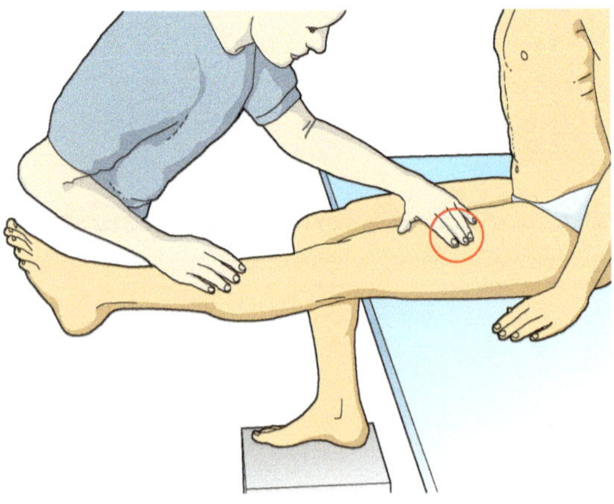

The rectus femoris can be palpated on the anterior surface of the thigh in the central part; the vastus intermedius is positioned too deep to be palpated; the vastus lateralis can be palpated on the lateral surface of the thigh in the central part; the vastus medialis can be palpated on the medial surface of the thigh in the distal part. The entire muscle group of the quadriceps femoris can be palpated above the tibial tuberosity, at the level of the patellar ligament.

In case of contracture of the hamstring muscles, an attempt should be made to extend the trunk to reduce the tension of the fibers during the movement. The patient can perform the same movement of leaning the trunk backwards to stretch the rectus femoris and increase its contribution to the knee extension movement.

Without gravity

Extension of the knee through the entire range of joint motion starting from the lateral decubitus position on the unexamined side, with the examiner holding the lower limb under examination with one hand, with the thigh in anatomical position and the knee flexed, and with the other hand stabilizing the thigh.

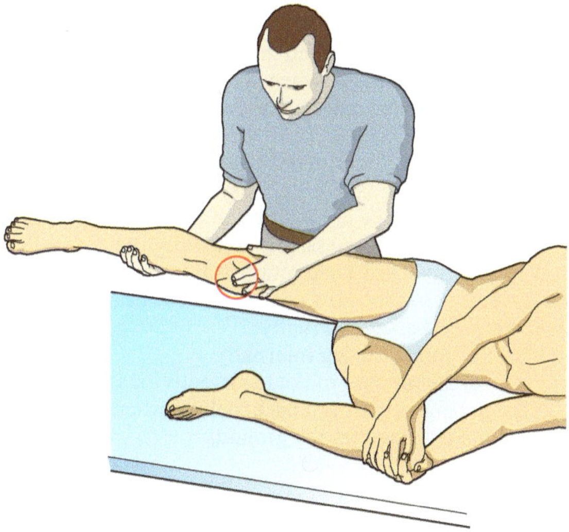

Functional aspects of the muscles of the knee

Flexor muscles of the knee

- The popliteus and the short head of the biceps femoris are the only monoarticular flexor muscles of the knee (they move only the leg):
  - the action of the popliteus as flexor of the knee is negligible
  - its main function is to rotate the leg internally when it begins to flex, thus unblocking the knee joint
  - when loads are transported while walking downhill, the activity of the popliteus is increased in order to stabilize the knee in the central part during the support phase of the foot
  - when a squatting position is assumed (for example, to lift an object from the ground), the popliteus contracts in order to avoid the forward movement of the femur relative to the tibia
- The majority of the flexor muscles of the knee are biarticular muscles (which can also move the thigh or foot):
  - the gastrocnemius flexes the leg and controls its hyperextension
- The action of the flexor muscles of the knee is exemplified by the seated position in which the ankle is supported on the contralateral thigh or by the position with the legs crossed at the level of the ankles
- The knee flexor muscles also contract when the flexion of the knee is forced at the end of the excursion, as happens, for example, when we put on a sock
- During upright position, the flexor muscles of the knee contract, for example, when the sole of the foot is examined
- During walking or running, the flexor muscles of the knee contract eccentrically to decelerate the leg that is extended to take a step forward
- Going up stairs does not require the contraction of the flexor muscles of the knee, since the flexion of the knee is carried out passively following the active flexion of the hip
- The flexor muscles of the knee also have rotary action on the leg (with the exception of the gastrocnemius):
  - the biceps femoris rotates the leg externally
  - the other flexor muscles rotate the leg internally
  - they initiate and control the rotation of the leg in activities such as running and turning
  - they are also active during squatting and kneeling when the trunk and upper limbs cause movements of the leg fixed on the ground.

Extensor muscles of the knee

- The rectus femoris acts on the thigh and leg and is most effective as an extensor of the knee when the hip is extended and its fibers are stretched:
  - the thigh must be stabilized in order for the rectus femoris to fully act as an extensor of the knee
- The vastus medialis contracts along with the vastus lateralis and vastus intermedius during the extension of the knee for the entire range of joint motion:
  - the inferior oblique fibers of the vastus medialis act in the final phase of the extension of the knee in order to prevent the displacement of the patella in a lateral direction (the patella is pulled medially)

Two principal patterns of movement are carried out at the level of the lower limb during the execution of the main activities of daily life:

- the first comprises the flexion of the hip, the flexion of the knee and the dorsiflexion of the foot:
  - in this pattern of movement, the extensor muscles of the knee contract eccentrically in order to control its flexion (an example is provided by activities during which the foot is fixed on the ground and the body is lowered, as in squatting to lift an object, sitting on a chair or going down stairs)
- the second comprises the extension of the hip, the extension of the knee and the plantar flexion of the foot:
  - in this pattern of movement, the extensor muscles of the knee contract concentrically in order to extend the leg (an example is provided by activities such as getting up from a chair, jumping, going up stairs and getting up to exit the bathtub)

- When the foot is not supported, the extensor muscles of the knee contract if the extension is carried out against resistance, which may also be represented by the weight of the limb
- Examples of functional activities that require the contraction of the extensor muscles of the knee are kicking a ball, putting on pants, breaststroke swimming.

Palpation of the knee

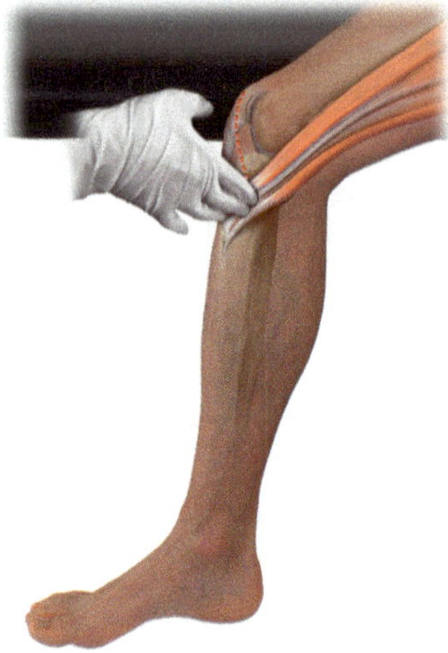

Goose's foot

The patient is seated with the knee flexed. The examiner begins palpation from the patella, then moves downward to look for the tibial tuberosity. From here continue in a medial direction until palpation of a soft structure (pad): this is the flat surface of the goose's foot.

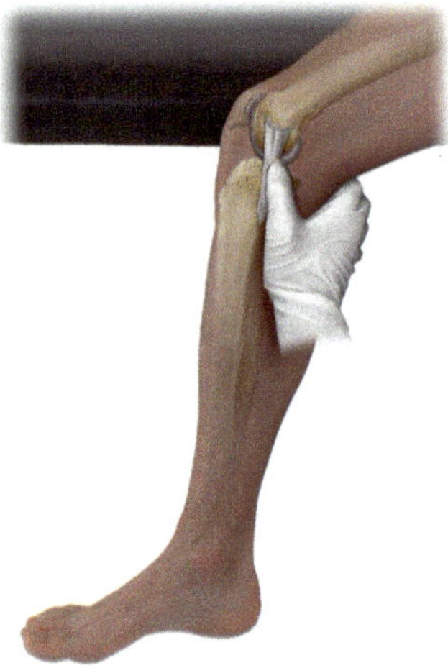

Tibial collateral ligament

The patient is seated with the knee flexed. The articular interline between the femoral and tibial condyles is identified, just medial to the patella and patellar ligament. Here a cavity of about 5 mm is appreciated, at the bottom of which a body of hard and elastic consistency is palpated: the meniscus. Continuing in a medial direction, the sensation of palpating a cavity is lost and a very consistent and superficial structure is found, with a thickness of approximately 5 mm, which hides the articular interline: it is the tibial collateral ligament. It is possible to follow it up to the femoral and tibial entheses.

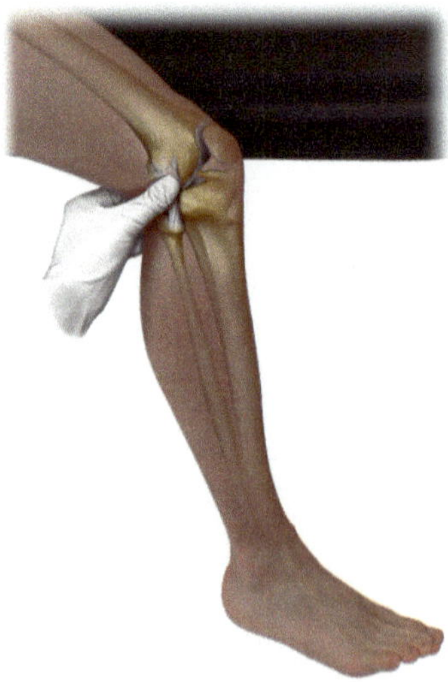

Fibular collateral ligament and tendon of the popliteus

The patient is seated with the knee flexed. The articular interline between the femoral and tibial condyles is identified, just lateral to the patella and patellar ligament, where a cavity is appreciated. Continuing in a lateral direction, after 2-3 cm the iliotibial tract is found first, and then the fibular collateral ligament. The patient is then asked to perform some isometric external rotations of the foot: in this way the tendon of the popliteus can be seen going up and down.

Patellar ligament

The patient is in the supine position, with the knee slightly flexed and resting on a cushion placed below the popliteal fossa. An imaginary line is drawn connecting the anterior inferior iliac spine to the patella and corresponding to the course of the rectus femoris. Palpation is performed following the muscle belly up to the patellar insertion and from here it is continued distally to the tibial tuberosity, detecting the presence of the patellar ligament 3-4 cm wide.

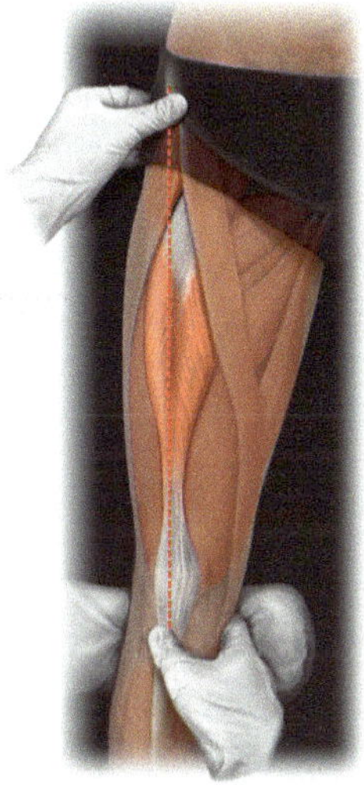

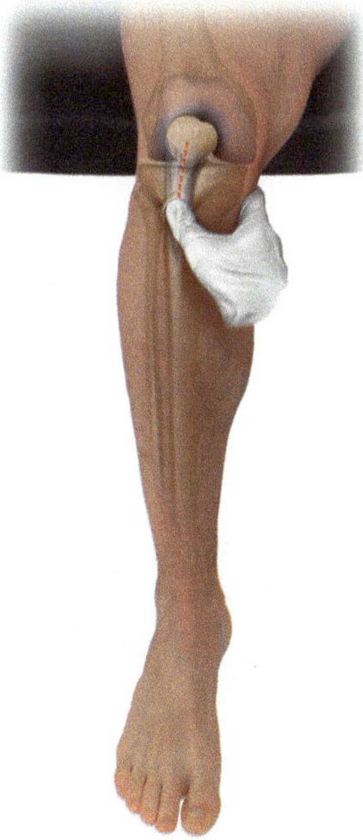

Tibial tuberosity

The patient is seated with the lower limbs flexed off the examination table. Once the apex of the patella is identified, palpation is performed distally and centrally for 8-10 cm, until reaching the bony protuberance of the tibial tuberosity. Keeping the fingers on the tibial tuberosity, the patient is asked to slightly extend the knee, to stretch the patellar ligament and identify its insertion point.

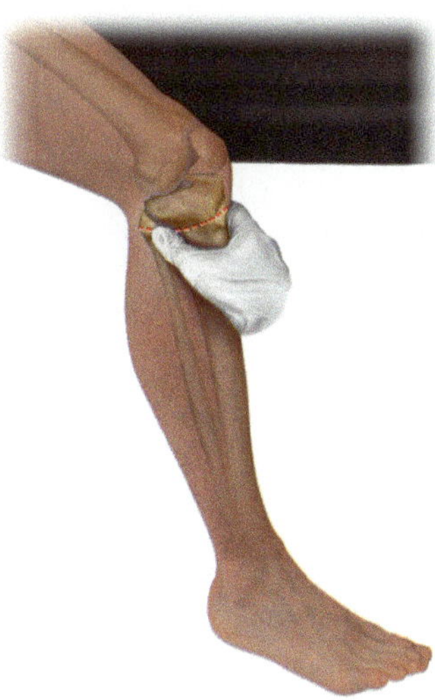

Head of the fibula

The patient is seated with the knee flexed. Palpation begins at the level of the tibial tuberosity, located distal to the patella, over the shaft (body) of the tibia. From here the fingers slide laterally towards the end of the leg for about 8-10 cm until finding, 2-3 cm from the lateral articular groove, a protuberance: the head of the fibula.

Medial meniscus

The patient is seated with the knee flexed at 90° and the foot off the ground so that the weight of the leg opens the joint line, facilitating palpation. The thumb is used to identify the joint space under the patella and, inside it, the medial superior articular surface of the tibia. With the other hand, the patient's leg is slowly brought in internal rotation, so that the meniscus is pushed forward, towards the thumb that performs the palpation.

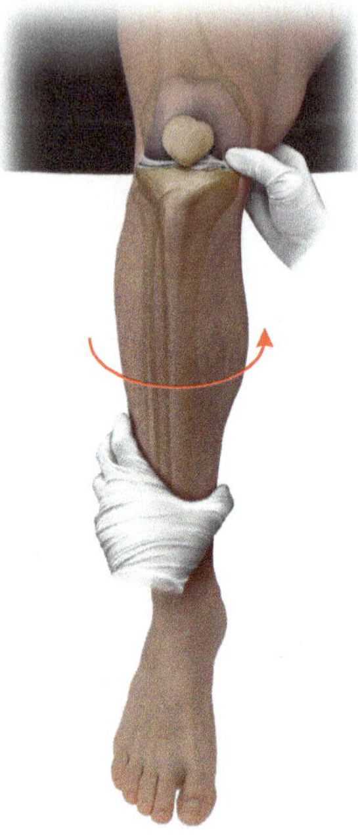

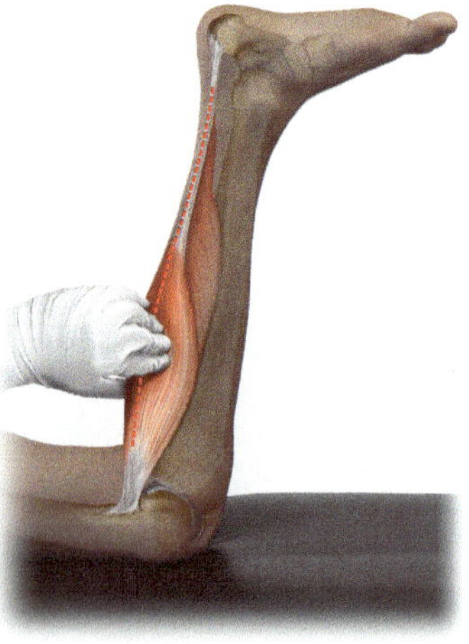

Gastrocnemius

The patient is in the prone position. The palpation fingers are rested at the level of the knee crease, which is then flexed to 90° to allow palpation of the tendons of the gastrocnemius. By sliding distally, the bulky belly of the gastrocnemius, which is located superficially, can be easily identified. Palpation continues caudally until the muscle fibers merge with the calcaneal tendon (Achilles tendon).

Anatomical landmarks on the surface of the knee

1	Greater trochanter of the femur: when the tip of the thumb is placed at the center of the iliac crest, the tip of the middle finger, pointing distally on the lateral surface of the thigh, rests on the superior border of the greater trochanter
2	Patella: large, triangular-shaped sesamoid bone on the anterior surface of the knee, with proximal base and distal apex
3	Patellar ligament: extends from the apex of the patella to the tibial tuberosity; its borders are palpable when the knee is extended
4	Tibial tuberosity: bony prominence at the proximal extremity of the anterior border of the tibia, to which the patellar ligament is inserted
5	Medial and lateral condyles of the tibia: to the two sides of the patellar ligament, the superior borders of the glenoid cavities of the medial and lateral condyles of the tibia are located in depressions formed by soft tissue; following the contours of the glenoid cavities medially and laterally, the articular fissure of the knee joint can be identified
6	Head of the fibula: rounded bony prominence on the lateral surface of the leg at the level of the tibial tuberosity
7	Anterior border of the tibia: subcutaneous bony crest along the anterior surface of the leg

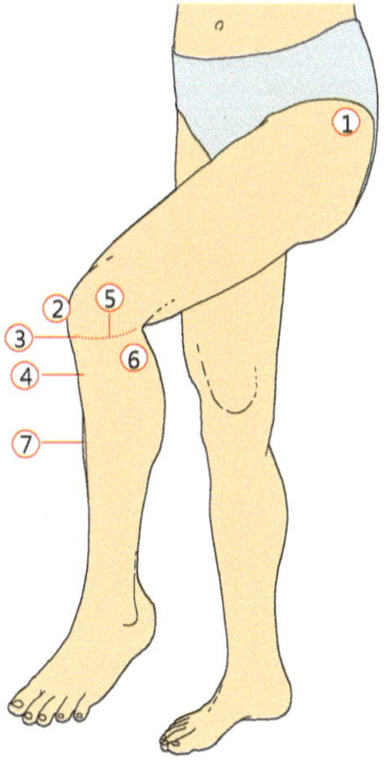

Inferior extremity of the tibia

- Base of the inferior extremity – anteroposteriorly concave articular surface, divided into two sides (corresponds to the trochlea of the talus) by a sagittal ridge
- Medial malleolus → protrusion of the inferior extremity (medial)
  - medial surface → furrowed by the tendons of the flexor muscles (corresponds to the teguments)
  - lateral surface → flat sagitally oriented articular surface (corresponds to the medial surface of the talus)
- Lateral surface of the inferior extremity – articular surface for the fibula (fibular notch)

(For the body and superior extremity of the tibia, see Chapter 11 "Knee").

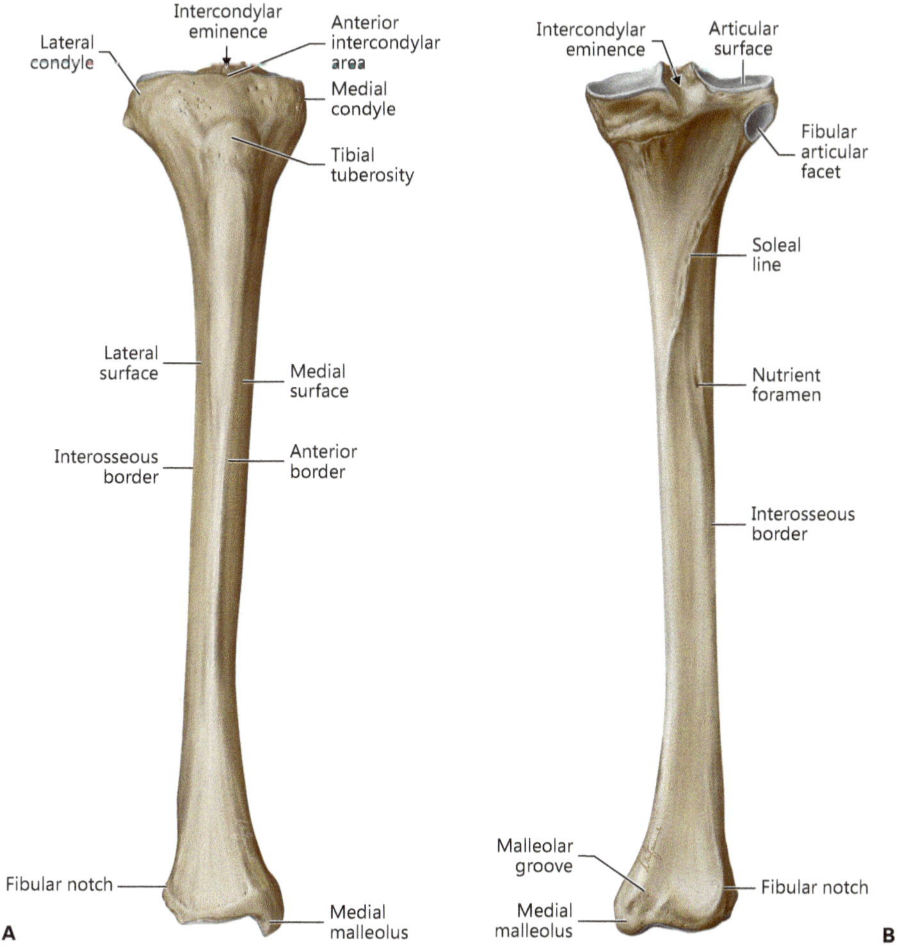

Anterior (**A**) and posterior (**B**) surfaces of the right tibia.

Inferior extremity of the fibula

- Lateral malleolus:
  - medial surface of the lateral malleolus → corresponds:
    - above, to the articular surface of the fibular notch of the tibia
    - below, to the lateral surface of the talus
    - posteriorly, to the insertion of the posterior talofibular ligament
  - lateral surface → corresponds to the integuments:
    - the sagittal groove in the posterior region (tendons of the fibularis muscles)

(For the shaft or body and the superior extremity of the fibula, see Chapter 11 "Knee").

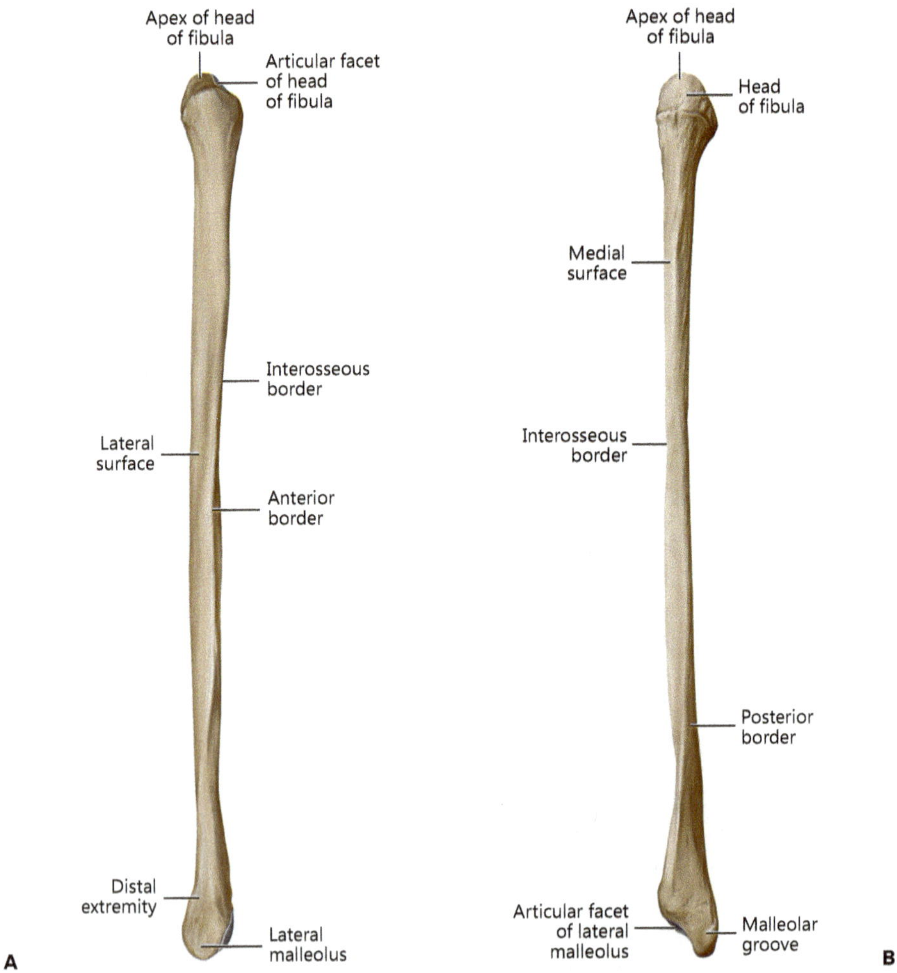

Anterior (**A**) and posterior (**B**) surfaces of the right fibula.

Tarsus

- Talus – interposed between the tibia and fibula above, the calcaneus below and behind, and the navicular to the front
- Calcaneus – under the talus

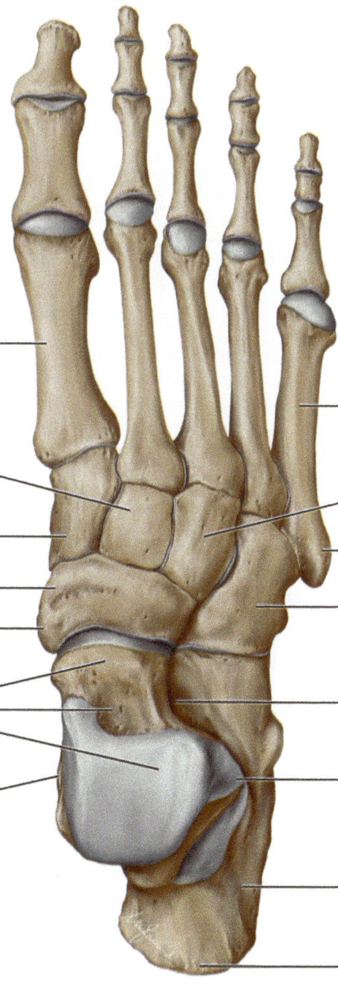

Right foot, skeleton seen from the dorsal surface. At the posterior and lateral part of the tarsus the tarsal sinus is delimited between the talus and the calcaneus.

- Cuboid – in front of the calcaneus, next to the navicular and the lateral cuneiform, behind the 4th and 5th metatarsals
- Navicular – in front of the talus, medially to the cuboid, behind the three cuneiforms
- Cuneiforms – in front of the navicular, medially to the cuboid.

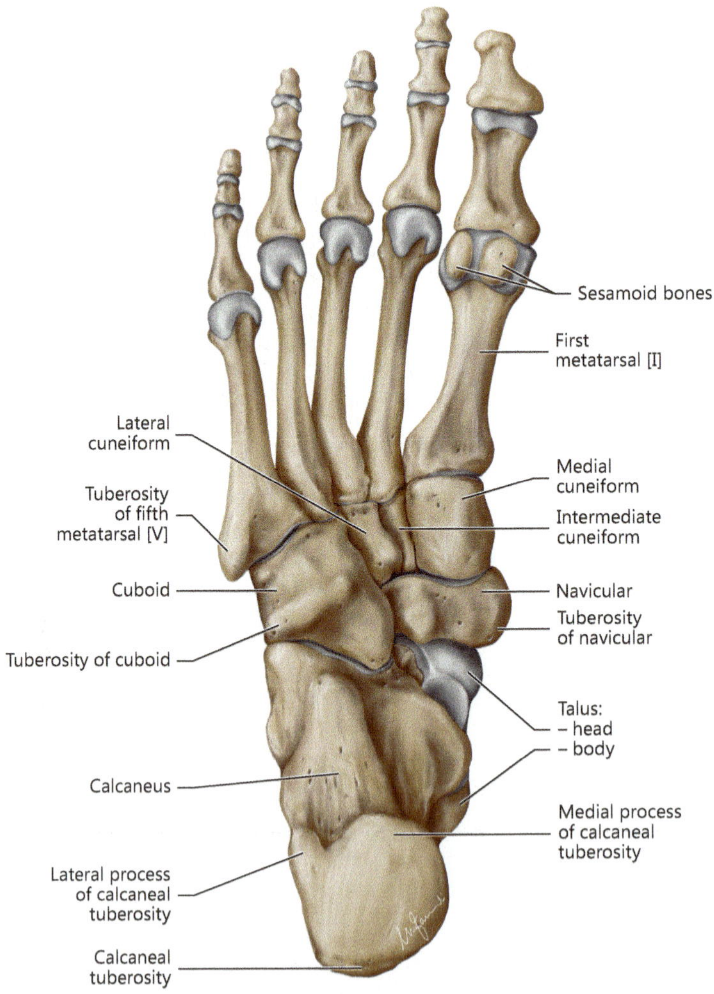

Right foot, skeleton seen from the plantar surface. In relation to the distal extremity of the 1st metatarsal, and in proximity to the metatarsophalangeal joint, there are two sesamoid bones.

Talus

In the talus, also called astragalus, three parts (in an anteroposterior direction: head, neck and body) and six surfaces can be distinguished:

- superior – trochlea of the talus (central groove with two sides) → corresponds to the base of the inferior extremity of the tibia
- inferior – two flat articular facets for the joint with the calcaneus (posterolateral and anteromedial – the latter divided into two facets: anterior and medial); between the posterolateral and anteromedial facets – the sulcus tali, which forms the tarsal sinus opposing the calcaneal sulcus
- medial – medial malleolar facet (corresponds to the lateral surface of the medial malleolus of the tibia)
- lateral – lateral malleolar facet (corresponds to the medial surface of the lateral malleolus of the fibula in its lower part)
- posterior – sagittal groove delimited by the medial and lateral tubercles of the talus
- anterior – head of the talus (articulates with the navicular).

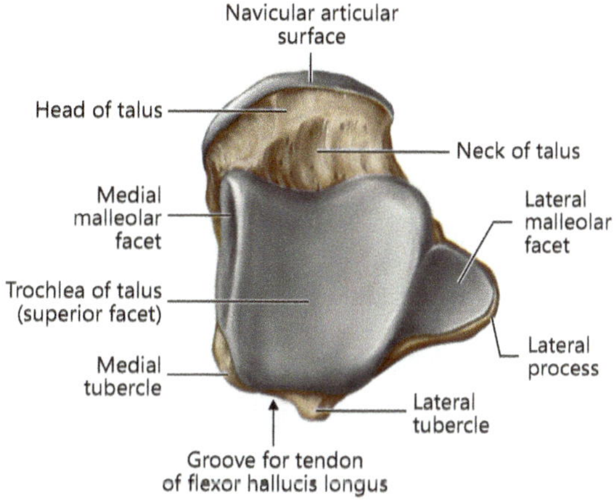

Dorsal surface of the right talus. Between the head and the trochlea there is a narrowing in the neck of the talus. On the sides of the trochlea two articular surfaces have been outlined: the lateral and medial malleolar facets.

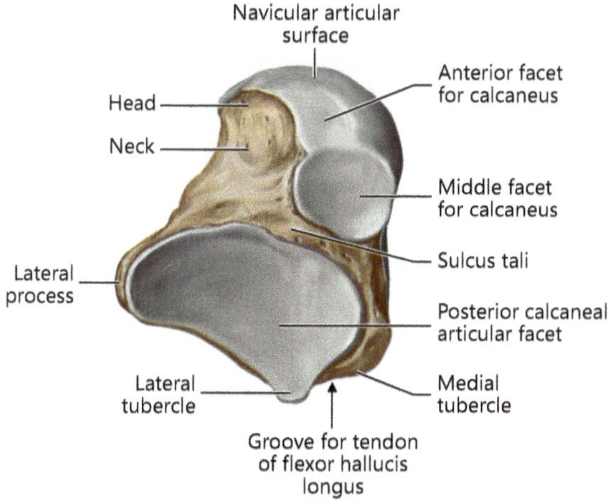

Plantar surface of the right talus. Much of this surface is occupied by the articular surfaces for the calcaneus. The sulcus tali is involved in the delimitation of the tarsal sinus.

Calcaneus

Six surfaces:

- superior – corresponds to the inferior surface of the talus (anterior, middle and posterior articular surfaces for the talus and calcaneal groove which, opposing the sulcus tali, form the tarsal sinus)
- inferior:
  - anterior tuberosity
  - posterior tuberosity
  - medial and lateral tubercles
- lateral:
  - fibular trochlea – between the anterior third and middle third
- medial:
  - medial calcaneal sulcus delimited:
    - posteriorly by the medial tubercle
    - anteriorly by the sustentaculum tali or talar shelf (head whose superior surface corresponds to the middle talar articular surface)
- anterior – articular surface (vertically concave and transversally convex) corresponding to the cuboid
- posterior – heel (insertion of the calcaneal tendon or Achilles tendon).

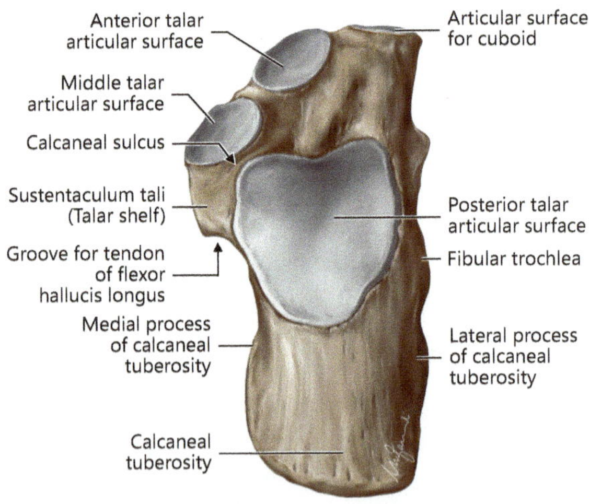

Dorsal surface of the right calcaneus. The posterior part of the bone rises into the robust posterior tuberosity.

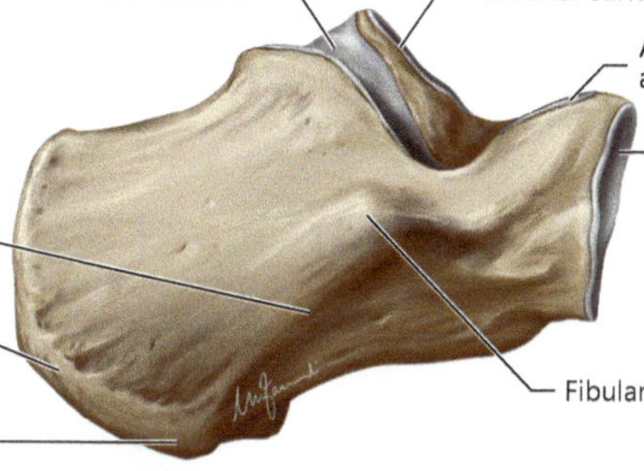

Lateral surface of the right calcaneus. The three articular surfaces for the talus are located on the anterior and superior part of the bone.

Cuboid

- Posterior surface – corresponds to the anterior surface of the calcaneus
- Medial surface – articular surface for the lateral cuneiform
- Anterior surface – medial and lateral articular surfaces; for the bases of the 4th and 5th metatarsals.

Navicular

- Posterior surface – glenoid cavity that articulates with the head of the talus
- Anterior surface – three flat facets that articulate with the three cuneiforms.

Cuneiforms

Medial, intermediate and lateral cuneiforms:

- articulate with each other, anteriorly with the bases of the first three metatarsals, laterally (lateral cuneiform) with the cuboid and posteriorly with the navicular.

Regions of the foot

Forefoot → metatarsals (1st, 2nd, 3rd, 4th and 5th) and phalanges
Midfoot → tarsal bones (navicular, cuboid and medial, intermediate and lateral cuneiforms)
Hindfoot → tarsal bones (talus and calcaneus)

Functions

- Forefoot:
  - locomotor thrust
- Midfoot:
  - cushion the support of the foot on the ground
- Hindfoot:
  - impact with the ground (first and rapid contact with the ground during walking)
  - receives all the load of the body through articular impact of the tibia and fibula with the talus, which transfers it to the calcaneus, which in turn transmits it to the entire foot (key point of foot function).

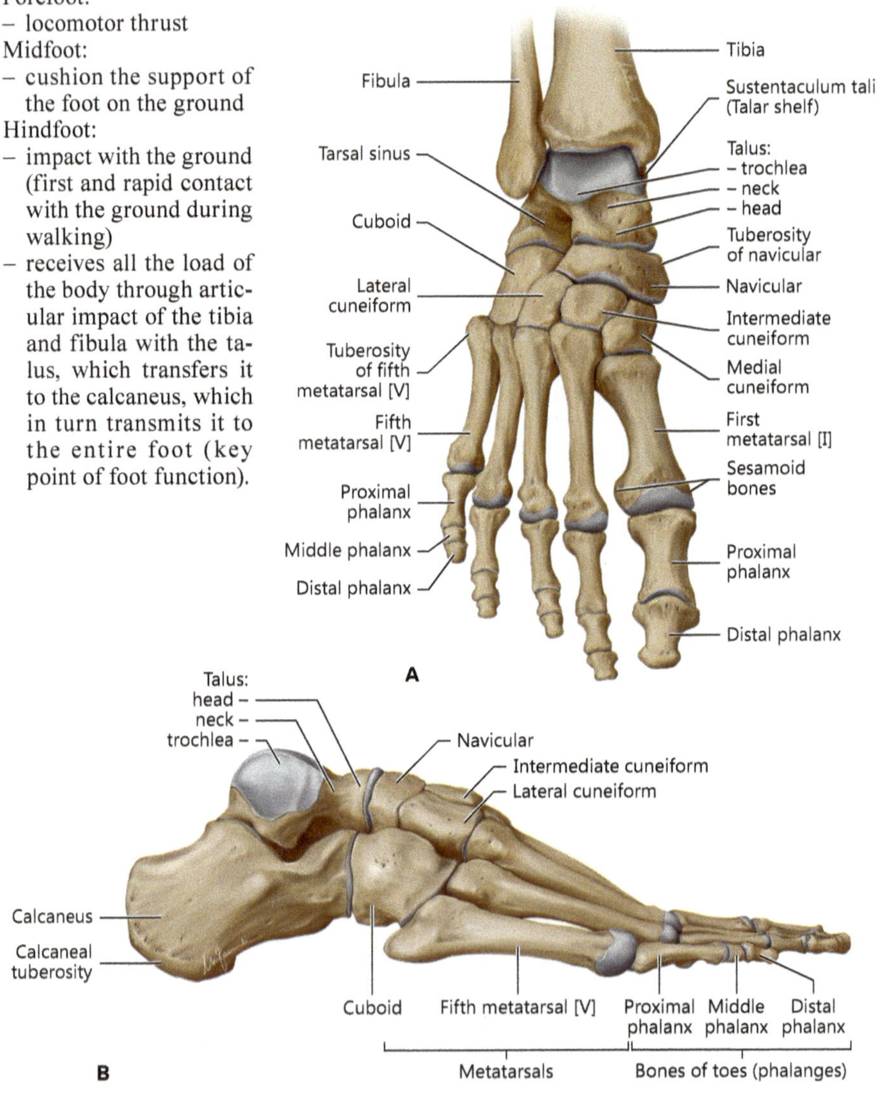

Skeleton of the right foot viewed from the dorsal (**A**) and lateral (**B**) surfaces.

Metatarsals and phalanges

Metatarsus

1st, 2nd, 3rd, 4th and 5th metatarsals:
- articulate with each other (2nd, 3rd, 4th and 5th metatarsals), posteriorly with the three cuneiforms (1st, 2nd, 3rd and 4th metatarsals) and with the cuboid (4th and 5th metatarsals).

Phalanges

2nd, 3rd, 4th and 5th toe – phalanges:
- proximal
- medial
- distal

1st toe (great toe) – phalanges:
- proximal
- distal.

Osteoarticular columns

Osteoarticular column – metatarsal + proximal, medial (except the 1st toe) and distal phalanges.

Metatarsal arch

It is formed by the heads of the metatarsals (anterior part of the transverse arch of the foot).

Arches of the foot

- Longitudinal:
  - internal
  - external
- Transverse

The internal longitudinal arch is formed by:
- talus
- navicular
- medial, intermediate and lateral cuneiforms
- 1st, 2nd and 3rd metatarsals

The external longitudinal arch is formed by:
- calcaneus
- cuboid
- 4th and 5th metatarsals

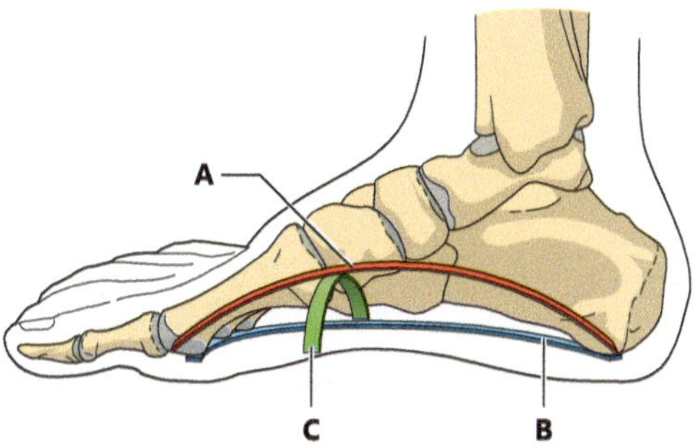

Outline of the three plantar arches. **A**, Internal longitudinal arch; **B**, external longitudinal arch; **C**, transverse arch.

The transverse arch (orthogonal to the longitudinal arches) is formed by:
- medial, intermediate and lateral cuneiforms and cuboid
- 1st, 2nd, 3rd, 4th and 5th metatarsals (metatarsal arch at the level of the heads).

Foot arch supports

Internal longitudinal arch:

- anterior support – on the sesamoid bones of the 1st toe and, partially, on the head of the 2nd metatarsal
- posterior support – on the calcaneus

External longitudinal arch:

- anterior support – on the head of the 5th metatarsal and, partially, on the heads of the 3rd and 4th metatarsals
- posterior support – on the calcaneus.

The arches of the foot absorb the load and the various pressures. During the upright position, both the external longitudinal and transverse arches (which therefore have a greater supporting function) undergo variations, while the internal longitudinal arch remains unchanged. In particular, the transverse arch flattens when the foot is loaded, with downward rotation of the intermetatarsal articular surfaces.

Hallux valgus

Outward deviation of the great toe, with superposition over the other toes.

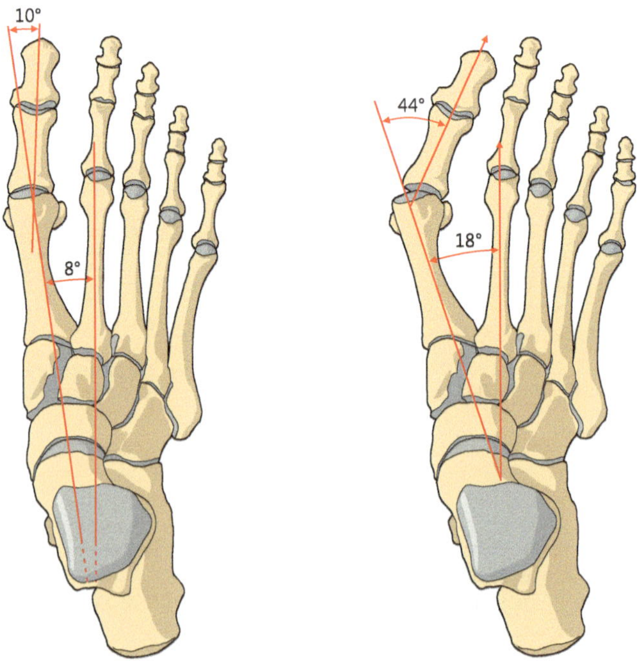

Joints of the ankle and foot

Joints of the ankle

- Distal tibiofibular
- Ankle (or talocrural).

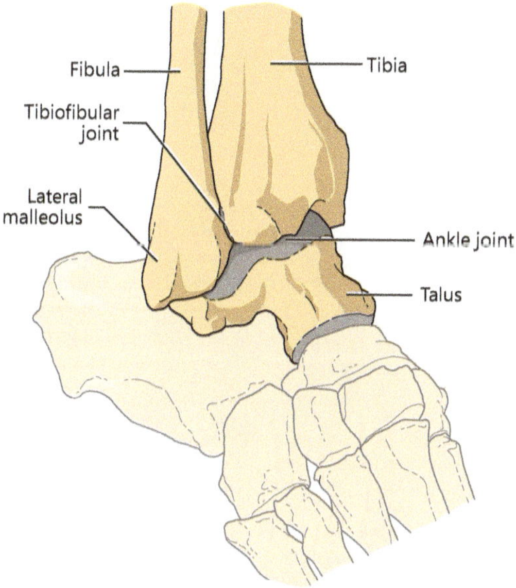

Joints of the foot

Tarsal joints (act simultaneously):

- subtalar (talocalcaneal)
- transverse tarsal or Chopart (between the bones of the proximal and distal tarsal rows):
  - medial or talonavicular – between the talus and the navicular
  - lateral or calcaneocuboid – between the calcaneus and the cuboid
- between the bones of the distal tarsal row
  - cuboideonavicular – between the cuboid and the navicular
  - cuneocuboid – between the cuboid and the lateral cuneiform
  - intercuneiform – between the medial and intermediate cuneiforms and between the intermediate and lateral cuneiforms
  - cuneonavicular – between the navicular and the cuneiforms

Metatarsal joints:

- tarsometatarsal (Lisfranc):
  - between the 1st metatarsal and the medial cuneiform
  - between the 2nd metatarsal and the medial, intermediate and lateral cuneiforms
  - between the 3rd metatarsal and the lateral cuneiform
- intermetatarsal

Phalangeal joints:
- metatarsophalangeal
- interphalangeal

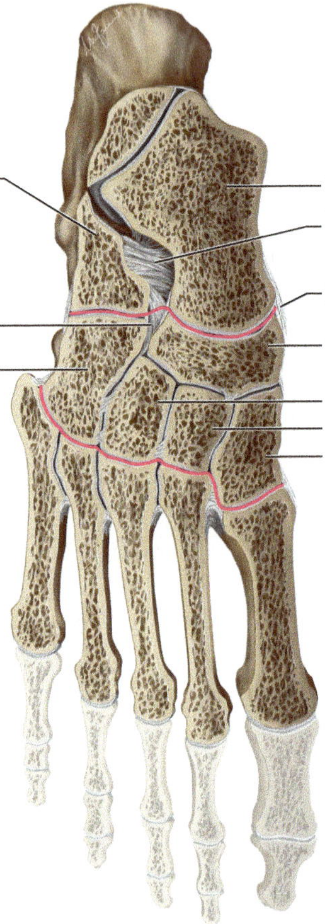

Right tarsal joints. The horizontal section plane, seen from above, shows the tarsal and tarsometatarsal joints. The two red lines, proximal and distal, indicate the transverse tarsal joint (Chopart joint) and tarsometatarsal joints, respectively.

Distal tibiofibular joint

- Synarthrosis between the inferior extremities of the tibia (fibular notch) and of the fibula (the superior part of the medial surface of the lateral malleolus); in this case the articular surfaces are covered by the periosteum

or

- Plane joint, dependent on the ankle joint, when the articular surfaces are covered by cartilage.

Ankle joint

<table>
<tr><td>Type of joint</td><td>Hinge joint</td></tr>
<tr><td>Articular surfaces</td><td>
Base of the inferior extremity of the tibia (concave surface with sagittal crest)
Lateral surface of the medial malleolus (plane joint type articular surface)
Inferior surface of the medial surface of the lateral malleolus (plane joint type articular surface)

The articular surfaces of the tibia and fibula form a notch called the tibiofibular mortise.

Trochlea of the talus (convex surface with sagittal cavity – talar neck)
Medial surface of the talus (plane joint type articular surface)
Lateral surface of the talus (plane joint type articular surface)

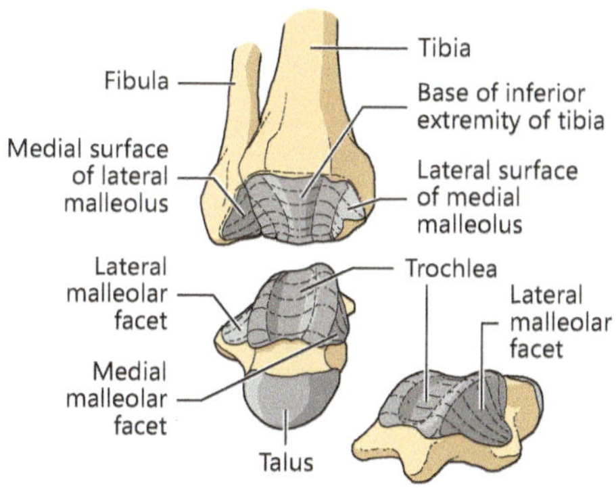

The trochlea of the talus is wider anteriorly and less posteriorly.

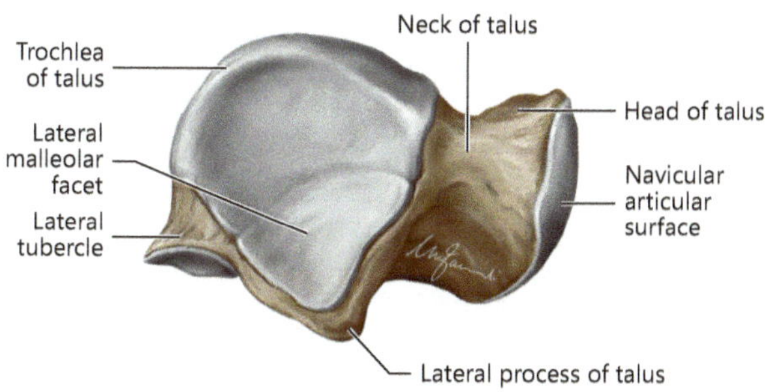

</td></tr>
</table>

(continued)

(continued)	This morphology determines a good concordance of the articular surfaces and a discrete myoligamentous tension in the presence of angles of approximately 90° between the leg and the foot, ensuring maximum stability to the ankle joint. Greater angles (for example, in the upright position in forefoot loading that occurs when wearing shoes with high heels) give instability to the ankle, accentuated by the reduction of the support base and by the elevation of the center of gravity. In this case, however, the greater space available for the talus allows for small lateral and rotational movements of the foot. In addition to the trochlea, the talus has two other characteristics: • it receives all the body weight, transmitting it to the foot • it has no muscular insertions These factors provide greater stability to the talus.
Movements	Flexion-extension (1 degree of freedom)

Subtalar (talocalcaneal) joint

Type of joint	Pivot joint
Articular surfaces	Posterior calcaneal articular facet of the talus Posterior talar articular surface of the calcaneus 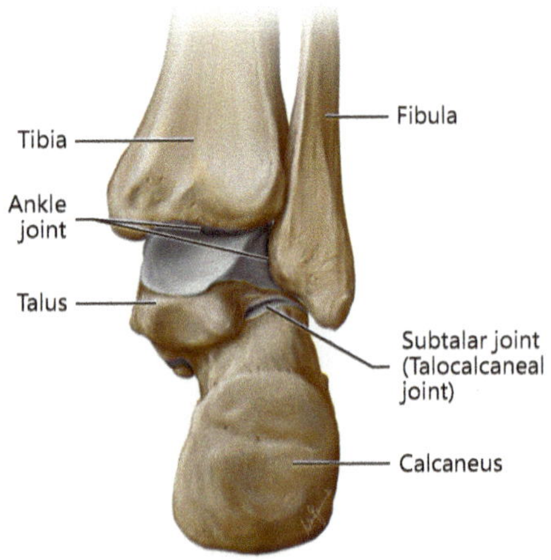
Movements	Eversion and inversion of the foot (1 degree of freedom) Through the subtalar joint, the load to which the talus is subjected is transmitted to the calcaneus.

Transverse tarsal joint

<table>
<tr><td>Type of joint</td><td>Ball and socket joint (between talus, calcaneus and navicular)
Diarthrosis saddle joint (between calcaneus and cuboid)</td></tr>
<tr><td>Articular surfaces</td><td>Talocalcaneonavicular joint, medial part of the transverse tarsal joint: head of the talus (navicular articular surface and convex anterior articular surface for the calcaneus) and posterior articular surface of the navicular (or articular surface for the talus) and medial and anterior articular surfaces for the talus of the calcaneus

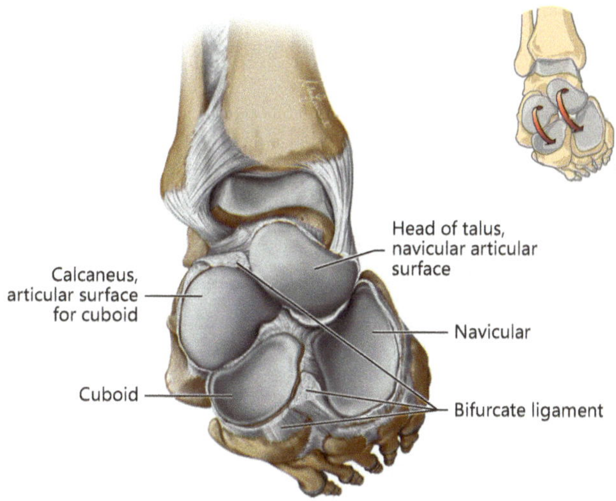

Calcaneocuboid joint, lateral part of the transverse tarsal joint: anterior surface of the calcaneus (articular surface for the cuboid, vertically concave and transversely convex) and posterior surface of the cuboid (articular surface for the calcaneus, vertically convex and transversely concave)

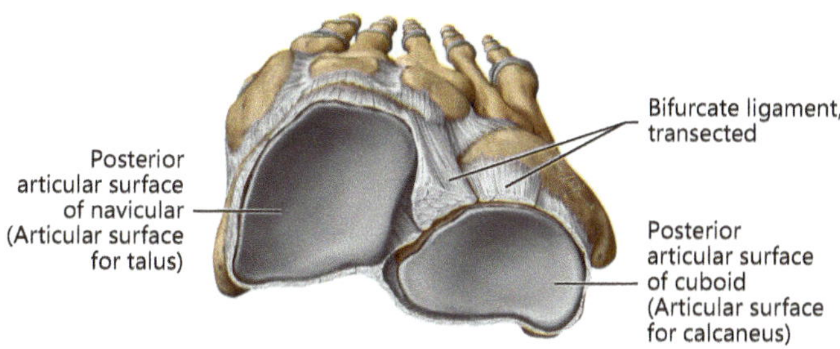
</td></tr>
<tr><td>Movements</td><td>Internal and external rotation of the foot</td></tr>
</table>

12

Joints between the bones of the distal tarsal row

Due to the shape of their articular surfaces, they are can be classified as plane joints and allow only small sliding movements.

- Cuboideonavicular joint – between the cuboid and the navicular
- Cuneocuboid joint – between the cuboid and the lateral cuneiform
- Intercuneiform joints – between the medial and intermediate cuneiforms and between the intermediate and lateral cuneiforms
- Cuneonavicular joint – between the navicular and the three cuneiforms.

Tarsometatarsal joints

Type of joint	Plane joints
Articular surfaces	Distal articular surfaces of the medial, intermediate and lateral cuneiforms Bases of the 1st, 2nd and 3rd metatarsals Articular surface of the cuboid Bases of the 4th and 5th metatarsals
Movements	Very modest sliding movements similar to flexion-extension (first and fourth osteoarticular column) and abduction-adduction (first osteoarticular column) movements.

Intermetatarsal joints

Between the bases of the last four metatarsals. They are plane joints and allow only small sliding movements.

Metatarsophalangeal joints

Type of joint	Condylar joints
Movements	Flexion-extension and abduction-adduction (2 degrees of freedom)

Interphalangeal joints

Type of joint	Hinge joints
Movements	Flexion-extension (1 degree of freedom)

Ligaments of the ankle and foot joints

Distal tibiofibular joint

Ligaments:
- fibrous interosseous
- anterior tibiofibular
- posterior tibiofibular.

Ankle joint

- Medial ligament (deltoid ligament) – originates from the medial (tibial) malleolus and is formed by the following parts:
  - tibionavicular
  - tibiocalcaneal
  - anterior tibiotalar
  - posterior tibiotalar
- Lateral ligament – originates from the lateral (fibular) malleolus and is formed by the following ligaments:
  - calcaneofibular
  - posterior talofibular
  - anterior talofibular.

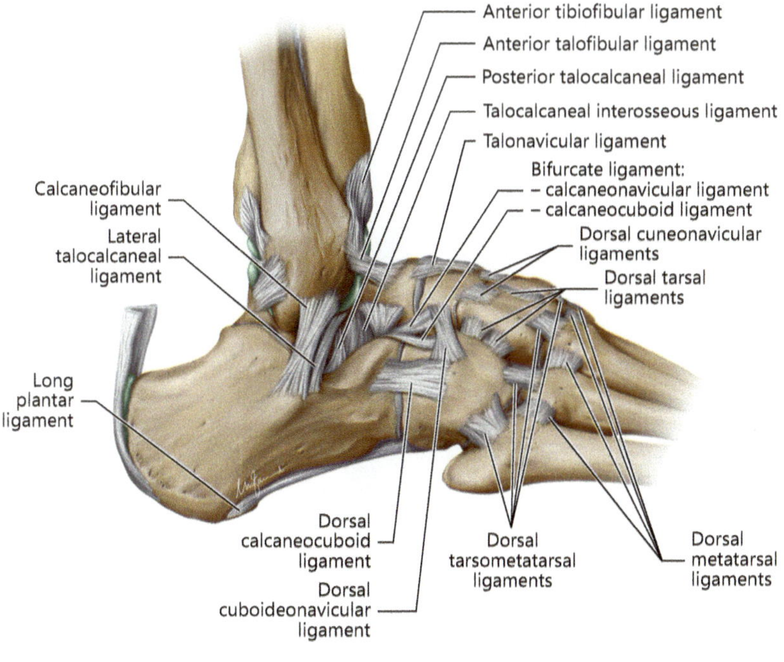

Ankle and tarsal joints on the right side. The means of union of the various joints are shown here laterally.

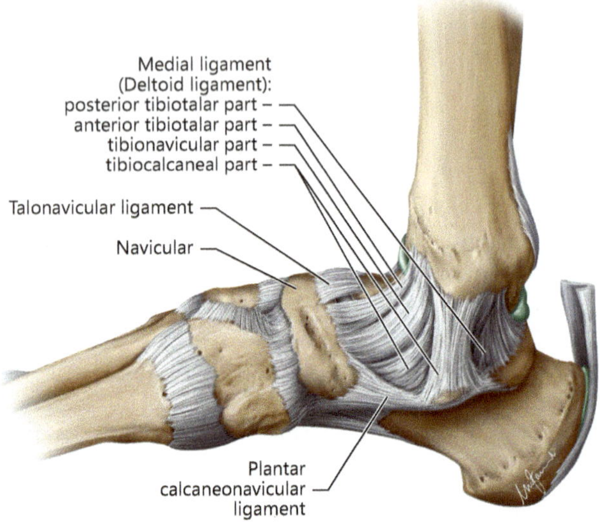

Ankle and tarsal joints on the right side. The means of union of the various joints are shown here medially.

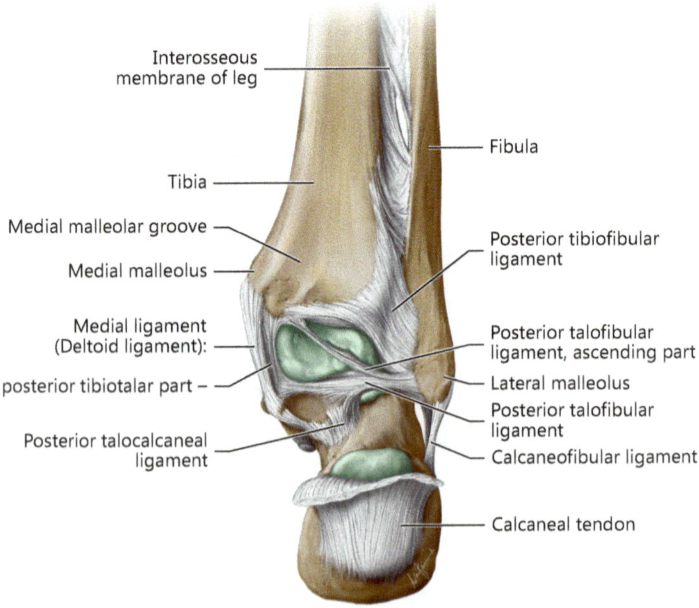

Ankle and subtalar (talocalcaneal) joints on the right side, seen from behind, with the foot in flexion. The joint capsule has been removed to show the reinforcing ligaments and part of the articular surface of the talus.

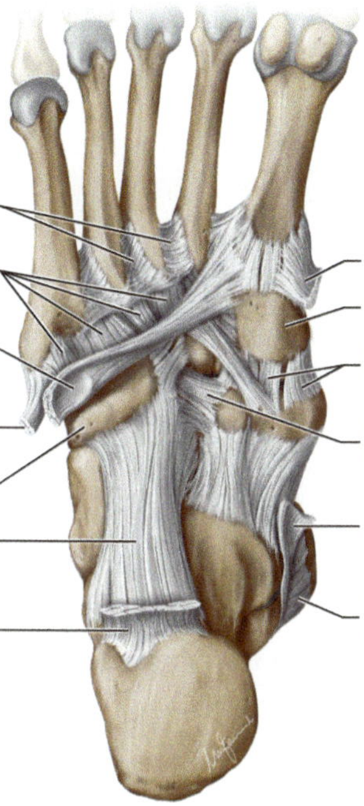

Ligaments of the sole of the right foot.

Subtalar (talocalcaneal) joint

- Talocalcaneal ligaments:
  - anterior
  - posterior
  - medial
  - lateral
  - interosseous (runs within the tarsal sinus and is therefore called interosseous).

Transverse tarsal joint

12

Ligaments:
- bifurcated (common or Y-shaped) – between the calcaneal process and the cuboid and navicular (calcaneonavicular and calcaneocuboid parts)
- dorsal talonavicular
- plantar calcaneonavicolar
- dorsal calcaneocuboid
- internal calcaneocuboid
- plantar calcaneocuboid
- long plantar.

Joints between the bones of the distal tarsal row

Ligaments:
- dorsal cuboideonavicular
- plantar cuboideonavicular
- interosseous cuboideonavicular
- interosseous cuneocuboid
- dorsal cuneocuboid
- plantar cuneocuboid
- dorsal intercuneiform
- plantar intercuneiform
- interosseous intercuneiform
- dorsal cuneonavicular
- plantar cuneonavicular.

Tarsometatarsal joints

Ligaments:
- dorsal tarsometatarsal
- plantar tarsometatarsal
- interosseous cuneometatarsal (the most important of these is the Lisfranc ligament, between the medial cuneiform and the base of the 2nd metatarsal).

Intermetatarsal joints

Ligaments:
- transverse of the heads of the metatarsals – joins the heads of the metatarsals
- intermetatarsal:
  - dorsal of the bases of the metatarsals
  - plantar of the bases of the metatarsals
  - interosseous.

Metatarsophalangeal and interphalangeal joints

Ligaments:
- plantar
- collateral.

Bursa of the calcaneal tendon

- Between the calcaneus and the calcaneal tendon (Achilles tendon).

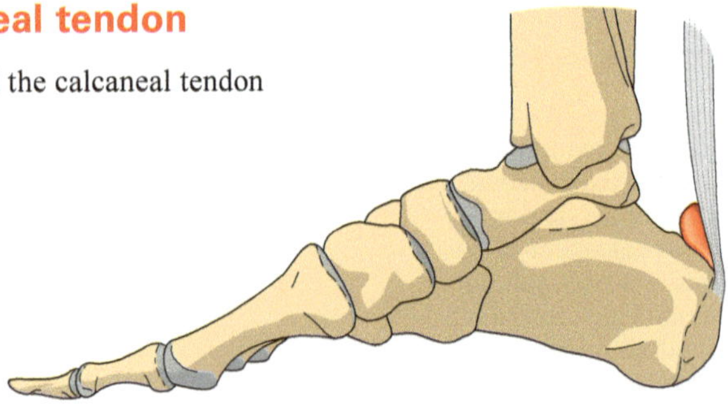

Movements of the ankle and foot joints

Ankle joint

Flexion-extension of the ankle

- Flexion of the ankle (of the foot):
  - movement of the dorsum of the foot towards the tibia (dorsiflexion of the foot)
  - amplitude: **30-35°**

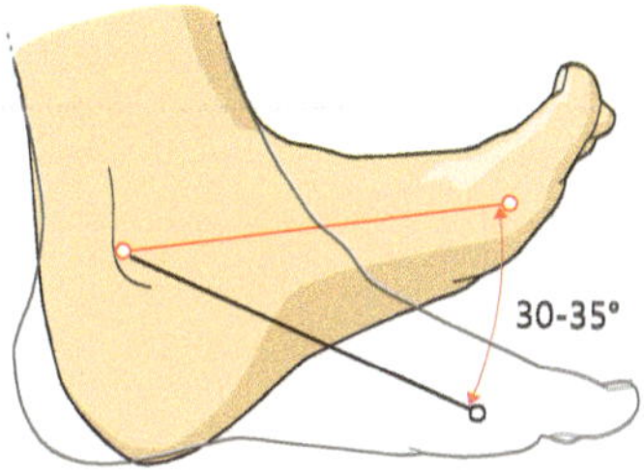

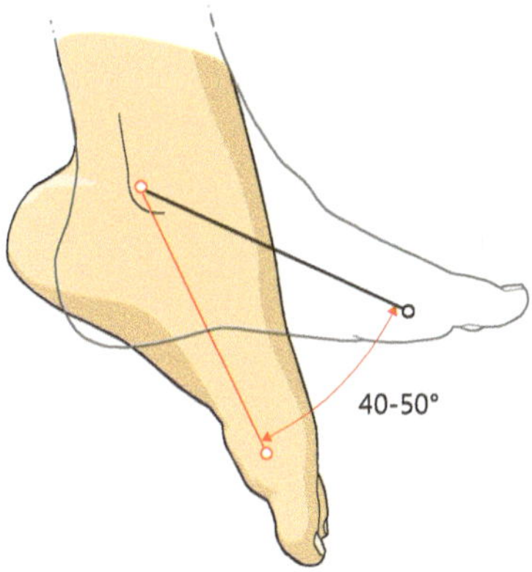

- Extension of the ankle (of the foot):
  - movement of the foot in the opposite direction in relation to the tibia (ventral flexion of the foot)
  - amplitude: **40-50°**

Axis of movement

- Frontal axis passing through the medial (tibial) and lateral (fibular) malleoli; there is actually no connection between this axis and the frontal plane, since the fibular malleolus is located further back and further down in relation to the tibial malleolus, so during dorsiflexion of the foot partial movements of supination, abduction and inversion of the foot occur in succession.

Reference position
- Angle of 90° between the axis of the foot and the axis of the leg.

> During flexion-extension of the foot, the talus moves together with the calcaneus, forming a single body.

Subtalar (talocalcaneal) joint

Adduction of the foot

The tip of the foot is brought inward (towards the median plane of symmetry).

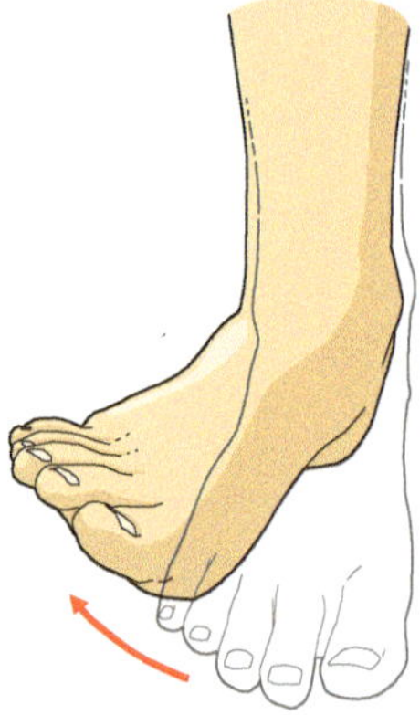

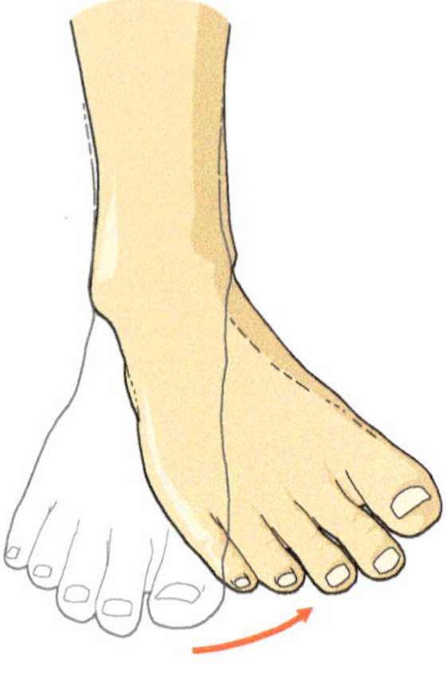

Abduction of the foot

The tip of the foot is brought outward (away from the median plane of symmetry).

The total amplitude of the abduction-adduction movements of the foot varies from 35 to 45°.

Supination of the foot

Rotation of the foot with inward exposure of the sole of the foot.

The amplitude of the supination movement of the foot is approximately 30-40°.

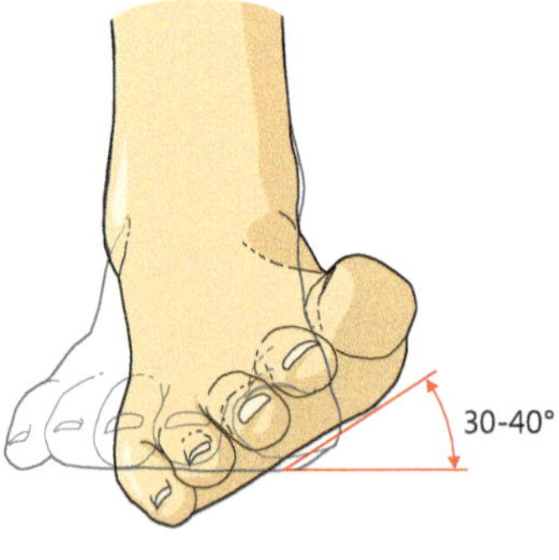

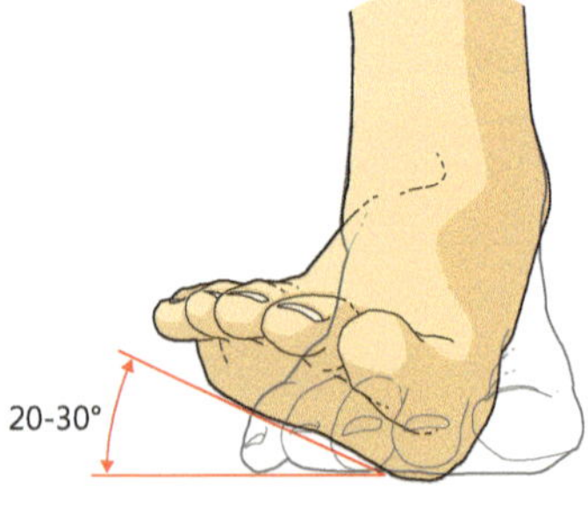

Pronation of the foot

Rotation of the foot with outward exposure of the sole of the foot.

The amplitude of the pronation movement of the foot is 20-30°.

The movements of adduction, abduction, supination and pronation, in relation to the mode of organization of the joints of the foot, do not occur individually, but are associated with one another and with the dorsal and plantar flexion of the foot, giving rise to movements of eversion and inversion of the foot.

Inversion and eversion of the foot

- Inversion – compound movements of adduction, supination and plantar flexion of the foot which lead to the inward movement of the sole of the foot.

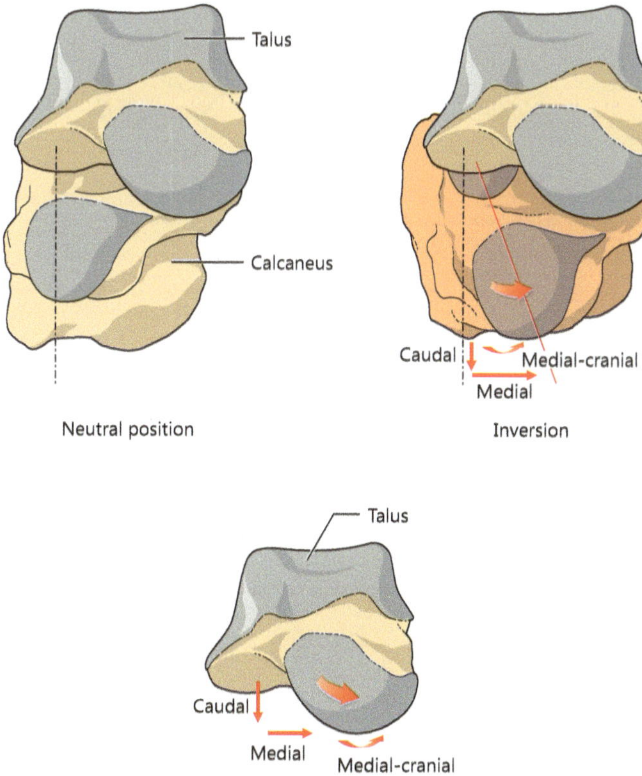

Sliding of the navicular in relation to the talus during inversion.

- Eversion – compound movements of abduction, pronation and dorsiflexion of the foot which lead to the outward movement of the sole of the foot.

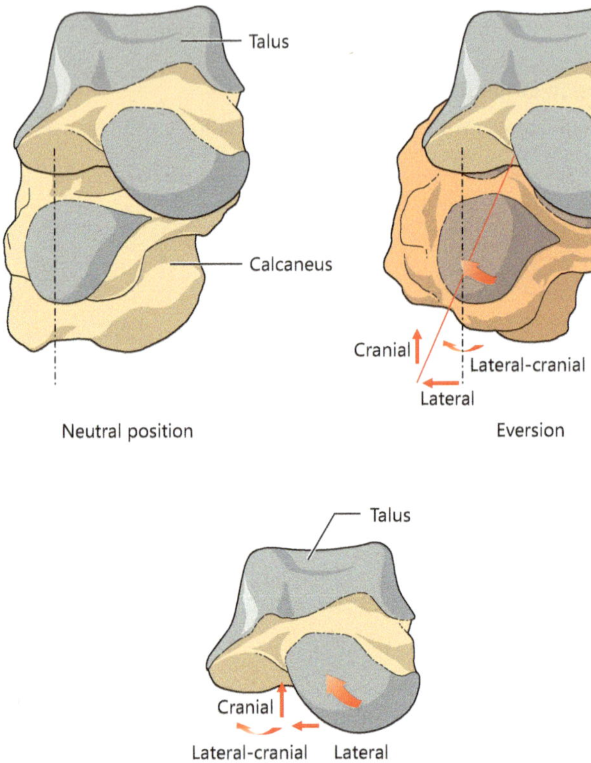

Sliding of the navicular in relation to the talus during eversion.

Axis of movement

- Between the posterior calcaneal tuberosity and the surface of the trochlea of the talus in the anteromedial position (this is an indicative axis, since individual movements occur, each around its own axis, which are added up together)
- In oblique direction from back to front, from lateral to medial and from bottom to top.

> During eversion and inversion of the foot, the talus is fixed between the tibia and the fibula, allowing the calcaneus to move with the rest of the foot.

Transverse tarsal joint (medial or talonavicular and lateral or calcaneocuboid joints)

Eversion and inversion of the foot.
Axis of movement:
- sagittal (passing between the navicular and the cuboid).

Joints between the bones of the distal tarsal row and tarsometatarsal and intermetatarsal joints

Sliding movements of the tarsometatarsal joints.
Movements that fix the forefoot:
- in pronation, when the hindfoot is in supination
- in supination, when the hindfoot is in pronation.

> These fixation movements occur both in static load and during locomotion, in order to adapt the position of the forefoot to that of the hindfoot.

Metatarsophalangeal joints

Flexion-extension and abduction-adduction of the proximal phalanges.
Reference axes:
- flexion-extension – frontal, passing through the center of the heads of the metatarsals
- abduction-adduction – vertical, passing through the center of the heads of the metatarsals.

> The movement of extension is broader than that of the corresponding joints of the hand (metatarsophalangeal), as is the plantar flexion of the foot compared to extension of the hand (these movements at the level of the foot facilitate upright position and walking). On the other hand, the movements of abduction and adduction of the proximal phalanges are reduced and difficult to control voluntarily (for these movements, the reference finger is the second finger).

Interphalangeal joints

Flexion-extension of the middle and distal phalanges (these movements are limited by the dorsal, plantar, medial and lateral ligaments, which also prevent lateral movements).

Assessment of the passive joint mobility of the ankle and foot

Dorsiflexion and plantar flexion of the ankle

Dorsiflexion of the ankle

Starting position	Supine, with the knee slightly flexed (20-30°, by the interposition of a rolled towel between the knee and the examination table) and the foot in anatomical position (0°, perpendicular to the lower leg)
Movement	Movement of the dorsum of the foot towards the anterior surface of the leg to the limit of dorsiflexion of the foot (20°) (the examiner holds, with one hand, the plantar surface of the forefoot moving the dorsum of foot towards the leg, while the other hand stabilizes the leg) 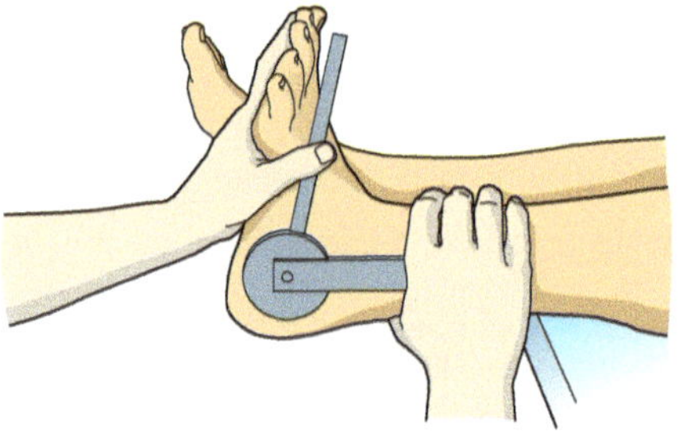

Plantar flexion of the ankle

Starting position	Supine, with the knee slightly flexed (by the interposition of a rolled towel between the knee and the examination table) and the foot in anatomical position (perpendicular to the lower leg)
Movement	Movement of the talus and calcaneus downward to the limit of plantar flexion of the foot (50°) (the examiner holds the dorsum of the foot with one hand, placing the radial border of the index finger on the anterior surface of the talus and the calcaneus, while the other hand stabilizes the leg) 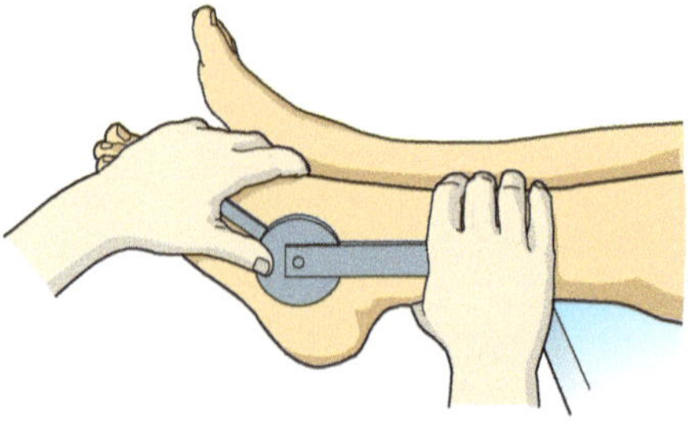

Inversion and eversion of the foot

Starting position	Supine, with the foot in anatomical position
Movement	Inward movement of the calcaneus to the limit of the inversion movement, and outward to the limit of the eversion movement (the examiner holds the posterior part and the sides of the calcaneus with one hand, while the other hand stabilizes the talus in front and below the malleoli) 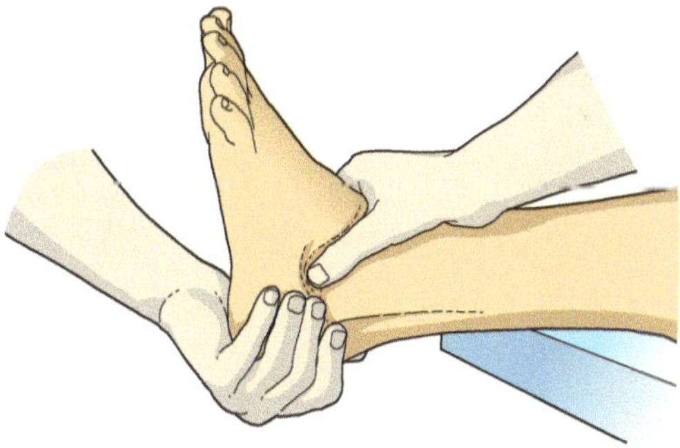 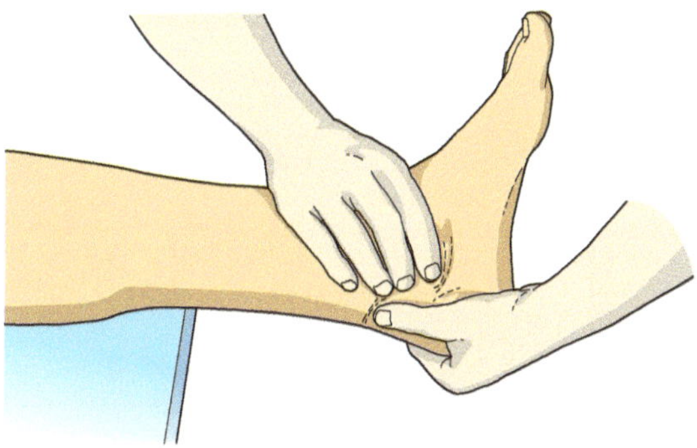

Metatarsophalangeal flexion and extension of the proximal phalanges

Starting position	Supine, with the foot and toes in anatomical position
Movement	The examiner moves the proximal phalanx of the examined toe to the limit of metatarsophalangeal flexion (45° for the great toe, 40° for the other toes) (first) and extension (70° for the great toe, 40° for the other toes) (then), after stabilizing the metatarsal of the examined metatarsophalangeal joint 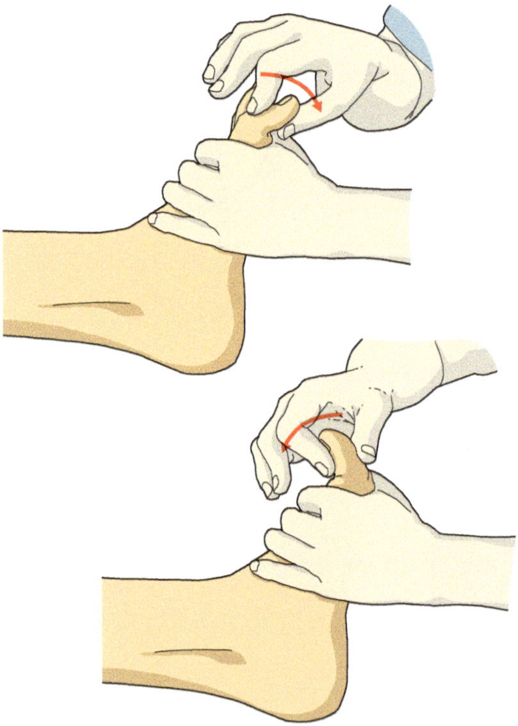

Metatarsophalangeal abduction and adduction of the great toe

Starting position	Supine, with the foot and great toe in anatomical position
Movement	The examiner moves the proximal phalanx of the great toe by traction and abduction and adduction of the great toe. Stabilization is on the first metatarsal 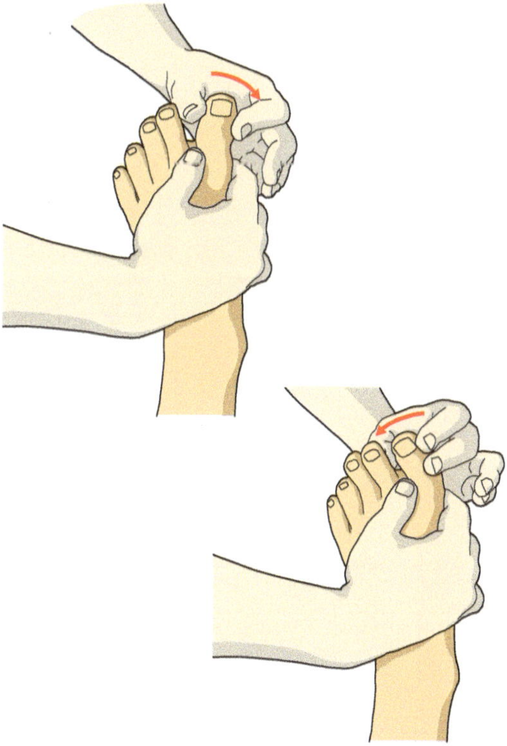

Interphalangeal flexion-extension of the great toe

Starting position	Supine, with the foot and great toe in anatomical position
Movement	The examiner moves the distal phalanx of the great toe to the limit of metatarsophalangeal flexion (first) and extension (then), after stabilizing the proximal phalanx. **Note**: in the metatarsophalangeal flexion-extension, the proximal phalanx will move stabilizing the first metatarsal 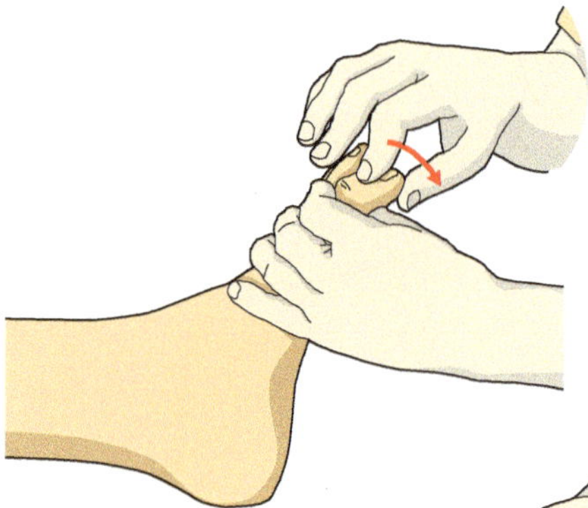 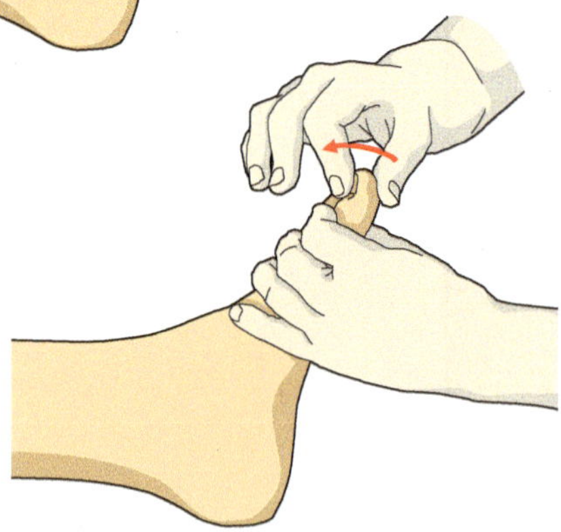

Functional aspects of the ankle and foot joints

Function of the foot

- Flexible support base for adapting to ground irregularities
- During the stance phase, the foot and the ankle lift the body
- When the body weight is supported by the foot, the metatarsophalangeal joints allow the movement of the rigid foot relative to the toes
- Cushioning function linked to the transmission of forces between the ground and the leg
- Rigid lever during the final phase of the stance phase of the gait cycle
- When off the ground it can be used to modify the formation, transformation or transmission of forces.

Mobility of the ankle

- Dorsiflexion:
  - a maximum amplitude between 14° and 27° is needed for climbing stairs
  - a maximum amplitude between 21° and 36° is needed for descending stairs
  - getting up from a seated position requires a considerable amplitude of movement, on average equal to 28°
- Plantar flexion:
  - the entire amplitude may be needed to climb, jump or stand on tiptoe
  - less mobility may be sufficient for activities such as stepping on the accelerator of a car or the pedals of a piano or for wearing high-heeled shoes
  - a maximum amplitude between 23° and 30° is needed for climbing stairs
  - a maximum amplitude between 24° and 31° is needed for descending stairs.

Mobility of the foot

- The active mobility of the subtalar (talocalcaneal) joint is 5°, both when inverted or everted, in the absence of movements of the forefoot:
  - can be increased, through movements of the forefoot, up to 35° and 15°, respectively
- Full mobility of the subtalar (talocalcaneal) joint, transverse tarsal joint and the joints of the forefoot is necessary to allow the foot to adapt to the different irregularities of the ground
- Only a few degrees of flexion of the great toe are required to perform the majority of daily activities
- Values close to the maximum amplitude of extension of the proximal phalanx of the great toe, equal to 90°, are necessary to carry out many daily activities
- The extension of the great toe and the other four toes is essential for activities such as rising up on the toes to reach objects placed up high of squatting
- In upright position, the proximal phalanges are extended at least 25° due to the downward inclination of the metatarsals
- The abduction and adduction of the proximal phalanges are negligible.

Muscles of the ankle and foot

Muscle	Action	Origin	Insertion	Innervation
Tibialis anterior	Dorsiflexion, inversion and adduction of the foot	Lateral condyle of the tibia, proximal half of the lateral surface of the shaft of the tibia; anterior surface of the interosseous membrane	Medial and inferior surfaces of the medial cuneiform; medial surface of the base of the first metatarsal	Deep fibular nerve [L4, L5, S1]
Gastrocnemius	Plantar flexion, inversion and abduction of the foot; flexion of the knee	*Medial head*: proximal and posterior surfaces of the medial condyle of the femur posteriorly to the adductor tubercle *Lateral head*: lateral and posterior surfaces of the lateral condyle of the femur; lower part of the supracondylar line	Calcaneal tuberosity, through the calcaneal tendon (Achilles tendon)	Tibial nerve [L4, L5, S1-S3]
Soleus	Plantar flexion and inversion of the foot	Posterior surface of the head and proximal quarter of the shaft of the fibula; soleal line and middle third of the medial border of the tibia	Calcaneal tuberosity, through the calcaneal tendon (Achilles tendon)	Tibial nerve [L4, L5, S1-S3]
Tibialis posterior	Plantar flexion, inversion and adduction of the foot	Upper two-thirds of the posterolateral surface of the tibia, below the soleal line; posterior surface of the interosseous membrane, medial surface of the proximal two-thirds of the fibula	Tuberosity of the navicular, with tendinous expansions directed to the plantar surface of the three cuneiforms	Tibial nerve [L4, L5, S1-S3]

(*continued*)

Muscles of the ankle and foot *(continued)*

Muscle	Action	Origin	Insertion	Innervation
Fibularis longus	Plantar flexion and eversion of the foot	Head and upper two-thirds of the lateral surface of the fibula; some fibers originate from the lateral condyle of the tibia	Lateral surface of the base of the first metatarsal and medial and intermediate cuneiforms	Superficial fibular nerve [L5, S1, S2]
Fibularis brevis	Plantar flexion and eversion of the foot	Lower two-thirds of the lateral surface of the fibula	Tuberosity of the fifth metatarsal	Superficial fibular nerve [L5, S1, S2]
Flexor hallucis brevis	Metatarsophalangeal plantar flexion of the great toe; adduction and abduction of the great toe, through the lateral and medial heads of the muscle, respectively	Plantar surface of the medial and intermediate cuneiforms	The muscular fascicles divide into a medial head, that inserts at the medial sesamoid bone of the metatarsophalangeal joint of the great toe, and into a lateral head, that partially merges with the adductor hallucis, and inserts at the lateral sesamoid bone of the metatarsophalangeal joint of the great toe	Medial plantar nerve [S2, S3] to the medial head and lateral plantar nerve [S2, S3] to the lateral head
Flexor hallucis longus	Interphalangeal plantar flexion of the great toe	Distal two-thirds of the posterior surface of the fibula; posterior surface of the interosseous membrane	Plantar surface of the base of the distal phalanx of the great toe	Tibial nerve [L4, L5, S1-S3]

(continued)

Muscles of the ankle and foot *(continued)*

Muscle	Action	Origin	Insertion	Innervation
Flexor digitorum longus	Distal interphalangeal plantar flexion of the lateral four toes	Posterior surface of the middle three-fifths of the tibia, below the soleal line	Plantar surface of the bases of the distal phalanges of the last four toes	Tibial nerve [L4, L5, S1-S3]
Flexor digitorum brevis	Proximal interphalangeal plantar flexion of the lateral four toes	Medial process of the calcaneal tuberosity; plantar aponeurosis	Medial and lateral surfaces of the middle phalanges of the last four toes	Medial plantar nerve [S2, S3]
Flexor digiti minimi brevis	Metatarsophalangeal plantar flexion of the little toe	Medial part of the plantar surface of the base of the fifth metatarsal; sheath of the fibularis longus	Lateral surface of the base of the proximal phalanx of the little toe	Lateral plantar nerve [S2, S3]
Lumbricals	Flexion of the proximal phalanges and extension of the medial and distal phalanges of the last four toes	First lumbrical: medial surface of the tendon of the flexor digitorum longus; from the second to the fourth lumbricals: adjacent sides of the tendons of the flexor digitorum longus	Medial surfaces of the dorsal digital expansion or aponeurosis on the proximal phalanges of the last four toes	First and second lumbricals: medial plantar nerve [S1, S2]; third and fourth lumbricals: lateral plantar nerve [S2, S3]
Abductor hallucis	Abduction and plantar flexion of the great toe	Medial process of the calcaneal tuberosity; flexor retinaculum and plantar aponeurosis	Medial surface of the base of the proximal phalanx of the great toe	Medial plantar nerve [S2, S3]
Abductor digiti minimi	Abduction and flexion of the little toe	Medial and lateral processes of the calcaneal tuberosity and part of the bone between the two processes; plantar aponeurosis	Lateral surface of the base of the proximal phalanx of the little toe	Lateral plantar nerve [S2, S3]

(continued)

Muscles of the ankle and foot (*continued*)

Muscle	Action	Origin	Insertion	Innervation
Dorsal interossei	Abduction of the second, third and fourth toe and flexion of the metatarsophalangeal joints	Adjacent sides of the metatarsals	First dorsal interosseous: medial surface of the base of the proximal phalanx of the second toe; from the second to the fourth dorsal interossei; lateral surface of the bases of the proximal phalanges of the second, third and fourth toes; dorsal digital expansion or aponeurosis	Lateral plantar nerve [S2, S3]
Plantar interossei	Adduction of the third, fourth and fifth toe and flexion of the metatarsophalangeal joints	Bases and medial surfaces of the third, fourth and fifth metatarsals	Medial surfaces of the bases of the proximal phalanges of the third, fourth and little toes; dorsal digital expansion or aponeurosis	Lateral plantar nerve [S2, S3]
Adductor hallucis	Adduction of the great toe	*Oblique head*: bases of the second, third and fourth metatarsals; sheath of the fibularis longus *Transverse head*: plantar ligaments of the metatarsophalangeal joints of the third, fourth and little toes and deep transverse metatarsal ligaments of the same toes	Both heads: lateral sesamoid bone of the first metatarsophalangeal joint and base of the proximal phalanx of the great toe	Lateral plantar nerve [S2, S3]
Extensor hallucis longus	Interphalangeal extension of the great toe	Middle two-quarters of the medial surface of the fibula; anterior surface of the interosseous membrane	Dorsal surface of the base of the distal phalanx of the great toe	Deep fibular nerve [L4, L5, S1]

(continued)

12

Muscles of the ankle and foot *(continued)*

Muscle	Action	Origin	Insertion	Innervation
Extensor digitorum longus	Extension of the metatarsophalangeal and interphalangeal joints of the last four toes	Lateral condyle of the tibia; proximal three-quarters of the medial surface of the fibula; anterior surface of the interosseous membrane	Dorsal surface of the base of the middle phalanx of the last four toes; dorsal surface of the base of the distal phalanx of the last four toes	Deep fibular nerve [L4, L5, S1]
Extensor digitorum brevis	Extension of the phalanges of the second, third and fourth toes	Distal part of the superolateral surface of the calcaneus, immediately in front of the tarsal sinus	Tendons that join the lateral surface of the tendons of the extensor digitorum longus for the second, third and fourth toes	Deep fibular nerve [L4, L5, S1]
Fibularis tertius	Dorsiflexion and eversion of the foot	Lower third of the medial surface of the fibula and corresponding part of the interosseous membrane	Dorsal surface of the base of the fifth metatarsal	Deep fibular nerve [L4, L5, S1]
Plantaris	Plantar flexion and inversion of the foot	Lateral condyle of the femur and posterior surface of the capsule of the knee joint	Medial part of the posterior surface of the calcaneus	Tibial nerve [L4, L5, S1-S3]
Quadratus plantae	Flexion of the middle phalanges of the last four toes	Lateral and medial borders of the inferior surface of the calcaneus	Laterally to the tendon of the flexor digitorum longus, before its division into four terminal tendons	Lateral plantar nerve [S2, S3]

Topographical classification of the muscles of the leg

(with action on the ankle and foot)

- Anterior:
  - tibialis anterior
  - extensor digitorum longus
  - extensor hallucis longus
  - fibularis tertius
- Lateral:
  - fibularis longus
  - fibularis brevis

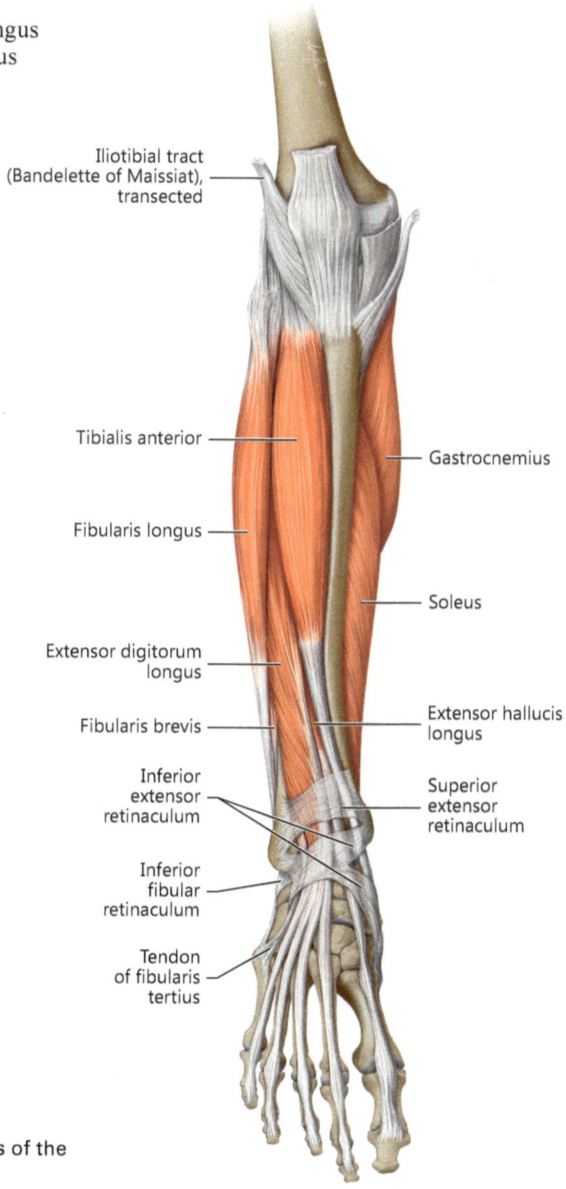

Anterior and lateral muscles of the right leg.

- Posterior:
  - gastrocnemius
  - soleus
  - plantaris
  - tibialis posterior
  - flexor digitorum longus
  - flexor hallucis longus

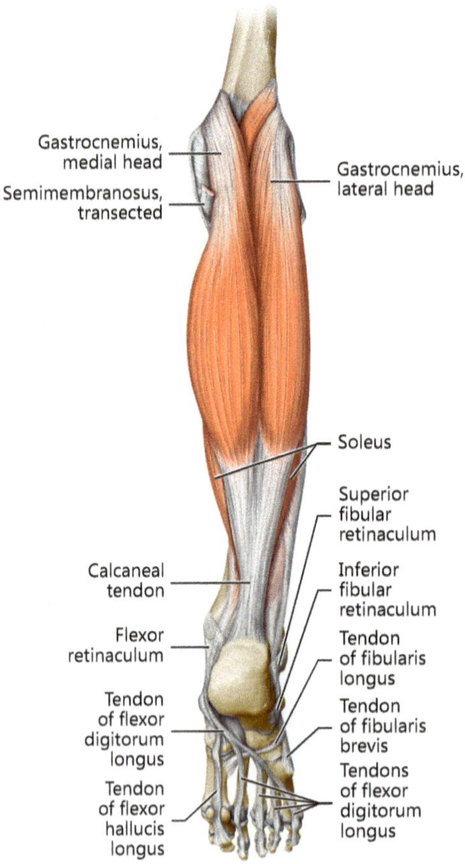

Posterior muscles of the right leg: superficial layer.

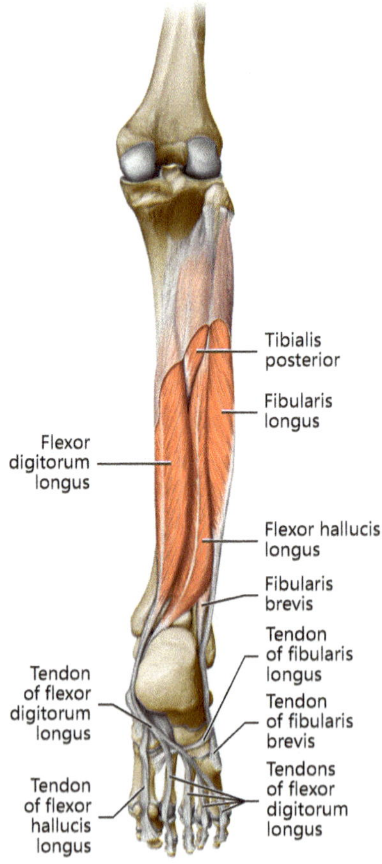

Posterior muscles of the right leg: deep layer.

Topographical classification of the muscles of the foot

- Dorsal:
  - extensor digitorum brevis
- Plantar:
  - medial:
    - abductor hallucis
    - flexor hallucis brevis
    - adductor hallucis
  - lateral:
    - abductor digiti minimi
    - flexor digiti minimi brevis
    - opponens digiti minimi
  - intermediate:
    - flexor digitorum brevis
    - quadratus plantae
    - lumbricals (1st, 2nd, 3rd and 4th)
    - interosseous:
      - plantar (1st, 2nd, 3rd)
      - dorsal (1st, 2nd, 3rd and 4th)

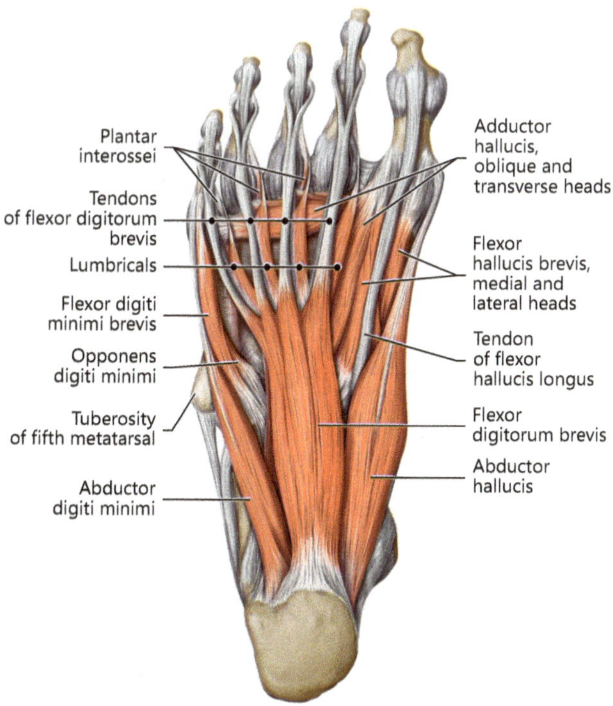

Plantar surface of the right foot.

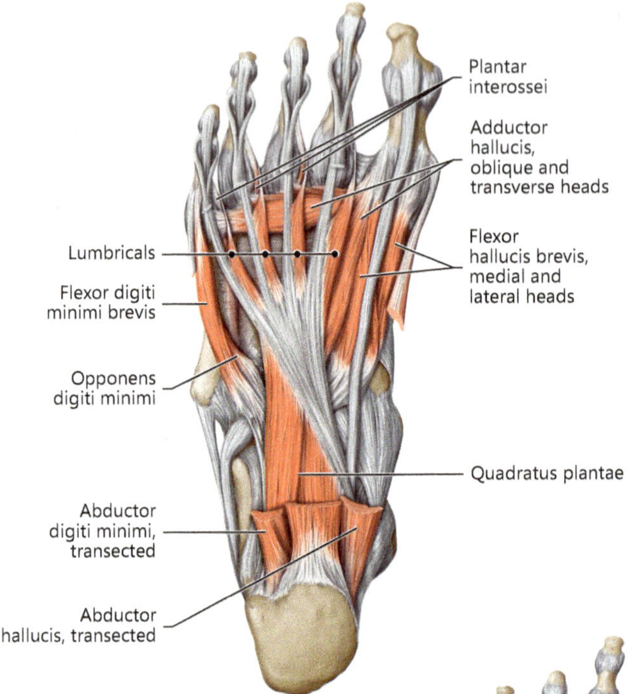

Intermediate layer of the plantar muscles of the right foot.

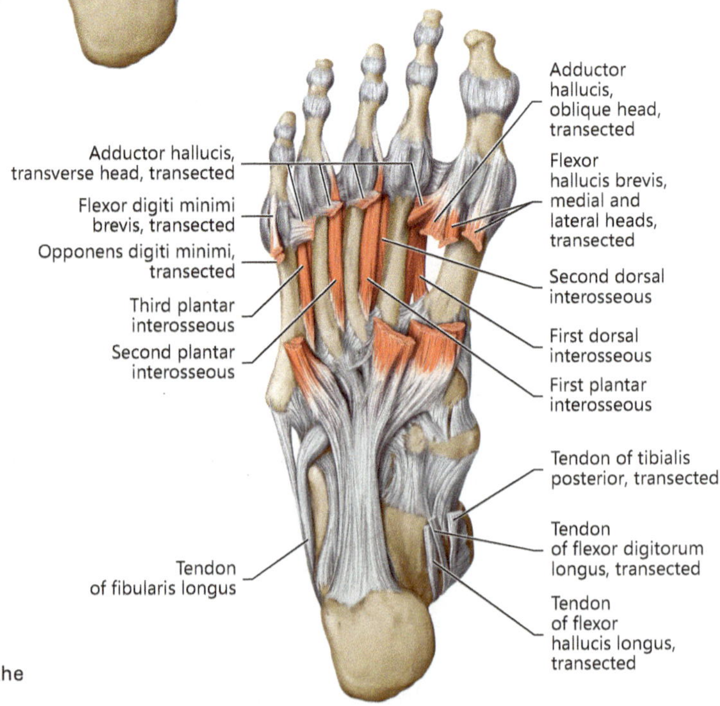

Deep muscles of the sole of the foot.

Action of the muscles in the movements of the ankle and foot

Plantar flexion of the ankle

Plantar flexor muscles of the foot:
- triceps surae: gastrocnemius and soleus
- flexor hallucis longus
- fibularis longus
- fibularis brevis
- plantaris
- flexor digitorum longus
- tibialis posterior.

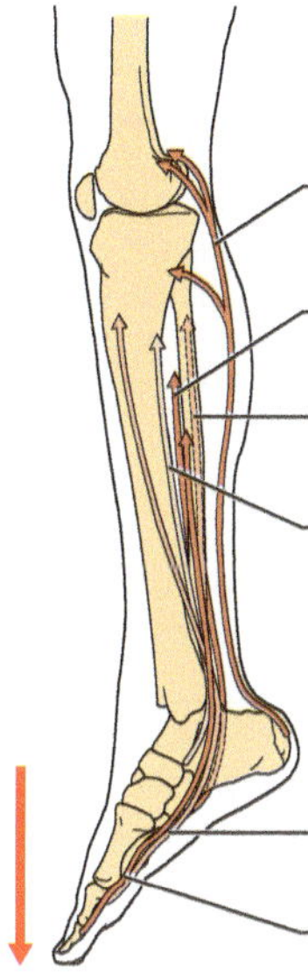

Action of the plantar flexor muscles of the foot

Gastrocnemius

- Strong plantar flexor of the foot (the action of the muscle is favored by the extension of the leg)
- Supination of the foot
- Strong flexor of the knee, especially in the initial phase of movement, when the knee is extended
- Fixes the knee to the tibia
- Supports the longitudinal arches of the foot.

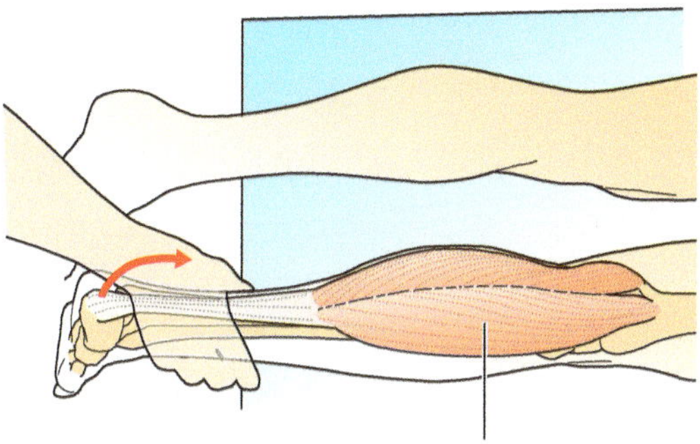

Soleus

- Plantar flexor of the foot
- Abduction of the foot
- Supination of the foot
- Supports the longitudinal arches of the foot.

The gastrocnemius and soleus, which together form the triceps surae, carry out a common action of plantar flexion of the foot when particular muscular force is required, and also play an important postural role.

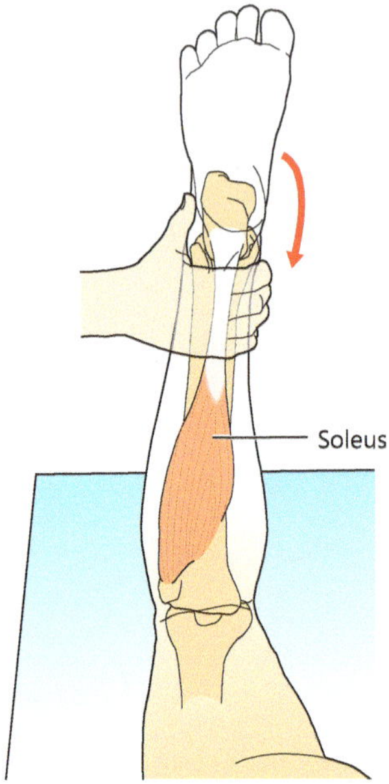

Flexor hallucis longus

- Plantar flexion of the great toe
- Supination of the foot
- Contributes to the plantar flexion of the foot
- Supports the longitudinal arches of the foot.

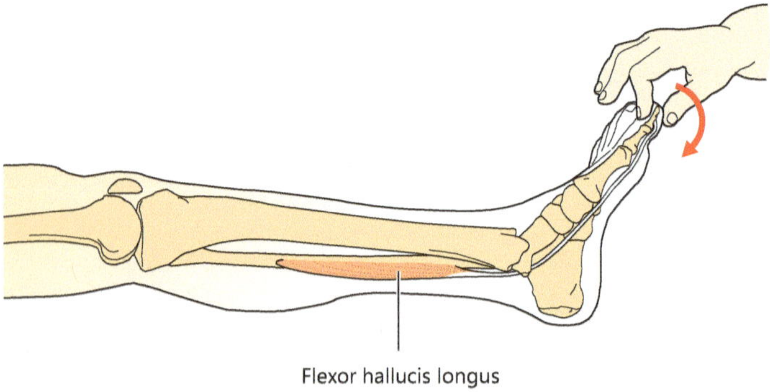

Fibularis longus

- Pronation of the foot
- Contributes to the plantar flexion of the foot
- Supports the transverse arch of the foot.

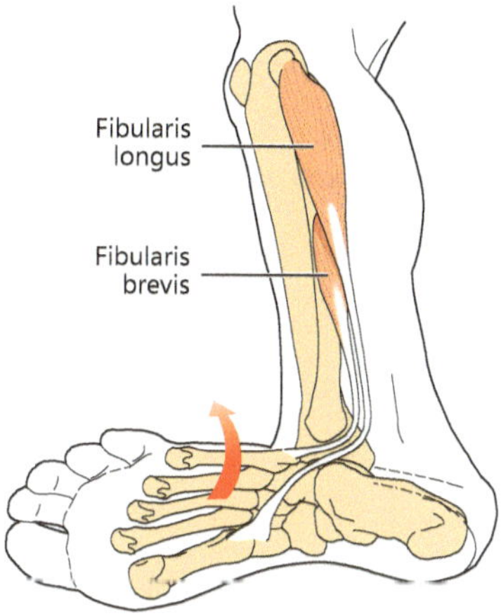

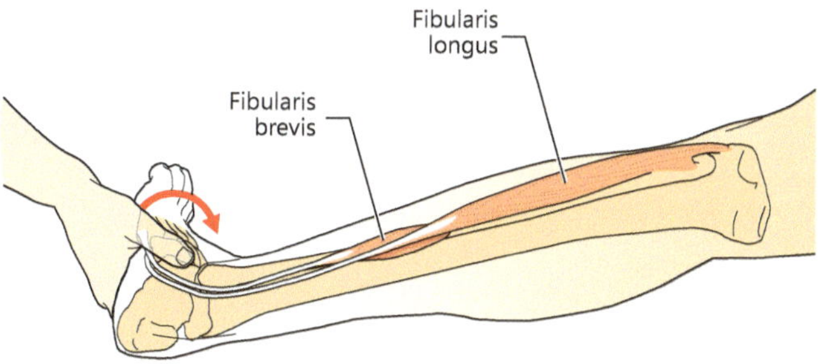

Fibularis brevis

- Action similar to that of the fibularis longus.

Plantaris (not always present)

- Modest plantar flexion of the foot
- Modest supination of the foot.

Flexor digitorum longus

- Flexion of the last four toes
- Contributes to the plantar flexion of the foot
- Contributes to the supination of the foot
- Supports the longitudinal arches of the foot.

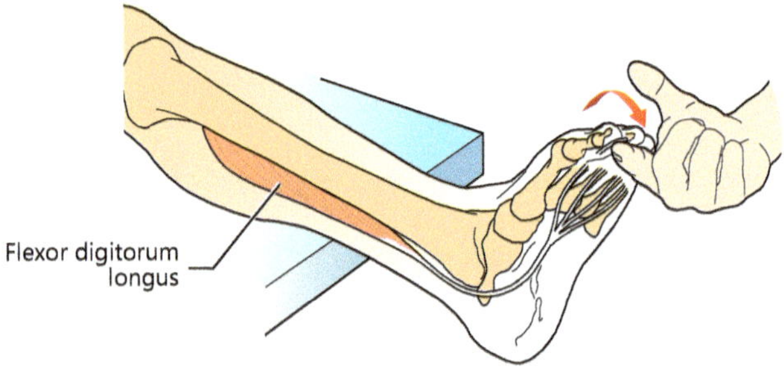

Tibialis posterior

- Plantar flexion of the foot
- Adduction of the foot
- Supination of the foot
- Supports the medial longitudinal and the transverse arches of the foot.

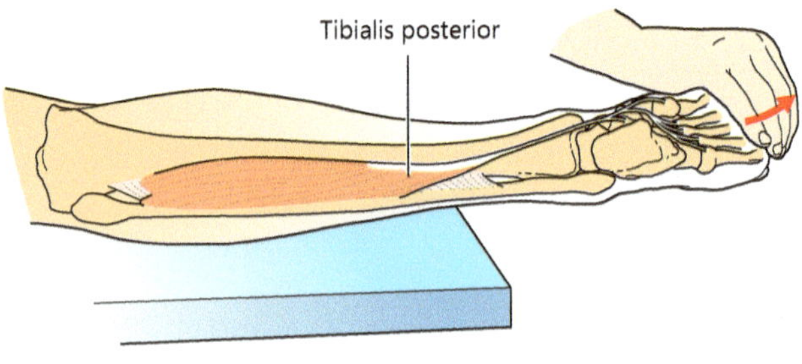

Dorsiflexion of the ankle

Dorsal flexor muscles of the foot:

- tibialis anterior
- extensor digitorum longus
- extensor hallucis longus
- fibularis tertius (located laterally to the extensor digitorum longus with which it is sometimes fused).

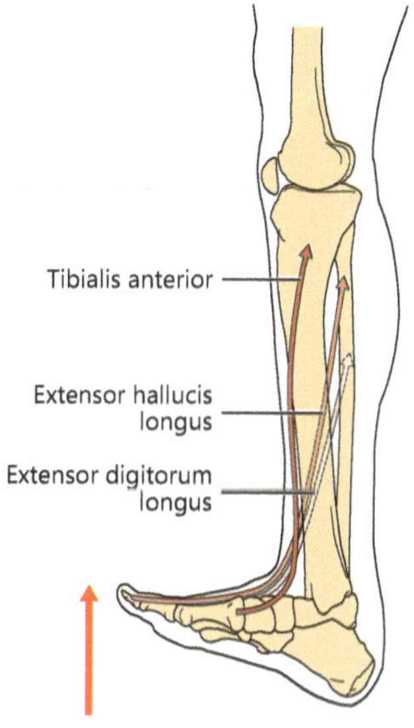

Action of the dorsal flexor muscles of the foot

Tibialis anterior

- Principal dorsal flexor muscle of the foot
- Adduction of the foot
- Supination of the foot
- Contributes to the support of the longitudinal arches of the foot.

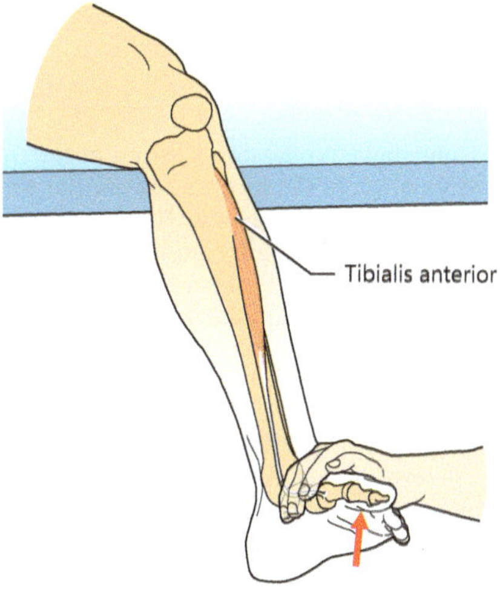

The action of the tibialis anterior is markedly greater than that of the other three dorsal flexor muscles of the foot, both for its muscular dimensions and its function, which involves the entire foot. With a fixed point on the foot, it brings the anterior surface of the leg towards the dorsum of the foot, an action that occurs particularly during fast walking.

Extensor digitorum longus

- Dorsiflexion of the foot (in agonist synergy with the tibialis anterior)
- Abduction of the foot (in antagonist synergy with the tibialis anterior)
- Pronation of the foot (in antagonist synergy with the tibialis anterior)
- With fixed point on the foot, it brings the anterior surface of the leg towards the dorsum of the foot.

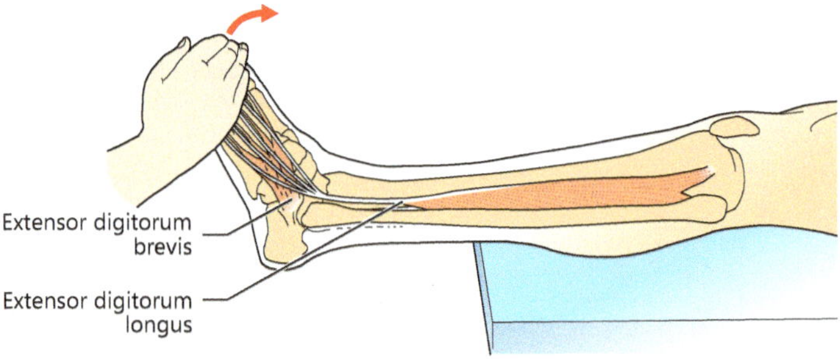

Extensor hallucis longus

- Dorsiflexion of the great toe
- Contributes to the dorsiflexion of the foot
- With fixed point on the foot, it brings the anterior surface of the leg towards the dorsum of the foot.

Fibularis tertius
(not always present)

- Contributes to the dorsiflexion of the foot
- Abduction of the foot (action similar to that of the fibularis longus and fibularis brevis, and of the extensor digitorum longus)
- Pronation of the foot (action similar to that of the fibularis longus and fibularis brevis, and of the extensor digitorum longus)

The fibularis tertius may be considered as a fifth terminal tendon of the extensor digitorum longus, inserted dorsally to the base of the fifth metatarsal.

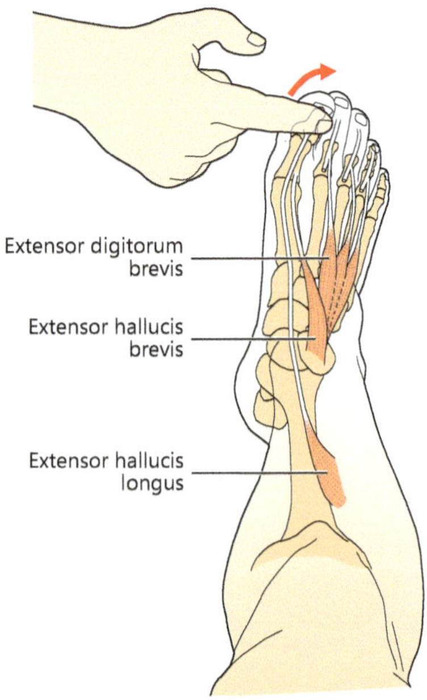

Inversion of the foot

(Adduction + supination + plantar flexion and of the foot)

Muscles:
- triceps surae (gastrocnemius and soleus) (see "Plantar flexion of the ankle", page 605)
- tibialis posterior (see "Plantar flexion of the ankle", page 605)
- flexor hallucis longus (see "Plantar flexion of the ankle", page 605)
- flexor digitorum longus (see "Plantar flexion of the ankle", page 605)
- tibialis anterior (see "Dorsiflexion of the ankle", page 609)
- plantaris (see "Plantar flexion of the ankle", page 605)

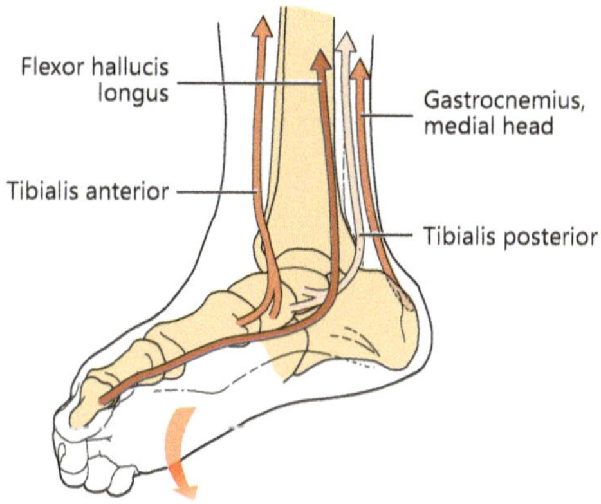

Contributions to the inversion movement of the foot:
- triceps surae (greater contribution) – plantar flexion and supination
- tibialis anterior – adduction and supination
- tibialis posterior, flexor hallucis longus and digitorum longus, plantaris – plantar flexion and supination.

Eversion of the foot

(Abduction + pronation + dorsiflexion of the foot)

Muscles:
- fibularis longus (see "Plantar flexion of the ankle", page 605)
- fibularis brevis (see "Plantar flexion of the ankle", page 605)
- extensor digitorum longus (see "Dorsiflexion of the ankle", page 609)
- fibularis tertius (see "Dorsiflexion of the ankle", page 609)

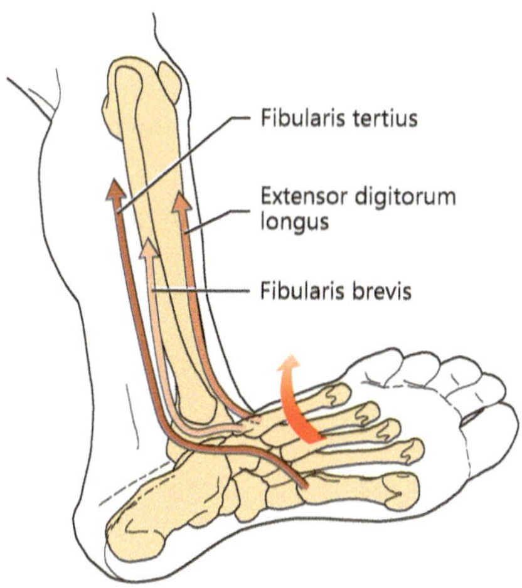

Contributions to the eversion movement of the foot:
- fibularis longus and fibularis brevis – abduction and pronation
- extensor digitorum longus and fibularis tertius – dorsiflexion, abduction and pronation of the foot.

Extension of the toes

Extensor muscles of the toes:
- extensor digitorum brevis
- extensor hallucis brevis.

Action of the extensor muscles of the toes

Extensor digitorum brevis
- Extends the second, third and fourth toes.

Extensor hallucis brevis
- Extends the great toe.

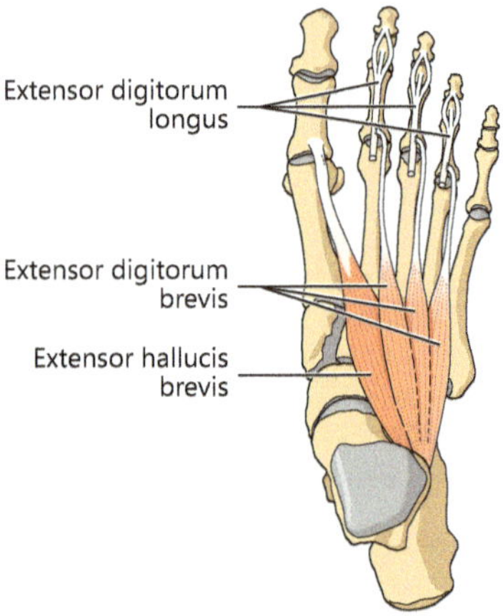

Flexion of the toes

Flexor muscles of the toes:
- flexor digitorum longus (see "Plantar flexion of the ankle", page 605)
- flexor hallucis longus (see "Plantar flexion of the ankle", page 605)
- flexor digitorum brevis
- flexor hallucis brevis
- quadratus plantae
- lumbricals.

Action of the flexor muscles of the toes

Flexor digitorum brevis
- Flexes the middle phalanges of the last four toes.

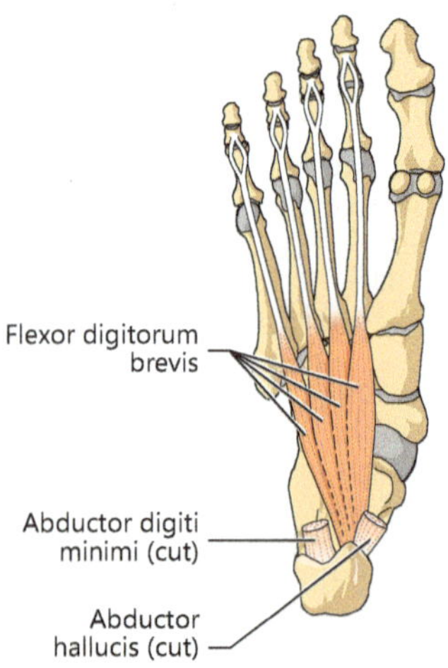

Flexor hallucis brevis

- Flexes the proximal phalanx of the great toe.

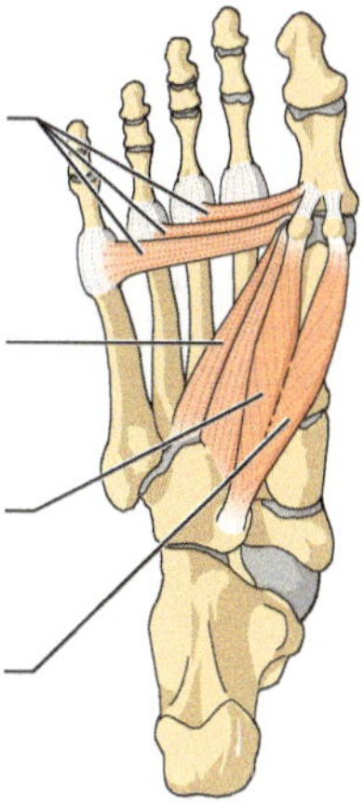

Quadratus plantae (flexor accessorius)

- Increases the flexor action of the middle phalanges of the last four toes carried out by the flexor digitorum longus.

Lumbricals

The lumbricals, four in number, originate individually from the internal and external borders of the tendons of flexor digitorum longus and insert at the base of the proximal phalanx and at the tendons of the extensor muscles of the second, third, fourth and fifth toes.
They are innervated by the medial plantar nerve [S1, S2] and by the lateral plantar nerve [S2-S3].

- Flex the first phalanx and extend the middle and distal phalanges of the last four toes.

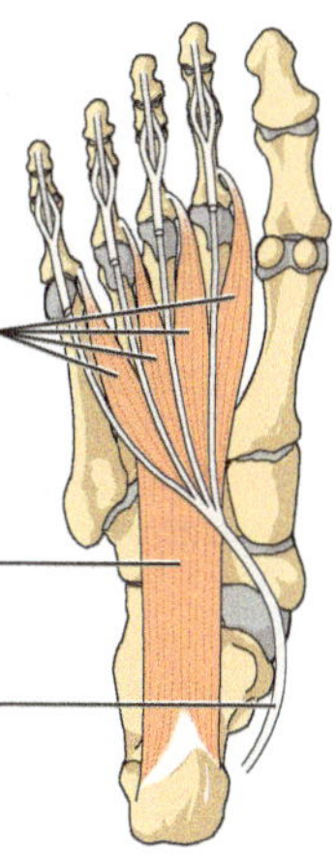

Abduction and adduction of the toes

> These movements occur only at the level of the metatarsophalangeal joints and therefore only involve the proximal phalanges of the toes.

Abductor muscles of the toes:
- abductor hallucis
- abductor digiti minimi
- dorsal interossei.

Adductor muscles of the toes:
- adductor hallucis
- plantar interossei.

Action of the abductor muscles of the toes

Abductor hallucis

- Abducts and slightly flexes the great toe.

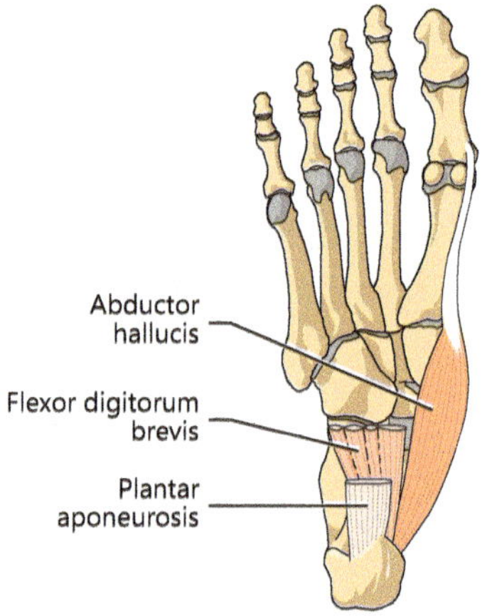

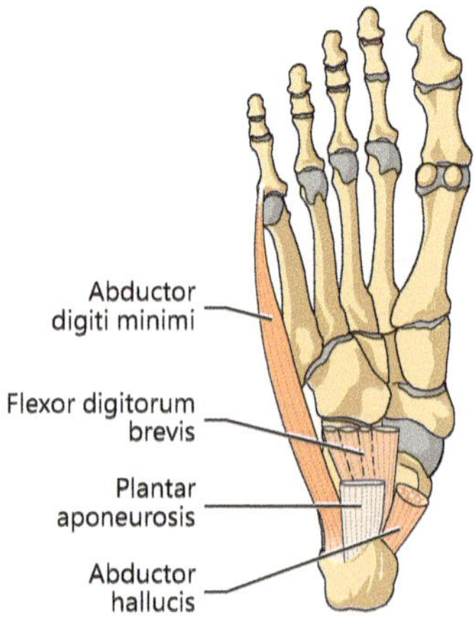

Abductor digiti minimi

- Abducts and flexes the little toe.

Dorsal interossei

- Second, third and fourth dorsal interossei → abduct (separate) the second, third and fourth toes from the great toe
- First dorsal interosseus → adducts (brings closer) the second toe to the great toe
- Flex the proximal phalanges and extend the distal phalanges.

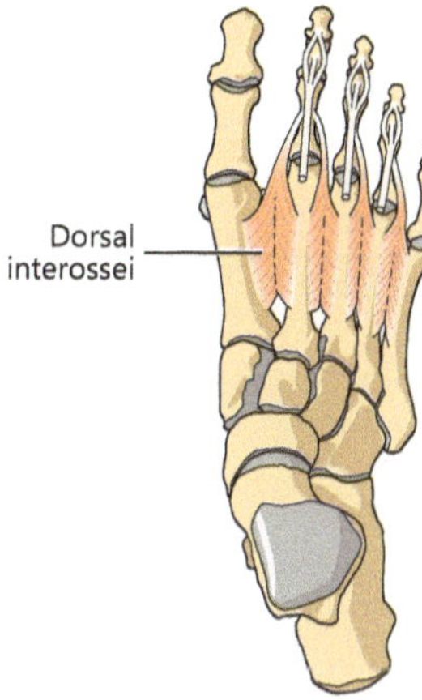

Adductor hallucis

- Moves the great toe in a medial direction and flexes its proximal phalanx
- Stretches the longitudinal arches of the foot (see image illustrating the flexor hallucis brevis, page 613).

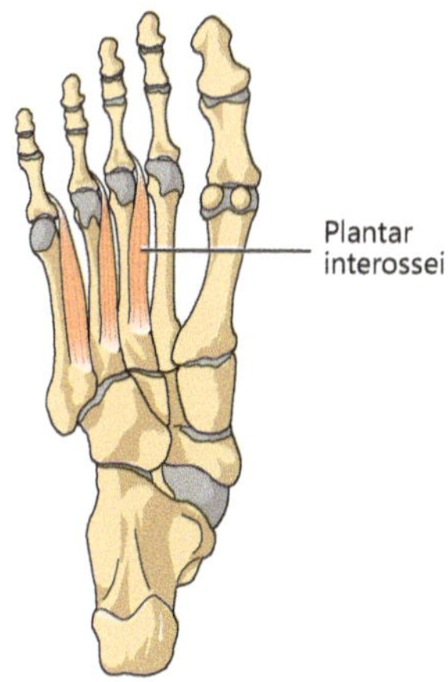

Plantar interossei

- Adduct (bring closer) the third, fourth and little toes to the second toe
- Flex the proximal phalanges and extend the distal phalanges (action in common with the dorsal interossei).

The following muscles can be added to the muscles of the foot mentioned so far:
- opponens digiti minimi (not always present)
  - flexes the 5th metatarsal
  - contributes to supporting the longitudinal arches of the foot
- flexor digiti minimi brevis (often fused with the abductor digiti minimi)
  - plantar flexion of the little toe

Assessment of the length of muscle fibers

Gastrocnemius

Starting position	Upright position with the lower limbs in anatomical position facing the examination table or a wall
Movement	The patient leans forward with the hands resting on the edges of the examination table or on the wall and bringing the unexamined leg forward of the examined leg (the foot of the examined limb should remain fully supported on the floor with the toes forward and the knee extended) 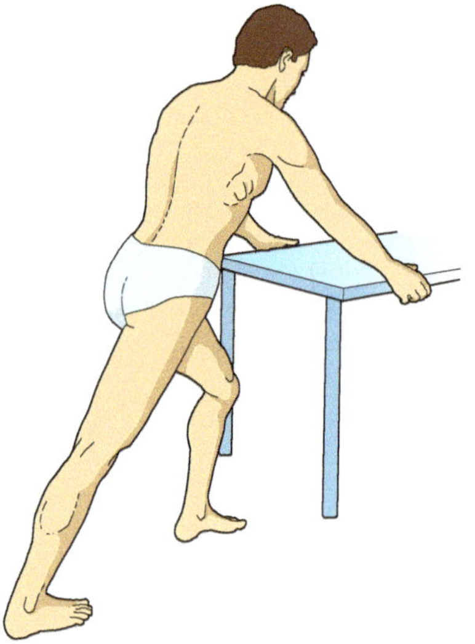 The fibers of the gastrocnemius are fully stretched while the patient leans forward. In the presence of muscle shortening, the movement of dorsiflexion of the ankle will be limited proportionally to the reduction of the length of the muscle. Since, during the test, the patient can flex the knee, which determines a reduction in the tension of the muscle fibers, the knee should be kept in extension 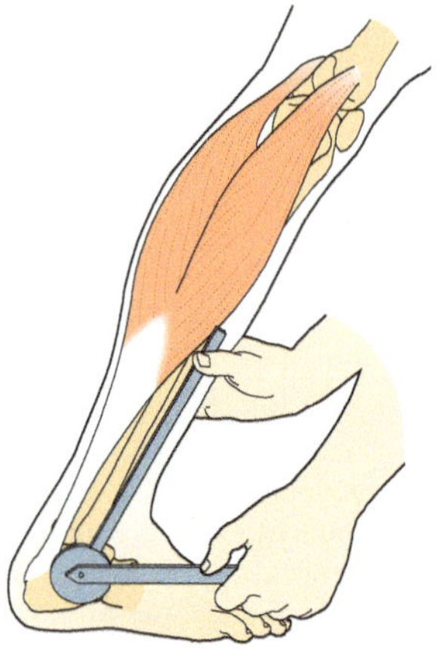

Alternative test

Starting position	Supine position with the knee extended
Movement	The examiner moves the foot with one hand to the limit of the dorsiflexion of the ankle, while with the other hand stabilizes the lower leg 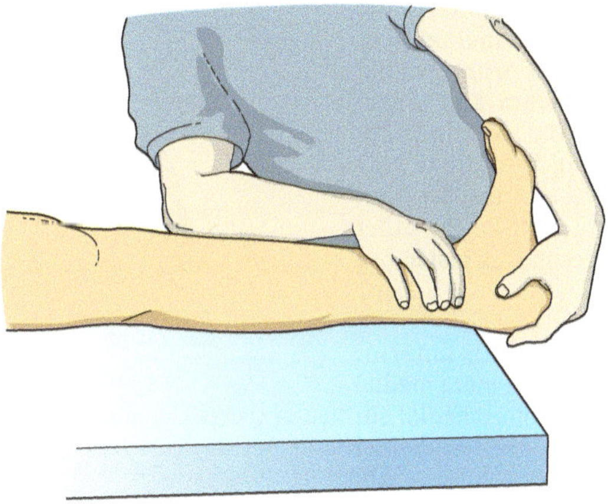

Assessment of the muscular force

Dorsiflexion of the ankle and inversion of the foot

Tibialis anterior

Against gravity

Dorsiflexion of the ankle and inversion of the foot through the entire range of joint motion from a seated position, with the foot in plantar flexion and slight eversion and the examiner applying resistance to the dorsomedial surface of the forefoot with one hand, while the other hand stabilizes the leg just above the ankle.

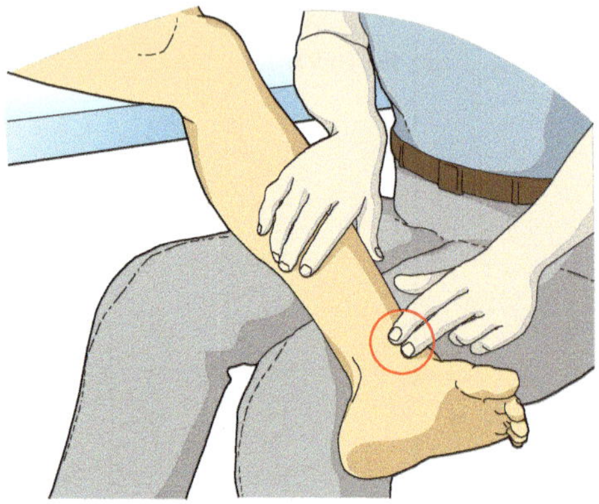

The tendon of tibialis anterior can be palpated in a more medial position on the anteromedial surface of the ankle, and always medially on the anterior border of the tibia.

Without gravity

Dorsiflexion of the ankle and inversion of the foot through the entire range of joint motion from the lateral decubitus position on the examined side, with the leg flexed to determine a reduction in tension of the gastrocnemius fibers and the foot in plantar flexion and slight eversion, while the examiner stabilizes the lower leg just above the ankle.

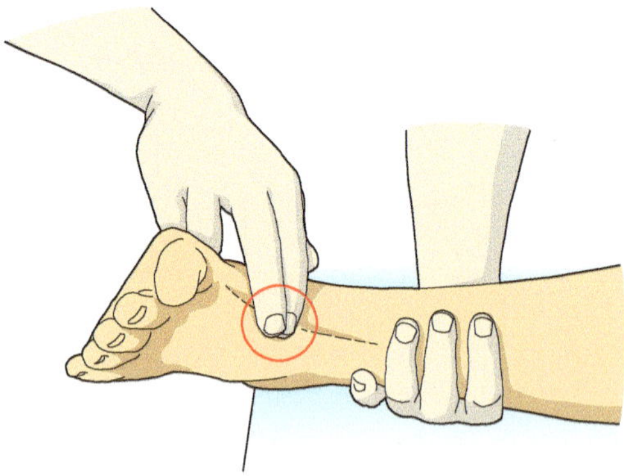

Plantar flexion of the ankle

Gastrocnemius and soleus

The strength of the gastrocnemius and soleus is assessed with the ankle in plantar flexion and the knee extended. Since the activity of the gastrocnemius and the isometric force exerted during plantar flexion of the ankle are reduced as knee flexion increases, and more significantly when the knee is flexed at an angle greater than 45°, a more specific assessment of the strength of the soleus can be obtained with flexion of the knee of at least 45°, thereby reducing the tension of the gastrocnemius fibers.

Against gravity

Gastrocnemiuse: plantar flexion of the ankle through entire range of joint motion from the prone position with the knee extended and the feet off the edge of the examination table.

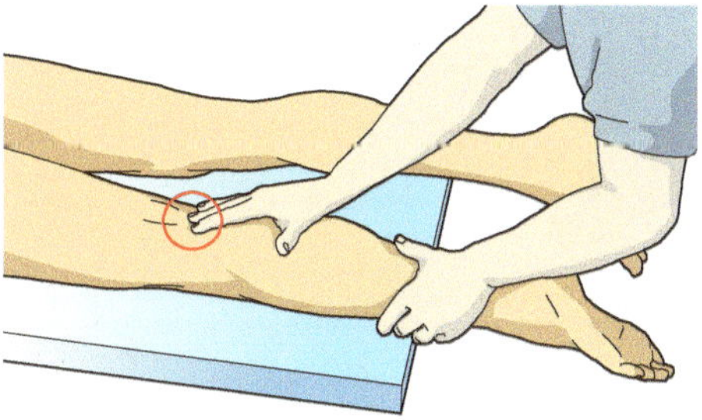

Soleus: knee flexed at 90° (soleus), with dorsiflexion of the ankle, while the examiner applies resistance to the posterior surface of the heel with one hand and stabilizes the lower leg just above the ankle with the other hand.

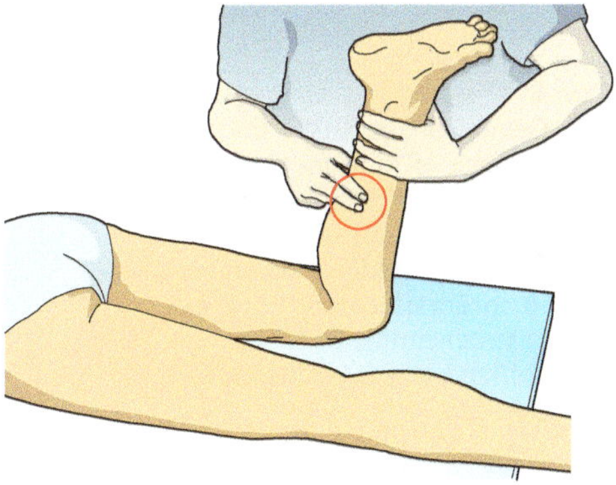

The gastrocnemius can be palpated at the medial and lateral borders of the popliteal fossa just below the knee, while the soleus can be palpated on both sides of the gastrocnemius, in the middle of the calf.

Alternative test

Plantar flexion of the ankle from the upright position with the foot of the unexamined limb off the ground, the foot of the examined side fully supported on the ground and the leg extended (gastrocnemius) or flexed (soleus), while the examiner acts as a support for the patient's hands and the resistance is given by the body weight.

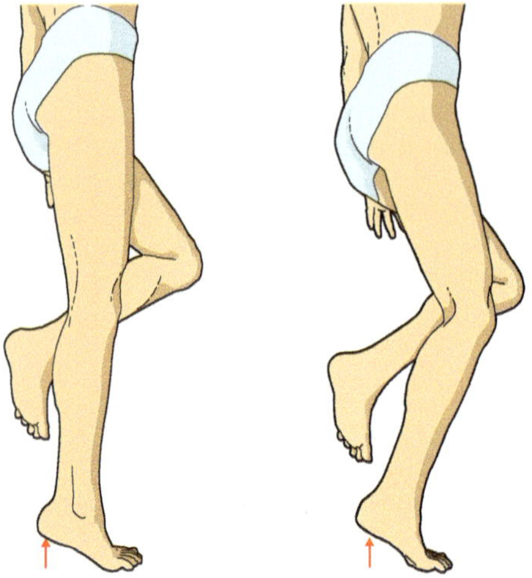

Grades of muscle strength

Grade 5 is attributed if the patient is able to completely detach the calcaneus from the ground for more than 6 times, grade 4 if he/she is able to completely detach the calcaneus from the ground for 3-5 times, grade 3 if he/she is able to completely detach the calcaneus from the ground only 1-2 times.

Without gravity

Plantar flexion of the ankle through the entire range of joint motion from the lateral decubitus position with the unexamined lower limb flexed at the hip and knee, the ankle of the examined limb in dorsiflexion, knee extended (gastrocnemius) or flexed (soleus), stabilized and held just above the ankle.

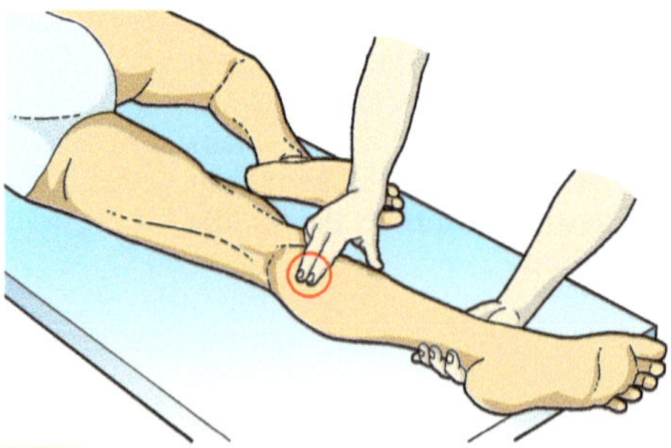

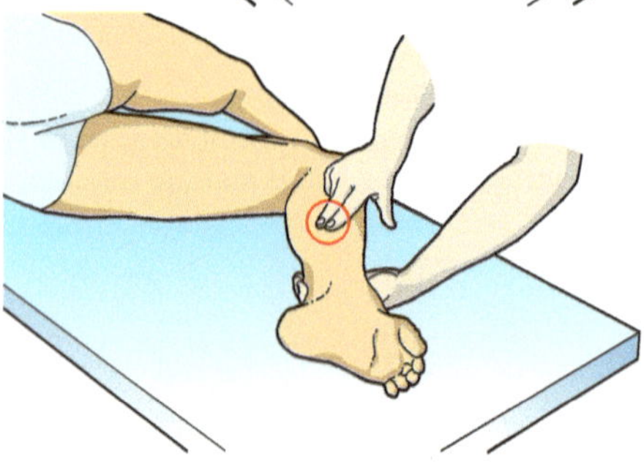

Inversion of the foot

Tibialis posterior

Against gravity

Inversion of the foot through the entire range of joint motion, also performing a slight plantar flexion, from the lateral decubitus position on the examined side with the knee slightly flexed and the foot off the edge of the examination table, in an intermediate position between inversion and eversion, to exclude the contribution of the tibialis anterior, which causes the inversion of the foot only between the eversion and intermediate positions. The examiner applies resistance to the medial border of the forefoot with one hand, while the other hand stabilizes the lower leg just above the ankle.

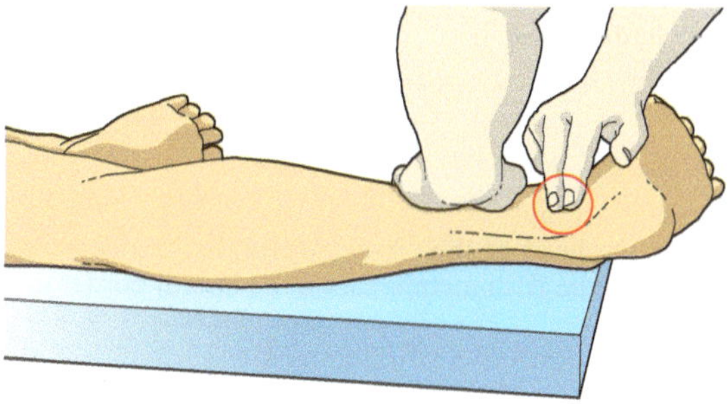

The tibialis posterior can be palpated between the apex of the medial malleolus and the navicular or just above and posteriorly to the medial malleolus.

Without gravity

Inversion of the foot through the entire range of joint motion, also performing a slight plantar flexion, from a supine position with the calcaneus off the edge of the examination table and the foot in an intermediate position between inversion and eversion, while the examiner stabilizes the lower leg just above the ankle.

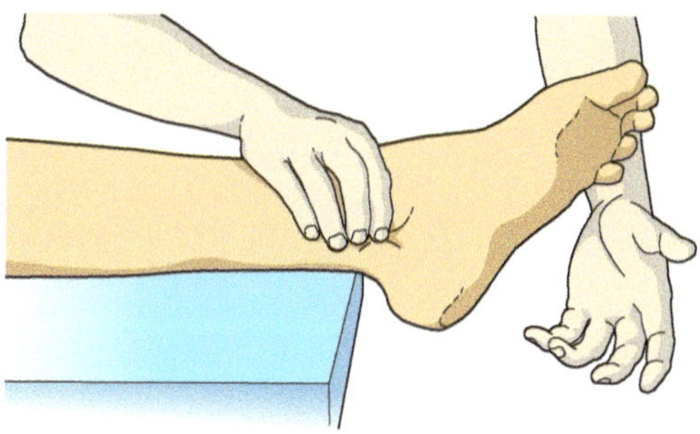

Eversion of the foot

Fibularis longus and fibularis brevis

Against gravity

Eversion of the foot through the entire range of joint motion, from the lateral decubitus position on the unexamined side, with the foot in plantar flexion and inversion off the edge of the examination table, while the examiner applies resistance to the lateral border of foot and to the plantar surface of the head of the first metatarsal with one hand and stabilizes the leg just above the ankle with the other hand.

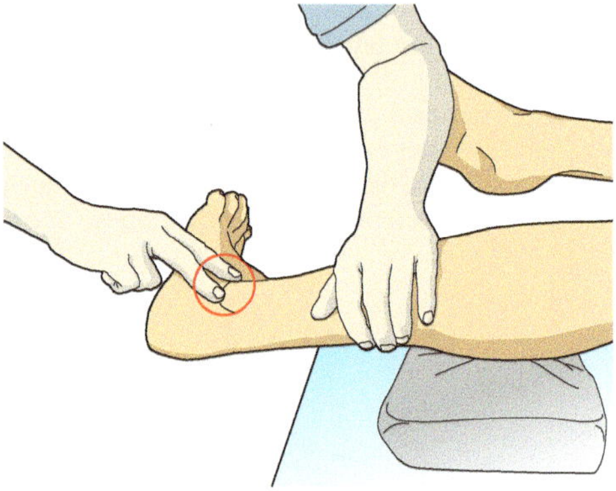

The fibularis longus can be palpated posteriorly to the lateral malleolus or just below the head of the fibula, while the peroneus brevis muscle can be palpated behind the base of the fifth metatarsal on the lateral border of the foot.

Without gravity

Eversion of the foot through the entire range of joint motion, from the supine position with the calcaneus off the edge of the examination table and the foot in inversion, while the examiner stabilizes the lower leg just above the ankle.

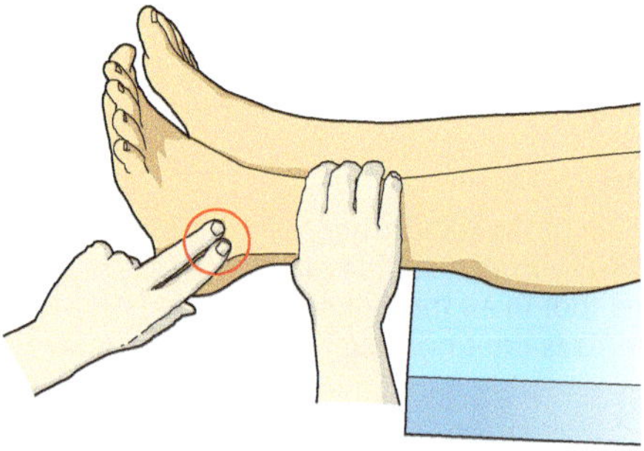

Movements of the toes

Gravity does not significantly influence the toe muscle strength test.

Flexion of the proximal phalanges

Flexor hallucis brevis (great toe) and lumbricals (last four toes)

Flexion of the proximal phalanges while keeping the corresponding middle and distal phalanges extended, from the supine position, with the foot and toes in anatomical position, while the examiner applies resistance to the plantar surface of the proximal phalanges with one hand and stabilizes the metatarsals with the other hand. The great toe is examined individually with respect to the other toes.

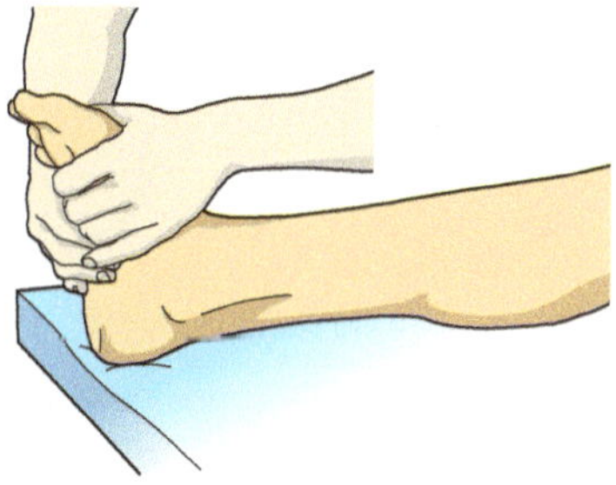

The lumbricals are not palpable, while the flexor hallucis brevis can be palpated on the medial border of the sole of the foot.

Flexion of the middle and distal phalanges

Flexor hallucis longus (flexion of the distal phalanx of the great first toe); flexor digitorum longus (flexion of the distal phalanges of the last four toes); flexor digitorum brevis (flexion of the middle phalanges of the last four toes)

Flexion of the distal phalanx of the great toe (which is examined individually with respect to the other four toes) and the middle and distal phalanges of the last four toes through the entire range of joint motion from the supine position, with the foot and the toes in anatomical position, while the examiner applies resistance to the plantar surface of the middle and distal phalanges with one hand and stabilizes the metatarsophalangeal joints of the toes with the other hand.

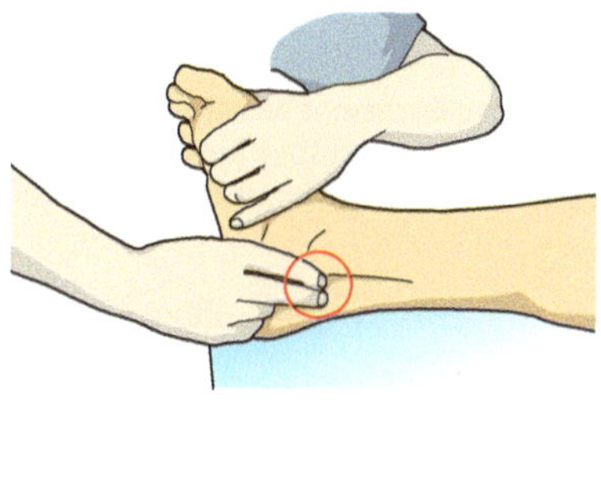

The flexor hallucis longus can be palpated on the plantar surface of the proximal phalanx of the great toe or inferiorly to the medial malleolus, the flexor digitorum brevis cannot be palpated, while the flexor digitorum longus can be palpated on the plantar surface of the proximal phalanges in some subjects.

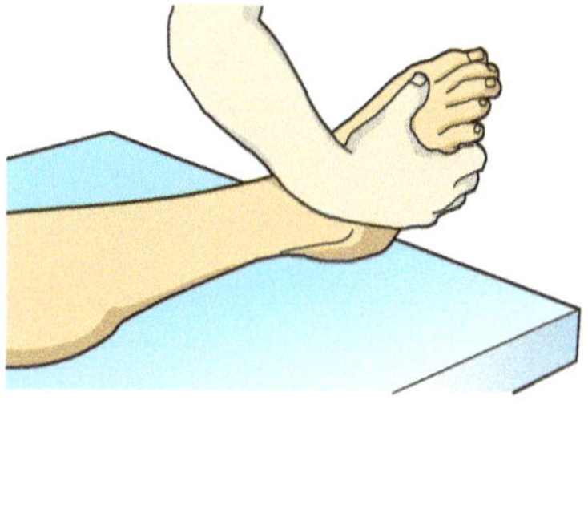

Abduction of the proximal phalanx of the great toe

Abductor hallucis

Abduction of the great toe through the entire range of joint motion, accompanied by a certain degree of flexion (the abductor hallucis simultaneously abducts and flexes the metatarsophalangeal joint), from the supine position with the foot and toes in anatomical position, while the examiner applies resistance to the medial surface of the proximal phalanx of the great toe with one hand and stabilizes the first metatarsal with the other hand.

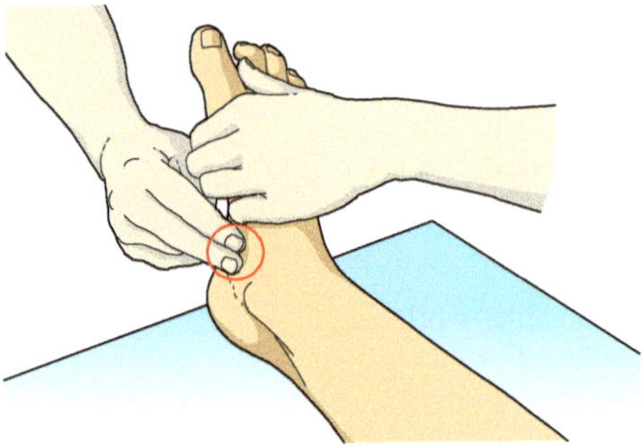

The abductor hallucis can be palpated on the medial border of the foot superficially up to the first metatarsal.

Abduction of the proximal phalanges of the last four toes

Abductor digiti minimi and dorsal interossei

These muscles cannot be assessed separately. Their function is determined by observing the abduction of the last four toes. This movement is associated with the flexion of the proximal phalanges, while the examiner stabilizes the great toe.

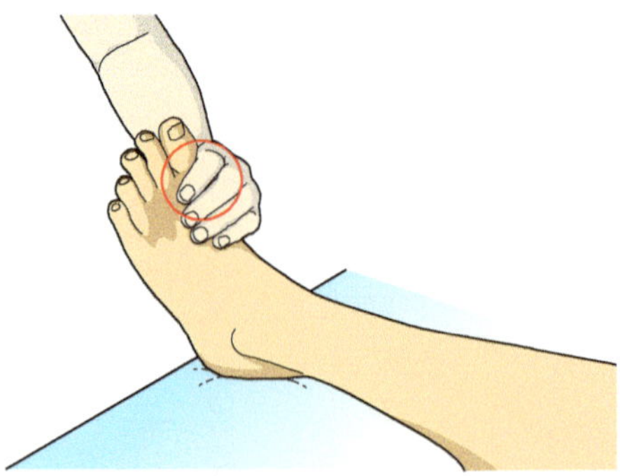

Extension of the proximal and distal phalanges

Extensor hallucis longus (extension of the distal phalanx of the great toe); extensor digitorum brevis (extension of the phalanges of the three intermediate toes and extension of the proximal phalanx of the great toe); extensor digitorum longus (extension of the phalanges of the last four toes)

Extension of the great toe through the entire range of joint motion and then of the other four toes from the supine position with the foot in an intermediate position and the toes flexed, while the examiner applies resistance to the dorsal surface of the distal phalanx of the great toe with one hand (extensor hallucis longus and extensor hallucis brevis) and to the dorsal surface of the four lateral toes (extensor digitorum longus and extensor digitorum brevis) and stabilizes the metatarsals with the other hand.

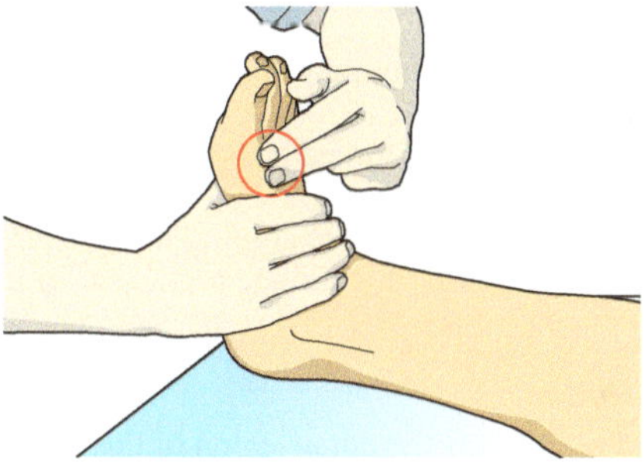

The extensor hallucis longus can be palpated on the dorsal surface of the first metatarsophalangeal joint or on the anterior surface of the ankle laterally to the tibialis anterior; the extensor digitorum brevis can be palpated on the dorsolateral surface of the foot anteriorly to the lateral malleolus; the extensor digitorum longus can be palpated on the dorsal surface of the metatarsals of the last four toes or on the anterior surface of the ankle laterally to the tendon of the extensor hallucis longus.

Since the extensor digitorum brevis does not insert on the little toe, a lesser degree of extension of this toe indicates a weakness of the extensor digitorum longus. The extension of the proximal phalanx of the great toe is due to the part of the extensor digitorum brevis that inserts at the base of the proximal phalanx of the great toe.

Functional aspects of the muscles of the ankle and foot

Plantar flexion of the ankle

- The gastrocnemius acts as a plantar flexor of the ankle:
  - when the foot is already in the position of plantar flexion
  - when a strong contraction is required
  - when the knee is extended
- The soleus is principally active during plantar flexion of the ankle:
  - when the ankle is flexed dorsally
  - when a minimal contraction is required
- The tibialis posterior, flexor hallucis longus, flexor digitorum longus, fibularis longus and fibularis brevis act as accessory plantar flexors
- The actions of the plantar flexor muscles are exemplified by activities in which the ankle is in plantar flexion against resistance, such as:
  - rising on toes
  - jumping
  - pressing the accelerator of an automobile
- The plantar flexor muscles of the ankle:
  - also contract when the movement is forced at extreme degrees of plantar flexion, such as in the action of putting on a sock
  - control the dorsiflexion of the ankle while coming down stairs when the foot is fixed
  - contract during the pushing phase of walking, participating mostly during deambulation.

Dorsiflexion of the ankle

- The tibialis anterior, which initiates the dorsiflexion of the ankle, and the extensor hallucis longus are dorsal flexor muscles stronger than the extensor digitorum longus and fibularis anterior
- The dorsal flexor muscles of the foot:
  - keep the foot under dorsiflexion during activities such as cutting toenails or tying shoelaces
  - control the plantar flexion of the foot when it is lowered against the ground, as happens when the foot is slowing pressed against the ground or in response to the load during the gait cycle
  - stabilize the tibia on the tarsus when getting up from the seated position to the upright position with the feet supported on the floor
  - are active in almost all gait phases (stance on the heel, midstance phase up to heel off and in nearly all of the swing phase).

Inversion and eversion of the foot

- The tibialis posterior is the main invertor muscle in the foot
- The gastrocnemius and soleus cause the inversion of the calcaneus during the plantar flexion of the foot
- The tibialis anterior and the flexor muscles of the last four toes act as weak invertors of the foot from the position of eversion to the intermediate position
- The tibialis anterior only acts as an invertor muscle when the medial border of the foot is lifted during the inversion movement
- The action of the invertor muscles of the foot is exemplified by activities such as bringing the foot to the contralateral thigh in a sitting position in order to look at the sole or walking on uneven ground, contributing in this latter case to the stabilization of the foot.

- The fibularis longus and fibularis brevis, assisted by the extensor digitorum longus and by the fibularis tertius, are responsible for the eversion of the foot:
  - the action of these muscles is also carried out during walking on uneven ground.

Flexion and extension of the toes

- The flexor muscles of the great toe are comprised of:
  - flexor hallucis longus
  - flexor hallucis brevis
  - abductor hallucis, which flexes the proximal phalanx and extends the distal phalanx of the great toe
- The flexor digitorum longus and flexor digitorum brevis flex the last four toes
- The flexor digiti minimi and abductor digiti minimi also contribute to the flexion of the little toe
- The flexor muscles of the toes:
  - act in such a way that the great toe presses firmly on the ground and the other toes hold on the ground, facilitating the maintenance of balance during unilateral support of the foot or standing on the tiptoes
  - contract eccentrically in order to control the passive extension of the toes, which occurs when bending down to pick up an object from the ground or while walking
- The extensor system of the foot is analogous to that of the hand:
  - the extensor muscles of the great toe are comprised of:
    - the extensor hallucis longus
    - the extensor hallucis brevis
    - the abductor hallucis
- The extensor digitorum longus and extensor digitorum brevis extend the proximal phalanges of the last four toes:
  - the extensor digitorum brevis does not reach the little toe; however, fibers coming from the abductor digiti minimi and the flexor digiti minimi brevis attach to the dorsal digital expansion of the little toe, favoring its extension
- The lumbricals and interossei flex the proximal phalanges and simultaneously extend the middle and distal phalanges of the last four toes
- The extensor muscles of the toes contract during walking and when climbing the stairs:
  - the action of these muscles is exemplified by the extension of the toes when cutting the toenails.

Intrinsic muscles of the foot and support of the arches of the foot

- A function of the intrinsic muscles of the foot is to stabilize the foot during its forward thrust
- The main intrinsic muscles of the foot (abductor hallucis, flexor hallucis brevis, flexor digitorum brevis and abductor digiti minimi) constitute the most significant muscular support of the arches of the foot, exerting a strong flexion of the forefoot and helping to stabilize the transverse tarsal joint
- The intrinsic muscles of the foot contract to stabilize the foot when the weight is transferred onto the forefoot while rising on toes or when going up or down stairs
- The triceps surae, fibularis longus, fibularis brevis, tibialis anterior and tibialis posterior contract along with the intrinsic muscles of the foot to stiffen the foot during activities such as running or climbing.

Palpation of the ankle and foot

Plantar aponeurosis

The patient is in the supine position. The examiner palpates the plantar aponeurosis starting from the enthesis over the calcaneus and moving towards the toes: observe how the aponeurosis widens in a V-shape, is stiffer in the central part and softer laterally and medially. It is important to palpate the entire surface both longitudinally and transversely. When passively flexing and extending the toes, you can feel how the tension of the plantar aponeurosis changes in relation to the movement.

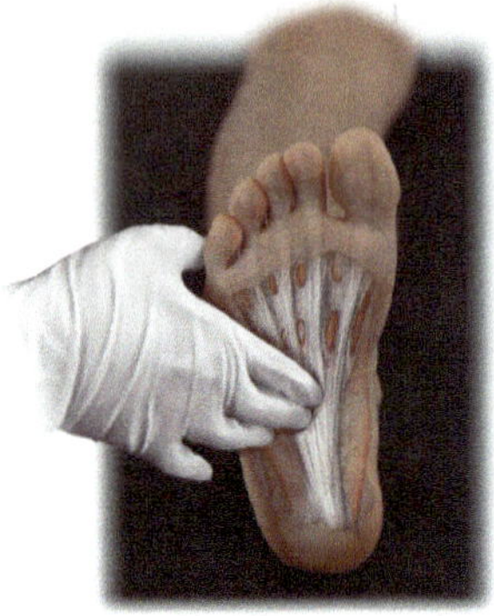

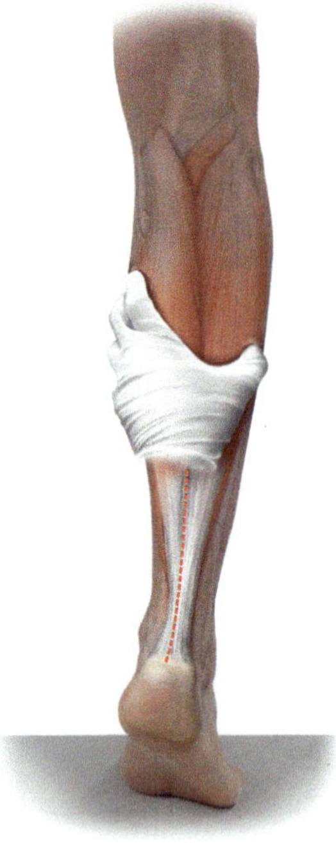

Calcaneal tendon (Achilles tendon)

The patient is in the upright position, with hands resting on the examination table to easily maintain balance while standing on tiptoes, to highlight the triceps surae. The examiner begins palpation of the muscle mass, in particular the gastrocnemius which is located on the surface. From here the palpation continues in a distal direction, until the fleshy muscle bellies transform into the harder, denser tissue of the calcaneal tendon (Achilles tendon). By descending along the tendon, it is possible to explore its medial and lateral borders.

Bursa of the calcaneal tendon

The patient is seated. The examiner identifies the calcaneal tendon (Achilles tendon) and follows it distally to its insertion into the calcaneus, slightly compressing the skin: bursae may be evident in case of inflammation.

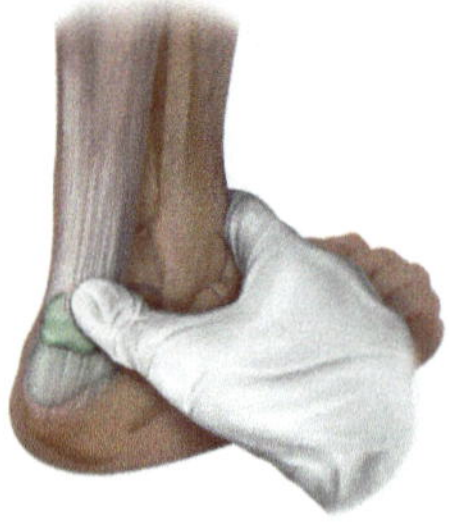

Metatarsals

The patient is seated. The examiner with both hands examines the metatarsals running superficially over the dorsum of the foot, from the base to the head. The interdigital spaces can also be easily explored over the dorsum of the foot.

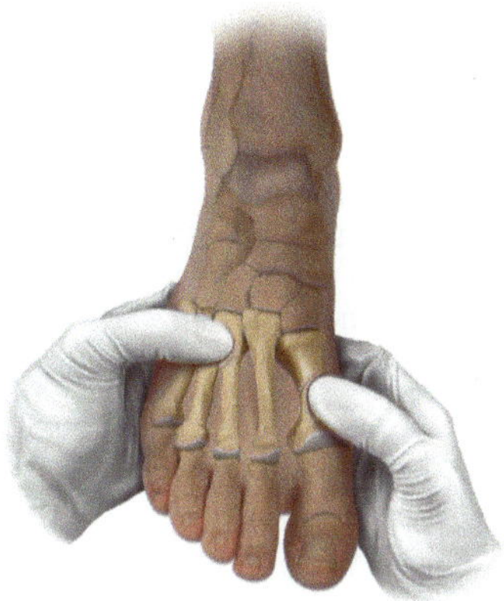

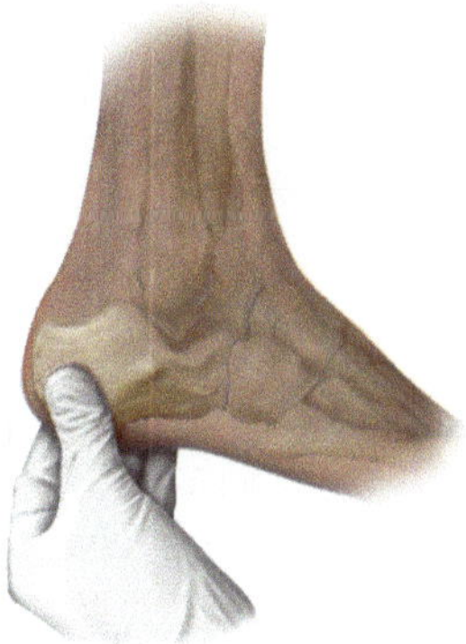

Calcaneal tuberosity

The patient is seated. Palpation starts from the malleoli and continues in a caudal direction following the bulky body of the calcaneus: the calcaneal tuberosity is the rounded structure that can be palpated on the posterior surface of the calcaneus.

Tuberosity of the navicular

The patient is seated. In the medial region of the foot, the examiner identifies the first metatarsal and from here continues palpation in a proximal direction. After crossing the surface of the medial cuneiform, the navicular is reached: its tuberosity, located about 3-5 cm distal to the medial malleolus, is usually the most protruding structure of the medial part of the foot.

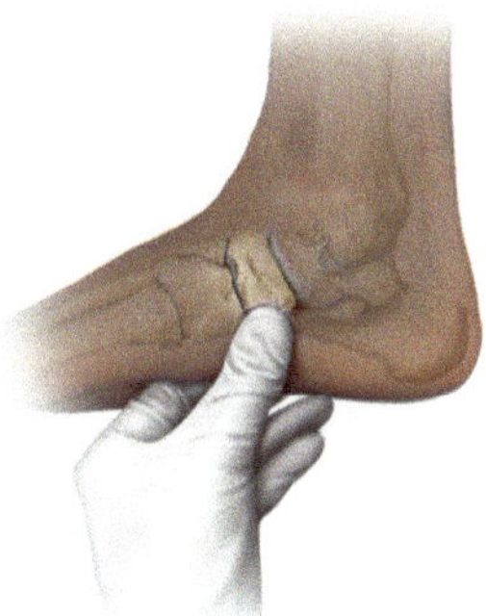

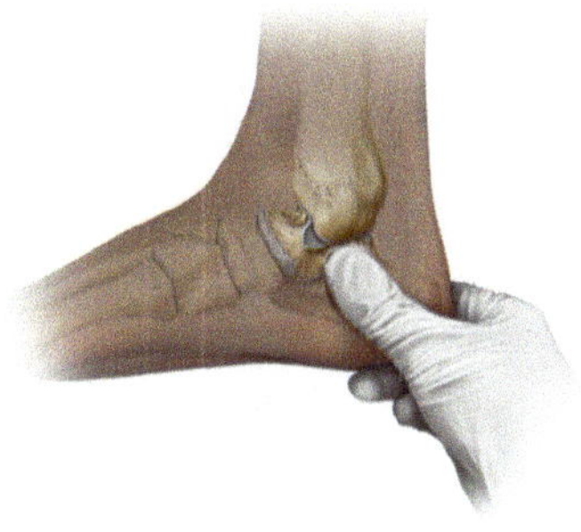

Talus

The patient is seated. The medial malleolus is identified and from here it continues in an anteroposterior direction, following an imaginary line inclined at about 45°. Here the posterior part of the talus with its medial tubercle is found. When performing passive plantar flexions and dorsiflexions, the sliding of the tubercle around the medial malleolus can be felt.

Trochlea of the talus

The patient is in the supine position. The medial and lateral malleoli are identified, and an imaginary horizontal line is drawn between the two structures. Starting from the center of this line, descend slightly looking for a bony protrusion. The trochlea lies deep beneath the tendinous structures and is slightly more prominent near the lateral malleolus.

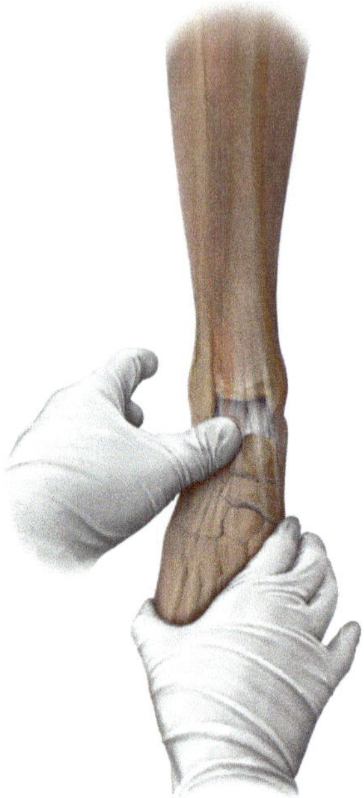

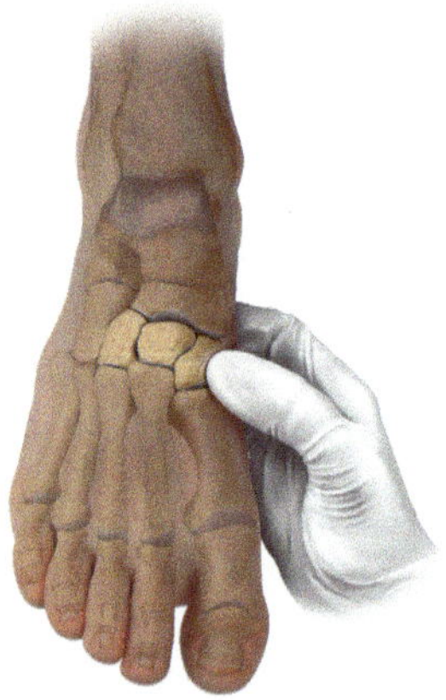

Cuneiforms

The patient is in the supine position. The examiner exerts traction on the first metatarsal to widen the articular line; sliding over this bone in a proximal direction, palpate its base, then a small depression corresponding to the first tarsometatarsal joint and finally reach the medial cuneiform, whose medial and dorsal surfaces can be explored. Continuing along the dorsum of the foot in a lateral direction, it is possible to identify the intermediate cuneiform and then the lateral cuneiform. Some flexion-extension movements of the metatarsals allow widening of the articular interline, facilitating palpation.

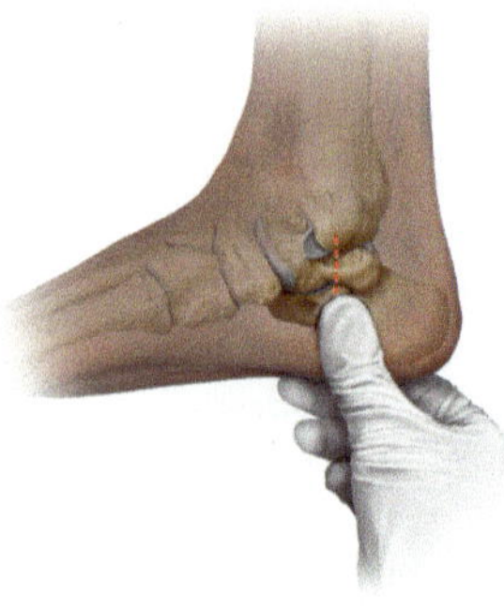

Sustentaculum tali (talar shelf)

The patient is seated. After identifying the medial malleolus, continue distally for about 2 cm until the small extremity of the sustentaculum tali is found. Palpation can be facilitated by passive supination of the foot.

Sesamoid bones

The patient is in the supine position. On the dorsal part of the foot, the head of the first metatarsal is identified and from here palpation moves to the corresponding plantar surface. With the palpating fingers, the small sesamoid bones are sought on the surface, passively flexing the great toe to relax the surrounding tissues.

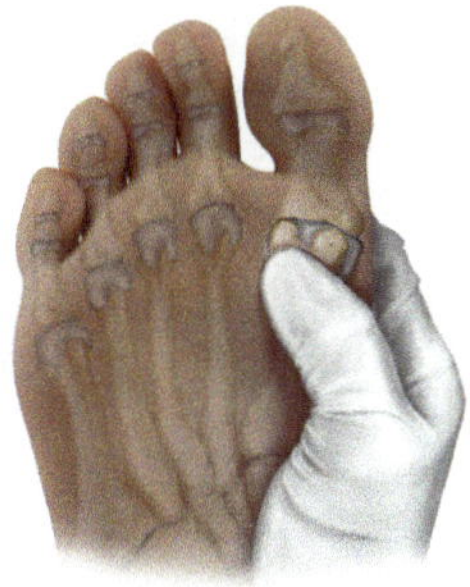

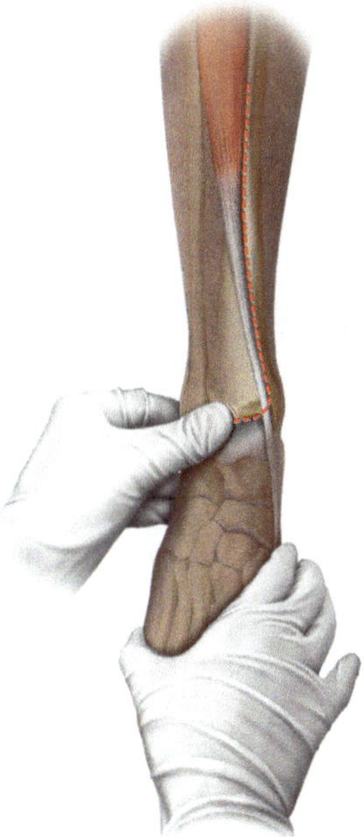

Ankle joint

The patient is seated. The examiner follows the anterior border of the tibia to its distal extremity and places the palpation finger slightly beyond this border. With the other hand bring the patient's foot in extension to relax the musculature and move the tendon of the tibialis anterior to palpate deeper, in contact with the bone. The articular line can be followed medially and laterally.

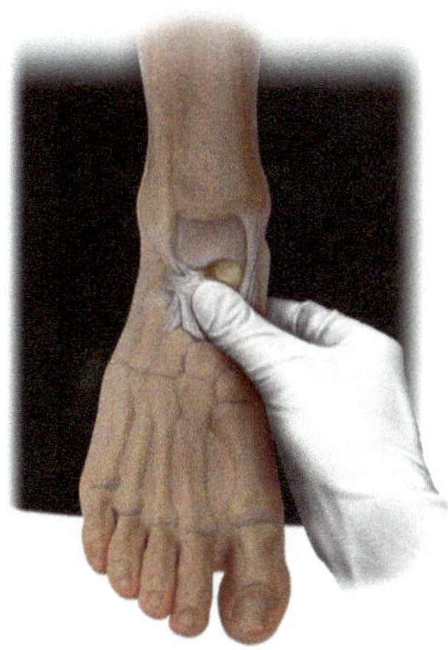

Transverse tarsal joint

The patient is seated, with the extended foot resting on the examination table. Once the head of the talus has been identified, the examiner proceeds with palpation in a distal direction until contact with the navicular, preceded by the joint space. It is possible to follow the articular line both medially and laterally, beyond the dorsum of the foot.

Metatarsophalangeal joint of the great toe

The patient is seated. The examiner identifies the metatarsal on the medial and dorsal part of the foot, which is more accessible than the plantar part that is covered by a thick muscular layer. Palpation continues distally until the first metatarsophalangeal joint is reached, which can be identified more easily by pulling on the great toe and rotating it.

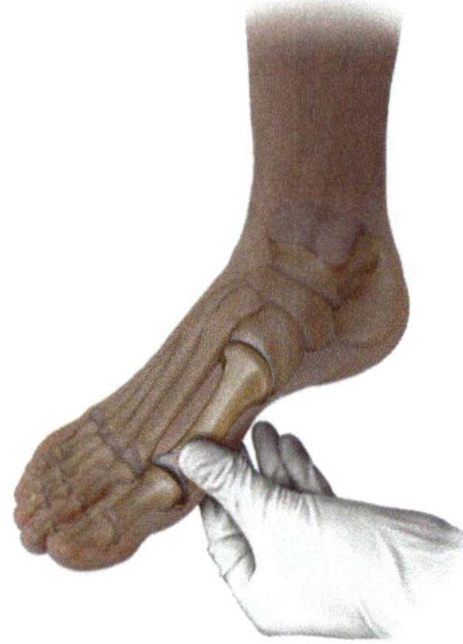

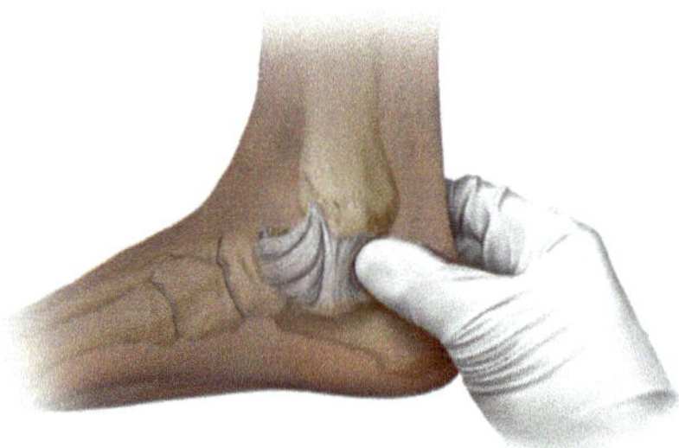

Medial ligament (deltoid ligament)

The patient is seated. The medial malleolus and the sustentaculum tali, located about 2 cm distally, are identified: by sliding the finger between these two points, a part of the fibers of the deltoid ligament is identified. From here the palpation continues by bringing the calcaneus in valgus to be able to perceive the fibers of the deltoid ligament that fan out from the medial malleolus.

Anterior talofibular ligament

The patient is seated. The examiner places his fingers on the distal extremity of the lateral malleolus, at the limit with the dorsal border of the tarsal sinus. At the same time, passive inversion movements of the foot are performed to stretch and relax the ligament and to facilitate its palpation, which occurs transversely with respect to its course.

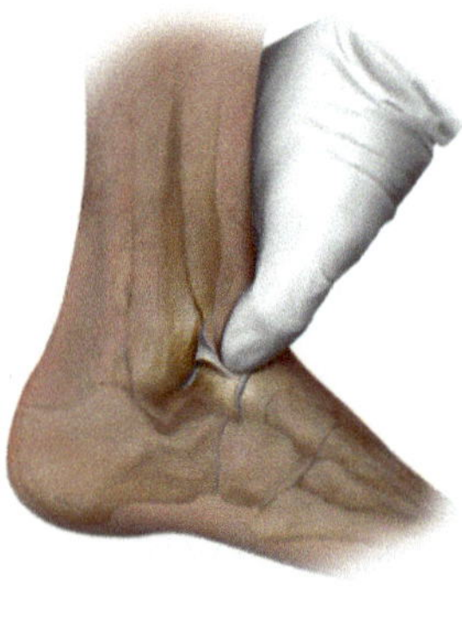

Dorsal calcaneocuboid ligament

The patient is seated, with the foot resting on the examiner's open palm, so that the palpating thumb is over the fifth metatarsal. Following the bone in a proximal direction, you first reach a bony protuberance that protrudes laterally on the surface, the tuberosity of the fifth metatarsal, then you reach the dorsal calcaneocuboid ligament: by forefoot supination and adduction it is possible to put it in tension to facilitate palpation.

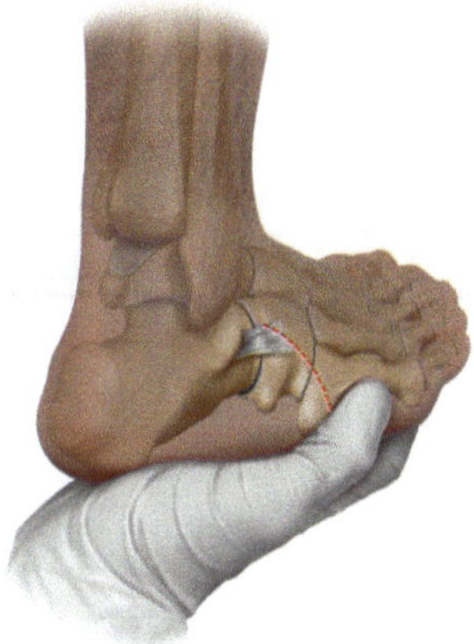

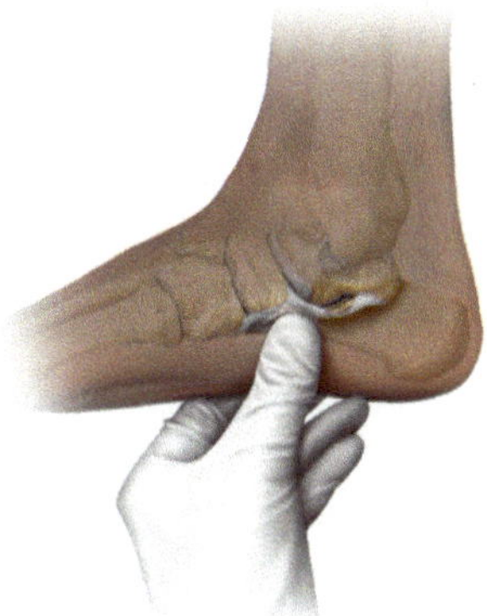

Plantar calcaneonavicular ligament

The patient is seated. The examiner performs a passive supination of the foot to stretch the surrounding tissue to identify the sustentaculum tali and the navicular. By palpating with a finger between these two structures it is possible to identify the rigid medial border of the plantar calcaneonavicular ligament.

Anatomical landmarks on the surface of the ankle and foot

1	Head of the fibula: rounded bony prominence on the lateral surface of the leg at the level of the tibial tuberosity
2	Anterior border of the tibia: subcutaneous bony crest along the anterior surface of the leg
3	Calcaneal tendon (Achilles tendon): prominent crest on the posterior surface of the ankle; the margins of the tendon are palpable just above the posterior surface of the calcaneus
4	Medial malleolus: distal extremity of the tibia protruding on the medial surface of the ankle
5	Lateral malleolus: distal extremity of the fibula protruding on the lateral surface of the ankle
6	Tuberosity of the navicular: approximately 2.5 cm inferiorly and anteriorly to the medial malleolus
7	Base of the fifth metatarsal: small bony prominence in the middle of the lateral border of the foot
8	Head of the first metatarsal: rounded bony prominence on the rounded medial part of the foot, at the base of the great toe
9	Calcaneus: posterior part of the tarsus

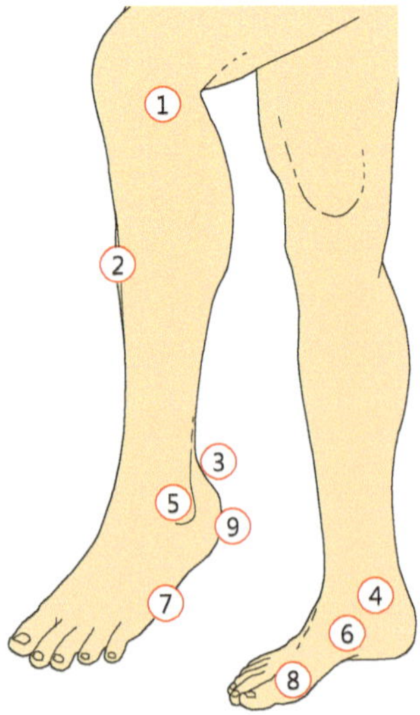

Upright position (orthostatism)

Definition: positioning of the body segments that allows the line of equilibrium, which passes through the body's center of gravity, to fall within the support polygon.

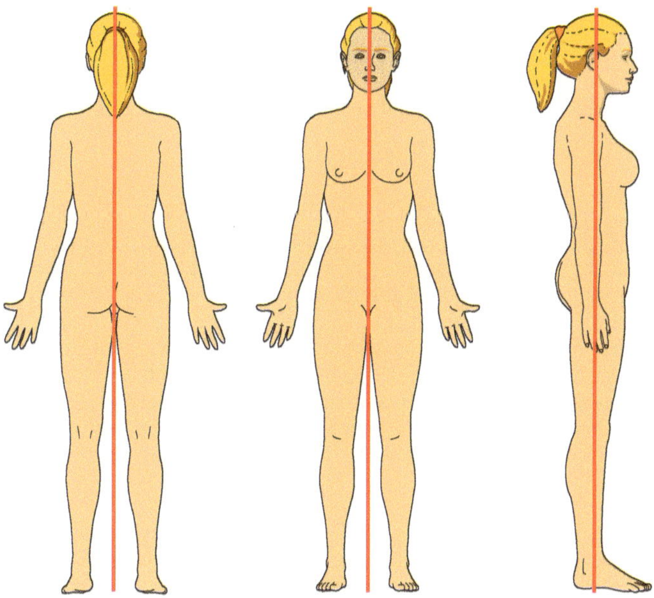

Upright position.

The line of equilibrium (or gravity) is the vertical on which the force of gravity acts (identified by tracing the vertical from the center of gravity to the support base).

The support polygon is an area delimited:
- laterally by the lateral perimeter of the feet
- anteriorly by the line joining the distal phalanges
- posteriorly by the line joining the heels

(See sections "Center of gravity" and "Balance" in Chapter 2 "Movement and biomechanics").

In the upright position, the body segments balance each other in such a way to prevent the body from falling.

Functional aspects of the upright position

- Makes walking possible
- It is more ergonomic (less energy expenditure) compared to the quadruped position (if the upright position is maintained without a particular posture – relaxed upright position – such as those resulting from hypertension of paravertebral muscles – attention position – or from the flexion of the trunk, the activity of the muscles of the lower limbs and pelvis is limited and the activity of the muscles supporting the trunk and head is low), so the resulting fatigue (over time) does not depend so much on muscular effort but rather on factors such as:
  - circulatory disorders of the lower limbs and vertebral column and alterations in load distribution
  - pressures of the intervertebral discs and vertebral zygapophysial joints
  - tension of the ligaments and joint capsules and abnormal pressures on the joint capsules (with pain in the first case and a reduction in articular space and arthritic phenomena in the second case) caused by rotation and translation of these structures following passive muscular, ligamentous and fascial tractions resulting from specific postures: indeed, in the upright position without the acquisition of specific postures, the horizontal axes of the differemt body segments (joint axes) and the segmental lines of gravity (lines passing through the centers of gravity of the body segments) cross perpendicularly with moments of force equal to zero (correct posture in orthostasis with the line of equilibrium falling within the support polygon); with the assumption of certain postures, the alignment of certain body segments is lost, with crossings that are no longer orthogonal and moments of force different from zero (the assumption of these postures depends on individual morphological characteristics, influences derived from the environment, age-related factors and lifestyle, which also influence circulation and load distribution).

The upright posture (as well as other postures) is never completely immobile, but is characterized by **oscillations** on the frontal and sagittal planes, due to variations in the pressure exerted on the ground by the different components of the sole of the foot, as a consequence of micromovements of the body segments necessary to maintaining **balance** (produced by mild stimuli that, at the pelvis and lower limb level, alternatively affects the gluteus muscles, quadriceps femoris, hamstring muscles, tibialis anterior, triceps surae, etc.).

Postural oscillations in the upright position are due to a continuous search for balance (see section "Balance" in Chapter 2 "Movements and biomechanics") that depends on two contradictory requirements:

- keeping the head in a position with the eyes horizontal in space (this position implies a forward movement of the center of gravity of the atlanto-occipital joint in relation to the horizontal axis, which destabilizes the ankle joint)
- stabilizing the ankle joint (this position produces head movements that compromise the horizontal position of the eyes).

Through postural oscillations, there are also thrusts that act on the venous circulation, favoring the return of blood to the heart.

The upright position involves a greater effort by the following muscles:

- psoas major and psoas minor, which reduce the load on the anterior ligaments of the hip joint (iliofemoral and pubofemoral ligaments)
- quadriceps femoris, gluteus muscles, hamstring muscles and adductors, which stabilize the femur
- triceps surae (gastrocnemius and soleus) in relation to the anterior muscles of the leg, due to the location of the line of gravity anteriorly to the ankle joint.

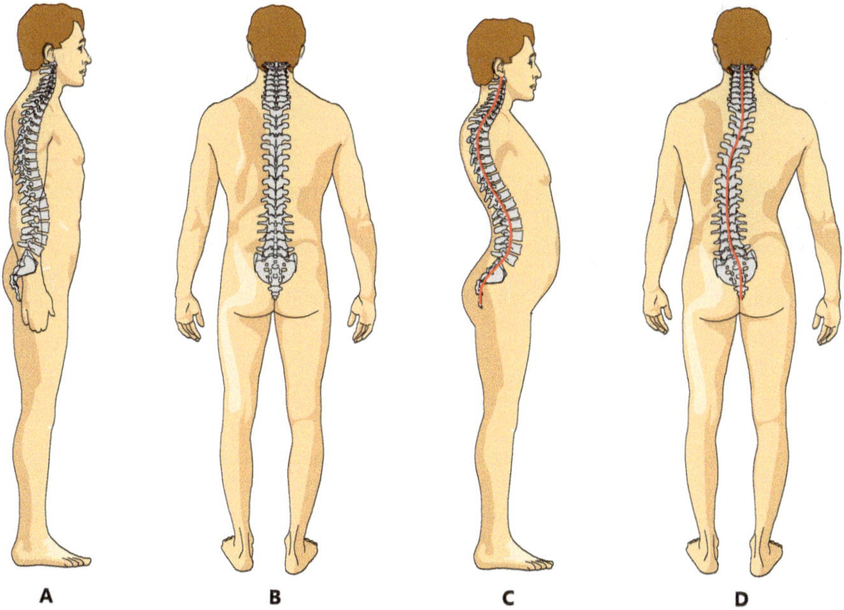

Upright position and posture. In **A** and **B**, the discrete alignment of the body segments allows a relative resetting of the moments due to the almost orthogonal crossing of the line of gravity with the horizontal axes of the various segments (head, vertebral column, pelvis, femur, leg, foot, etc.). In **C** and **D**, on the other hand, the non-orthogonal crossing produces rotations and translations that involve, above all, the ligaments and joint capsules (with the possibility of tension, pain and exhaustion) and the joint cartilage (with abnormal and asymmetrical pressures that may lead to reduction of articular spaces and arthrosis).

Posturography (stabilometry)

The maintenance of balance in the upright position depends on vestibular, visual and somatosensory information whose integration at the central level allows the body's center of gravity to be kept within the support polygon. It is possible to assess balance during the upright position (efficiency of the sensory systems and quantification of postural performance) with the use of a stabilometric platform (posturographic, stabilometric or orthostatic examination), whose surface is characterized by weight sensors or load cells that acquire posturographic signals, i.e., pressure variations of the different components of the sole of the foot in orthostatism (force platform). Through an interface, the conversion of this analog data into digital data is obtained and sent to a computer that processes it by providing numerous parameters.

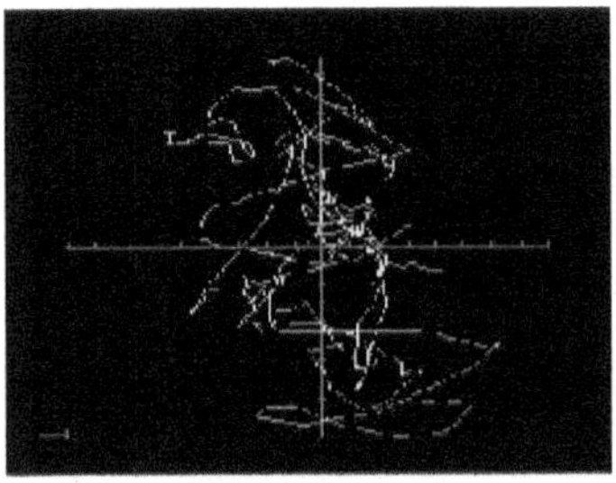

Statokinesigram: represents the actual displacement of the center of gravity referred to the plantar support. The platform provides the coordinates of the center of gravity at any time, which represented on the x- and y-axes provide the movement of the point of the center of gravity. This displacement is called "ball" (in relation to the movement trace memory) and corresponds to the oscillations on the platform.

Processing of the statokinesigram data:

- the average of the points identifying the displacement of the center of gravity (center of the curve) makes it possible to detect the deviation of the patient's center of gravity with respect to the theoretical center (corresponding in the graph to the intersection of the axes) (see section "Reference system" in Chapter 2 "Movements and biomechanics")
- the mean value of the x-coordinate represents the midpoint of the oscillations on the frontal plane
- the mean value of the y-coordinate represents the midpoint of the oscillations on the sagittal plane (the mean x and y values quantify the deviations from the axis of the body, which are related to the vestibulospinal tracts)
- the length of the center of gravity's movement can be analyzed as a function of the supporting surface, providing an evaluation of the energy expended for the maintenance of balance (indeed, in two different examinations, the value of the supporting surface remains constant, while the length of the movement varies)
- the x and y values (oscillations on the frontal and sagittal planes) can be analyzed as a function of time (therefore, a fundamental frequency of oscillation, of approximately 0.02 Hertz, is detected for both the x-function and the y-function, with which the visual, proprioceptive and vestibular afferences that determine the postural corrections are detected; a different value of this fundamental frequency may have a pathological significance).

Other data acquired through the stabilometric platform are represented by:

- the area of the support polygon
- isobaric zones
- areas corresponding to different pressure levels
- centers of gravity of the left and right feet
- plantar surfaces under load of both feet
- weight supported by each foot (also as a percentage of the total weight).

Walking

Definition: succession of alternating rhythmic movements of the lower limbs, pelvis, trunk, upper limbs and head which, by determining a forward displacement of the body's center of gravity, cause, through a series of rotations and translations of all the joint segments involved, the forward progression of the body.

Gait cycle

Stride: distance between two consecutive strikes of the same heel.

Characteristics of a stride:
- length (distance between two consecutive strikes of the same heel), equal to 80-90% of the body's height
- width (distance between the most protruding point of the heel – center of the heel – and the line of gait progression), equal to approximately 5-6 cm
- angle (between the longitudinal axis of the foot – externally rotated – and the line of gait progression), equal to approximately 15°.

With the increase in speed, the width tends to increase and the angle to decrease.

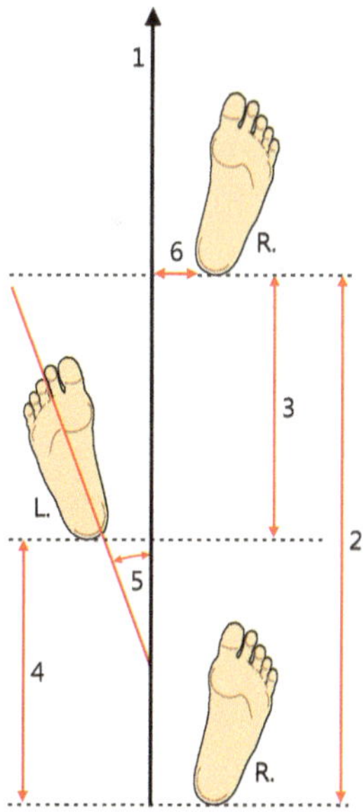

Gait cycle: transverse plane. **1**, Line of gait progression; **2**, stride; **3**, step or right anterior step; **4**, step or left anterior step; **5**, stride angle; **6**, stride width.

Step (single step – right anterior or left anterior – or step): distance between consecutive strikes of the two different heels.

During the physiological gait, the duration of the right anterior step is equal to that of the left anterior step. In general, in central nervous system diseases, there is a difference in duration and length between two steps, while in peripheral nervous system diseases there is only a difference in length (the step of the deficient limb has a shorter length than the step of the healthy limb).

Phases of the gait cycle

Two phases: stance and swing.

Stance (or support) phase

Phase included between heel support and push off.

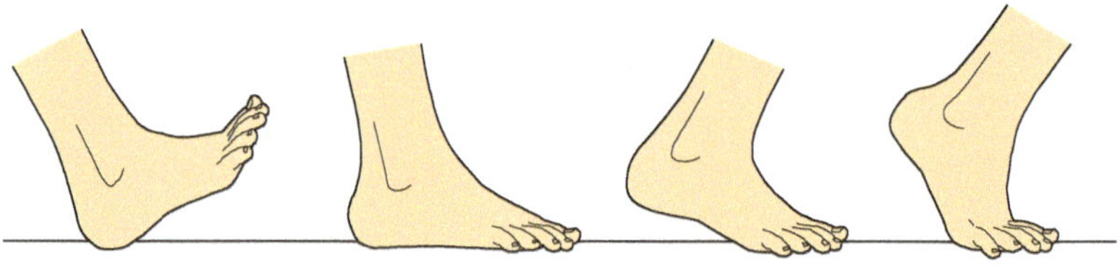

Five subphases (referring to one of the two feet, for example, the right foot):

- heel contact (or heel strike) – support of the right heel (in this subphase the left foot, placed behind the right heel, initiates the thrust on the forefoot; the first double stance phase takes place)
- foot flat (or extended foot stretched) – the sole of the right foot adheres to the ground (the left foot, pushed off from the ground, swings forward towards the right foot)
- midstance – the sole of the right foot is always in contact with the ground (the left foot, at the end of the swing, is at the level of the right foot; this is the moment of greatest instability of balance during gait, with the body weight resting on the supporting limb)
- push off
  - heel off – the right foot is still partially supported on the ground (the second phase of double support begins with the strike of the left heel)
  - toe off – push off on the right forefoot and push off from the ground (single support of the left foot).

Braking period: the first three subphases of the stance phase.
Propulsive period: the last two subphases of the stance phase.

Swing (oscillating or suspended) phase

Two periods (referring to one of the two feet, for example, the right foot):

- acceleration (or midswing) period – begins with the separation of the toes of the right foot and ends when the right foot is in correspondence with the left foot in the midstance phase
- deceleration period – moment preceding contact of the right heel with the ground (heel contact).

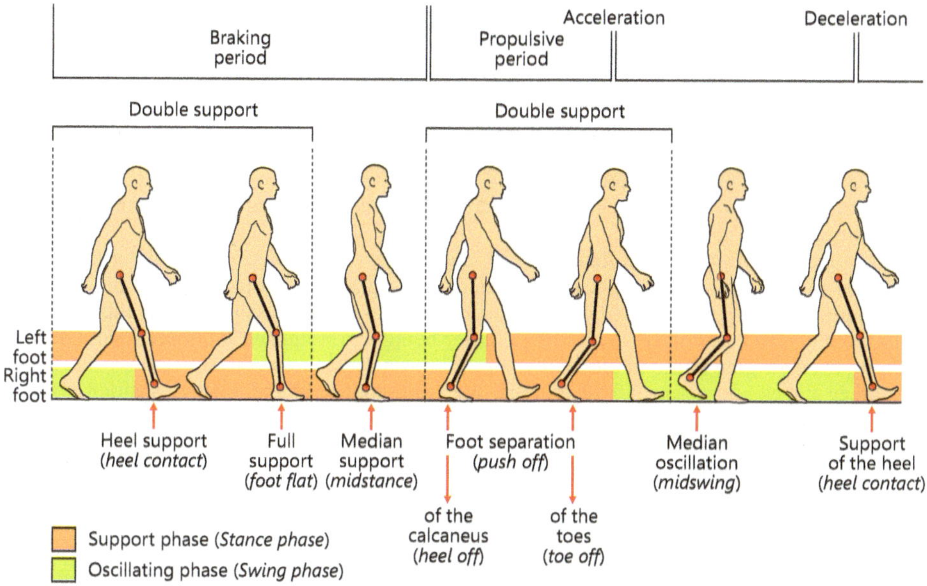

Gait cycle (gait phases): the right lower limb has been taken into account. Double support occurs in phases 1 and 4.

Cadence (or walking rate): number of steps in a unit of time:

- increase in cadence – reduction of the duration of the two double support phases (they disappear as one starts to run)
- decrease in cadence – increase in the duration of the two double support phases.

Gait speed

Stride length × walking rate (number of steps in a unit of time).

Percentage distribution of the duration of the normal step in the different phases

The duration of a normal step (a little more than 1 second) can be broken down as follows:

- 60-65% stance phase (25% double support and 35-40% single support) of which:
  - 12% heel
  - 60% sole
  - 28% forefoot
- 40-35% swing phase.

13

Ontogeny

The importance of the human gait is "discovered" between the first and third month of life only if the baby is placed with its feet resting on the edge of a table and held by an adult by the trunk which is pushed with a modest forward flexion.
In response, in fact, the lower limbs are distended and, alternating with flexion, perform the so-called "primary automatic gait".
However, until 6 or 7 months of life, the child does not achieve conscious perception of the lower limbs.
This recognition, which is simultaneous with the gradual reduction of flexor hypertonia of the limbs and the initial development of muscular strength, allows the child to stand up, at about 8 months, holding himself/herself up with both lower limbs (assisted by an adult) and, at 10 months, even with only one limb, the latter being a prerequisite for successively performing the swinging phase of gait.
The other stages are, at around 12 months, the maintenance of the upright position with extended base and without assistance.
From this moment on, true walking begins, which, in the healthy subject, may take place at 10 months or may be delayed until 14 months.
All movements of the limbs, trunk and pelvis reach their physiological level between 3 and 5 years of age and are considered refined by the age of 10 years.
However, the complete maturity of walking is reached between 15 and 17 years of age. In addition, the child performs spatial movements at 7 or 8 months with "crawling" and at 9 or 10 months in quadruped position.
This last stage can often be skipped without developmental problems, although recent research suggests that lack of crawling performance may, in some predisposed subjects, promote dyslexia.

Neurological aspects of human locomotion

"Telencephalization", i.e., the addition of the cerebral hemisphere to the primitive brain during phylogenesis, has allowed human beings to obtain advantages in both refinement and lower energy expenditure when walking compared to the locomotion of other mammals; although humans, when they suffer major CNS injuries, almost always have greater difficulties and need more time to recover a "potential" gait than most animals.
In fact, the latter, possessing a simpler nerve structure, manage (even in a very short time) to build new, imperfect and more wasteful forms of locomotion (due to anomalous compensations), but which allow them easier and faster ways of moving.
Gait, in its most basic form, is carried out by stimulations coming from the spinal cord through the so-called central patter generators (CPGs).
For their functioning, these CPGs can dispense with both the modulatory motor afferents from the supraspinal centers and the sensory afferents from the proprioceptors, tactile receptors, exteroceptors and teleceptors.
Their function, in a way, can be compared to the respiratory stimulators, which are also located in the spinal cord at the level of the second cervical vertebra, whose injury almost always leads to arrest of respiratory function.
In animals, the mere presence of the CPGs is usually sufficient, with the contribution of peripheral sensitivity, to allow a normal walking rhythm.
In humans, on the other hand, the organizational process of movements (carried out in areas 4 and 6 of the cerebral cortex) and the simultaneous, prior and successive interventions of

the subcortical centers of the brainstem, the basal ganglia and the cerebellum can make gait more complex, making its eventual recovery more difficult.

Gait kinematics

From the point of view of joint excursions, gait can be viewed globally by simply evaluating the displacements of the body's center of gravity which, as already mentioned, reaches maximum vertical displacements going up and down, respectively, when the swinging limb is at the level of the supporting foot (midstance-midswing) and when the two lower limbs are in the double support.

The center of gravity, observed on the sagittal plane, describes a pseudo-sinusoidal line. The more modest these vertical displacements of the center of gravity, the lower the muscular energy expenditure.

On the other hand, in cases where the joint excursions of the body segments during the phases of gait require more detailed assessment, the problem becomes much more complex, it nevertheless seems more important to evaluate first the displacements on the three body planes of the thigh, the leg and foot, as well as an assessment, albeit more concise, of the excursions of the pelvis, trunk, upper limbs and head.

Evaluation of the displacements of the center of gravity

As mentioned above, the step or gait cycle is represented by the forward movement of the entire body (in physics we speak of "variations of the position of a body from a point, called position 0, to another point called position 1 and so on").

The stride consists of the advance of two steps from a double support position; therefore, the stride is constituted by the sum of two steps.

Each stride has a stance phase in which one of the two lower limbs is in partial or full contact with the ground and the other is suspended, i.e., in swing phase. When both feet are in contact with the ground, we speak of double support: this phase is obviously the most stable for the body and is usually taken as the starting and final position for the evaluation of the gait cycle.

Having referred to some fundamental parameters of gait, before continuing with this mode of kinematic evaluation, some additional knowledge needs to be established.

The center of gravity (physicists prefer to call it "center of mass") of an adult person in the upright position is located just in front of the second sacral vertebra. It can be found at approximately 55% of the body height measured from the ground.

The segmental centers of gravity, i.e., those specific to each body segment, can be verified in the graphs on page 644.

In order to be able to walk physiologically, i.e., with the least expenditure of energy, humans instinctively use all those forms of response to the outside world that initiated and acquired during the first 18 months of life. Specifically, they use balance reactions, as well as straightening reactions and muscular adaptations.

Due to the need to maintain the line of the center of gravity within the support polygon, the subject, at the moment he/she starts walking and during its development, prepares his/her own body segments (head, trunk, pelvis, upper and lower limbs) in a position of moderate imbalance.

This imbalance, which is repeated rhythmically because the gait must adapt to the stimuli coming from the CNS, is responded to with the known modalities of balance reactions that bring the body's line of gravity to a more stable position. Gait tends to be characterized as a sequence of losses and recoveries of balance.

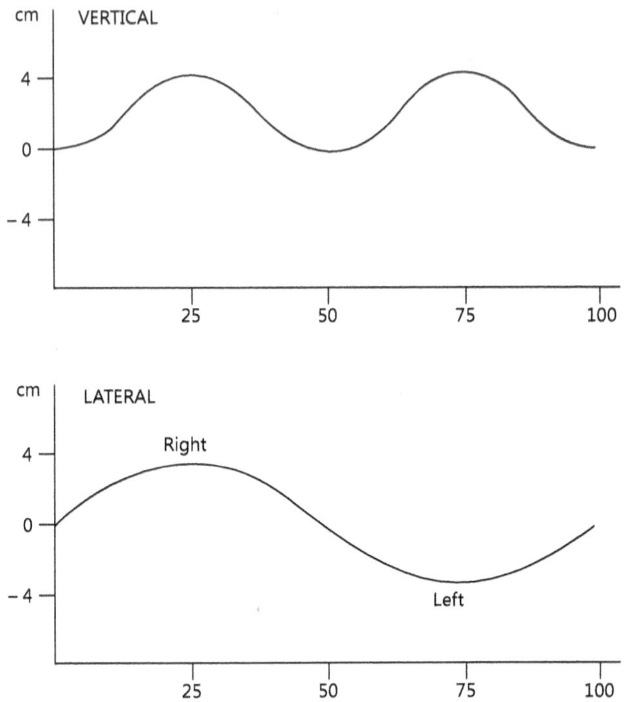

Trajectory of the body's center of mass during gait: above on the sagittal plane, below on the horizontal plane.

The displacements of the center of gravity occur both on the sagittal direction, which is the common direction of all human and animal gait, and on the lateral direction. The latter displacement is related to the need to transfer the load from one limb to the other.

In its displacement on the sagittal plane, the center of gravity rises and falls and can be graphically described as a sinusoid.

Similar, although slightly smaller, lateral displacements can be described graphically on the horizontal plane.

In practice: when, for example, the left, posteriorly positioned lower limb begins to move forward after the foot of this limb has pushed off the ground (swing phase), the center of gravity moves forward and laterally in a smaller support polygon of a single foot, in this case the right one. This ensures stability.

Subsequently, as soon as the foot of the left lower limb contacts the ground, the center of gravity moves to the left and forward. As already mentioned, during these changes of position, the center of gravity undergoes elevations and descents.

The center of gravity is lower when the double support occurs and it is also less laterally displaced; instead, it reaches its maximum height in the phase called full support (midstance), i.e., when the suspended, advancing limb is in correspondence with the supporting limb: here its lateral displacement is maximum.

The characterization of gait as successive phases of the loss and recovery of balance is produced both by the elevations, descents and lateral movements of the center of gravity, as well as by the displacements of the body segments.

In fact, it is a modest flexion of the trunk forward and toward the supporting limb that causes the forward movement of the suspended limb, as occurs (see ontogeny section, page 642) in the newborn (automatic gait) when these same movements are passively provoked by the adult.

The loss of balance due to flexion of the trunk causes the suspended limb to move forward with the main objective of regaining its stability, exactly as stated by Nashner in his second strategy for reacting to loss of balance.

In this way, as soon as the suspended foot contacts the ground, the line of gravity moves laterally towards the new stable point, the other limb begins the suspension, and the scheme is repeated contralaterally.

In summary: the forward movement is ensured by the thrust that the posterior foot begins to make as soon as the heel of the other foot comes into contact with the ground; by the frontal and lateral movements of the trunk (and of the other body segments) which, by increasing the frontal and lateral translation of the center of gravity, make the lower limb accelerate its movement to regain balance; finally, by the force of gravity which first limits the movement in the thrust phase and then facilitates the fall towards the support of the lower limb.

Visually, the displacements of the center of gravity can be deduced by observing the head during walking: it will be possible to note, on the sagittal plane, the elevations and descents of the head corresponding to the different phases of gait.

On the frontal plane, lateral displacements can also be seen, while, always on this plane, vertical displacements will be better evidenced if the observation is performed on several subjects while they move towards the observer, each subject being in a different phase of gait.

The first research dates to 1887 and is the Marey study reported by McMahon.

During normal walking, the vertical displacements of the center of gravity are equal to 3-4 cm and the lateral displacements are about 4-5 cm.

As already mentioned, the graphical representation of the center of gravity trajectories is similar to a sinusoid where the highest point of the sinusoid on the sagittal plane indicates the moment when the lower limb in suspension is, in its swing, approximately at the height of the limb in support, while the center of gravity is lower during double support.

The lateral excursion of the center of gravity can be evidenced by the plantar footprint.

At the beginning of the walk, and when the subject is standing with the lower limbs parallel to the line of gravity (LoG) placed between the two feet, approximately aligned with Chopart line, there is a small displacement backwards and in a lateral direction of the LoG towards the foot that will move first, e.g., the right (displacement perhaps due to the modest thrust on the ground that the "flat" foot must make before pushing off), then the LoG moves clearly to the left "passing" the foot from back to front until the left foot pushes off and the LoG moves contralaterally.

The evaluation of the kinematics of the center of gravity is important because an excess of vertical and lateral displacements leads, on the one hand, to stiffer and less harmonic motion and, on the other hand, to an increase in muscular work.

Since several authors have recognized that there is a natural tendency in humans to seek a gait in which the sinusoid that characterizes the sagittal displacements of the center of gravity is as linear as possible, it is also understood why when it is necessary to increase the speed this is done by increasing the stride length to a lesser extent with respect to its frequency.

An excessive increase in stride length would, in fact, lead to excessive elevations and descents of the center of gravity with a considerable expenditure of muscular energy. In fact, the problem is solved by a mediation between the increase of the stride length and the increase of its frequency. First Saunders and then Inma and collaborators have emphasized the importance of modest displacements of the center of gravity during walking, highlighting the existence of six factors resulting from the structure of the human skeleton, in particular the so-called "lower body" (sum of the lower limbs and pelvis) that contribute to this end.

The six factors are:
- rotation of the pelvis around the vertical axis of the body
- inclination of the pelvis to the side of the suspended limb
- flexion of the knee in the stance phase
- ankle movements
- movements of the joints of the foot
- coordinated movements of the knee and the ankle.

Evaluation of the displacements of the body segments

Kinematics on the sagittal plane

It is the most described, since it evaluates the gait on the plane in which the progression occurs (figure on next page).

The movement of the three joints of the lower limbs will be analyzed in detail: ankle, knee and hip and brief remarks will follow on the positions of the other body segments during gait.

Three different phases can be identified:
- stance phase up to the midstance
- midstance to heel off
- toe off to the end of the swing phase (deceleration phase).

Phase I: from the beginning of the stance phase to midstance

In relation to the ankle:
- at the heel contact: the foot-ankle angle is 90°; the leg-ground angle is 100-120°; the thigh-ground angle is 120-130°
- from heel contact to foot flat: plantar flexion of approximately 15° is observed
- at foot flat: the ankle has an angle of almost 90° with the leg and thigh
- at midstance: dorsiflexion of the ankle is observed due to the closure of the angle by the leg of a few degrees.

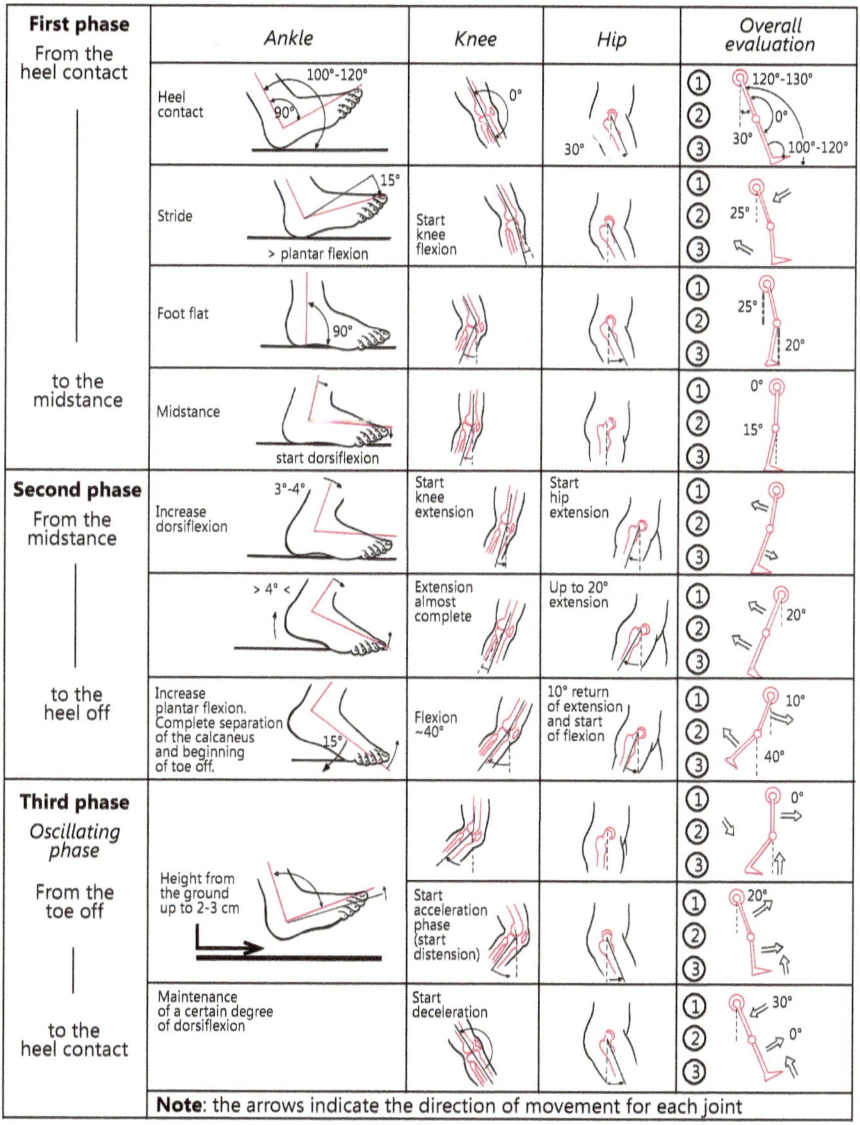

1, Hip joint; **2**, knee joint; **3**, ankle joint.

Gait kinematics on the sagittal plane (ankle, knee and hip joints).

In relation to the knee:
- at the heel contact: the knee begins to flex (an instant before touching the ground it was extended = 0°)
- at foot flat: flexion is approximately 20° and the extension begins
- at midstance: flexion is approximately 15° and the extension continues.

In relation to the hip:
- at the heel contact: the hip is flexed 30° and the extension begins
- at foot flat: the hip is flexed approximately 25°
- at midstance: the hip is in neutral position.

Phase II: from midstance to heel off

For the ankle:
- at midstance: dorsiflexion of 3-4° tends to increase
- at heel off: dorsiflexion goes from 4° to 15°
- at the end of heel off and the start of toe off: it goes from 15° of dorsiflexion to 20° of plantar flexion.

For the knee:
- at midstance: from 15° of flexion, the knee begins to extend
- at heel off: extension is almost complete (177-178°)
- at the start of toe off: the knee flexes to approximately 40°.

For the hip:
- at midstance: it begins its extension from neutral position
- at heel off: goes from 10° to 20° of extension
- at the start of toe off: extends approximately 10° and flexion begins.

Phase III: swing

For the ankle:
- from toe off to heel contact: a certain degree of dorsiflexion is maintained.

For the knee:
- after toe off (and up to the beginning of the accelerating swing phase): the flexion of the knee concludes (60-70°)
- at the start of the acceleration phase: the distension of the knee begins
- at the start of the deceleration phase: the distension is completed.

For the hip:
- after toe off: flexion begins
- acceleration phase: flexion of the hip of approximately 20°
- at midswing: the hip is flexed approximately 30-35°
- at the deceleration phase: the hip is flexed approximately 30°.

Other body segments

In kinematics on the sagittal plane, the *pelvis* tends to maintain a relatively fixed position. There is a rotation around the femur that leads to a slight anteversion after heel contact with the ground.
When the length of the stride is particularly wide, it seems that the pelvis accentuates this anteversion.
The trunk maintains its position due to compensation to the lower limbs.
The head presents vertical displacements of 3-4 cm from the lowest position (double support) to the highest (midstance and midswing).
The upper limbs have reciprocity of movement in relation to the lower limbs. When the right upper limb swings forward, the right lower limb swings backward and the left lower limb swings forward.
Obviously, the forearm has a wider swing (it is lighter) and an internal rotation in its anterior movements.

Kinematics on the frontal and horizontal plane

Observation on the frontal and horizontal plane allows the trajectory of the following body parts to be evaluated: first the foot and, together, the legs, thigh and pelvis.
The foot, in the stance phase, shows heel support, first external with inversion and supination, and immediately afterwards, internal with pronation (the latter for stabilizing purposes).
In particular, the subtalar (or talocalcaneal) and transverse tarsal (Chopart) joints allow these movements also favored by the possibility of lateralization and medialization of the tibiofibular mortise for the trochlea of the talus.
Then there is an additional forward displacement (cuboid, fifth-fourth-third metatarsals and toes) of the load on the external side of the foot and, finally, on the internal side (second and first metatarsals, second toe and great toe with supination of the forefoot).
When the heel is lifted, eversion and pronation of the forefoot begins with the separation of the last three toes and the fourth and fifth metatarsals, the second toe and, finally, the great toe.
During the swing phase, the foot is oriented in eversion and supination, moving forward and laterally, concluding its itinerary with the support as just explained (it must be remembered that the heel elevation is normally placed between 2.5 and 3 cm, while the axis of the foot, when parallel to the ground, reaches approximately 1 cm in height).

The leg, thigh and pelvis rotate internally in the first 15 hundredths of the cycle, at heel strike, and then reduce their rotation until approximately 60-70 hundredths of the gait cycle when the external rotation reaches its peak.
Then, the internal rotation begins, which reaches its peak at approximately 15 hundredths of a second from the moment of heel strike.
During the swing phase, the leg and thigh rotate externally. While the leg presents a range of 9-10 degrees for each rotation, the thigh does not exceed 8 degrees.

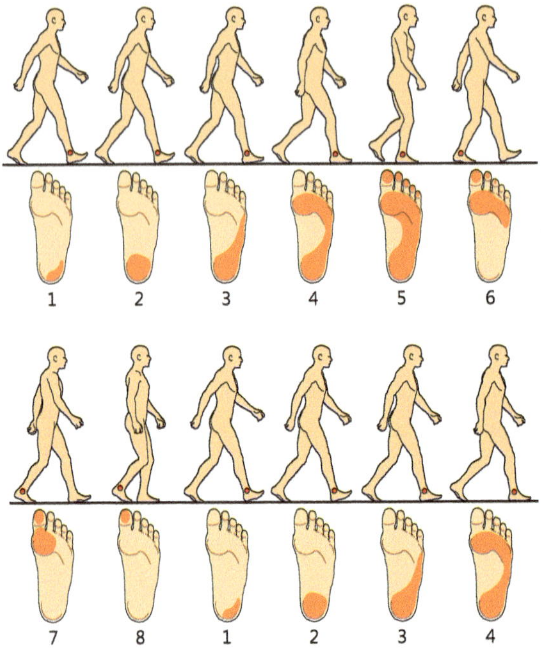

Classic theory of the zones of plantar support. From the initial support of the heel (support 1 - stabilization 2) to the final support of the great toe (8).

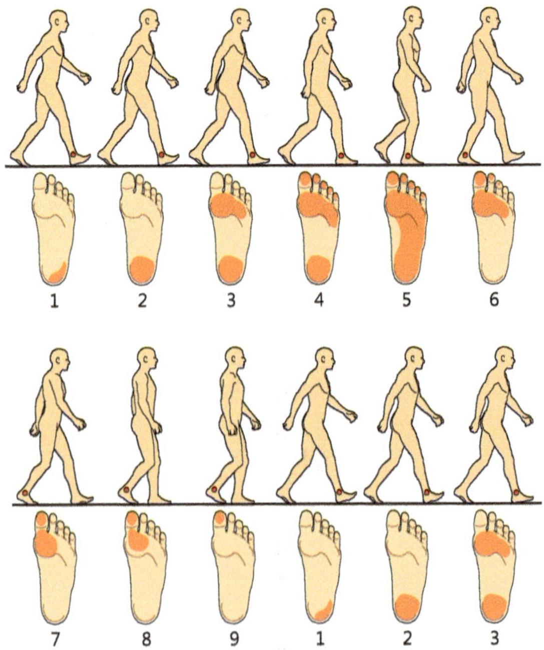

Theory of "mediated" support, from the outer edge.

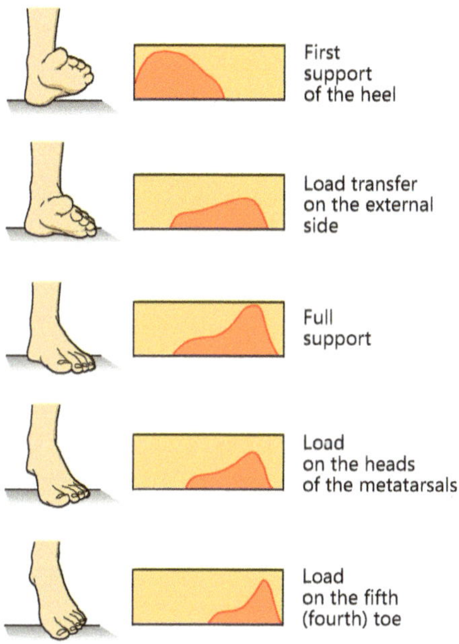

Movements of the foot on the frontal plane during the stance phase.

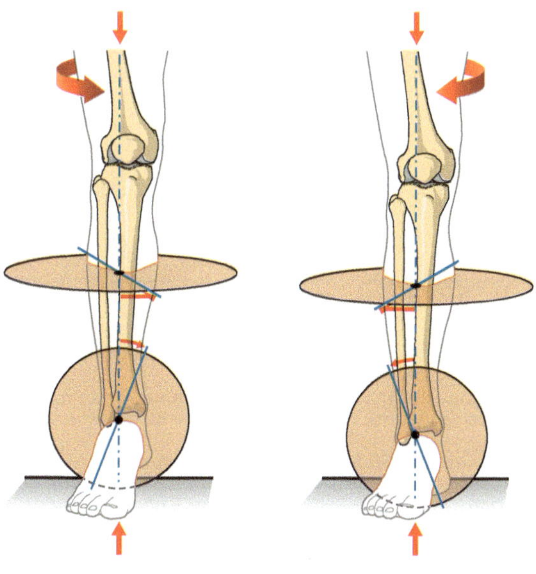

Movements of the thigh, leg and foot on the frontal plane and on the transverse plane during the stance phase.

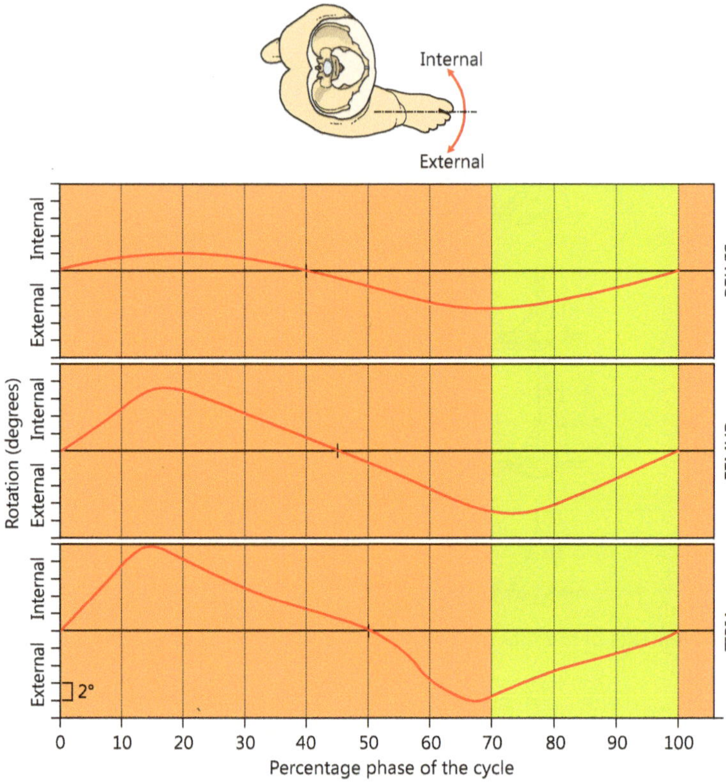

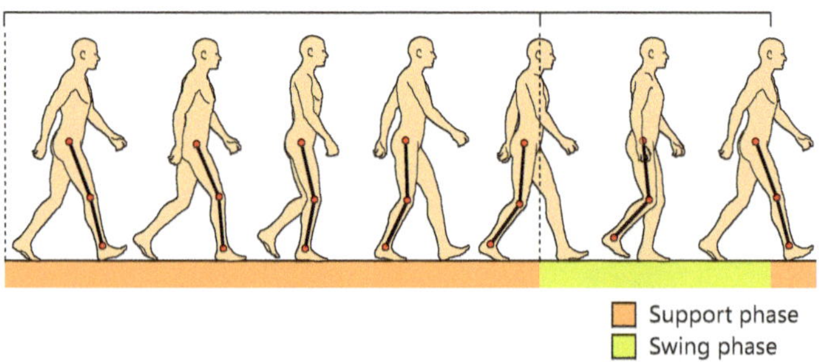

Rotations on the horizontal plane of the tibia, femur and pelvis. They maintain internal rotation, but begin to rotate externally until the thrust phase (~ 60% of the cycle) where the true external rotation begins.

- The tibia rotates internally up to ~ 15-20% of the stance phase cycle
- The femur rotates internally up to ~ 15-20% of the stance phase cycle
- The pelvis rotates internally up to ~ 15-20% of the stance phase cycle

In summary: the reduction of the total joint excursion of the center of gravity of ~ 10 cm is obtained in three ways: on the frontal plane as a result of the 1st, 2nd, 3rd, 4th and 5th factors; on the frontal plane due to the effect of the frontal rotation of the pelvis (inclination in the midswing phase, lowers the center of gravity) and the 6th factor is related to the displacements of the center of gravity on the horizontal plane (see page 646 for the six factors).

Muscles of the trunk and lower limb involved during walking

Trunk and vertebral column

Rotation of the trunk

The forward rotation of the pelvis by the suspended limb is associated with the forward rotation of the upper trunk on the opposite side to reduce body motion during the gait cycle.

Intrinsic muscles of the vertebral column

At the beginning and end of the stance phase, the contraction of the contralateral paravertebral muscles occurs in the supporting limb to prevent the trunk from falling forward due to the flexion moment created at hip of the supporting limb.

Muscles of the abdomen

These are not usually active during walking.

Pelvis and thigh

- The **hamstring** muscles (semimembranosus, semitendinosus and biceps femoris) and the **gluteus maximus** – contract at the end of the swing phase and at the beginning of the stance phase to decelerate the forward swing of the suspended limb and to extend the hip at the initial contact with the ground and in response to the load
- **Tensor fasciae latae** – contracts at the beginning of the stance phase to neutralize the posterior displacement of the iliotibial tract produced by the contraction of the gluteus maximus (which inserts on the iliotibial tract)
- **Hip abductor** muscles, **gluteus medius** and **gluteus minimus** – contract on the side of the supporting limb in the swing phase, when the pelvis is not supported contralaterally by the suspended limb, preventing the pelvis from falling on the unsupported side
- **Hip flexor** muscles, **iliopsoas, rectus femoris** and **tensor fasciae latae** – contract at the end of the stance phase and at the beginning of the swing phase, initiating the movement of the hip flexion
- **Hip adductor** muscles – contract during the swing phase to keep the suspended limb on the midline and contribute to the flexion of the hip at the end of the swing phase.

Leg

- The **flexor** and **extensor** muscles **of the knee** – contract simultaneously to stabilize the knee in extension and prepare the heel for the initial contact with the ground
- **Quadriceps femoris**:
  - contracts eccentrically during the first part of the stance phase to prevent the flexion of the knee at the initial moment of heel contact with the ground and in response to the load when the weight is transferred onto the supporting limb
  - can contract or not, extending the knee, from the moment of the response to the load up to the middle of the stance phase
  - can contract during fast walking to prevent excessive knee flexion and begin extension at the beginning of the swing phase
- **Hamstring** muscles – contract eccentrically at the end of the swing phase to reduce the forward displacement speed of the oscillating limb
- **Sartorius** – is active throughout the swing phase, contributing to the flexion of the hip necessary for the toes push off from the ground and to the external rotation of the hip with forward rotation of the pelvis on the oscillating side

- **Gracilis** – contracts at the end of the stance phase and at the beginning of the swing phase
- **Popliteus** – rotates the tibia internally, maintaining this position from the middle of the swing phase to the end of the stance phase and at the beginning of the swing phase.

Foot

- **Dorsiflexor** muscles **of the ankle** – contract at the beginning of and during the swing phase of the gait cycle to allow the foot to detach from the ground
- **Tibialis anterior**, **extensor hallucis longus** and **extensor digitorum longus** – contract:
  - at first concentrically, with the dorsiflexion of the ankle from the end of the stance phase to the middle of the swing phase
  - secondly isometrically, to kept the foot in the reached position
  - eccentrically, to control the descent of the foot to the ground at the end of the swing phase, from the initial contact until the end of the response to the load during the stance phase
- **Gastrocnemius** and **soleus** – contract:
  - eccentrically from the load response until the end of the stance phase, controlling the dorsiflexion of the ankle caused by the forward movement of the tibia with respect to the foot fixed to the ground
  - concentrically at the end of the stance phase and at the beginning of the swing phase, together with the fibularis longus, fibularis brevis and flexor hallucis longus, at heel off
- **Fibularis longus** – controls balance during normal gait
- **Intrinsic** muscles **of the foot** – contract during the stance phase, at the moment of the gait cycle when maximum foot stability is required.

Gait biomechanics

Forces acting during gait:
- internal – muscular forces
- external – frictional, gravitational and inertia forces

The propulsive force of the muscles acts mainly in the phases of:
- start of the gait
- the thrust on the forefoot
- deceleration.

Variations in balance and displacements of the body's center of gravity during walking

The following displacements of the center of gravity occur during the gait:

- forward
- vertical

The center of gravity reaches:

- the highest point in the acceleration of the swing phase and in the midstance phase (when the foot of the oscillating limb is in correspondence with the foot of the supporting limb)
- the lowest point in the two double support phases.

Energy expenditure associated with walking

During the thrust on the forefoot that occurs in the separation phase of the foot (at the end of the stance phase), produced by the action of the muscular forces of the foot (muscular work), the trunk flexes slightly forward, with leverage on the supporting foot. Through this flexion (which moves the center of gravity forward), the forward movement of the suspended limb is facilitated, due to the slight loss of balance, which is already recovered at the end of the acceleration period of the swing phase (when the suspended foot is in correspondence with the supporting foot). The propulsion of the suspended foot in the deceleration period of the swing phase (during the descent to the ground) occurs by inertia (deceleration) of the preceding propulsion, until the suspended limb is supported.

The forward displacement of the center of gravity and the consequent loss of balance, followed by the more central repositioning of the line of gravity with respect to the support polygon (with recovery of balance), are accomplished by the action of the gravitational and inertia forces.

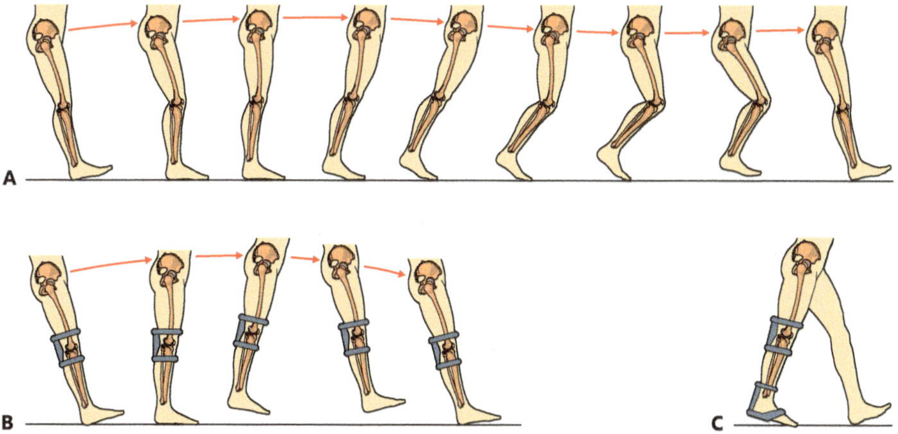

Variations in oscillation of the hip joint in normal human gait (**A**), in a gait with the extension of the knee locked (**B**) and with the ankle in neutral position (90°) (**C**).

The energy expenditure associated with walking is very low, being related to the muscular work during the phase of separation of the foot:

- with the vertical displacement of the center of gravity, which is of modest degree (the lower the energy expenditure, the smaller the vertical displacement of the center of gravity); in fact, the hip, knee and ankle joints, through their reciprocal movements, prevent excessive vertical displacements of the center of gravity; if there were a single center of joint rotation at the hip level, with the knee locked in extension and the ankle locked in an intermediate position between dorsiflexion and plantar flexion, the vertical excursion of the center of gravity would be greater, with significant additional muscular work required to raise and lower the trunk and recover the loss of balance.
- with the muscular work in the deceleration period, which is eccentric (isotonic contraction with lower energy expenditure; see section "Type of muscle contraction" in Chapter 1 "Bones, joints and muscles") and, therefore, modest.

Frictional forces

- The vertical component of the load (transmitted to the foot) must be greater than the horizontal component, otherwhise slippage would occur (especially in the heel's stance phase) (see section "Frictional forces" in Chapter 2 "Movement and biomechanics")
- The vertical or counterthrust component of the ground reaction (see section "Action and reaction" in Chapter 2 "Movement and biomechanics") must be effective for the movement, ensuring good propulsion (in the forefoot thrust phase), and this is only possible if the ground is sufficiently rigid.

Gait analysis

- Visual recording of gait
- Measurement of the temporal parameters of gait
- Measurement of foot pressure
- Measurement of gait movements
- Force platform
- Electromyography.

Visual recording

Visual recording of gait before the aplication of any instrument (electromyographic electrodes, footswitches, movement markers, etc.) that could alter gait characteristics. Images are obtained through two video cameras, one placed anteriorly and the other laterally. Visual documentation of gait is useful in cases of discrepancy of movement data from the examiner's visual observation.

Measurement of the temporal parameters

Typical measurement parameters:

- cadence of the stride
- duration of the gait cycle
  - duration of the stance phase
  - duration of the swing phase
  - duration of single support
  - duration of double support

If the measurements are made over a defined distance, it is possible to calculate:
- average walking speed
- stride length.

Instruments
- Footswitches – thin soles placed between the sole and the shoe which contain an electrical circuit through which every variation of pressure exerted on specific contact areas on the heel, 1st and 5th metatarsals and great toe can be recorded
- Gait mats – mats containing electrical circuits that record the contacts due to foot pressure (in this case, the calculation of the temporal parameters of gate is added to that of the spatial parameters, made possible thanks to the knowledge of the geometric characteristics of the mat).

Measurement of foot pressure

Measurement of plantar pressure through electrical transducers. The data obtained include:
- areas of increased compression at the level of the plantar surface
- gait lines
- force and pressure as a function of time
- integrals of force and pressure/time ratio
- detailed analysis of specific areas.

Instruments
- Pressure mats – mats that record foot pressure variations (placed along the line of gait progression and function as force platforms)
- Pressure insoles – soles that record variations in foot pressure (allowing measurement over several gait cycles).

Measurement of movements

Kinematic measurements:
- speed and acceleration of the lower limb segments:
  - determination of kinetic measurements
    - joint movements
    - forces.

Instruments
- Electrogoniometers – electromechanical devices attached to the proximal and distal body segments of the joint whose movements are to be measured (the electrogoniometer voltage variation is proportional to the angular variation between the two body segments, assuming that the traction is exerted on the midline of the body segment)
- Three-dimensional visual recording of the joint movements – computerized analysis of the displacement of the various movement markers located on the lower limb (a series of video cameras provides the movement data of each marker which, processed by the computer, provide the three-dimensional coordinates; at least three markers are applied to each body segment).

Force platform

Measurement of the reaction forces of the ground to the thrusts exerted on it through the strides during walking:

- vertical and horizontal force components
- displacement of the center of gravity during walking

(The visual recording of the movement together with the force platforms allows the moments and joint forces to be determined, through computerized analysis of kinetic data, that require the knowledge of the ground reaction forces).

Instruments

- Force platform – a raised platform in relation to the surrounding floor, separated from the support surface through the interposition of force transducers positioned near the angles of the platform.

Electromyography

The of electromyography applied to gait analysis provides a precise picture of how the muscles contribute, through their activity, to gait changes observed and measured with other instruments (see section "Electromyography" in Chapter 1 "Bones, joints and muscles").

Running

Parameters that differentiate running from walking:
- phases
- reciprocal duration of the different phases
- length and width of stride
- energy expenditure
- kinematics
- kinetics.

The walking speed ranges from a few hundred meters per hour to 7-8 km per hour. Between 8 and 15 km per hour, energy expenditure is no longer proportional to the increase in speed, making running more convenient. Running begins when walking speed exceeds 15 km per hour (at this speed it is no longer possible to maintain a double support; this corresponds to 90 strides per minute, for a stride length of 150 cm).

Phases of the running cycle

(referring, for example, to the right foot)

- Right foot support
- Double suspension
- Left foot support
- Double suspension

The double support of the gait cycle (which occurs during the heel strike and heel off phases) is replaced in running by double suspension, so that, in this case, the load is carried on one foot, first the right foot and then the left foot.

Duration of the running cycle

The duration of the single support phases (support of the right foot and support of the left foot) is approximately two-thirds of the double suspension phases (i.e., the two double suspension phases correspond to one-third of the cycle duration, and this is because the shorter the double suspension, the bigger the thrusts made on the ground, and faster the run will be).

Running speed

While running, the speed depends on the stride length and its rate (speed = stride length × number of strides in a unit of time), as in walking, which is increased following an increase in these parameters, but also by the impact modes of the foot with the ground. In fact,

- the support on the forefoot or on the sole of the foot (in comparison to the heel strike when walking) and the greater forward flexion of the trunk that occurs when running (with the line of gravity placed approximately at the level of the thrusting foot) reduce the horizontal component of the foot's thrust and, consequently, the horizontal component of ground reaction force (or deceleration component) compared to walking; additionally, the impact of the foot with the ground is greater, so there is an increase in the vertical component of the foot's thrust and, consequently, in the vertical component of ground reaction (with greater thrust to propulsion).

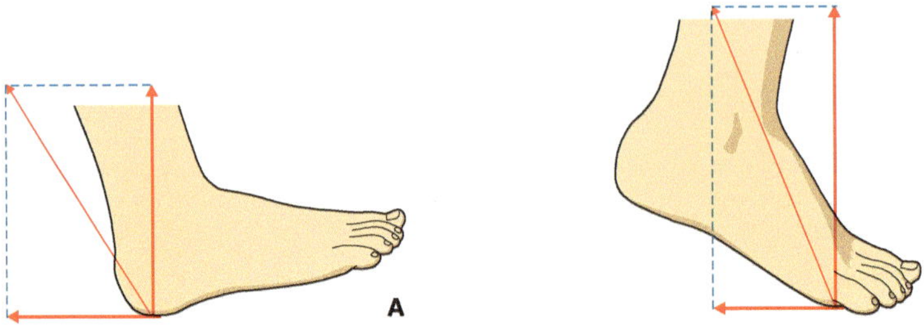

Reduction of the horizontal component of the backward ground reaction (deceleration) when running (**B**), in comparison to walking (**A**), (red arrow) due to the effect of the support on the forefoot and the greater inclination of the trunk that brings the line of gravity to the supported foot.

During running, the body's center of gravity is located lower in relation to walking as a result of greater flexion of the knee, hip and trunk.

Characteristics of running strides

Length: ≥ 3 m (up to twice or more the walking length)
Width: decreases until it is canceled (the frequency of the stride width during running exceeds that of walking by 50%).

Running kinematics

Stance phase of the foot

- Start (foot in contact with the entire sole in slow running); foot in contact only with the forefoot in sprinting:
  - trunk flexed 50-60° in the initial phase (flexion of the trunk is reduced to 15-25° in sprinting)
  - hip flexed to a greater extent than in walking
  - knee slightly flexed
- Central phase:
  - hip flexed
  - knee flexed
  - slight plantar or dorsiflexion of the ankle
  - extended metatarsophalangeal joints
- Thrust:
  - hip extended
  - knee extended
  - ankle mostly in plantar flexion.

Suspension phase

- Initially:
  - hip extended
  - knee flexed (the heel is in corrispondence with the gluteus muscles)
- Subsequently:
  - hip flexed
  - knee less flexed and at the end extended (anticipation of the stance phase).

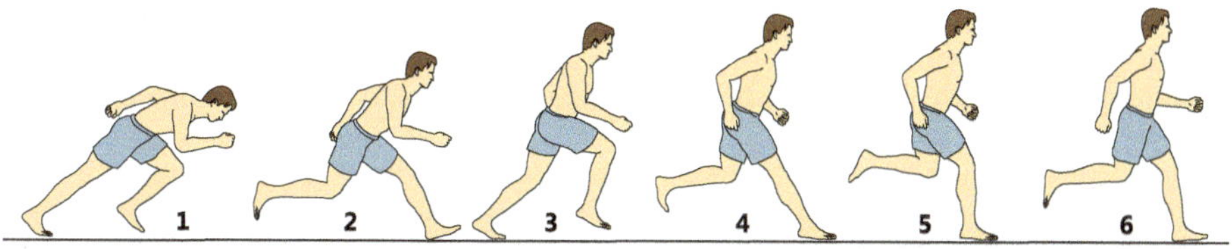

Phases of the sprint. **1**, Start; **2**, acceleration; **3-4**, full speed; **5-6**, deceleration.

Phases of the sprint

- Start
- Acceleration
- Full speed
- Deceleration

Joint motion

Flexion and extension of the hip

- Sprinting (1600 meters/7.5 minutes):
  - maximum hip flexion of 31° at the midpoint of the suspension phase
  - maximum extension of the hip of 11° during the thrust of the foot stance phase

Flexion of the knee

- Sprinting (1600 meters/7.5 minutes)
  - from 103° flexion at the midpoint of the suspension phase to 11° flexion at the end of the suspension phase

Dorsiflexion and plantar flexion of the ankle

- Running (slow or sprint)
  - from 17° dorsiflexion at the beginning of the stance phase to a maximum of 32° plantar flexion at the beginning of the suspension phase.

Running kinetics

The most important factor is muscular force, which is obviously related to body weight.

The most active muscles during running are:
- intrinsic muscles of the foot
- flexor muscles of the toes
- triceps surae (gastrocnemius and soleus)
- hamstring or ischiocrural (semimembranosus, semitendinosus and biceps femoris)

With respect to gait, the muscles that play the most important role are:
- gluteus maximus
- iliopsoas

Muscles of the upper limb mainly involved:
- deltoid
- flexors of the forearm.

Jumping

Definition: overcoming a distance through a flight phase that occurs due to the thrust exerted by one or both feet.

Use of jumping:
- in the practice of sports activities
- to strengthen the extensor muscles of the limbs (standing vertical jump)

Standing high jump

There are four phases:
- impulse – squat position (low center of gravity):
  - lower limbs: flexion of hips, knees, ankles and metatarsophalangeal joints
  - upper limbs: extension of the shoulders and flexion of the elbows (stretching of the antagonist muscles – hip and knee extensor muscles and plantar flexor muscles of the ankle and toes – which facilitate the movements of the next phase)
- thrust – of the upper and lower limbs (with movements that affect first the proximal muscles and then the distal muscles, creating a contraction wave that allows the muscles to express their full potential):
  - lower limbs: extension of the hips and knees and plantar flexion of the feet (facilitated by the stretching of the musculature performed in the preceding phase and by the ground reaction to the extensor muscle work)
  - upper limbs: flexion of the shoulders and extension of the elbows (with increased upward and forward trunk displacement as a result of the coordinated thrust of the upper and lower limbs and the locking of the upper limbs as soon as the feet leave the ground)
- flight – the trajectory depends on the force exerted and the direction and cannot be modified (high center of gravity); segmental movements can modify the flight height
- fall – the cushioning of the fall, which makes the impact less violent (the speed of the fall cannot be modified), and the maintenance of balance can be obtained by lengthening the flight time through increasing the distance (assuming a squat position in the descent phase, swinging, oblique descent).

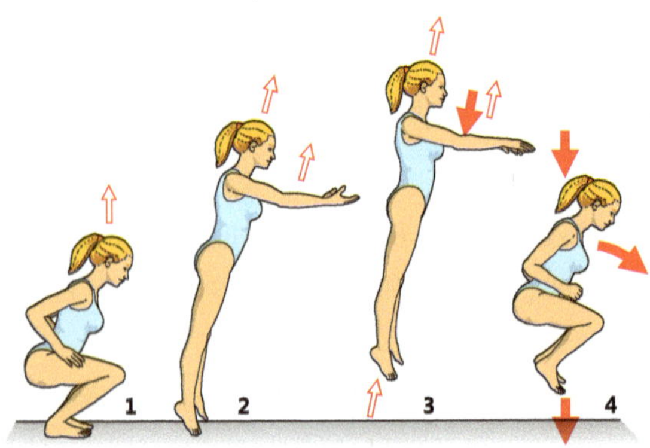

Standing high jump. **1**, Impulse; **2**, thrust; **3**, flight; **4**, fall.

Kicking

Definition: movement of a lower limb directed against an object (which is pushed, struck or thrown) while the contralateral lower limb and the rest of the body fix the muscles in order to maintain balance and make the gesture more precise.

Phases of kicking

- Preparation – the lower limb which remains in support (constituting the pivot of the action) is brought forward the body
- Load – while the trunk is flexed, in the lower limb performing the action:
  - the hip is extended
  - the knee is flexed
  - the ankle is in plantar flexion
- Acceleration – the lower limb performing the action is brought forward:
  - flexing the knee
  - flexing the hip
  - extending the knee
  - with the foot in plantar flexion
- Impact with the object:
  - extension of the trunk with rotation on the opposite side to that of the limb performing the action, together with the pelvis (in order to maintain balance)
  - anterior translation of the upper limb on the same side of the limb performing the action; in the latter:
    - the knee ends its extension
    - the foot flexes dorsally
- Deceleration – in the lower limb that has performed the action:
  - increases hip flexion
  - initiates knee flexion
  - decreases hip flexion
  - initiates knee extension
- Recovery of the double support
  - support on the floor of the limb that has performed the action, at the level of the contralateral limb or posterior to it.

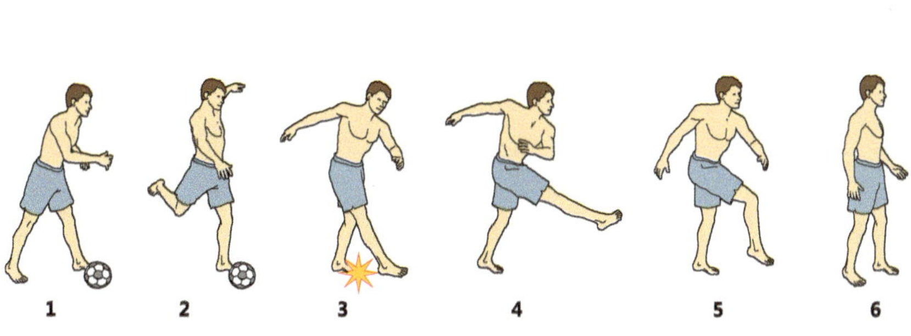

Kicking. **1**, Preparation; **2**, load; **3-4**, acceleration and impact; **5**, deceleration; **6**, recovery of the double support.

Throwing

Definition: oscillation of the upper limb that gives an object a more or less long trajectory in space.

Launch mode:
- overarm
- underarm
- sidearm

The center of rotation of the upper limb is represented by the shoulder joint and the propulsive action is given by the entire upper limb.

Compared to kicking, in throwing there is a greater:
- amplitude of movement
- angular velocity (2 times that of kicking)
- kinetic energy (4 times that of kicking).

Phases of throwing

- Preparation – searching for the best body position; the weight is distributed:
  - first on both feet
  - then on the side where the shoulder movement begins
- Load:
  - posterior translation of the trunk and the shoulder, elbow, wrist and hand of the throwing upper limb (stretching of the musculature used for propulsion and positioning of the upper limb at a distance, before the thrust, to reach the release of the object with maximum acceleration)
  - the shoulder is abducted, extended and externally rotated (by the action of the supraspinatus, infraspinatus, teres minor and deltoid, whose work decreases at the end of the loading phase, when the work of the rotator cuff muscles increases, which reduces the tension in the anterior part of the joint capsule of the shoulder caused by the thrust of the head of the humerus)

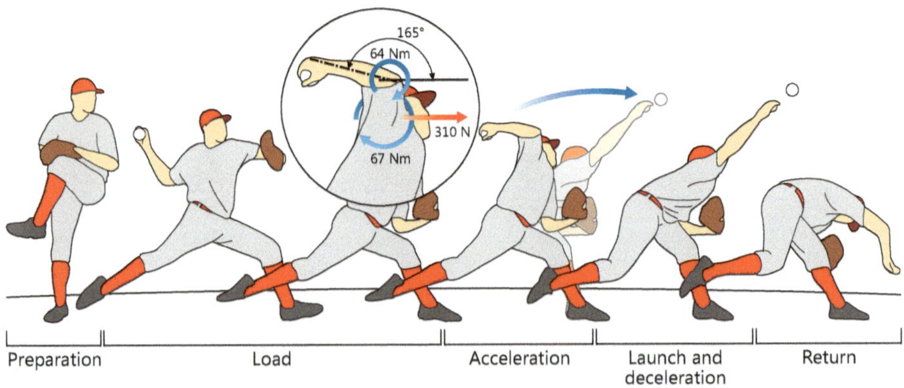

Throwing in baseball.

  - the elbow is flexed with slight pronation of the forearm
  - the wrist is flexed dorsally
- Acceleration:
  - rapid transition from the external to internal rotation of the shoulder (first advancement of the trunk and shoulder and then of the forearm and hand, with recruitment first of the proximal and then of the distal body segments) after activation of the subscapularis, pectoralis major and latissimus dorsi (moderate activation of the rotator cuff muscles continues to stabilize the shoulder joint; the rotator cuff muscles along with the biceps brachii are used mainly by untrained throwers, while trained throwers use almost exclusively the subscapularis)
- Launch – after the hand and the object are no longer in contact:
  - there is a deceleration phase, with the relaxation of the internal rotator muscles and contraction of the external rotator muscles; the latter reduces the stretching of the posterior part of the capsule, protecting the joint and the soft parts of the shoulder
- Return – variable according to the type of launch.

Recommended readings

Anastasi G, Gaudio A, Tacchetti C & Estomih Mtui (Editor English Edition). Human Anatomy - Atlas. Milan, Edi.Ermes, 2022.

Brotzman SB, Wilk KE. Clinical Orthopaedic Rehabilitation. 2nd Edition. Mosby, 2003.

Clarkson HM. Musculoskeletal assessment - Joint range of motion and manual muscle strength. 2nd Edition. Philadelphia, Lippincott Williams & Wilkins, 2000.

Faletti C, Castagna A. Spalla. Turin, UTET, 2002.

Francesconi K, Gandini G. L'intelligenza nel movimento - Percezione, propriocezione, controllo posturale. Milan, Edi.Ermes, 2015.

Morroni M & Estomih Mtui (Editor English Edition). Functional Anatomy and Imaging - Locomotor System. Milan, Edi.Ermes, 2024.

Niel-Asher S. The Concise Book of Trigger Points. Lotus Publishing and North Atlantic Books, 2005.

Pirola V. Cinesiologia: Il movimento umano applicato alla rieducazione e alle attività sportive. 2nd Edition. Milan, Edi.Ermes, 2017.

Pirola V. La gestione della medicina riabilitativa e le sue linee guida. 2nd Edition. Villasanta (MI), Ed. Le Scienze Motorie, 2000.

Pirola V. Patologie del cammino: analisi del movimento e riabilitazione. Origgio (MI), Novartis Farma SpA, 2002.

Pirola V. Riabilitazione oncologica: compendio pratico di clinica e riabilitazione dei tumori. Villasanta (MI), Ed. Le Scienze Motorie, 2001.

Pirola V. Rieducazione delle scoliosi e delle lombalgie. Milan, Edi.Ermes, 2009.

VV. AA. & Estomih Mtui (Editor English Edition). Human Anatomy - Topographic Approach. Milan, Edi.Ermes, 2022.

VV. AA. & Estomih Mtui (Editor English Edition). Treatise on Human Anatomy. Milan, Edi.Ermes, 2022.

Index

Page numbers followed by the letter f refer to figures in the text. Numbers followed by the letter t refer to tables.

G

H

U

V

W

Z